This book was purchased with money generously donated by the Nuffield Oxford Hospitals Fund

Bone repair biomaterials

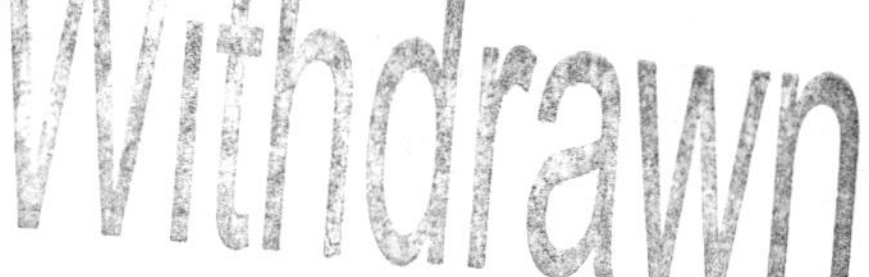

Related titles:

Orthopaedic bone cements
(ISBN 978-1-84569-376-3)
Bone cements are widely used in orthopaedic applications to bond an implant to existing bone and in remodelling following bone loss. *Orthopaedic bone cements* is an authoritative review of research focused on improving the mechanical and biological performance of bone cements. The first section of the book discusses the use of bone cements in medicine in addition to commercial aspects and delivery systems. Bone cement materials are reviewed in the second part of the book, while their mechanical properties are discussed in part three. In the final section, techniques to enhance bone cements are considered, for example antibiotic loading and bioactive cements.

Bioceramics and their clinical applications
(ISBN 978-1-84569-204-9)
Bioceramics are potentially suitable for a wide range of important applications within the medical device industry. *Bioceramics and their clinical applications* provides an authoritative review of this highly active area of research, written by leading academics from around the world. Chapters in the first section of the book discuss issues of significance to a range of bioceramics, such as their structure, mechanical properties and biological interactions. The second part reviews the fabrication, microstructure and properties of specific bioceramics and glasses, concentrating on the most promising materials. The final group of chapters reviews the clinical applications of bioceramics.

Shape memory alloys for biomedical applications
(ISBN 978-1-84569-344-2)
Shape memory metals are suitable for a wide range of biomedical devices including applications in dentistry, bone repair, urology and cardiology. This book provides a thorough review of shape memory metals and devices for medical applications. The first part of the book discusses the materials, primarily Ti-Ni based alloys; chapters cover the mechanical properties, thermodynamics, composition, fabrication of parts, chemical reactivity, surface modification and biocompatibility. Medical and dental devices using shape memory metals are reviewed in the next section, with chapters covering stents, orthodontic devices and endodontic instruments. Finally, future developments in this area are discussed including alternatives to Ti-Ni based shape memory alloys.

Details of these and other Woodhead Publishing materials books can be obtained by:

- visiting our web site at www.woodheadpublishing.com
- contacting Customer Services (e-mail: sales@woodheadpublishing.com; fax: +44 (0) 1223 893694; tel.: +44 (0) 1223 891358 ext. 130; address: Woodhead Publishing Limited, Abington Hall, Granta Park, Great Abington, Cambridge CB21 6AH, UK)

If you would like to receive information on forthcoming titles, please send your address details to: Francis Dodds (address, tel. and fax as above; e-mail: francis.dodds@woodheadpublishing.com). Please confirm which subject areas you are interested in.

Bone repair biomaterials

Principal editor: Josep A. Planell

Section editors: Serena M. Best, Damien Lacroix and Antonio Merolli

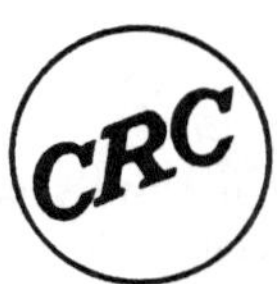

CRC Press
Boca Raton Boston New York Washington, DC

WOODHEAD PUBLISHING LIMITED
Oxford Cambridge New Delhi

Published by Woodhead Publishing Limited, Abington Hall, Granta Park, Great Abington, Cambridge CB21 6AH, UK
www.woodheadpublishing.com

Woodhead Publishing India Private Limited, G-2, Vardaan House, 7/28 Ansari Road, Daryaganj, New Delhi – 110002, India
www.woodheadpublishingindia.com

Published in North America by CRC Press LLC, 6000 Broken Sound Parkway, NW, Suite 300, Boca Raton, FL 33487, USA

First published 2009, Woodhead Publishing Limited and CRC Press LLC

British Library Cataloguing in Publication Data
A catalogue record for this book is available from the British Library.

Library of Congress Cataloging in Publication Data
A catalog record for this book is available from the Library of Congress.

Woodhead Publishing ISBN 978-1-84569-385-5 (book)
Woodhead Publishing ISBN 978-1-84569-661-0 (e-book)
CRC Press ISBN 978-1-4398-0195-6
CRC Press order number: N10044

The publishers' policy is to use permanent paper from mills that operate a sustainable forestry policy, and which has been manufactured from pulp which is processed using acid-free and elemental chlorine-free practices. Furthermore, the publishers ensure that the text paper and cover board used have met acceptable environmental accreditation standards.

Typeset by Replika Press Pvt Ltd, India
Printed by TJ International Limited, Padstow, Cornwall, UK

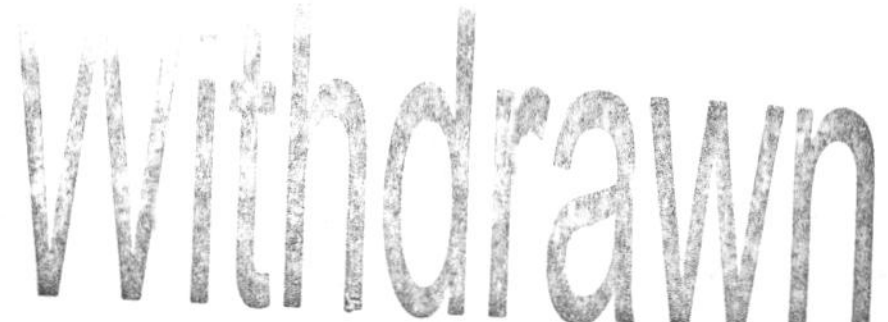

Contents

Contributor contact details

(*= main contact)

Chapter 1

Josep A. Planell* and Melba Navarro
Institute for Bioengineering of Catalonia (IBEC)
Technical University of Catalonia
CIBER-BBN
C/Baldiri Reixac 10–12
08028 Barcelona
Spain

Email: japlanell@ibec.pcb.ub.es
mnavarro@ibec.pcb.ub.es

Chapter 2

Robyn K. Fuchs and Stuart J. Warden
School of Health and Rehabilitation Sciences
Department of Physical Therapy
Indiana University
Indianapolis
Indiana 46202
USA

and

Charles H. Turner*
Indiana University-Purdue University Indianapolis, Department of Biomedical Engineering
Indiana University School of Medicine, Department of Orthopaedic Surgery
Indianapolis
Indiana 46202
USA

Email: turnerch@iupui.edu
rfuchs@iupui.edu
sjwarden@iupui.edu

Chapter 3

Nicola Baldini,* Elisabetta Cenni, Gabriela Ciapetti, Donatella Granchi and Lucia Savarino
Laboratorio di Fisiopatologia degli Impianti Ortopedici
Istituto Ortopedico Rizzoli
via di Barbiano 1/10
40136 Bologna
Italy

Email: nicola.baldini@ior.it

Chapter 4

Damien Lacroix
Institute for Bioengineering of Catalonia (IBEC)
C/Baldiri Reixac 13
08028 Barcelona
Spain

Email: dlacroix@ibec.pcb.ub.es

Chapter 5

Ashley A. White and Serena M. Best*
Department of Materials Science and Metallurgy
University of Cambridge
Pembroke Street
Cambridge
CB2 3QZ
UK

Email: ashley.ann.white@gmail.com
smb51@cam.ac.uk

Chapter 6

José Luis González-Carrasco
Centro Nacional de Investigaciones Metalúrgicas (CENIM-CSIC)
Avda Gregorio del Amo n°8
28040 Madrid
Spain

E-mail: jlg@cenim.csic.es

and
Centro de Investigación Biomédica en Red: Bioingeniería
Biomateriales y Nanomedicina
CIBER-BBN
Spain

Chapter 7

María Vallet-Regí* and Antonio J. Salinas
Departamento de Química Inorgánica y Bioinorgánica
Facultad Farmacia
Universidad Complutense
28040 Madrid
Spain

Email: vallet@farm.ucm.es
salinas@farm.ucm.es

and
Centro de Investigación Biomédica en Red: Bioingeniería
Biomateriales y Nanomedicina
CIBER-BBN
Spain

Chapter 8

Miguel Angel Mateos-Timoneda
Institute for Bioengineering of Catalonia (IBEC)
CIBER-BBN
C/Baldiri Reixac 15-21
08028 Barcelona
Spain

Email: mamateos@ibec.pcb.ub.es

Chapter 9

Roberto De Santis,* Vincenzo Guarino and Luigi Ambrosio
IMCB-CNR Institute of Composite and Biomedical Materials - National Research Council
P.le Tecchio, 80
Naples 80125
Italy

Email: rosantis@unina.it
vguarino@unina.it
ambrosio@unina.it

Chapter 10

Maria-Pau Ginebra
Department of Materials Science and Metallurgical Engineering
Technical University of Catalonia (UPC)
CIBER-BBN
Av. Diagonal 647
08028 Barcelona
Spain

Email: maria.pau.ginebra@upc.edu

Chapter 11

G. Helary and Véronique Migonney*
Laboratoire de Biomatériaux et Polymères de Spécialité
LBPS/CSPBAT-FRE CNRS
Institut Galilée
Université Paris 13
99 Avenue Jean-Baptiste Clément
93430 Villetaneuse
France

Email: veronique.migonney@univ-paris13.fr

Chapter 12

David Taylor
Trinity College Dublin
College Green
Dublin 2
Ireland

Email: dtaylor@tcd.ie

Chapter 13

Antonio Merolli*
Orthopaedics and Hand Surgery
The Catholic University in Rome
Complesso 'Columbus'
via Moscati 31
00168 Rome
Italy

Email: antonio.merolli@rm.unicatt.it

Paolo Tranquilli Leali
Orthopaedic Surgery
University of Sassari
viale San Pietro 43
07100 Sassari
Italy

Email: tranquilli@uniss.it

Chapter 14

Matteo Santin
School of Pharmacy and Biomolecular Sciences
University of Brighton
Cockcroft Building Lewes Road
Brighton
BN2 4GJ
UK

E-mail: m.santin@brighton.ac.uk

Chapter 15

Anders Palmquist* and Peter Thomsen
Department of Biomaterials
Sahlgrenska Academy at University of Gothenburg
Box 412, 405 30
Göteborg
Sweden

Email: anders.palmquist@biomaterials.gu.se
peter.thomsen@biomaterials.gu.se

Rickard Brånemark
Department of Orthopaedics
Sahlgrenska Academy at University of Gothenburg
Göteborg
Sweden

Email: richard.branemark@orthop.gu.se

Håkan Engqvist
Department of Materials Science
Ångström Laboratory at Uppsala University
Uppsala
Sweden

Email: hakan.engquist@angstrom.uu.se

Jukka Lausmaa
Department of Chemistry and Materials Technology
SP Technical Research Institute of Sweden
Box 857
SE-501#15 Borås
Sweden

Email: jukka.lausmaa@sp.se

Chapter 16

Leen Trommelmans* and Kris Dierickx
Centre for Biomedical Ethics and Law
Katholieke Universiteit Leuven
Kapucijnenvoer 35/3 Box 7001
3000 Leuven
Belgium

Email: Helena.Trommelmans@med.kuleuven.be
Kris.Dierickx@med.kuleuven.be

Joseph Selling
Faculty of Theology
Katholieke Universiteit Leuven
Sint-Michielsstr 6
3000 Leuven
Belgium

Email: Joseph.Selling@theo.kuleuven.be

Part I

Introduction

1
Challenges of bone repair

J. A. PLANELL and M. NAVARRO,
Institute for Bioengineering of Catalonia (IBEC), Spain

Abstract: Musculoskeletal problems, including bone and joint pathologies are among the main causes of chronic pain, physical disability, and work absenteeism in both developed and developing countries, and they affect millions of people worldwide. This is the reason why biomaterials play a key role in bone repair and regeneration. In this chapter, the societal impact of musculoskeletal diseases, as well as other bone problems is discussed in terms of their costs and the degree of physical disability that they generate. In addition, some of the most relevant clinical challenges in bone repair are presented.

Key words: musculoskeletal diseases, societal impact, economical impact, quality of life, bone diseases, clinical challenges in bone repair.

1.1 Introduction

Musculoskeletal problems, including bone and joint pathologies that lead to tissue degeneration and inflammation, are among the main causes of chronic pain, physical disability and work absenteeism in both developed and developing countries and they affect millions of people worldwide, especially those aged over 50 years. Present forecasts state that the percentage of target population affected by these diseases will double by 2020. Thus, it is expected that the demand and development of new caring techniques and treatments for these problems will also largely increase in these next few years. Musculoskeletal ailments frequently require surgery, including bone substitution and total joint replacement. Furthermore, the treatment of most bone traumatisms and malfunctions require the use of different devices. This is the reason why biomaterials play a key role in bone repair and regeneration. In this chapter, the societal impact of musculoskeletal diseases as well as other bone problems are discussed in terms of their costs and the degree of physical disability that they generate. In addition, some of the most relevant clinical challenges in bone repair are presented.

1.2 Social and economical impact of musculoskeletal disease

Bone and joint degenerative and inflammatory problems affect millions of people across the world. In fact, musculoskeletal conditions, namely joint pathologies, fractures related to osteoporosis, back pain, serious injuries and different sorts of bone diseases and disabilities are among the most common causes of hundreds of millions of people worldwide suffering severe long-term pain and becoming physically handicapped or crippled.

It has been reported that over 100 million Europeans suffer chronic musculoskeletal pain, while in the USA musculoskeletal problems affect over 40 million people aged 45 years or older and are projected to affect more than 60 million persons, or 22% of the population, by the year 2030. While mortality from these conditions is low, they have a major effect on disability, medical costs and patient quality of life (Murray and Lopez, 1996; White and Harth, 1999).

The two most commonly reported causes of pain worldwide are back pain and arthritis. These two conditions represent a third of all reported causes. Low-back pain is the most common problem, affecting approximately 4–33% of the population. Although back pain affects almost everyone at some point in life, it seems to be more prevalent in men and in younger people. Arthritis, a pathology that involves damage to and inflammation of the joints, is the most frequent cause of pain in women and in older people. In fact, it has been estimated that osteoarthritis affects nearly 10% of men and 18% of women aged over 60 years, while rheumatoid arthritis, which is a more severe disease, affects 0.3–1% of the general population and is more prevalent among women and in developed countries (Elliott *et al.*, 1999; Woolf and Pfleger, 2003). Moreover, it has been estimated that approximately 40% of arthritic adults suffer from osteoarthritis of the knee, 80% of people with osteoarthritis have limitation of movement and 25% cannot perform their major daily activities (Brooks, 2002).

Osteoporosis and, particularly, fractures caused by this illness are another of the most common problems affecting contemporary society. Osteoporosis has been defined as a condition in which BMD (bone mass density) is 2.5 standard deviations or more below the mean seen in young healthy subjects (WHO, 1994). Osteoporotic fractures primarily result from low BMD. However, microstructural changes in bone, especially of trabecular bone, also contribute significantly by increasing trabecular brittleness. This fragility is translated in an increase of vertebra, wrist and hip fractures (Kanis and Melton, 1994; Bonjour *et al.*, 1996).

The prevalence of osteoporosis in the USA only is estimated to increase from ten million to more than 14 million people by 2020. This is a significant increase in population with a high risk of falls and fractures (National Osteoporosis Foundation, 2002). Indeed, fractures related to osteoporosis have almost doubled in number in the last decade and it is foreseen that 40% of all women over 50 years will suffer from an osteoporotic fracture (Bone and Joint Decade's Musculoskeletal Portal, 2001). Although osteoporosis is less prevalent in men than in women, it is estimated that 30% of all hip fractures occur in men (Campion and Maricic, 2003). In addition, studies have shown that the fracture-related morbidity rate is higher in men than in women (Olszynski *et al.*, 2004). As in the case of arthritis and other musculoskeletal diseases, osteoporosis is a functional abnormality and an important clinical syndrome leading to many problems with respect to quality of life (Yilmaz *et al.*, 2008).

Hip and vertebral fractures are the most common fractures among individuals suffering osteoporosis. In osteoporotic women, low BMD particularly at the femoral neck, increases the risk of hip fractures two- to-threefold (Cummings *et al.*, 1985).

Hip fractures constitute a major and growing health care problem in the Western world and an emerging problem in the developing countries (Cummings *et al.*, 1985; WHO, 1994). It has been estimated that the worldwide annual number of hip fractures in 1990 was 1.66 million (Cooper *et al.*, 1992b). If current demographic and incidence trends continue, the worldwide annual number of hip fractures will increase to 6.26 million by year 2050 (Cooper *et al.*, 1992b; Melton, 1993). They are associated with considerable disability, loss of independence and diminished quality of life, but more importantly with a 20% reduction in expected survival (Cummings *et al.*, 1990; Kannus *et al.*, 1996; Melton, 1993; Richmond *et al.*, 2003). Additionally, hip fractures constitute a significant economic burden for modern medical care, both directly during fracture treatment and indirectly particularly during the first year after the fracture (Lauritzen, 1996; Sernbo and Johnell, 1993). Thus, as measured by their frequency, influence on quality of life and economic cost, hip fractures are a public health problem of crisis proportions.

Vertebral fractures and deformities affect approximately 20% of postmenopausal women and are the hallmark of osteoporosis (O'Neill *et al.*, 1996; Fechtenbaum *et al.*, 2005). Postmenopausal women with previous or incident vertebral fractures are at higher risk of both vertebral and non-vertebral fractures than women without previous vertebral fractures, independent of bone density (Klotzbuecher *et al.*, 2000; Kotowicz *et al.*, 1994; Burger *et al.*, 1994). In contrast to other major osteoporotic fractures, the majority of vertebral deformities do not come to clinical attention (Kanis and McCloskey, 1992; Cooper *et al.*, 1992a; Cooper and Melton, 1992).

Vertebral fractures may cause local pain for three years or more, although they may be presented asymptomatically (Ross, 1997). Clinical vertebral fractures are associated with increased back pain, kyphosis, height loss, impaired functional capacity in daily life, sleep problems, mood changes and reduced general health, with recent fractures having the greatest impact and causing greater health care utilization, including increased numbers of physician visits (Armstrong *et al.*, 1992; Cooper and Melton, 1992; Ettinger *et al.*, 1992; Leidig *et al.*, 1990; Huang *et al.*, 1996). Social isolation and depression have been also reported in patients with vertebral fractures. All together, these factors have an important impact on patients' health-related quality of life (QOL) (Kanis *et al.*, 1992).

Severe trauma caused by accidents is also noteworthy among the most important musculoskeletal conditions that affect contemporary society. The severe injuries caused by traffic accidents and war produce a tremendous demand for preventive and restorative help. It is anticipated that 25% of the health expenditure of developing countries will be spent on trauma-related care by the year 2010. Recent world health statistics from the WHO revealed that road traffic accidents will emerge as the fifth leading cause of death by the year 2030 (WHO, 2008). Thus, it is expected that severe bone trauma related to this cause will also increase during this period of time.

1.3 Economic burden of musculoskeletal disease

The costs of illness are generally divided into three categories: direct costs, indirect costs and intangible costs. Direct costs include expenditure for medical care and related items. These include expenditure for physician visits, diagnostic tests, prescription and over-the-counter medications, hospital stays, aids and devices, and outpatient surgical procedures.

Indirect costs are those resulting from lost function in one's usual activity, including work disability, sick leave or reduced productivity associated with a reduction in work hours or a need to change the nature of one's work to reduce pain and improve physical function. A number of studies have shown the significant effect of musculoskeletal conditions on employment (Blyth *et al.*, 2001). Depending on the specific condition, the indirect costs of musculoskeletal conditions may equal, or even exceed, the direct costs.

Intangible costs are those associated with loss of function, increased pain and reduced quality of life. As observed, disability is a significant outcome of musculoskeletal diseases. The limitations associated with these conditions include limitations of the activities of daily living, reduction in leisure and community activities, chronic pain and psychological problems, including depression and anxiety, and reduced general health.

1.3.1 Direct costs of musculoskeletal conditions

The direct costs associated with musculoskeletal conditions are substantial, especially among persons with arthritis. The reason behind these increased direct medical costs is mainly due to the increasing number of higher cost drug therapies. Other medical treatment with attendant high costs include total joint replacement surgery, which is common among persons with rheumatoid arthritis and osteoarthritis, and it is expected to increase over the coming decades with the growing prevalence of musculoskeletal disease in an ageing population.

The specific musculoskeletal condition results in different direct costs. In the USA and Europe, rheumatoid arthritis alone is estimated to cost US$1–2 billion per year (Yelin, 1996; Allaire *et al.*, 1994; Yelin and Wanke, 1999; Fautrel and Guillemin, 2002; Reginster, 2002).

Several studies on rheumatoid arthritis carried out in the USA revealed that the average direct costs ranged from US$2299–8500 (Yelin *et al.*, 1999; Yelin and Callahan, 1995). Total annual costs were US$8500, with hospitalizations accounting for between 55 and 62–68% of all expenditure. In Canada, it has been reported that total costs for patients with rheumatoid arthritis averaged US$2299 (Lubeck, 2003).

For osteoarthritis, a less severe arthritic condition, total costs ranging from US$3.4–13.2 billion per year, with almost half associated with direct medical expenditure, have been reported (Leigh *et al.*, 2001). The total medical costs for people under 65 years of age were found to be twice as high when compared with similar individuals without the condition. Among those individuals with osteoarthritis over the age of 65 years, expenditure was 50% higher than for those without the condition. Much of the difference was due to the costs of hospitalization (MacLean *et al.*, 1998). Osteoarthritis and related conditions accounted for more than half of all total hip replacements and 85% of all total knee replacements a decade ago and the cost for these replacements was over $300 million (Praemer *et al.*, 1992).

The economic impact of musculoskeletal diseases and chronic pain associated with them not only involves the direct, indirect and intangible costs previously mentioned, they also have a deep effect on the economic burden related with work absenteeism and lower performance. It has been estimated that the impact of arthritis on lost productive work time amounted to US$7.11 billion, but with 66% if this attributed to the 38% of workers with pain-related disabilities (Ricci *et al.*, 2005).

Furthermore, musculoskeletal conditions are the most common medical cause of long-term sickness absence (Woolf and Pfleger, 2003). In the UK, for instance, 3000 people go on to the incapacity benefit scheme every week and approximately 300 never return to work (Frank and Chamberlain, 2001). In Germany, musculoskeletal conditions cost employers US$30.8 million and are considered to be the largest single contributor to lost productivity (Phillips, 2006). In France, a study of nearly 2000 professionals suffering from acute pain showed that approximately 50% of them suffered musculoskeletal related pain; the average number of sick days resulting from their disability was 9 days/year (Autret-Leca *et al.*, 2001).

1.3.2 Economic impact of osteoporosis and related fractures

Current direct medical costs of osteoporosis in the USA have been estimated at US$13.7–20.3 billion. This burden is projected to grow by approximately 50% by 2025. A similar situation is expected to take place in other developed countries (Day, 1996; Ray *et al.*, 1997; Hoerger *et al.*, 1999; Chrischilles *et al.*, 1994).

In the USA, it has been estimated that total cost of incident fractures will rise from US$209 billion during 2006–2015 to US$228 billion for 2016–2025. Some interesting predictions about fracture sites and race/ethnicity of the affected population in USA have been reported. Across fracture types, the largest changes are predicted for pelvic fractures, where incidence increases by 56% and costs are predicted to rise by 60% between 2005 and 2025. By race/ethnicity, the proportion of fractures and costs among the non-white population will increase from 14% and 12% in 2005, respectively, to 21% and 19% in 2025. The most rapid increase is projected to occur in the Hispanic and other subpopulations. The annual costs for Hispanics are estimated to grow from US$754 million in 2005 to over US$2 billion per year by 2025 for an increase of 175%. Similarly, the other population shows cost increases of 175%, starting from a smaller 2005 total of US$502 million and rising to more than US$1.38 billion per year in 2025 (Burge *et al.*, 2007).

1.3.3 Costs of cancellous bone grafting versus alternative methods in trauma surgery

At present, one of the most popular and used techniques for substituting bone in those conditions where bone replacement is required is the use of autologous bone. Autologous bone grafts are prescribed in numerous cases such as defect pilon tibial, osteomyelitis, arthodesis, juvenile bone cysts, fracture, ventral spondylodesis, tibial plateau fractures and non-unions (Lohmann *et al.*, 2007). The main advantages of autologous bone are its biological nature which avoids possible disease transmission or host rejection and also its osteoconductive, osteoinductive and osteogenetic properties.

Cancellous bone grafting is currently the most frequent method for replacement of bone tissue. Worldwide, in 10% of all orthopaedic operations, a bone substitute is necessary. In Germany, 125 000 bone grafts are harvested per year (Bischo, 1995). Owing to the easy access and high transplant quantity, autogenous bone is predominantly taken from the iliac crest. However, the use of autologous bone as a bone graft or replacement also presents several disadvantages, such as deep infection, prolonged wound drainage, nerve injuries and chronic pain.

Allogenic bone material has been predominantly taken from the femoral head during hip arthroplasty. The harvested bone material had to be processed and stored in expensive bone banks. The allogenic bone is osteoconductive but has only reduced osteostimulative affectivity owing to the production process. Owing to the remaining high risk of disease transmission, this method is disregarded. In recent years, several alternative therapeutic approaches such as synthetic bone substitutes, local growth factors and composites have been developed.

It has been calculated from clinical data that, in the USA, the average direct costs relating to the use of cancellous bone grafts account for approximately US$4000 (St John *et al.*, 2003). The use of synthetic materials and growth factors is usually considered as rather expensive alternatives in comparison with autologous bone; however, according to a study performed by Lohmann *et al.* (2007), the costs of alternative methods are comparable and even cheaper than using cancellous bone grafts for bone replacement. Furthermore, given the complications associated with harvesting bone tissue, total costs, especially follow-up costs, increase when using cancellous bone grafts in comparison to bone replacement biomaterials.

Although autogenic bone grafting is associated with a considerable complication rate and secondary morbidity (Younger and Chapman, 1989; Arrington *et al.*, 1996), it is still the gold standard for bone replacement. Introduction of synthetic materials has opened up a wider range of available material during the last 10 years. Nonetheless, the question of an optimal bone substitute is still unsolved.

Given the numerous complications caused by bone harvesting at the donor site, follow-up costs play a key role in medical decision making. Thus, since the direct costs for alternative bone materials are comparable to the costs for autologous bone grafting, surgeons are urged to take these materials into account for the benefit of their patients and the health care system.

1.4 Social aspects of dental and maxillofacial conditions

Oral diseases such as dental caries, periodontal disease, tooth loss, oropharyngeal cancers and orodental trauma are major public problems worldwide. The experience of pain, problems with eating, chewing, smiling and communication caused by missing, discoloured or damaged teeth have a major impact on people's daily lives and well-being. Furthermore, oral diseases restrict activities at school, at work and at home, causing millions of school and work hours to be lost each year throughout the world (Petersen *et al.*, 2005). Because the nature of most dental problems is not life-threatening, but acute and normally are easily managable, their impact on well-being is not obvious and is often minimized in the context of other more serious chronic conditions (Reisine, 1998).

Within oral conditions, those involving tooth loss are among the ones with a greater impact in society. Tooth loss in adult life may also be attributable to poor periodontal health and more specifically to the presence of periodontitis and gingivitis conditions. Severe periodontitis is found in 5–20% of most adult populations worldwide, especially adults between 35–44 years old, whereas most children and adolescents present signs of gingivitis (WHO, 2004).

Dental erosion which consists of a progressive, irreversible loss of dental hard tissue owing to chemical etching of its surface is a growing problem among the population of several countries, affecting 8–13% of adults (Cate and Imfeld, 1996). Other oral conditions affecting people worldwide are related to developmental disorders such as congenital diseases of the enamel or dentine of teeth namely amelogenesis imperfecta, problems related to the number, size and shape of teeth, and craniofacial birth defects such as cleft lip and palate (Poulsen *et al.*, 2008; WHO, 2004).

The current global distribution of oral disease is very variable and highly dependent on the living conditions, lifestyles and the implementation of preventive oral health systems in different countries. However, it is expected that with the growing consumption of tobacco in developing countries, the risk of periodontal disease and tooth loss is likely to increase. Periodontal disease and tooth loss are also linked to chronic diseases such as diabetes mellitus; the growing incidence of diabetes may have a negative impact on the oral health of people in several countries. Thus, public health problems related to tooth loss and weakened oral function are expected to increase, particularly in many developing countries (Petersen *et al.*, 2005)

One of the most important developmental disorders involving both dental and craniomaxillofacial problems is the cleft lip and palate. The medical condition of patients with cleft lip and palate problems is very complex as it involves hearing, speech, learning, nutrition and socialization problems as well as frequent surgery and prolonged difficult dental care (Waite and Waite, 1996). The incidence of cleft lip and palate varies enormously from one country to another. Native Americans show the highest incidences at 3.74 per 1000 live births, whereas a uniform incidence of 1:600 to 1:700 live births is reported among Europeans. The incidences appear high among Asians (0.82–4.04 per 1000 live births), intermediate in Caucasians (0.9–2.69 per 1000 live births) and low in Africans (0.18–1.67 per 1000 live births) (WHO, 2002).

Orodental trauma is another source of dental problems. Although there is a lack of reliable data about the distribution and severity of this condition, there are some studies reporting that most dental trauma relates to sports, unsafe playgrounds or schools, traffic accidents or violence. Some studies have reported dental trauma in about 15% of school children in Latin American countries and around 5–12% in some Middle East countries. Moreover, it seems that there is an increasing tendency towards traumatic injuries in some developed countries where the percentages of affected people range between 16–40% among 6-year-old children and from 4–33% among 12–14 year-old children (Andreasen and Andreasen, 2002)

Maxillofacial trauma has a high social impact, specifically from the psychological point of view. The psychological consequences of facial injury can persist long after the injury has taken place and the low self-esteem resulting from patients' perception of their deformity may limit their ability to perform their economic and social activities to the full. According to some studies, the proportion of maxillofacial trauma in relation to all types of trauma reported from accident and emergency departments varies from 9.1% to 33% (Ribeiro *et al.*, 2004). Furthermore, it has been reported that in the UK, each patient who needs care for maxillofacial injuries costs the NHS approximately £733, whereas in California, USA, a total of US$34 million is spent on maxillofacial care per year (Lowry, 1990; Azevedo *et al.*, 1998).

1.5 Some clinical challenges of bone repair

Although new technologies and advances in orthopaedic surgery have significantly contributed to improving musculoskeletal conditions and to enhancing bone repair during the last decades, there are still some cases where problems related to improper bone healing need to be solved. One of the most important problems is related to fracture non-unions and delayed-unions. Under normal conditions, the fracture healing process should be driven by mesenchymal stem cells which migrate to the injury site and differentiate into osteoblastic cells leading to bone repair. However, some fractures do not succeed in healing and become non-unions, which may lead to morbidity and functional disability for patients.

There are some types of non-unions where there is minimal callus formation (oligotrophic non-unions) or where the body is not able to make a new callus and to bridge the fracture gap (atrophic non-unions). In this particular case, bone ends are avascular and in some instances they also show resorption. In these cases where these two types of non-unions are present, a special treatment is required to boost the bone osteogenic potential in order to fill the gap between both ends. There are also cases where a non-union stabilizes into a fibrous union. Alternatively cartilaginous tissue and fluid may occupy the interval between fracture ends creating a pseudarthrosis (false joint) (Keene, 1999; Pacheco *et al.*, 2004).

The current approach to overcoming the non-union problem involves the use of autologous bone grafts. Autografts are the gold standard, given that they provide an excellent osteoconductive matrix, osteoinductive factors and cells capable of building new bone tissue. However, as previously commented, autologous bone, as well as allogenic and xenogenic grafts, present some well-known limitations. Thus, non-union of fractures remains a challenging and important problem in orthopaedic surgery and new approaches to improve bone bridging when oligotrophic or atrophic non-union problems at present are required (Pacheco *et al.*, 2004; Wraighte and Scammell, 2007).

New materials for the elaboration of structures for tissue engineering and cell/drug delivery systems able to guide bone repair, to release an adequate dose of osteoinductive signals and to supply or attract cells capable of responding to these signals and differentiating into osteogenic cells are currently under development (Cole *et al.*, 2007; Corsi *et al.*, 2007).

In the case of fractures related to osteoporosis, one of the major challenges is the inadequate strength of the bone that must be used to anchor the fixation device. Osteporosis affects metaphyseal bone and, therefore, most osteoporotic fractures are in the metaphyseal site. This type of fracture is usually treated by internal fixation; however, owing to the low bone density, the use of screws to provide a stable fixation is not always possible. In response to this problem, research and technological development have focused on three approaches to improve surgery results. These include improved anchoring techniques, improved load distribution between the bone and the implants and the augmentation of the strength of the host bone to improve anchorage. Prosthetic replacement is a fourth approach that is also applicable to many osteoporotic fractures (Cornell, 2005).

Hence, once more a material able to induce bone formation to reinforce the host bone and improve anchorage is required. The development of new low modulus metallic alloys and polymeric devices with mechanical properties similar to those of osteoporotic bone are also required in order to get a uniform distribution of loads between the bone and the implants and avoid further resorption of the bone.

Even more challenging than non-unions are problems related to lack of bone strength and other bone loss defects, found with diseases such as osteoporosis, osteonecrosis and osteogenesis imperfecta where increased bone mass, increased bone density, or bone regeneration may be required at multiple sites. In these cases, biomaterials carriers for genes, cells or drugs may be very helpful, including biomaterial-mediated gene delivery systems where a gene carrier is applied directly to cells in culture (*ex vivo* therapy) or applied to the damaged tissue (*in vivo* therapy), or biomaterial-mediated drug delivery (Gersbach *et al.*, 2007).

Another problem of paramount importance when talking about musculoskeletal conditions is infection. Musculoskeletal infections are common, they can affect all parts of the musculoskeletal system, and can be dangerous and even life threatening. A significant number of bone fractures are affected by infection problems. In fact, a very common focus of infections is non-unions. An infected fracture non-union is a disastrous complication.

Management of this type of infection is difficult, prolonged and not always successful. Thirty per cent of non-unions are infected and 70% follow open fractures. The most common site is the tibia which accounts for approximately 60% of cases (Skinner, 2006; Motsitsi, 2008).

During infection, bacteria can gain entry into the body from direct penetrating trauma, by hematogenous spread from adjacent or remote sites of infection, or during surgical exposures leading eventually to severe osteomyelitis conditions. Bacteria may migrate through adjacent gaps in the endothelium and adhere to the bone matrix. Infection can also track through soft tissues giving place to secondary septic arthritis. Thus, the hip joint is particularly susceptible to secondary infection arising from a spreading osteomyelitis of the femoral head or neck (Skinner, 2006).

It has been reported that all biomaterials commonly used for total joint arthroplasty increase the incidence of *Staphylococcus aureus* infections. In fact, it has been reported that in the case of hip fractures, deep infection around the implant occurs in about 1–3% of cases, with a mortality of up to 50% (Parker, 2007).

In the specific case where polymethylmethacrylate cements are used, *Escherichia coli* and *S. epidermidis* infections seem to be very common. Adherence of bacteria to the surface of implants is promoted by a polysaccharide biofilm called glycocalyx which acts as a barrier against host defence mechanisms and antibiotics. In order to avoid this problem, the incorporation of antibiotics such as vancomycin and gentamicin to methacrylate cement is used to lower the risk of infection and eliminate surface bacteria before they can produce glycocalyx (Skinner, 2006).

Other materials that are prone to elicit infection are the ones used for sutures. Some natural suture materials, such as silk, may act as infection nuclei. Although synthetic suture materials such as nylon and polyglycolic acid are less likely to facilitate wound infection than the natural ones, there are also chances for infections to take place. In this regard, superior sutures in preventing infection must be designed.

Significant infection has been also observed after implantation of small amounts of allograft bone and connective tissue. When big osteoarticular allografts are used, the infection risk can be increased considerably (8–12%). Fresh and fresh-frozen allograft bone and soft tissue harvested and processed into implants in an aseptic manner are implicated in clostridium infections because of problems with not detecting contaminated donors and not sterilizing the tissue for spores. In 2001, approximately 875 000 of these implants were used in the USA, with a rate of infection with properly selected donors and treated tissues of much less than 0.1% (Skinner, 2006). Thus, there is a clear need to develop new implants whose surfaces are able to release properly drugs against infection as well as biomaterial-mediated drug delivery systems able to act with high specificity in targeted sites.

With respect to maxillofacial conditions, few procedures are more challenging than the surgical repair of patients with craniomaxillofacial deformities, not only because of the technical implications but also because of the psychological ones. These deformities are usually the outcome of trauma, cancer, infection, or congenital anomalies and involve both bone and overlying soft tissue. Regardless of the etiology, it is a surgeon's task to restore the functionality and correct the aesthetic defect. When treating patients who have undergone tumour resection or suffered severe facial trauma, both the surgeon and the patient must understand that the patient will probably never function or appear as they did prior to their trauma or tumour surgery (Keene, 1999).

One of the greatest challenges that exist today in oral and maxillofacial surgery is the reconstruction with augmentation material of the cavities and bone defects of the maxillae. The aesthetic and functional possibilities that osteointegrated implants represent has led to an increased use of bone augmentation procedures and to an increasing interest in bone regeneration techniques and the use of a variety of osteoinductive materials to cope with clinical conditions such as alveolar clefts, elevation of the sinus or the nasal pit for the insertion of osteointegrated implants, apicectomies, cystectomies, odontogenic or bone tumours excision, and to post-extraction alveolus, pre-prosthesis and periodontally treated crest defects (Infante-Cossio *et al.*, 2007)

Materials destined for bone augmentation purposes should reinforce the resistance of the maxilla, re-establish its continuity and provide support for dental prostheses or osteointegrated implants. In addition, the bone regeneration period should be shortened significantly. From the biological point of view, bone autograft remains the best option in spite of its limitations. Although nowadays there is a wide range of materials for this application, they lack the osteoinductive potential that autograft possesses. Therefore, more work on the development of new biomaterials, surface treatments and the design of new biomolecules to induce bone formation must be done in order to overcome the limitations of present materials.

An important procedure within the dentistry field is the restoration of posterior teeth. Within this context, efficient enamel–dentine adhesives play an important role in modern dentistry. The development of resin-based materials has successfully substituted amalgams during the last decades. Materials aimed at this type of restoration must endure a harsh environment which varies from patient to patient. Mastication forces, occlusal habits, abrasive foods, chemically active foods and liquids, temperature fluctuations, humidity variation, bacterial byproducts and salivary enzymes are part of uncontrollable factors that affect composite restoration durability (de Gee *at al.*, 1996; Sarrett *et al.*, 2000).

In spite of the numerous advances that composite science has achieved recently, clinical data indicate that the two main challenges are secondary caries and bulk fracture. Although there is only sparse literature related to this issue, there seems to be a general consensus about the implications that polymerization shrinkage of dental composites has in the fracture of cusps and in the predisposition of teeth to secondary caries and postoperative pain.

Hence, it is envisioned that future composite materials for teeth restoration applications will contain agents that suppress bacterial activity at the tooth–composite interface and avoid the appearance of caries (Ebi *et al.*, 2001; Imazato, 2003). It is further suggested that research into improving the fracture resistance of composite be continued to avoid further fractures and any bacterial effects. Research focused on improving the usability of the material will allow dentists to place higher quality restorations with fewer flaws; this should increase restoration durability. Furthermore, the future for all restorative materials development should be bioactive materials that inhibit plaque collection, inhibit caries-producing bacteria and mitigate the effects of decreased pH during cariogenic activity (Shen *et al.*, 1994).

There are some bone disorders caused by variations in bone mineral density and mineralization, such as hypercalcaemia, hypocalcaemia, osteopetrosis, osteonecrosis and Paget's disease of the bone. Although some of them are very rare diseases that do not affect high percentages of people worldwide, they are noteworthy since they also represent important clinical challenges that require the use of biomaterials.

Hypocalcaemia in bone is normally associated with the 'hungry bone syndrome', an excessive calcification of the bone that occurs postoperatively, after thyrotoxicosis or hyperparathyroidism conditions. A rapid increase in bone remodelling takes place when the stimulus is removed (thyroid hormone or parathyroid hormone). Hypocalcaemia can occur if the rate of skeletal mineralization exceeds the rate of osteoclast-mediated bone resorption. This syndrome can be associated with severe and diffuse bone pain. Hypercalcaemia is another metabolic-related condition that may affect the mineral composition and resistance of bone. Hypercalcaemia is characterized by a considerable increase of Ca levels in blood and one of the causes is high concentrations of calcium being released from bones.

Osteopetrosis, also known as the marble bone disease, is an inherited bone remodelling disorder in which there is a defect in bone resorption by osteoclasts. Thus, there is an increase in skeletal mass owing to abnormally dense bone and the formation of very brittle bones that have a propensity to fracture (Fudge *et al.*, 2007). Osteopetrosis has been reported in 1:20 000–500 000 in its dominant form and 1:200 000 in the recessive form (Tolar *et al.*, 2004). The consequences of this condition include pathological fractures, coxa vara, long-bone bowing, back pain, arthritis and osteomyelitis (Shapiro, 1993). In addition to the problems previously mentioned, fracture treatment of marble bones is very difficult because of their hardness. In these cases, special tools made of tungsten carbide are required (Ramiah *et al.*, 2006).

Osteonecrosis, also known as ischaemic necrosis of bone, aseptic necrosis or avascular necrosis (AVN), is due to a loss of the blood supply in the bone tissue. This pathology affects approximately 20 000 new patients per year in the USA. Although any age group may develop osteonecrosis, most patients are between 20 and 50 years old, with the average age in the late thirties. Patients over the age of 50 are likely to have developed osteonecrosis either by a fracture of the hip or, more rarely, in association with disease of the major blood vessels of the lower leg.

When a section of the bone has died, it does not heal spontaneously. Thus, one approach to this problem is to remove the dead bone surgically and fill the empty space with bone graft that is either taken from the patient or from the bone bank. The success of this approach depends upon the quantity of bone that has died. The use of synthetic biomaterials is a potential alternative to the use of autografts and allografts. In cases where osteonecrosis attacks larger areas such as joints, total joint replacement procedures must take place.

Paget's bone disease, also regarded as the osteoclasts disease, is a more common disease affecting 1–2% of white adults older than 55 years. The disease is characterized by an increased bone turnover that affects one or more sites throughout the skeleton. The most common affected sites are the pelvis (70% of cases), femur (55%), lumbar spine (53%), skull (42%) and tibia (32%) (Kanis, 1992). The prevalence of Paget's disease increases substantially with age. Studies performed in the UK suggest that the disease affects about 8% of men and 5% of women by the eighth decade of life (Van Staa *et al.*, 2002). There are large variations in the prevalence of this disease depending on the ethnicity and geographic location of people. It has been reported that the UK has the highest prevalence of Paget's disease of the bone in the world.

The rapid rate of bone turnover in Paget's disease leads to the production of bone that has a disorganized architecture and reduced mechanical strength, leading to an increased risk of developing deformities and pathological fractures. In this sense, surgical intervention is frequently required for the management of complications caused by Paget's disease. The most common indication for surgical treatment is joint replacement for osteoarthritis, but others include fracture fixation, osteotomy to correct bone deformity, surgery to correct spinal stenosis and prophylactic surgery in patients with painful pseudofractures (Redden *et al.*, 1981). The fixation of Pagetic fractures can be technically challenging because of bony enlargement, deformity, hard bone and increased vascularity (Kaplan, 1999).

1.6 Conclusions and future trends

From the socioeconomical point of view, it is expected that by 2020, the percentage of persons over 50 years will double in Europe and the USA. As the average age of the population rises, the impact of musculoskeletal conditions on society will also increase. Indeed, it is predicted that by 2025, the number of annual fractures and costs will increase by 50%. The way in which musculoskeletal disease affects an individual depends on several variables like the severity of the condition, the characteristics of the individual and the length of time with the condition. Other factors more related to the patient such as age, gender, race/ethnicity and lifestyle also affect strongly the outcome of the disease. Recent studies have shown the importance of performing more profound studies to identify growing unrecognized needs from different population sectors (Burge *et al.*, 2007)

The disability associated with certain musculoskeletal conditions, such as arthritis, the most prevalent musculoskeletal condition, osteoporosis and its related fractures, severe trauma and crippling diseases and deformities affects society in a significant way; most of the time, the individuals' quality of life is considerably affected. In the worst cases, the individual is not able to have a fully independent lifestyle (Yilmaz *et al.*, 2008). As a consequence, employers and society have to deal, not only with healthcare expenses associated with the treatment and recovery from the musculoskeletal condition, but also with the costs associated with lost productivity and increased sick leave.

Thus, it is clear that more work is required to evaluate the costs of medical care in terms of effectiveness or benefit. Besides, it is necessary to identify cost effective treatments that have a durable response in terms of reduce disability or pain. In particular in the case of osteoarthritis, joint replacement surgery is a good example of such a treatment. Investment in effective interventions and programmes for pain relief and reductions in disability levels will generate both economic and social outcomes that more than repay the original investment.

The prevalence of bone and joint diseases, as well as severe trauma, has led to the development of biomaterials for both permanent and temporary devices aimed at overcoming these clinical conditions. Within this context, orthopaedic biomaterials have been developed and have evolved according to the specific demands required by each particular application. For instance, in the case of bone fractures, the need for rigid and mechanically resistant materials for the manufacture of bone fixation devices has led to the use of existing metals and the development of new metallic alloys which allow the design of new devices such as plates, pins, rods and external fixation systems.

In the case of arthritis and other clinical conditions where joints are severely injured and total joint replacement is required, there is the need for materials with high strength, but also with excellent corrosion resistance and low wear rates especially for materials used in articulating heads and cups of the prostheses. Certain ceramics and some ultra high molecular weight polyethylene have emerged as a solution to these needs and are currently combined with metals when designing and manufacturing joint prostheses.

Calcium phosphate ceramics, cements, glasses and glass-ceramics arose as a solution to the cases where bone substitutes were required to fill bone defects, as in pathologies where bone loss takes place, as well as in oral and craniomaxillofacial defects. The bioactive potential of some CaP ceramics and bioglasses have also been exploited to enhance the integration and binding between the implants and the surrounding tissue. The use of bioactive ceramics and glasses for coatings has come up as an answer to the implant loosening problems. In addition, the development of CaP cements loaded with specific drugs and antibiotics has resulted as an option for avoiding undesirable infection problems.

More recently, biodegradable materials and, more specifically, biodegradable polymers have been developed to overcome the numerous limitations presented by some metals and ceramics and for those cases where temporary devices are required. Furthermore, these polymers have been also used in the development of matrices for sophisticated drug delivery systems and in the development of novel three-dimensional (3D) porous scaffolds for bone regeneration. Synthetic scaffolds for bone tissue engineering are one of the most promising options to substitute for current bone grafts in bone replacement procedures.

Thus, from the biomaterials point of view, the variety of biomaterials and their possible applications have significantly expanded during recent decades. The development of new materials has allowed the design of novel devices for both regenerative and repair tasks, and therefore the spectrum of possible solutions for different musculoskeletal conditions has also increased considerably. In addition, the possibility of modifying and controlling the surface properties of materials, in particular their topography and surface chemistry, at the micro and nano level, represents a major breakthrough, since it opens up a complete new range of approaches aimed at improving the osteoinductive capacity of materials and stimulating other specific interactions with the biological environment.

The development of new surface treatments and materials able to stimulate specific biological responses is one of the latest strategies for implants aimed at regenerating bone tissue. Surface tailoring, together with the development of new 3D tissue engineering structures able to induce and differentiate stem cells into the osteogenic lineage *in vivo* or to act as cell carriers for *in vitro* cell differentiation inside a bioreactor and for further implantation, is one approach with more potential in regenerative medicine.

The use of biodegradable and smart polymers and the development of carriers for stem cells, drugs and genes which aim to act with high specificity are among the most promising strategies for avoiding infection or for attacking other specific bone disorders such as osteoporosis, osteopetrosis and Paget's disease of the bone, among others.

It is envisioned that already existing materials will continue to be used for numerous musculoskeletal conditions such as large fractures, large resections, joint malfunctions and spinal pathologies, although new materials designed to solve the problems of the current ones are under development. Besides, it is expected that advances in the regenerative medicine approach together with the appearance of new biomaterials may overcome numerous present limitations in orthopaedics.

More detailed information about the different biomaterials used and their applications in orthopaedics will be provided in later chapters of this book.

1.7 Sources of further information and advice

Woolf AD, Zeider H and Hagland U (2004), 'Musculoskeletal pain in Europe: its impact and a comparison of population and medical perceptions of treatment in eight European countries', *Ann Rheum Dis*, **63**, 342–7.
This work present the results of a survey of approximately 6000 people with pain and 1500 physicians to determine common management strategies and perceived advantages and disadvantages of treatment.

Arthritis Care (2006) *Arthritis Care Factsheet, the Impact of Arthritis 2007*, [online] available http://www.arthritiscare.org.uk/PublicationsandResources/Listedbytype/Factsheets, accessed August 2008.
This website provides valuable information about arthritis, its socioeconomical impact and its treatments.

National Osteoporosis Foundation (2008) Available at: http://www.nof.org, Accessed August 2008.
This website provides comprehensive data with respect to the osteoporosis pathology, its social and economic burden and current treatment.

1.8 References

Allaire S, Prashker M and Meenan R (1994), 'The cost of rheumatoid artritis', *Pharmacoeconomics*, **6**, 513–22.

Andreasen J O and Andreasen F M (2002), 'Dental trauma', in *Community Oral Health*, Pine C, ed., Elsevier Science Limited, London.

Armstrong A L, Thomas G, Wallace W A and Green D (1992), 'Vertebral fractures', *BMJ*, **304**, 1308.

Arrington E D, Smith W J, Chambers H G, Bucknell A L and Davino A (1996), 'Complications of iliac crest bone graft harvesting', *Clinic Orthop*, **329**, 300–9.

Autret-Leca E, Bertin P and Boulu P (2001), 'La doleur aiguë de ládulte en médicine générale. Enquête épidéiologique transversale nationale', *Rev Pract*, **16**, 648–52.

Azevedo A B, Trent R B and Ellis A (1998), 'A population-based analysis of 10,766 hospitalisations for mandibular fractures in California, 1991–1993', *J Trauma*, **45**, 1084–7.

Bischo V A (1995), 'Knochentransplantation', *Aktuelle Traumatologie*, **25**, 1–8.

Blyth F M, March L M, Brnabic A J, Jorm J R, Williamson M and Cousins M J (2001), 'Chronic pain in Australia: a prevalence study', *Pain*, **77**, 231–9.

Bone and Joint Decade's Musculoskeletal Portal, 2001. Available at: http://www.boneandjointdecade.org. Accessed August 2008.

Bonjour J P, Schurch M A and Rizzoli R (1996), 'Nutritional aspects of hip fractures', *Bone*, **18**, 139–44.

Brooks P M (2002), 'Impact of osteoarthritis on individuals and society: how much disability? Social consequences and health economic implications', *Curr Opin Rheumatol*, **14**, 573–577.

Burge R, Dawson-Hughes B, Solomon D H, Wong J B, King A and Tosteson A (2007), 'Incidence and economic burden of osteoporosis-related fractures in the United States, 2005–2025', *J Bone Miner Res*, **22**(3), 465–75.

Burger H, van Daele P L A, Algra D, Hofman A, Grobbee D E, Schutte H E, *et al.* (1994), 'Vertebral deformities as predictor of non-vertebral fractures', *BMJ*, **309**, 991–2.

Campion J M and Maricic M J (2003), 'Osteoporosis in men', *Am Fam Physician*, **67**, 1521–6.

Cate J M and Imfeld T (1996), 'Dental erosion, summary' *Europ J Oral Sci*, **104**, 241–4.

Chrischilles E, Shireman T and Wallace R (1994), 'Costs and health effects of osteoporotic fractures', *Bone*, **15**, 377–86.

Cole P A, Miclau T and Bhandari M (2007), 'What's new in orthopaedic trauma', *J Bone Joint Surg Am*, **89**, 2560–77.

Cooper C, Atkinson J A, O'Fallon W M and Melton L J (1992a), 'Incidence of clinically diagnosed vertebral fractures: a population-based study in Rochester, Minnesota 1985–1989', *J Bone Miner Res*, **7**, 221–7.

Cooper C, Campion G and Melton L J (1992b), 'Hip fractures in the elderly: a worldwide projection', *Osteopor Int*, **2**, 285–9.

Cooper C and Melton L J (1992), 'Vertebral fractures: How large is the silent epidemic?' *BMJ*, **304**, 793–4.

Cornell C H (2005), 'Fixation considerations in osteoporotic bone fractures', *Curr Opin Orthop*, **16**, 376–81.

Corsi K A, Schwarz E M, Money D J and Huard J (2007), 'Regenerative medicine in orthopaedic surgery', *J Orthop Res*, **25**, 1261–8.

Cummings S R, Kelsey J L, Nevitt M C, O'Dowd K J (1985), 'Epidemiology of osteoporotic fractures', *Epidemiol Rev*, **7**, 178–208.

Cummings S R, Rubin S M and Black D (1990), 'The future of hip fractures in the United States. Numbers, costs and potential effects of postmenopausal estrogens', *Clin Orthop Relat Res*, **252**, 163–6.

Day J C (1996), *Population Projections of the United States by Age, Sex, Race, and Hispanic Origin: 1995 to 2050*, US Government Printing Office, Washington, DC.

de Gee A J, Wendt S L, Werner A and Davidson C L (1996), 'Influence of enzymes and plaque acids on *in vitro* wear of dental composites', *Biomaterials*, **17**, 1327–32.

Ebi N, Imazato S, Noiri Y and Ebisu S (2001), 'Inhibitory effects of resin composite containing bactericide-immobilized filler on plaque accumulation', *Dent Mater*, **17**, 485–91.

Elliott A M, Smith B H, Penny K I, Smith W C and Chambers W A (1999), 'The epidemiology of chronic pain in the community', *Lancet*, **354**, 1248–52.

Ettinger B, Black D M, Nevitt M C, Rundle A C, Cauley J A, Cummings S R *et al* (1992), 'The study of osteoporotic fractures research group. Contribution of vertebral deformities to chronic back pain and disability', *J Bone Miner Res*, **7**, 449–56.

Fautrel B and Guillemin F (2002), 'Cost of illness studies in rheumatic diseases', *Curr Opin Rheumatol*, **14**, 121–6.

Fechtenbaum J, Cropet C, Kohtla S, Horlait S, Orcel P and Roux C (2005), 'The severity of vertebral fractures and health-related quality of life in osteoporotic postmenopausal women', *Osteopor Int*, **16**, 2175–9.

Frank A O and Chamberlain M A (2001), 'Keeping our patients at work: implications for the management of those with rheumatoid artritis and musculoskeletal conditions', *Rheumatology*, **40**, 1201–5.

Fudge S, Amirfeyz R, Dimond D and Gargan M (2007), 'Marble bone disease', *Curr Orthop*, **21**, 438–41.

Gersbach C A, Phillips J E and García A J (2007), 'Genetic engineering for skeletal regenerative medicine', *Annu Rev Biomed Eng*, **9**, 87–119.

Hoerger T J, Downs K E, Lakshmanan M C, Lindrooth R C, Plouffe L Jr, Wendling B, West S L and Ohsfeldt R L (1999), 'Healthcare use among U.S. women aged 45 and older: Total costs and costs for selected postmenopausal health risks', *J Womens Health Gend Based Med*, **8**, 1077–89.

Huang C, Ross P D and Wasnich R D (1996), 'Vertebral fracture and other predictors of physical impairment and health care utilization', *Arch Intern Med*, **156**, 2469–75.

Imazato S (2003), 'Antibacterial properties of resin composites and dentin bonding systems', *Dent Mater*, **19**, 449–57.

Infante-Cossío P, Gutiérrez-Pérez J L, Torres-Lagares D, García-Perla A, González-Padilla J D (2007), 'Bone cavity augmentation in maxillofacial surgery using autologous material' *Rev Esp Cir Oral y Maxilofac*, **29**(1), 7–19.

St John TAS, Vaccaro A R, Sah A P, Schaefer M, Berta S C, Albert T and Hilibrand A (2003), 'Physical and monetary costs associated with autogenous bone graft harvesting', *Am J Orthop*, **32**, 18–23.

Kanis J A (1992), *Pathophysiology and Treatment of Paget's Disease of Bone*, 1st edn, Martin Dunita, London.

Kanis J A and McCloskey E V (1992), 'Epidemiology of vertebral osteoporosis', *Bone*, **13**, S1–S10.

Kanis J A, Minne H W, Meunier P J, Ziegler R and Allender E (1992), 'Quality of life and vertebral osteoporosis', *Osteopor Int*, **2**, 161–3.

Kanis J A and Melton L J III *et al.* (1994), 'The diagnosis of osteoporosis', *J Bone Miner Res*, **9**, 1137–41.

Kannus P, Parkkari J, Sievanen H, Heinonen A, Vuori I and Jarvinen M (1996), 'Epidemiology of hip fractures', *Bone*, **18**, 57S–63S

Kaplan F S (1999), 'Surgical management of Paget's disease', *J Bone Miner Res*, **14** (suppl 2), 34–8.

Karlsson M K, Gerdhem P and Ahlborg H G (2005), 'The prevention of osteoporotic fractures', *J Bone Joint Surg*, **87B**, 1320–7.

Keene G S (1999), *Key Topics in Orthopaedic Trauma Surgery*, BIOS Scientific Publishers, Oxford, UK.

Klotzbuecher C M, Ross P D, Landsman P B, Abbott T A and Berger M (2000), 'Patients with prior fractures have an increased risk of future fractures: a summary of the literature and statistical sinthesis', *J Bone Miner Res*, **15**, 721–39

Kotowicz M A, Melton L J III, Cooper C, Atkinson E J, O'Fallon W M and Riggs B L (1994), 'Risk of hip fracture in women with vertebral fracture', *J Bone Miner Res*, **9**, 599–605.

Lauritzen J B (1996), 'Hip fractures: incidence, risk factors, energy absorption, and prevention', *Bone*, **18**, 65S–75S.

Leidig G, Minne H W, Sauer P, Wüster C, Wüster J, Lojen M, Raue F and Ziegler R (1990), 'A study of complaints and their relation to vertebral destruction in patients with osteoporosis', *Bone Miner*, **8**, 217–29.

Leigh J P, Seavey W and Leistikow B (2001), 'Estimating the costs of job related arthritis' *J Rheum*, **28**, 1647–54.

Lohmann H, Grass G, Rangger C and Mathiak G (2007), 'Economic impact of cancellous bone grafting in trauma surgery', *Arch Orthop Trauma Surg*, **127**, 345–8.

Lowry J C (1990), 'Maxillofacial surgery: the economic aspect', *Br J Oral Maxillofac Surg*, **28**, 16–19.

Lubeck D P (2003), 'The costs of musculoskeletal disease: health needs assessment and health economics', *Best Practice and Research Clinical Rheumatology*, **17** (3), 529–39.

MacLean C H, Knigh K, Paulus H, Brook R H and Shekelle P G (1998), 'Costs attributable to osteoarthritis', *J Rheumatol*, **25**, 2213–18.

Melton L J (1993), 'Hip fractures: a worldwide problem today and tomorrow', *Bone*, **14**, 1–8.

Motsitsi N S (2008), 'Management of infected nonunion of long bones: The last decade (1996–2006)', *Injury, Int J Care Injured*, **39**, 155–60.

Murray J L and Lopez A D (1996), *The Global Burden of Disease: A Comprehensive Assessment of Mortality and Disability from Diseases, Injury and Risk Factors in 1990 and Projected to 2020*, Harvard University Press, Cambridge, MA.

National Osteoporosis Foundation (2002), *America's Bone Health: The State of Osteoporosis and Low Bone Mass in Our Nation*. National Osteoporosis Foundation, Washington, DC.

O'Neill T W, Felsenberg D, Varlow J, Cooper C, Kanis J A, Silman A J (1996), 'The prevalence of vertebral deformity in European men and women: the European Vertebral Osteoporosis Study', *J Bone Miner Res*, **11**, 1010–18.

Olszynski W P, Shawn Davison K, Adachi J D, Brown J P, Cummings S R, Hanley D A, Harris S T, Hodsman A B, Kendler D, McClung M, Miller P D and Yuen C K (2004), 'Osteoporosis in men: Epidemiology, diagnosis, prevention, and treatment', *Clin Ther*, **26**(1), 15–28.

Pacheco R J, Bradbury M D, Kasis A G and Saleh M (2004), 'Management of nonunion in trauma', *Trauma*, **6**, 225–47.

Parker M J (2007), 'Fractures of the hip' Orthopaedic V: injuries to the spine, pelvis and lower limbs, *Surgery*, **25**(10), 424–9.

Petersen P E, Bourgeois D, Ogawa H, Estupian-Day S and Ndiaye C (2005), 'The global burden of oral diseases and risks to oral health', *Bull World Health Org*, **83**, 661–9.

Phillips C J (2006), 'Economic burden of chronic pain', *Expert Rev. Pharmaeconomics Outcomes Res*, **6**(5), 591–601.

Poulsen S, Gjorup, Haubek D, Haukali G, Hintze H, Lovschall H and Errboe M (2008), 'Amelogenesis imperfecta–a systematic literature review of associated dental and oro-facial abnormalities and their impact on patients', *Acta Odontologica Scand*, **66**, 193–9.

Praemer A, Furner S and Rice D P (1992), *Musculoskeletal Conditions in the United States*. American Academy of Orthopaedic Surgeons, Park Ridge, IL.

Ramiah R D, Baker R P and Bannister G C (2006), 'Conversion of failed proximal femoral internal fixation to total hip arthroplasty in osteopetrotic bone', *J Arthroplasty*, **21**(8), 1200–2.

Ray N F, Chan J K, Thamer M, Melton L J III (1997), 'Medical expenditures for the treatment of osteoporotic fractures in the United States in 1995: Report from the National Osteoporosis Foundation', *J Bone Miner Res*, **12**, 24–35.

Redden J F, Dixon J, Vennart W and Hosking D J (1981), 'Management of fissure fractures in Paget's disease', *Int Orthop*, **5**, 103–6.

Reginster J Y (2002), 'The prevalence and burden of arthritis', *Rheumatology*, 41(supplement 1), 3–6.

Reisine S T (1998), 'The impact of dental conditions on social functioning and the quality of life', *Ann Rev Public Health*, **9**, 1–19.

Ribeiro M F, Mercenes W, Croucher R and Sheiham A (2004), 'The prevalence and causes of maxilofacial fractures in patients attending accident and emergency departments in Recife-Brazil', *Int Dental J*, **54**, 47–51.

Ricci J A, Stewart W F, Chee E, Leotta C, Foley K and Hochberg M C (2005), 'Pain exacerbation as a major source of lost productive time in US workers with arthritis', *Arthritis Care Res*, **53**, 673–81.

Richmond J, Aharonoff G B, Zuckerman J D and Koval K J (2003), 'Mortality risk after hip fracture', *J Orthop Trauma*, **17**, 53–6.

Ross P D (1997), 'Clinical consequences of vertebral fractures', *Am J Med*, **103**, 30S–43S.

Sarrett D C, Coletti D P and Peluso A R (2000), 'The effects of alcoholic beverages on composite wear', *Dent Mater*, **16**, 62–7.

Sernbo I and Johnell O (1993), 'Consequences of a hip fracture: a prospective study over one year', *Osteopor Int*, **3**, 148–53.

Shapiro F (1993), 'Osteopetrosis. Current clinical considerations', *Clin Orthop Relat Res*, **294**, 34–44.

Shen C, Sarrett D, Batich C D, Anusavice K J (1994), 'System for the pH-dependent release of a dye in model dental restorations', *J Dent Res*, **73**, 1833–40.

Skinner H (2006), *Current Diagnosis and Treatment in Orthopedics*, McGraw-Hill, Blacklick, OH, USA.

Tolar J, Teitelbaum S L and Orchard P J (2004), 'Osteopetrosis', *N Engl J Med*, **351**(27), 2839–49.

Van Staa T P, Selby P, Leufkens H G, Lyles K, Sprafka J M, Cooper C (2002), 'Incidence and natural history of Paget's disease of bone in England and Wales', *J Bone Miner Res*, **17**, 465–71.

Waite P D and Waite D E (1996), 'Bone grafting for the alveolar cleft defect', *Semen Orthod*, **2**, 192–6.

White K P and Harth M (1999), 'The occurrence and impact of generalised pain', *Ballieres Clin Rheumatol*, **12**, 379–89.

Woolf A D and Pfleger B (2003), 'Burden of major musculoskeletal conditions' *Bull World Health Org*, **81**, 646–56.

World Health Organization (1994), 'Assessment of fracture risk and its application to screening for postmenopausal osteoporosis', *World Health Org Tech Rep Ser*, **843**, 1–129.

World Health Organization (2002), *Global Strategies to Reduce the Health Care Burden of Craneofacial Anomalies*, World Health Organization, Geneva.

World Health Organization (2004), *Global Oral Health Data Bank*, World Health Organization, Geneva.

World Health Organization (2008), *World Health Statistics*, WHO Press, Geneva, Switzerland.

Wraighte P J and Scammel B E (2007), 'Principles of fracture healing: The foundation years', *Acute Care*, **3**(6), 243–51.

Yelin E (1996), 'The costs of rheumatoid arthritis: absolute, incremental, and marginal estimates', *J Rheumatol*, **23**(supplement), 47–51.

Yelin E and Callahan L F (1995), 'The economic costs and social and psychological impact of musculoskeletal conditions', *Arthritis & Rheumatism*, **38**, 1351–62.

Yelin E and Wanke L A (1999), 'An assessment of the annual and long-term direct costs of rheumatoid arthritis', *Arthritis & Rheumatism*, **42**, 1209–18.

Yelin E H, Trupin L S and Sebesta D S (1999), 'Transitions in employment, morbidity, and disability among persons ages 51–61 with musculoskeletal and non-musculoskeletal conditions in the US, 1992–94', *Arthritis & Rheumatism*, **42**, 769–79.

Yilmaz F, Sahin F, Ergoz E, Deniz E, Ercalik C, Yucel S and Kuran B (2008), 'Quality of life assessments with SF 36 in different musculoskeletal diseases', *Clin Rheumatol*, **27**, 327–32.

Younger E M and Chapman M W (1989), 'Morbidity at bone graft donor sites', *J Orthop Trauma*, **3**, 192–5.

2
Bone anatomy, physiology and adaptation to mechanical loading

R. K. FUCHS and S. J. WARDEN, Indiana University and Indiana University School of Medicine, USA and C. H. TURNER, Indiana University-Purdue University Indianapolis, and Indiana University School of Medicine, USA

Abstract: Bone is a specialized connective tissue designed primarily to provide mechanical support. It also plays a vital role in maintaining mineral homeostasis and hematopoiesis. This chapter provides an overview of skeletal anatomy and physiology in relation to these various functions. Details are provided for the macro and microscopic structure of bone tissue and the processes of bone growth, modeling and remodeling. In addition, the mechanical role of bone and its response to situations of loading, disuse and overuse are discussed.

Key words: bone adaptation to loading and unloading; bone morphology; bone remodeling and modeling; cell signaling in bone; inorganic and organic bone matrix.

2.1 Introduction

Bone is a specialized connective tissue consisting of cells, fibers and ground substance. Unlike other connective tissues, its extracellular components are mineralized giving it substantial strength and rigidity. This makes bone ideally suited to fulfilling its most recognized role within the body, that of mechanical support. Bone provides internal support, countering the force of gravity, forms specific cavities which serve to protect vital internal organs and provides attachment sites for muscles, allowing motion to occur at specialized bone-to-bone linkages. To fulfill these mechanical roles, bone needs to be stiff to resist deformation, yet flexible to absorb energy. In addition to meeting these contrasting mechanical demands, bone also needs to be able to meet the important auxiliary functions of maintaining calcium homeostasis and hematopoiesis. This chapter provides an overview of the anatomy and physiology of bone in relation to these functions, with particular reference to the mechanical role of bone and its response to mechanical stimuli.

2.2 Macroscopic bone anatomy

The anatomy or morphology of bone can be viewed hierarchically, starting at the gross, macroscopic level and progressing microscopically down to the nanoscale level (Fig. 2.1).

The human skeletal system contains over 200 unique bones, each of which have a different macroscopic appearance. To assist in simplifying the system, a number of classification methods have been used to categorize bones into groups. This has included grouping bones according to their type (long, short, flat or irregular), location (axial or appendicular) or predominant tissue composition (cortical or trabecular). The categorization of bones according to their type or location is convenient; however, greater information regarding bone function can be derived by identifying the predominant bone tissue type present within a specific bone or bone region. The skeleton can be divided macroscopically into two distinct types of bone tissue–cortical and trabecular (Fig. 2.2). These two tissue types have the same matrix composition; however, they differ substantially in terms of their structure and function, and relative distribution both between and within bones.

2.2.1 Cortical bone

Cortical (or compact) bone makes up approximately 80% of total skeletal tissue mass. It has a high matrix mass per unit volume and low porosity. These features endow cortical bone with great compressive strength, enabling it to contribute prominently to the mechanical role of bone. This is reflected in its distribution primarily within the long bones of the appendicular skeleton.

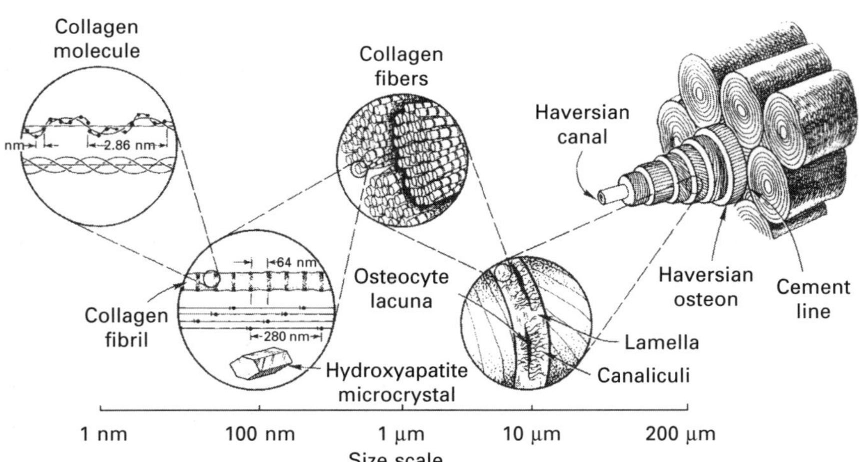

2.1 Hierarchical structure of cortical bone (reproduced with permission of Macmillan Publishers from Lakes[229]).

The appendicular or peripheral skeleton is predominantly made up of long and short bones, including all of the bones of the upper and lower limbs.

Long bones can be divided into three general regions – a relatively cylindrical shaft (diaphysis), two expanded ends (proximal and distal epiphyses) and a developing region called the metaphysis located in between the epiphyses at each end of the bone (Fig. 2.2). Cortical bone is particularly prominent within the diaphysis where it forms a thick cortical shell (cortex) that surrounds a medullary canal filled with bone marrow. This tube-like structural design distributes bone mineral away from bending axes, resulting in a substantial increase in bending resistance without a concomitant increase in bone weight. This endows long bones the strength and rigidity required for muscle action and weight bearing, yet the lightness required for energy efficient locomotion. Cortical bone thins towards the metaphyses and epiphyses of long bones where it plays a lesser, yet clinically significant mechanical role. The best example of this is at the femoral neck where cortical bone thickness and distribution are important variables influencing osteoporotic fracture risk.[1–3]

While cortical bone appears to be solid, it does contain microscopic pores (constituting approximately 10% of total cortical bone volume) which permit vascular and neural supply,[4] and the delivery of nutrients. This porosity is site-specific,[5] and can be influenced by age- and disuse-related bone loss,[6, 7] bone overuse injury,[8] and pharmacological interventions.[9, 10] The degree of porosity of cortical bone is important from a fracture standpoint as an increase in intracortical porosity can result in reduced bone strength and a concomitant increase in fracture risk.[11, 12]

Cortical bone does not appear to have a major role in hematopoiesis beyond skeletal maturity. The diaphyses of long bones have a medullary canal filled

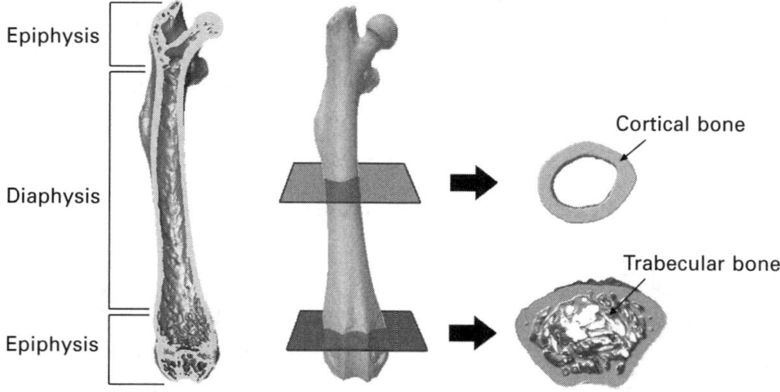

2.2 Macroscopic anatomy of a long bone. The relatively cylindrical shaft or diaphysis consists predominantly of cortical bone, whereas the expanded epiphyses have a greater proportion of trabecular bone enclosed within a relatively thinner cortical shell. Images are of a mouse femur acquired using microcomputed tomography.

with bone marrow. However, the content of the marrow transforms after birth from red (hematopoietic, metabolically active) into yellow (fatty tissue that is not metabolically active) marrow during skeletal maturation.[13–15]

2.2.2 Trabecular bone

In contrast to the low porosity of cortical bone, trabecular (or cancellous) bone has high porosity, with pores making up 50–90% of total trabecular bone volume. These pores are interspersed among an orderly arranged network of vertical and horizontal plate- and rod-like structural elements called trabeculae, which give trabecular bone a sponge-like appearance. The reduced matrix mass per unit volume and high porosity of trabecular bone reduces its compressive strength to approximately one-tenth that of cortical bone;[16] however, it has the function of providing increased surface area for red bone marrow, blood vessels and connective tissues to be in contact with bone. This facilitates the role of bone in hematopoiesis and mineral homeostasis.

Trabecular bone does not have the strength of cortical bone; however, it contributes to the mechanical role of bone by providing internal support. This supportive role facilitates the ability of bone to evenly distribute load and absorb energy, particularly in the vicinity of joints. It is also important during aging, as trabecular bone is lost earlier and at a greater rate than cortical bone.[17] This ultimately contributes to osteoporosis at skeletal sites rich in trabecular bone, such as the femoral neck and vertebral bodies. Bone strength at these sites is determined by the number, thickness, spacing, distribution and connectivity of trabeculae, with the later being particularly important.[18] For a given trabecular density, loss of connectivity has a more deleterious effect on bone strength than the presence of thin but well connected trabeculae.[19–21] This is supported by the finding that women with low bone mass and vertebral fractures have four times as many unconnected trabeculae as women without fractures, despite a similar bone mineral density.[22]

2.3 Microscopic bone anatomy

2.3.1 Bone coverings

The microscopic anatomy of bone is demonstrated in Fig. 2.3. The outer and inner surfaces of bone are covered by specialized connective tissues called the periosteum and endosteum, respectively. The periosteum serves as a transitional fibrous layer between cortical bone and the overlying soft tissue or musculature. It covers the external surfaces of most bones, except at articular surfaces, tendon insertions and the surfaces of sesamoid bones.[23] The periosteum can be divided into two distinct layers (Fig. 2.3F). The

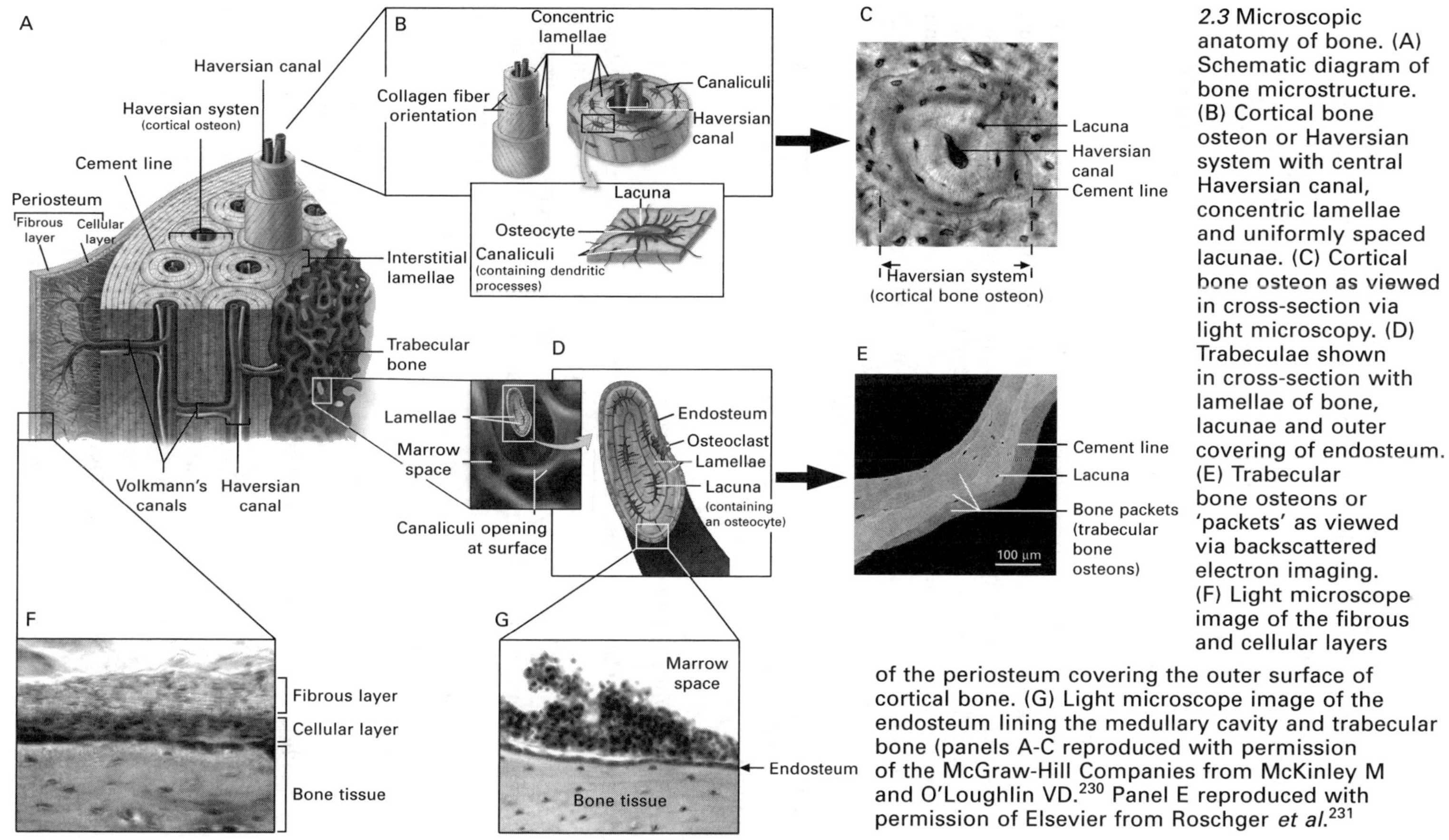

2.3 Microscopic anatomy of bone. (A) Schematic diagram of bone microstructure. (B) Cortical bone osteon or Haversian system with central Haversian canal, concentric lamellae and uniformly spaced lacunae. (C) Cortical bone osteon as viewed in cross-section via light microscopy. (D) Trabeculae shown in cross-section with lamellae of bone, lacunae and outer covering of endosteum. (E) Trabecular bone osteons or 'packets' as viewed via backscattered electron imaging. (F) Light microscope image of the fibrous and cellular layers of the periosteum covering the outer surface of cortical bone. (G) Light microscope image of the endosteum lining the medullary cavity and trabecular bone (panels A-C reproduced with permission of the McGraw-Hill Companies from McKinley M and O'Loughlin VD.[230] Panel E reproduced with permission of Elsevier from Roschger *et al.*[231]

outermost 'fibrous' layer is composed of fibroblasts, collagen and elastin fibers,[24] along with a distinctive nerve and microvascular network.[25] The inner 'cambium' or 'cellular' layer is positioned in direct contact with the bone surface. It contains mesenchymal stem cells (MSCs) which have the potential to differentiate into osteoblasts and chondrocytes,[26–28] and differentiated osteogenic progenitor cells, fibroblasts, microvessels and sympathetic nerves.[29] The localization of MSCs and osteoprogenitor cells within the cambium layer has made the periosteum a target for drug therapies and cell harvesting for tissue engineering purposes.

The endocortical or inner surface of a bone faces the medullary canal and is lined with a membranous sheath called the endosteum (Fig. 2.3G). The endosteum is lined with a single thin layer of bone lining cells (mature osteoblasts) and osteoblasts which form a membrane over endocortical and trabecular bone surfaces to enclose the bone marrow.[30] Osteoclasts can also be present in the endosteum in regions of active bone resorption. The endosteum contains osteoprogenitor cells, but does not appear to contain either MSCs or hematopoietic stem cells (HSCs). However, a portion of HSCs can be found next to the endosteum, suggesting reciprocal communication between cells within the endosteum and multipotent HSCs.[31] This forms a so-called 'stem cell niche' whereby the cells of the endosteum physically support and influence stem cell activity.[32, 33]

2.3.2 Microscopic bone structure

Cortical and trabecular bone are both composed microscopically of bone structural units (BSUs) or osteons. In cortical bone, the osteons are commonly referred to as Haversian systems (Fig. 2.3A–C). Haversian systems are cylindrical in shape and form an anastomosing network.[34] They contain a central Haversian canal housing blood vessels and nerves which are enveloped in concentric layers or lamellae of bone tissue. This arrangement gives each osteon an appearance of a tree trunk in cross-section with a circumferential cement line representing the tree's bark. The cement line represents the outermost boundary of an osteon and consists of a 5 μm ring of highly or similarly mineralized bone as contained within the osteon.[35] Uniformly spaced throughout the lamellae are lenticular cavities called lacunae. Radiating in all directions from each lacuna are branching canaliculae. These penetrate the lamellae of the interstitial substance and anastomose with canaliculae of neighboring lacunae to form a continuous network of interconnecting cavities. Interstitial bone fills the region between adjacent osteons and appears as short arched layers which are remnants of older partially resorbed osteons. In trabecular bone, osteons are referred to as a bone packets which are saucer shaped and consist of stacks or layers of lamellae (Fig. 2.3D,E). Adjacent packets in trabecular bone are separated by a cement line.

2.3.3 Woven and lamellar bone

Microscopic visualization of both cortical and trabecular bone reveals tissue that is either woven or lamellar in structure. Woven bone is characterized by bone tissue with a disorganized collagen fibril arrangement (Fig. 2.4A). It primarily develops embryonically and is gradually replaced between three and four years of age by lamellar bone. Woven bone is not frequently found in the adult skeleton, except in pathological conditions (such as Paget's disease and osteosarcoma) or following injury.[36–41] The disorganization of woven bone may result from the speed at which it forms, which precludes the orderly deposition of the collagen fibrils.[42] This disorganization provides woven bone with enhanced flexibility, at the cost of stiffness. This is functionally important during development because it allows a baby to pass safely through the birth canal without causing skeletal trauma. It is also valuable following bone injury as the rapid, early formation of woven bone enhances early restoration of skeletal mechanical integrity.[40, 41] This reparative woven bone is gradually resorbed and replaced by lamellar bone during later stages of healing.

Lamellar bone is characterized by the organized arrangement of collagen fibers into layers or lamellae, similar to the organization of plywood (Fig. 2.4B). This arrangement gives lamellar bone greater stiffness when compared to the disorganized nature of woven bone. Lamellae form osteons in cortical and packets in trabecular bone. Outer lamellae form first in cortical osteons, whereas in trabecular packets the first lamellae are formed towards the center of the trabeculae. Each successive lamella in a cortical osteon is laid concentrically inside the preceding one, while in trabeculae packets they are stacked in parallel layers away from the center of the trabeculae toward the bone surface.

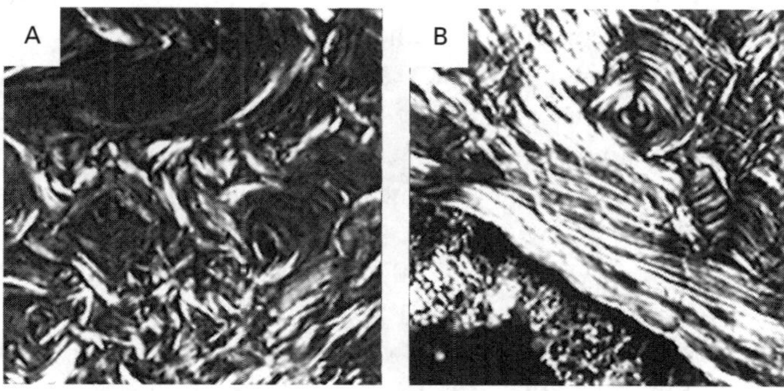

2.4 Microscopic visualization of (A) woven and (B) lamellar bone under polarized light reveals disorganized or organized collagen fibril arrangement, respectively.

2.3.4 Organic and inorganic bone matrix

Bone matrix is a composite material consisting of organic and inorganic components. The organic matrix makes up ~20% of the wet weight of bone and is comprised primarily of collagen. Collagen is the major structural component of the bone matrix, whereby the majority is type I collagen (~90%) with smaller amounts of collagen types III, V, X and XII.[43] Collagen is a fibrous protein that has a rope-like structure made up of ~1000 amino acids and is ~300 nm in length. A collagen fibril consists of two $\alpha 1$ and one $\alpha 2$ polypeptide chains that are synthesized within osteoblasts, creating a triple-helix pro-collagen molecule.[44, 45] The pro-collagen molecule is secreted from osteoblasts, after which individual collagen molecules converge together to create collagen fibrils. Individual collagen fibrils are then spontaneously grouped together to create a collagen fiber.[46, 47]

Collagen gives bone its flexibility, whereas the addition of mineral to the collagen network provides bone with its stiffness. Without the addition of mineral to collagen, bone tissue would be very flexible, with properties similar to a rubber band. Conversely, without collagen, bone is brittle like chalk. Thus, varying the amounts and distribution of collagen and mineral provides bone with its ability to balance its flexibility and stiffness requirements.[48] Alterations to the structure of collagen that occur from aging or genetic abnormalities such as osteogenesis imperfecta[49] can compromise the structural integrity of bone tissue resulting in a weaker structure with a greater than normal susceptibility to fracture.[46, 50]

In addition to collagen, 10% of the organic matrix is made up of non-collagenous proteins such as fibronectin, osteopontin, osteocalcin and bone sialoprotein,[51–53] along with proteoglycans such as decorin and biglycan. Bone sialoprotein and osteopontin constitute the majority of the non-collagenous proteins found in the bone matrix. While the non-collagenous proteins and proteoglycans only contribute a small amount to the total mass of the organic matrix, they serve several important functions during osteoblast differentiation, tissue mineralization, cell adhesion and bone remodeling.[51, 52, 54, 55]

The inorganic matrix contributes approximately ~65–70% of the wet weight of bone and serves as an ion reservoir storing approximately 99% of total body calcium, approximately 85% of phosphorus and between 40 and 60% of the body's sodium and magnesium.[43] These ions form crystalline structures surrounding and within the collagen fibers to give bone the majority of its stiffness. Bone crystals are ~200 Å and are predominantly in the form of calcium hydroxyapatite [$Ca_{10}PO_4OH_2$], the primary mineral found in the skeleton. Hydroxyapatite crystals can be found both on the surface and impregnated within hole zones (gaps) of the collagen fibrils.[56, 57]

2.3.5 Cellular elements

Cellular elements contribute only a small amount of the total mass of the skeleton, and are derived from either HSCs or MSCs (Fig. 2.5). HSCs and MSCs give rise to the principal cells that mediate bone resorption (osteoclasts) and formation (including osteoprogenitor cells, osteoblasts, osteocytes and bone lining cells), respectively.

The process of bone resorption is mediated exclusively by osteoclasts. Osteoclasts are large, multinucleate cells that create and occupy shallow concavities on the bone surface called Howship's lacunae. Osteoclastogenesis begins when a HSC is stimulated to generate mononuclear cells, which then become committed preosteoclasts and are introduced into the blood stream (Fig. 2.5A). This step requires expression of the Ets family transcription factor PU.1 and macrophage colony stimulating factor (M-CSF).[58, 59] The circulating precursors exit the peripheral circulation at or near the site to be resorbed and fuse with one another to form a multinucleated immature osteoclast. Fusion of the mononuclear cells into a polykaryon (immature osteoclast) requires the presence of M-CSF and the receptor activator of nuclear factor (NF) κB ligand (RANK-L).[60–62] Successful production of immature osteoclasts is associated with the initiation of tartrate-resistant acid phosphatase (Trap) expression, an enzyme that is used to assist with bone resorption in fully differentiated osteoclasts. The ability of an immature osteoclast to undergo differentiation only occurs in the continued presence of RANK-L and requires the expression of several genes, including the AP-1 member c-fos,[63, 64] micropthalmia-associated transcription factor (MITF)[65] and nuclear factor of activated T cells, calcineurin dependent 1 (NFAT-c1).[63, 66]

The signaling axis to which RANK-L belongs plays such a major role in osteoclast biology that it warrants further elaboration. For many years, researchers focused on identifying a specific factor produced by cells of the osteoblastic lineage which was required for osteoclastogenesis, as osteoclast differentiation *in vitro* from HSCs required co-culture with cells of mesenchymal origin.[67] This unknown factor turned out to be RANK-L and the receptor on osteoclasts and their precursors was subsequently identified as RANK (Fig. 2.6A).[68] RANK-L exists in both membrane-bound and soluble forms, but evidence suggests that the former is more potent.[69] This was reflected by the finding that physical contact with stromal cells, and not secretion of some soluble compound into the media by stromal cells, was required for osteoclastogenesis.[70, 71] At the same time as the identification of RANK-L, a soluble factor was found that inhibited the activity of RANK-L, which was identified as osteoprotegerin (OPG).[72] OPG is a soluble decoy for RANK-L and functions to reduce osteoclastogenesis by competitively occupying stromal RANK-L binding sites on precursor and later-stage osteoclasts (Fig. 2.6A).[73, 74] Consequently, cells of mesenchymal origin can

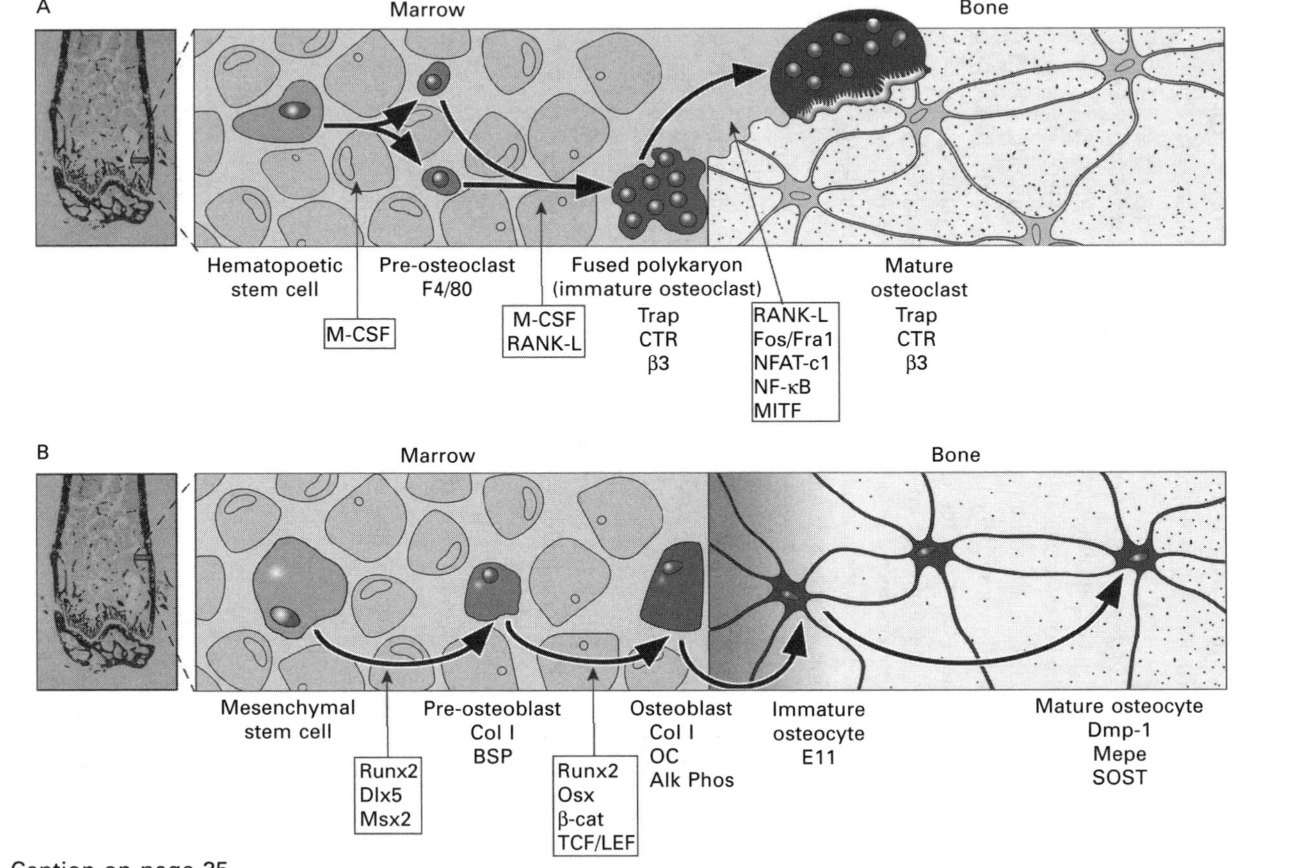

Caption on page 35

control osteoclastogenesis in a positive direction by increasing the expression of RANK-L and decreasing the expression of OPG, or conversely, the proportions can be reversed to decrease resorptive activity (Fig. 2.6C).

Once osteoclasts fully differentiate into mature cells, the bone-resorbing activity and survival of these cells is regulated by RANK-L. The mature osteoclast establishes a microenvironment between itself and the underlying bone by peripherally attaching to the matrix using integrins.[75] This creates a compartment between the ruffled basal border of the osteoclast and the bone surface that is isolated from the general extracellular space.[76] An electrogenic proton pump transports in H^+ ions to acidify the compartment which acts to mobilize the mineralized component of bone. This exposes the organic matrix which is subsequently degraded using proteases. The end result is the removal of bone matrix and the development of characteristic Howship's lacunae.

Osteoblast development follows a different course, beginning with the local proliferation of MSCs residing in the bone marrow stroma and periosteum (Fig. 2.5B). Expression of the transcription factors runt-related transcription factor-2 (Runx2), distal-less homeobox-5 (Dlx5) and msh homeobox homologue-2 (Msx2) are required to drive precursor cells toward the osteoblast lineage and away from the adipocyte, myocyte and chondrocyte lineages which are also derived by MSCs.[77–81] Once a precursor cell is committed to the osteoblast lineage, the immature osteoblasts (also called preosteoblasts) express type I collagen and bone sialoprotein (Bsp). Further differentiation of the preosteoblast into a mature, bone-forming osteoblast

---

2.5 Lineage of osteoclasts and osteoblasts. (A) Osteoclasts are derived from a hematopoeitic precursor in the bone marrow, spleen or liver. Proliferation of mononuclear cells from the precursor population requires M-CSF. The bloodborne preosteoclasts enter the circulation and arrive at the site to be resorbed. They will fuse together into a polykaryon only in the presence of M-CSF and RANK-L. The immature osteoclast begins to express Trap, calcitonin receptor (CTR), and the beta-3 (β3) integrin. RANK-L and a host of transcription factors are required to push the cell into a mature osteoclast phenotype, which maintains expression of many of the same immature osteoclast markers. (B) Osteoblasts are derived from a mesenchymal stem cell, which can also give rise to adipocytes, myoblasts and chondrocytes. Proliferating precursors are pushed toward the preosteoblast phenotype by the expression of Runx2, Dlx5 and Msx2. The preosteoblast expresses collagen I (Col I) and bone sialoprotein (BSP). Further, Runx2 expression, as well as osterix and members of the Wnt signaling cascade (b-catenin, TCF/LEF1) are required to achieve a mature, matrix-producing osteoblast phenotype (Col I, osteocalcin (OC) and alkaline phosphatase expression). Osteoblasts that become trapped in the matrix express E11, an early osteocyte marker, and eventually express DMP-1, Mepe and SOST, as the mature osteocyte phenotype is reached (reproduced with permission of the Annual Reviews from Robling *et al.*[112]).

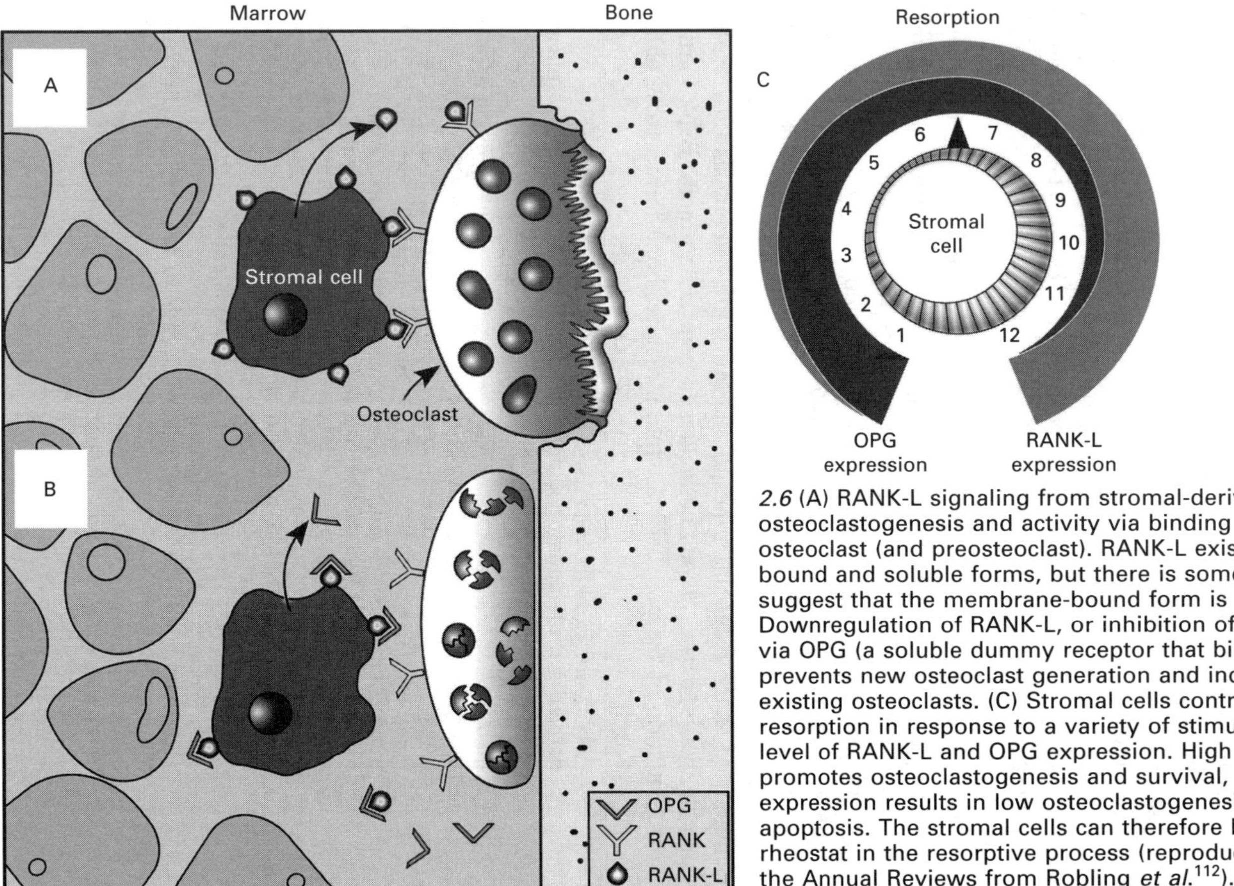

2.6 (A) RANK-L signaling from stromal-derived cells induces osteoclastogenesis and activity via binding to RANK on the osteoclast (and preosteoclast). RANK-L exists in both membrane-bound and soluble forms, but there is some evidence to suggest that the membrane-bound form is more potent. (B) Downregulation of RANK-L, or inhibition of RANK-L availability via OPG (a soluble dummy receptor that binds RANK-L release), prevents new osteoclast generation and induces apoptosis in existing osteoclasts. (C) Stromal cells control osteoclastic bone resorption in response to a variety of stimuli by adjusting the level of RANK-L and OPG expression. High RANK-L expression promotes osteoclastogenesis and survival, whereas high OPG expression results in low osteoclastogenesis and osteoclast apoptosis. The stromal cells can therefore be thought of as a rheostat in the resorptive process (reproduced with permission of the Annual Reviews from Robling *et al.*[112]).

phenotype requires the expression of Runx2, osterix (Osx), and several components of the Wnt signaling pathway.[78, 82–84] The mature osteoblast expresses the matrix proteins type I collagen (Col I) and osteocalcin (OC) and a key enzyme in the mineralization process, alkaline phosphatase (Alk Phos), as a row of active osteoblasts secretes unmineralized matrix (osteoid). These cells will either become bone lining cells or become incorporated into the bone matrix. Those cells that become incorporated into the matrix will gradually develop long cytoplasmic processes in order to remain in communication with surrounding cells and upregulate expression of E11, an early osteocyte marker.[85] At this point the cells are considered immature osteocytes. As the matrix matures and mineralizes, and the osteoid seam moves further away, the osteocyte becomes entombed in a bony matrix and begins to mature and express a new set of genes, including dentin matrix protein-1 (DMP-1), matrix extracellular phosphoglycoprotein (MEPE) and Sost.[86–90]

Osteocytes are the most numerous cells in bone and are found dispersed throughout the matrix where they occupy lacunae (Fig. 2.3B,C). Lacunae are interconnected by an elaborate network of thin tunnels called canaliculi through which osteocytes pass cytoplasmic or dendritic processes.[91] These processes connect individual osteocytes with neighboring cells via gap junctions to facilitate both the transport of nutrients for osteocyte viability and the conveyance of intercellular messages.[92, 93] Intercellular communication is also facilitated by the osteocytic release of signaling molecules into the extracellular fluid which flows through the lacuna–canalicular system.[94, 95] Osteocyte function remains unclear; however, their principal role appears to be the sensing of mechanical stimuli. Osteocytes have long been considered the mechanosensor in bone because of their sheer numbers, distribution and interconnectivity.[96] It is only recently that supportive data has been generated to implicate the osteocyte network as the primary mechanosensory cell type, to the exclusion of other bone cells.[97, 98] This evidence is discussed in greater detail later in this chapter. In addition to mechanosensation, recent evidence has also found osteocytes to have the capacity to regulate mineral metabolism and alter the properties of their surrounding matrix.[98–100]

2.4 Bone physiology

Bone is a dynamic tissue capable of altering its structure and mass in order to adapt to changing requirements. This is achieved via a number of different fundamental tissue-level activities, including repair, growth, modeling and remodeling.[101, 102] It is suggested that each of these activities have their own functions, mediator mechanisms and responses to drugs, hormones, mechanics and other agents.[101, 102] Bone growth, modeling and remodeling will be discussed below.

2.4.1 Bone growth

Bones are formed through two distinct developmental processes—intramembranous and endochondral bone formation. Intramembranous bone formation gives rise to the flat bones that comprise the cranium and medial clavicles, and begins with the condensation of mesenchymal cells which differentiate into osteoblasts and develop ossification centers by direct bone matrix deposition. This forms plates which expand during development, but do not fuse at their junctions with other cranial bones.[103] These junctions or sutures maintain separation between membranous bones and regulate expansive growth of the skull.

Endochondral bone formation gives rise to long bones that comprise the appendicular skeleton, facial bones, vertebrae and portions of the clavicles. As with intramembranous bone formation, endochondral bone formation also begins with the condensation of mesenchymal cells; however, during endochondral bone formation, the differentiation of these cells gives rise to a proliferating population of centrally localized type II collagen-expressing chondrocytes and more peripherally localized type I collagen-expressing perichondrial cells.[104] The chondrocytes produce a specialized extracellular matrix containing type II collagen which forms a cartilaginous template (or 'anlage'). Midway between the ends of this elongated template, chondrocytes exit the cell cycle (hypertrophy) and an ossification center forms by neovascularization of the initially avascular cartilaginous template. Osteoblasts that are associated with the newly developed vasculature begin secretion and mineralization of a type I collagen-containing extracellular matrix. As bones grow, this center of ossification propagates toward the two epiphyseal plates.

The epiphyseal growth plates allow longitudinal bone growth by a sequence of chondrocyte proliferation, differentiation to hypertrophy and cell death (apoptosis) (Fig. 2.7). Proximally (toward the end of a developing bone), a pool of chondrocytes (called the resting or reserve zone) supplies cells to a population of proliferating chondrocytes. Proliferating chondrocytes in turn differentiate to form a transient pool of prehypertrophic and then a more long-lived pool of hypertrophic chondrocytes. At the distal end of the epiphyseal growth plate, hypertrophic chondrocytes die by apoptosis and are replaced by trabecular bone. In this manner, hypertrophic chondrocytes provide a template for the formation of trabecular bone. Chondrocyte proliferation in this process is stopped by the negative influence of local fibroblast growth factor (FGF) signaling,[105] whereas the cytokine parathyroid hormone-related peptide (PTHrP) functions to stop chondrocyte differentiation to hypertrophy by signaling through its receptor.[106]

The determination of whether mesenchymal cells differentiate into either bone-forming osteoblasts for intramembranous bone formation or cartilage producing chondrocytes for endochondral bone formation is regulated

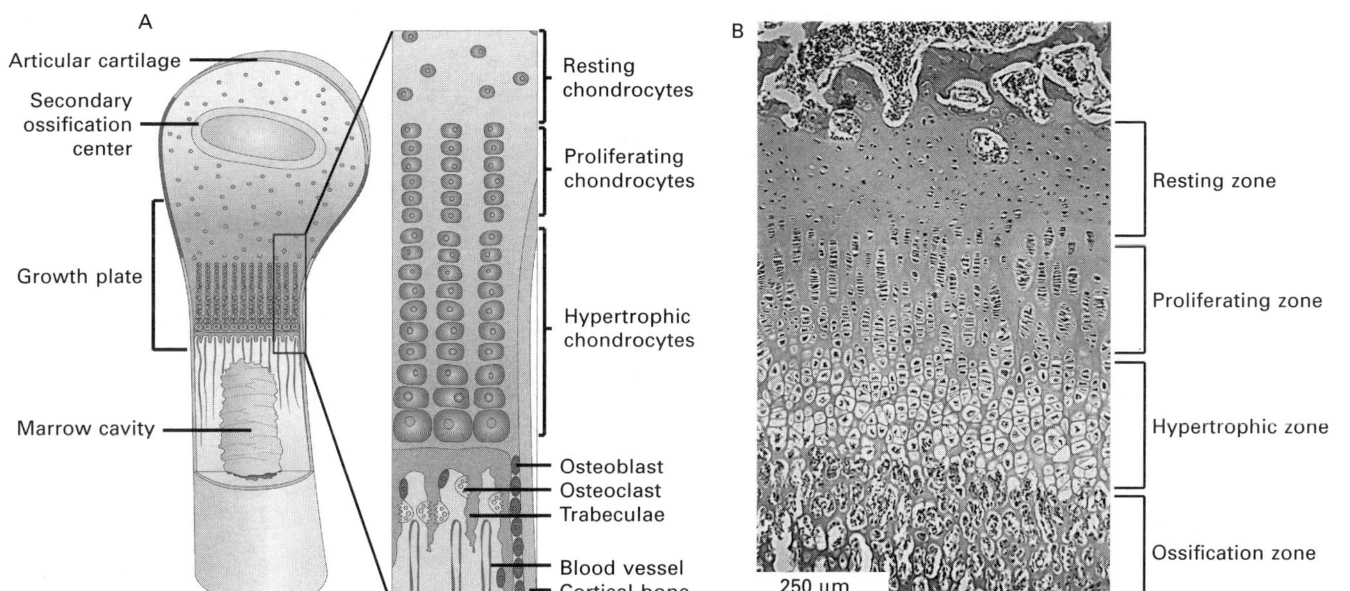

2.7 The epiphyseal growth plate shown (A) schematically and (B) via light microscopy. Growth plates allow longitudinal bone growth by a sequence of chondrocyte proliferation, differentiation to hypertrophy and cell death (apoptosis). Chondrocyte death is accompanied by vessel ingrowth and bone matrix production resulting in ossification of the cartilage scaffold (panel A reproduced with permission of Macmillan Publishers from Page-McCaw *et al.*[232] Panel B courtesy of the University of Kansas Medical Center [©2008]).

by the Wnt/β-catenin or canonical pathway (Fig. 2.8).[107, 108] In areas of intramembranous bone formation, Wnt signaling (induced in part by signaling through another cytokine, sonic hedgehog) results in high levels of β-catenin in MSCs.[83] This induces the expression of genes (including Runx2 and OSX) that are required for osteoblastic cell differentiation and inhibits transcription of genes needed for chrondrogenic differentiation. In contrast, during endochondral bone formation, there are low levels of β-catenin which results in upregulation of the transcription factors of SOX9 and other members of the SOX family.[109] This drives the mesenchymal cells toward chrondrogenic differentiation and away from osteoblastic differentiation.

2.4.2 Bone modeling

Bone modeling is a process that works in concert with bone growth and functions to alter the spatial distribution of accumulating tissue presented by growth.[110,111] The result is a change in the size, shape and position of a typical long bone cross-section which facilitates the ability of the skeleton to meet the rapidly evolving mechanical demands associated with growth.[112, 113] For instance, radial growth via periosteal bone apposition results in greater distribution of bone mineral away from bending axes and a consequential increase in bending resistance. To facilitate locomotion, periosteal apposition is often accompanied during growth by endocortical bone resorption which results in a concomitant increase in the medullary area without a significant impact on bone strength.

Bone modeling is accomplished by modeling drifts whereby bone tissue is selectively added or removed from an existing bone surface to alter bone geometry. This is achieved by the spatially independent actions of bone forming osteoblasts and bone resorbing osteoclasts. As bone formation and resorption during modeling do not occur at the same location, the two processes are said to be 'uncoupled'. When modeling activities are initiated on previously quiescent bone surfaces, either bone formation (F) or resorption (R) follows activation (A). Thus, modeling can be described as either A→F or A→R.[110, 114]

Bone modeling primarily occurs during growth and declines to a relatively trivial level once skeletal maturity is reached. However, renewed modeling in the adult skeleton can occur. Stimuli that potentiate this include increases in mechanical loading, administration of parathyroid hormone (PTH) and the withdrawal of estrogen.[115–120]

2.4.3 Bone remodeling

Remodeling represents bone reconstruction wherein discrete, measureable 'packets' of bone are removed and replaced by new bone. This occurs

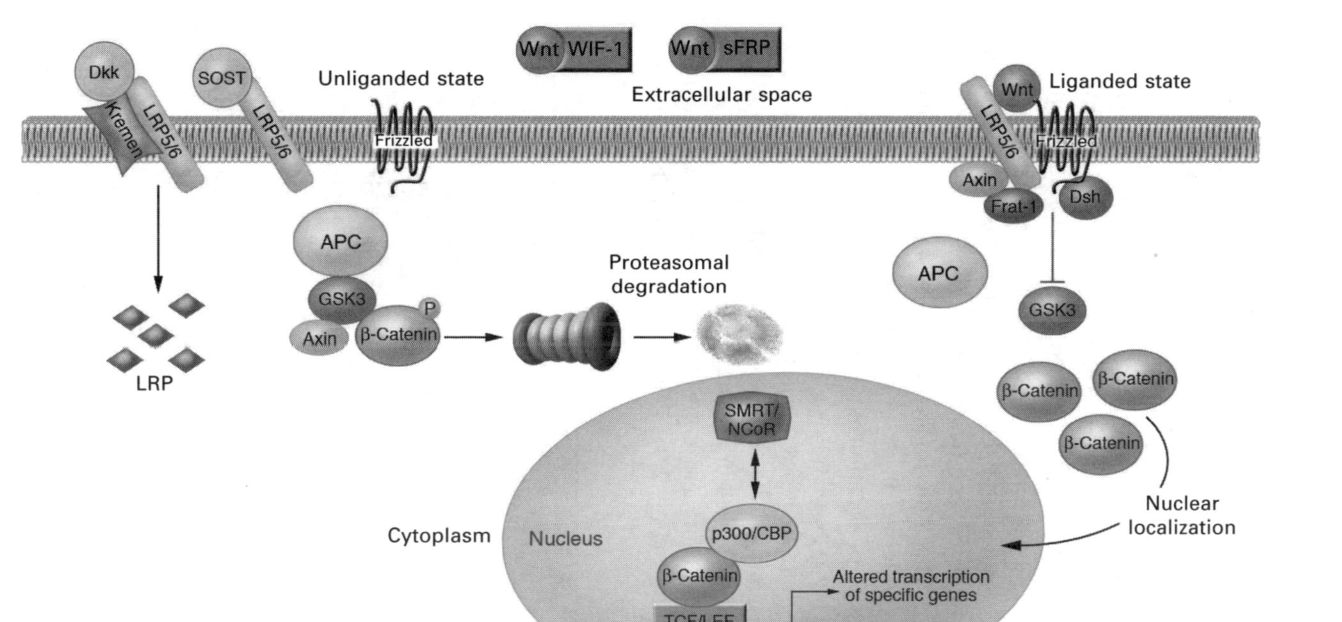

2.8 Elements of the Wnt/β-catenin or canonical pathway. Binding of members of the Wnt cytokine family to Frizzled receptors and low-density lipoprotein receptor-related protein 5 and 6 (LRP5/6) co-receptors inhibits glycogen synthase kinase 3 (GSK3) through mechanisms involving the Axin, Frat-1 and Disheveled (Dsh) proteins. β-catenin accumulates and is translocated to the nucleus where it binds to T cell factor/lymphoid enhancer binding factor (TCF/LEF) to cause displacement of transcriptional corepressors (i.e. silencing mediator of retinoid and thyroid receptors and nuclear receptor corepressor [SMRT/NCoR]) with transcriptional coactivators (i.e. p300 and cAMP response element-binding protein [p300/CBP]). Wnt signaling can be blocked by interactions of Wnt with inhibitory factors including Wnt inhibitory factor 1 (WIF-1) and members of the secreted frizzled-related protein (sFRP) family, or via interaction of LRP5/6 with the Dickkopf (Dkk)/Kremen complex or sclerostin (SOST gene product). The resultant phosphorylation of β-catenin by GSK3 stimulates β-catenin degradation (reproduced with permission of the American Society for Clinical Investigation from Krishnan *et al.*[233] Permission conveyed through Copyright Clearance Center, Inc).

continuously throughout life such that bone is constantly being remodeled in the growing, adult and senescent skeleton. In contrast to modeling, which involves activation and isolated bone resorption (A→R) or formation (A→F) at a bone locus, remodeling involves the temporally and spatially coordinated actions of osteoclasts and osteoblasts. These cells form teams collectively known as basic multicellular units (BMUs) which always remodel bone in a activation→resorption→formation sequence (A→R→F) (Fig. 2.9).

During activation, osteoclast precursors differentiate as previously described into multinucleate osteoclasts (Fig. 2.5A). Although the precise pathways directing osteoclast precursor recruitment are not fully understood, known triggers include mechanical forces, microscopic bone damage (microdamage) and systemic hormones.[121] Remodeling that occurs in response to mechanical forces and microdamage replaces specific packets of bone and is referred to as targeted remodeling.[122] This functions to maintain skeletal mechanical integrity. In contrast, remodeling in response to systemic hormones is apparently random in terms of location and, thus, is referred to as non-targeted remodeling.[122] This type of remodeling enables bone to fulfill its metabolic requirements, which includes the storage and release of minerals such as calcium and phosphorus. It has been estimated that roughly 30% of remodeling is targeted and that 70% in non-targeted.[122]

Resorption follows activation, and consists of an advancing front of actively resorbing osteoclasts (Fig. 2.9). During intracortical remodeling,

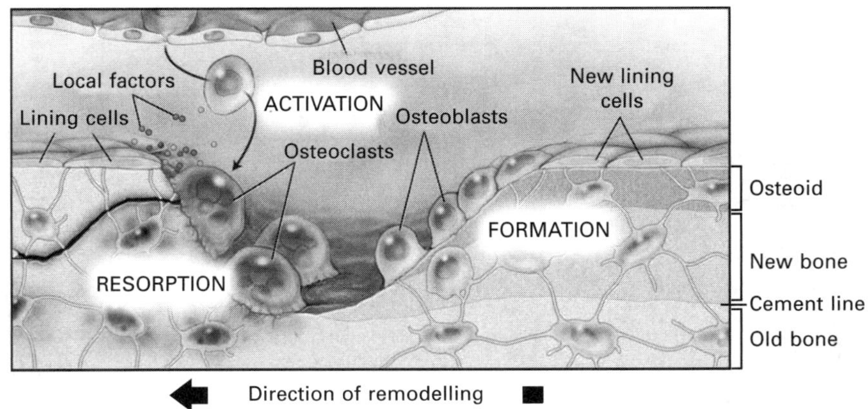

2.9 Bone remodeling by a basic multicellular unit (BMU). A stimulus activates osteoclast precursors to differentiate and form an advancing front of actively resorbing osteoclasts. The resorptive bay created by osteoclastic bone resorption is lined by mononuclear cells (not shown) prior to the formation of osteoid (unmineralized bone matrix) by osteoblasts (reproduced with permission of the Massachusetts Medical Society [©2007; all rights reserved] from Canalis *et al.*[234]).

these cells form a 'cutting cone' which excavates a tunnel roughly 250–300 μm in diameter in the direction of the longitudinal axis of a long bone diaphysis.[123, 124] In trabecular and endocortical bone remodeling, the advancing osteoclasts do not dig or tunnel, as with intracortical remodeling, rather they scallop a saucer-shaped packet of bone from the bone surface.[124] In both situations, a group of mononuclear cells closely follow the advancing front of osteoclasts to line the resorptive bay and probably smooth the surface in preparation for the deposition of a reversal or cement line.

Behind the mononuclear cells, rows of osteoblasts deposit layers of osteoid (unmineralized bone matrix) (Fig. 2.9). During intracortical remodeling, the osteoid is laid down centripetally such that the size of the remodeling space constricts as more concentric osteonal lamellae are deposited and mineralized. This deposition ceases at a specified point leaving a Haversian canal in the center of the newly formed osteon, with the osteon being surrounded circumferentially by a cement line (Fig. 2.3A–C). In trabecular and endocortical bone remodeling, the osteoid is deposited and mineralized in stacks, with the new packet of bone being separated from older packets by a newly laid cement line (Fig. 2.3E).

Remodeling is highly time-dependent with the speed with which a BMU travels through tissue space being referred to as the 'sigma period'. The sigma period quantifies the number of days it takes for a BMU completely to remodel a fixed two-dimensional slice through a region of bone. In human cortical bone, it takes approximately 120 days for the entire BMU to pass through a plane, leaving a new osteon behind.[125, 126] Roughly 20 days is spent initiating and increasing the diameter of the resorption cavity by the osteoclasts, followed by 10 days of reversal (relative quiescence) and finally 90 days of centripetal deposition of bone matrix by the osteoblast teams.

As osteoblasts always trail behind osteoclasts in BMUs and the entire structure moves as a unit, the resorption and formation processes are said to be coupled to one another. Coupling is a strictly controlled process in remodeling which ensures that where bone is removed new bone is deposited.[127] The net amount of old bone removed and new bone restored in the remodeling cycle is a quantity called the bone balance.[121] While coupling is rarely affected, bone balance can vary quite widely in many disease states. For instance, in osteoporosis, prolonged bed rest or hemi-, para- or quadri-plegia, resorption and formation are coupled but there is a negative bone balance such that more bone is resorbed than is replaced by the typical BMU. This results in a net loss of bone mineral which can be assessed clinically by performing non-invasive bone mass assessments. Logically, many pharmaceutical agents for the treatment of conditions wherein there is a net bone loss attempt to create a positive bone balance whereby bone formation exceeds resorption in a typical BMU. This results in a net gain of bone mineral and can be achieved either by inhibiting bone resorption (such as occurs with the administration of bisphosphonate therapies) or by stimulating osteoblasts to produce greater quantities of bone (such as occurs with the administration of PTH).[128]

2.5 Bone adaptation to mechanical loading

2.5.1 Mathematical models for predicting skeletal adaptation to mechanical loading

It has long been established that bone is mechanosensitive and adapts its mass, architecture and mechanical properties in response to mechanical loading. This phenomenon is often loosely referred to as 'Wolff's law', named after the German anatomist/surgeon Julius Wolff who suggested that the form of bone is related to mechanical stress by a mathematical law.[129] Although many basic tenets of Wolff's law have since been suggested to contain engineering and biological inaccuracies,[130, 131] the general concept that bone adapts to its mechanical environment is widely accepted and supported by an abundance of scientific evidence.

One of the key determinants directing the adaptive response of bone to mechanical loading is the level of internal strain experienced within the bone.[132, 133] Strain refers to the change in length per unit length of a bone. It is a unitless value; however, because it is very small for bone, it is often expressed in terms of microstrain ($\propto\varepsilon$). One thousand microstrain is equivalent to 0.1% of deformation or, in other words, a deformation of 0.1 mm for a 10 cm long bone. Bone strains typically range from 400 to 1500 $\propto\varepsilon$ during normal activities of daily living, although activities that involve high impact loads result in higher strains.[134] As complete bone fractures typically occur from single loads that generate strains in excess of 10 000 $\propto\varepsilon$, the safety factor between normal and failure strains is large.

The level of strain experienced within a moiety of bone contributes to one of four tissue-level outcomes: (1) net mineral loss, (2) mineral homeostasis, (3) net mineral gain, or (4) damage formation. Everyday mechanical strains have been predicted to fall between two effective strain levels—the minimum effective strain (MES), speculated to be in the vicinity of 1500–2500 $\mu\varepsilon$[135] and a lower effective strain level, suggested to be approximately 50–200 $\mu\varepsilon$.[136] The combination of these two strain levels created a 'physiological window' for bone adaptation to mechanical loading. When mechanical strains fell within this window, bone resorption during remodeling equaled formation, resulting in mineral homeostasis and no bone adaptation. When mechanical usage caused strain levels to fall outside the limits of the physiological window, an imbalance between bone resorption and formation was predicted. Bone loss (net mineral loss) was predicted for strains below the lower effective strain level (50–200 $\mu\varepsilon$), whereas bone gain (net mineral gain) was predicted for strains above the MES (1500–2500 $\mu\varepsilon$). For extremely high strains, microscopic trauma (microdamage) was predicted.

2.5.2 Factors affecting skeletal adaptation to mechanical loading

Strain magnitude is a key determinant of bone adaptation to a loading stimulus. Bone formation is initiated above a certain threshold strain and incremental increases in strain beyond the threshold result in further increases in formation activity.[133, 137–139] Thus, increasing strain magnitude is one step towards more effective application of mechanical forces to promote osteogenesis. However, there are a number of other important features of a loading stimulus that determine the adaptive response.

The cellular accommodation theory does not solely use strain magnitude to predict the adaptive response to a mechanical stimulus, but rather it uses strain stimulus.[140] The strain stimulus is the product of the strain magnitude and loading frequency.[141] In order for mechanical loading to induce adaptation, the load needs to be introduced dynamically. This follows teleologically given the dynamic nature of bone loading during typical normal functional use. Dynamic loading induces significantly greater adaptation than if the same strain magnitudes are held statically,[142–144] indicating that bone adaptation is not dependent on strain magnitude alone.

Features of dynamic loading that are important determinants of bone adaptation are loading frequency and strain rate.[145, 146] Loading frequency refers to the number of loading cycles per second, whereas strain rate is the product of strain magnitude and loading frequency. Loading has no effect on cortical bone formation unless it is applied at a frequency of 0.5 Hz or greater.[145] A positive relationship between loading frequency and cortical bone formation exists beyond this threshold, with increasing frequency generating progressively greater adaptation.[145–148] However, this relationship may not persist when loading frequencies exceed 10 Hz[149, 150] and may not hold true for trabecular bone, which has shown variable adaptive responses in response to increasing load frequencies.[151–153]

Further features of a loading stimulus that influence the skeletal adaptive response are the duration of the skeletal load and the length of rest between loading bouts. Extending the duration of skeletal loading does not yield proportional increases in bone mass.[154, 155] As loading duration is increased, the bone formation response tends to fade as the mechanosensitive cells accommodate to the prevailing environment (Fig. 2.10). The decline in adaptation with ongoing loading fits a logarithmic relationship, such that after only 20 loading cycles bone has lost more than 95% of its mechanosensitivity. This indicates that loading programs do not need to be long in order to induce adaptation. Similarly, it indicates that bone cells need to be able to resensitize when given a period of rest between loading bouts in order to be responsive to future loading bouts. This is indeed the case with resensitization occurring in seconds to hours, depending on the nature of the loading stimulus. For

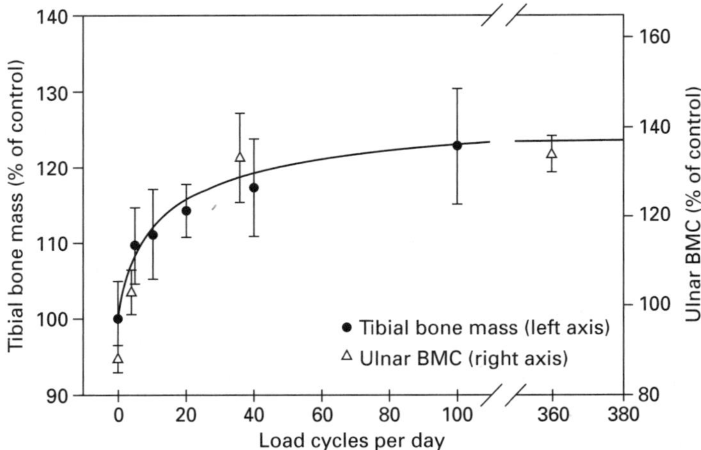

2.10 The bone formation response to a mechanical stimulus fades with increasing loading duration. Although bone mass in the ulna of turkeys (open triangles)[154] and tibia of rats (closed circles)[155] increases with mechanical loading, the anabolic effect saturates as the number of loading cycles increases. There is limited benefit of additional loading cycles above approximately 40 cycles/day (reproduced with permission of Elsevier from Burr *et al.*[235]).

instance, rests of a number of seconds between each consecutive load cycle result in greater bone adaptation than if the same strain stimulus is introduced in back-to-back cycles,[156, 157] whereas rests of a number of hours between consecutive loading bouts results in greater bone adaptation than if the same strain stimulus is introduced in back-to-back bouts.[158–160]

2.5.3 Site-specificity of the adaptive response of bone to mechanical loading

As the response of bone to mechanical loading is highly stimulus-specific, it follows that its adaptive response is also highly site-specific. Only those bones that are actually loaded undergo adaptation. This has most clearly been shown in racquet-sport players in whom the playing or racquet arm has significantly greater bone mass and size than in the contralateral, non-playing arm.[37, 161–163] Yet, the site-specific nature of bone adaptation to mechanical loading can be localized further than to the individual bone level. Long bones are curved such that they bend when axially loaded. Bending results in the exposure of different regions within the bone cross-section to different levels of microstrain. Only those regions within the bone that experience sufficient strain stimulus adapt. This can be clearly observed in the rodent ulna axial compression model (Fig. 2.11). The site-specific depositing of new bone is functionally important. It adds bone and increases bone strength where it is

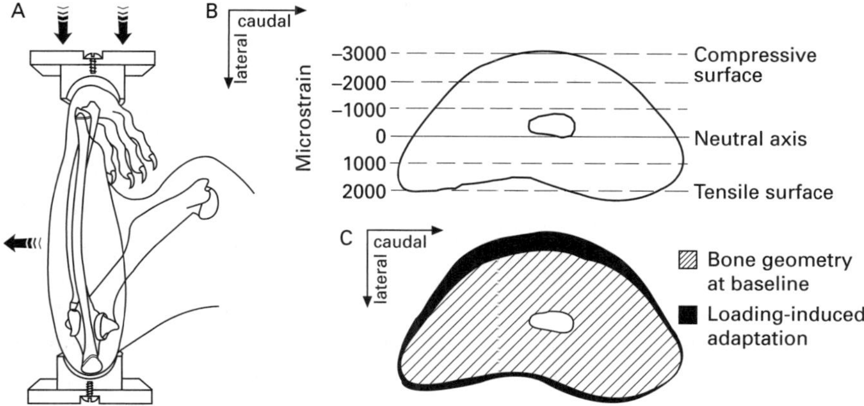

2.11 The adaptive response of bone to mechanical loading is site-specific such that only those regions within a bone that experience sufficient microstrain will adapt. (A) Schematic diagram of the rodent ulna axial compression model. The distal forelimb is fixed between upper and lower cups. When force is applied to one of the cups, the ulna is caused to bow laterally. (B) The bending of the ulna under axial compression generates medial surface compression and lateral surface tension at the midshaft. There is no strain along the axis through which the bone is bending (neutral axis). (C) Loading of rat ulnas for 16 weeks using the axial compression model causes new bone to be formed on surfaces of high strain (medial and lateral surfaces). There is minimal new bone formation near the neutral axis (caudal and cranial surfaces) where there is the least microstrain during loading.

needed most, in the direction of loading, while not overtly increasing the overall weight of the bone. This means for a small increase in bone mineral, much larger increases in bone strength can be generated. The implication of the site-specific response of bone to mechanical stimuli is that loading needs to be directed toward the bones and sites where promotion of osteogenesis is desired. To achieve this and induce the most functional adaptation, the loading should be in the same direction as the bone is loaded in function.

2.5.4 Bone response to disuse

Skeletal disuse results in profound bone loss. In growing bones the effect of disuse is most apparent at the periosteal surfaces of long bones, where normal appositional growth is suppressed. This results in bones of smaller cross-section. After skeletal maturity is achieved, disuse causes frank bone loss involving accelerated remodeling and bone resorption, with loss occurring mainly at endosteal and trabecular surfaces of long bones. Skeletal disuse results from a number of conditions, including prolonged bed rest,[164] space flight,[165] disease states (including spinal cord injury and stroke[166, 167]) and following injury.[168] The most pertinent of these in the current context are the bone changes that occur with prolonged bed rest and following injury.

Bed rest was first introduced as a medical treatment in the 19th century. During this time, any adverse complications associated with bed rest were attributed to the condition responsible for bed rest. It was not until the 1940s that it was questioned whether the increased calcium excretion associated with disease (predominantly polio at the time) was caused by the disease itself or the resulting inactivity. Dietrick *et al.*[169] explored this by placing otherwise healthy medical students on bed rest in lower body casts for 30 days. They showed that the disuse associated with bed rest resulted in increased calcium excretion and decreased lower extremity bone density, indicating for the first time that prolonged bed rest is detrimental to bone. Today it has been established that prolonged bed rest is associated with a 0.5–1% loss of bone density per month.[164] To counter this, most medical protocols currently encourage the least possible interruption to an individual's weight-bearing status.

Prolonged bed rest represents an extreme situation of disuse. A less extreme, yet more frequent scenario involves regional disuse caused by local injury or pathology. Local injury results in reduced mechanical loading within a region in an attempt to reduce tissue stresses and the subsequent provocation of symptoms. Combining this with the use of external supports to limit excessive motion and permit healing, and the introduction of any localized stress shielding resulting from the introduction of rigid internal fixation, there is localized disuse and a subsequent site-specific net loss of bone mineral. This is often temporary and reversed with the reintroduction of usual loads; however, it is not uncommon for residual deficits in bone mass to persist.[168]

2.5.5 Bone response to overuse

The safety factor between normal strains and those required for bone failure (fracture) is large. Thus, bone does not typically fail during everyday activities, such as walking and running. However, subfailure strains associated with these activities are capable of generating damage when introduced repetitively. As with other structural materials, a natural phenomenon in bone associated with repetitive strain (mechanical overuse) is the generation of damage (often termed microdamage). Microdamage was first described by Frost[170] and has since been categorized morphologically according to four types: (1) microcracks, (2) cross-hatching cracks, (3) diffuse damage and (4) microfractures (Fig. 2.12A).[171, 172] Microcracks are small linear cracks that take the form of planar ellipses, typically with major and minor axes of length of 400 μm and 100 μm, respectively.[173] They are most commonly

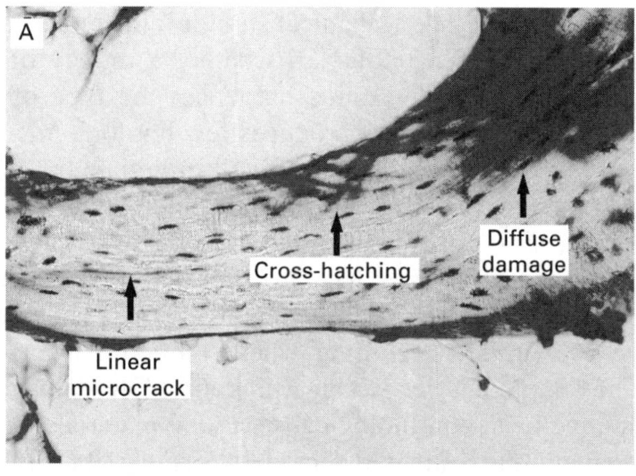

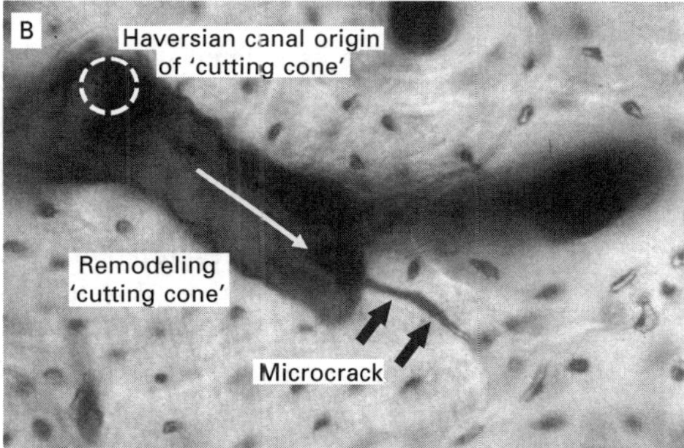

2.12 Microdamage in bone. (A) Trabecular bone strut stained with basic fuchsin demonstrating three types of microdamage. (B) Interstitial cortical microcrack that is the target of remodeling activity (panel A reproduced with permission of Elsevier from Fazzalari *et al.*[236] Panel B courtesy of Dr. David B. Burr, Indiana University School of Medicine).

found in cortical interstitial lamellae and are frequently limited by osteonal cement lines. Diffuse damage is more frequently found in trabecular bone and is identified by an intensely stained mineralized matrix which represents areas containing many small cracks each of the order of a micrometer in size.[173] Also, common in trabecular bone are intermediate-sized cracks arranged in a cross-hatched pattern (cross-hatched cracks) and completely fractured trabecular struts (microfractures).[174]

Microdamage is a mechanically related phenomenon. Its formation is both strain magnitude and rate dependent, with increases in either beyond threshold levels resulting in increased damage formation.[175–178] Damage is also influenced by the total number of bone loading cycles, with its formation occurring at physiological strains in response to pure cyclic overloading.[179]

In addition to these features of the mechanical stimulus, the mode of loading influences damage formation. In particular, whether a moiety of bone is exposed to compressive or tensile strains influences the type of damage that forms.[180, 181] Compressive loading produces few but long microcracks, suggesting that cracks in compression are difficult to initiate but propagate easily.[181] They are thought to result from the shearing of longitudinally oriented osteons.[182] In contrast, tensile loading primarily produces diffuse damage, which suggests that cracks in tension have a lower initiation threshold but do not readily propagate.[181]

Questions have been raised regarding whether microdamage in bone is good or bad. The simple answer is that it is both. Microdamage can be good, as bone is unique from non-biological structural materials in that it is capable of self-repair through targeted remodeling (Fig. 2.12B). This was demonstrated by Burr and colleagues[183, 184] who found new bone BMUs to be four- to six-times more likely to be associated with fatigue-induced microcracks than by chance alone. Furthermore, when bone remodeling is suppressed by treatment with bisphosphonates, the amount of microdamage significantly increases.[185–187] Thus, damage serves as a stimulus that activates bone remodeling, with the initiating stimulus possibly being osteocyte apoptosis.[188, 189] The remodeling response ensures relative homeostasis between damage formation and its repair and maintains skeletal mechanical competence. It also enables a bone to adapt over time to its mechanical environment such that it can meet increasing levels of loading.

On the other hand, microdamage in bone may be bad as it has been associated with a pathology continuum that includes stress fractures and complete bone fractures.[190–192] Damage serves as a stimulus that activates bone remodeling which normally removes damage approximately as fast as it occurs. However, remodeling is time dependent with the time required to reach a new equilibrium following the development of damage being in the order of one remodeling period (approximately 3–4 months).[125, 126] If insufficient time is given to adapt to a mechanical stimulus, further damage may occur with additional loading. Although a remodeling reserve exists that allows increased activation of remodeling units in response to increases in damage formation, an increase in the number of active remodeling units removes bone temporarily, reducing bone mass and potentially increasing the chance for damage initiation when loading is continued. This feed forward results from the fact that resorption precedes formation in the remodeling process so that an increase in the number of currently active remodeling units is associated with an increase in bone porosity. This reduces the elastic modulus of the bone, which in turn increases strain and, subsequently, the rate of damage formation. Thus, microdamage can be viewed as bad as it can be associated with a progressive loss of stiffness and strength as microcracks coalesce forming larger macrocracks until eventual fatigue failure is reached.

2.5.6 Mechanisms for bone adaptation to mechanical loading

The mechanosensitivity of the skeleton has long been established; however, the precise mechanisms underlying this response remain uncertain. It is logical to assume that the process involves some form of mechanotransduction, which refers to the conversion of a biophysical force into a cellular response.[193] It is a generic process whose role is to enable living organisms to respond to their mechanical environment. A model for mechanotransduction in bone is illustrated in Fig. 2.13.

Osteoblasts, bone-lining cells and osteocytes have all been shown to respond to mechanical stimulation; however, it is the osteocyte that appears anatomically to be the best positioned to sense and convey changes in the local mechanical environment.[96] This results from the sheer numbers and distribution of osteocytes throughout the bone matrix and their high degree of interconnectivity.[94] Recent evidence investigating the role of an osteocyte-specific protein (sclerostin, the protein product of the SOST gene) supports osteocytes as the primary mechanosensory cell, to the exclusion of the other bone cell types (i.e. osteoblasts and bone lining cells).[97]

Even though osteocytes are thought to be mechanosensors, there is little conclusive data to show how mechanical loading is sensed by these cells. One of the more accepted forms is the flow of bone interstitial fluid driven by extravascular pressure in combination with applied mechanical loading.[194, 195] This theory has support from studies demonstrating mechanically enhanced transport within the lacunar–canalicular system of bone.[95] Fluid flow along cell bodies or processes produces drag force, fluid shear stress and an electrical potential called a streaming or stress-generated potential. Each of these signals may activate bone cells, although cell culture experiments suggest that cells are more sensitive to fluid forces than they are to electrical potential.[195, 196] Fluid shear stresses on osteocytes appear to deform the cells within their lacunae and the cellular dendrites within the canaliculi.[195] It may also influence the primary cilium that projects extracellularly from the osteocyte cell body.[197]

Following detection of a local mechanical stimulus, the signal needs to be translated into a cellular response by the sensor. Mechanical deformation of a cell membrane by fluid shear stresses may have a direct influence on the cellular translation of mechanical stimuli.[198, 199] The phospholipid membrane of bone cells contains membrane spanning glycoproteins called integrins. Extracellularly, these integrins connect with the collagen of the organic matrix via specific receptors for extracellular matrix proteins.[199, 200] Intracellularly, they attach to the intracellular cytoskeleton which, in turn, connects to the nuclear membrane and other cytoplasmic constituents.[201] The result is the formation of a continuous network called the extracellular matrix–integrin–cytoskeleton

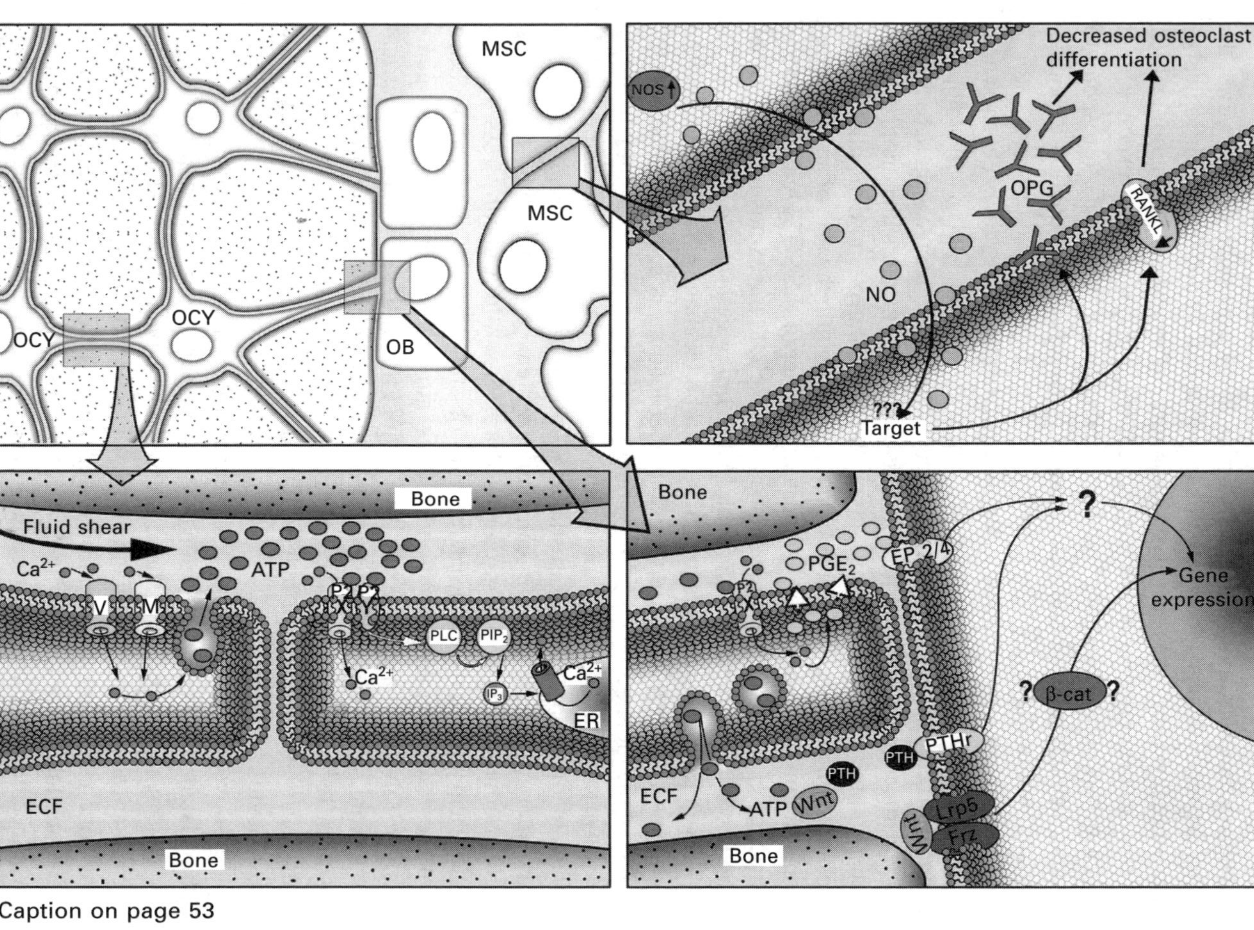

Caption on page 53

axis which connects the extracellular matrix directly to the nucleus and cytoplasmic constituents of the cell. As the cytoskeleton continually generates an internal tensile force, the extracellular matrix–integrin–cytoskeleton axis is constantly under tension.[202, 203] Consequently, deformation of the cell membrane away from its extracellular anchors may increase cytoskeleton tension and transmit fluid shear stresses directly to the internal environment of the cell in order to alter protein synthesis and gene expression.[193, 198]

Cell membrane deformation by fluid shear stresses is putatively involved in biochemical coupling; however, it is possible that the extracellular matrix–integrin–cytoskeleton axis simply acts as an amplifier of mechanical signals, rather than an actual mechanotransducer.[204] Instead, it is possible that biochemical coupling is primarily mediated by influences on transmembrane–membrane ion channels. Bone cells respond to fluid shear stresses with a rapid increase in intracellular Ca^{2+} which is dependent on extracellular Ca^{2+} entry and intracellular Ca^{2+} release.[205] Rapid Ca^{2+} entry into a cell requires the activation of multiple ion channels. One of these, the mechanosensitive cation-selective channel (MSCC), is activated by membrane deformation.[206, 207] When this channel is blocked by a non-specific blocker (gadolinium [Gd^{3+}]), the fluid shear-induced increase in intracellular Ca^{2+} is significantly reduced, confirming the channel's contribution to biochemical coupling.[205, 208–210]

Once a mechanical stimulus has been converted into a biochemical response by the sensor cells, these cells need to convey a signal to the cells responsible for generating bone adaptation. One of the first steps in transmission appears to be Ca^{2+} dependent vesicular release of ATP into the extracellular milieu.[211]

2.13 Model for mechanotransduction in bone. Fluid shear on osteocytes (OCY) induces an influx of extracellular Ca^{2+} via voltage-sensitive (V) and perhaps mechanosensitive (M) channels. Shear stress also enhances ATP release, which binds to the purinergic receptors P2X (ionotropic) and P2Y (metabotropic). Signaling through P2Y is required for Ca^{2+} release from intracellular stores via a G_q–PLC–PIP_2–IP_3 pathway. ATP release causes PGE_2 release through signaling downstream of the $P2X_7$ receptor. PGE_2 binds and signals through one of the EP receptors, probably EP4 and/or EP2, and ultimately results in enhanced bone formation. PTH signaling also appears to be required for mechanotransduction to occur, but the intracellular pathways involved are not well understood (?). Wnt signaling through the Lrp5 receptor, which acts through beta catenin (β-cat) translocation to the nucleus, also appears to be important in mechanically induced bone formation. Pressure in the marrow cavity and/or fluid shear forces on marrow stromal cells (MSC) may stimulate nitric oxide synthase (NOS) activity and nitric oxide (NO) release. NO is a strong inhibitor of bone resorption and probably acts by inhibiting RANK-L expression, while increasing osteoprotegerin (OPG) production (RANK-L enhances osteoclast differentiation, whereas OPG suppresses this process). OCY = osteocyte; OB = osteoblast; MSC = marrow stromal cell (reproduced with permission of the Annual Reviews from Robling *et al.*[112]).

Once released, ATP binds with purinergic (P2) receptors, which can be divided into two families – metabotropic G protein-linked P2Y receptors and ionotropic P2X receptors.[212] Activation of these receptors results in an increase in intracellular Ca^{2+}.[213, 214] P2Y receptor activation increases intracellular Ca^{2+} levels by stimulating the release of Ca^{2+} from intracellular stores via a phospholipase C (PLC)–phosphatidylinositol bisphosphate (PIP_2)–inositol triphosphate (IP_3) pathway, whereas P2X receptors are ligand-gated ion channels which form pores within the cell membrane allowing permeation of extracellular Ca^{2+}.[112]

Activation of the P2 receptors, and in particular the $P2X_7$ receptor, influences the adaptive response of bone to mechanical loading. In particular, as much as 73% of the osteogenic response to loading *in vivo* has been linked to the $P2X_7$ receptor.[215] The downstream mechanism/s by which P2 activation and the increase in intracellular Ca^{2+} results in signal transmission required for bone adaptation is not yet resolved. However, it has been shown that P2 signaling modulates cyclooxygenase-2 (COX-2) expression[216] and prostaglandin release.[217, 218] COX-2 is the rate limiting enzyme in the conversion of arachidonic acid to prostaglandins. Prostaglandins have effects on bone formation and resorption, which are mediated through the proliferation and differentiation of osteoblasts and the regulation of osteoclast differentiation.[219] The upregulation of COX-2 and subsequent release of prostaglandins following mechanical loading is important in regulating an effector response, as inhibition of COX-2 reduces the prostaglandin response[220, 221] and suppresses mechanically induced bone adaptation.[222, 223]

The signal is transmitted to the bone surface where it stimulates the differentiation of precursor cells into osteoblasts to elicit a response. The timing of a response following mechanical loading is similar among different models of mechanical loading. Studies in avian ulna compact bone have shown that a single loading exposure transformed the periosteal cellular layer from a quiescent to an osteogenic cell layer within five to seven days.[224, 225] In the rat tibia, mineral apposition rate was highest over a similar period, five to eight days after a single loading bout.[226, 227] This increased bone formation is believed to result from the activation of discrete packets of osteoprogenitor cells which differentiate and synthesize osteoid.[227] Two days following a single loading bout, osteoblast surface length increases with a peak on day 3.[228] From days 5–12, bone formation rate is increased largely owing to increases in bone forming surface.[227] Nine days after a single loading session, osteoblast surface length returns to normal.

2.6 Conclusions

In this chapter we presented details of the structure and function of bone tissue in a hierarchical format, starting at the gross macroscopic level and extending down to the microscopic cellular level. Understanding the basic biology of bone tissue is essential for a detailed understanding of how bone responds to its environment, including how it repairs with both surgical and non-surgical interventions, and how it interacts with biomaterials.

2.7 References

1. Beck TJ, Oreskovic TL, Stone KL, Ruff CB, Ensrud K, Nevitt MC, Genant HK and Cummings SR (2001). 'Structural adaptation to changing skeletal load in the progression toward hip fragility: the study of osteoporotic fractures', *J Bone Miner Res*, **16** (6), 1108–19.
2. Duan Y, Beck TJ, Wang XF and Seeman E (2003). 'Structural and biomechanical basis of sexual dimorphism in femoral neck fragility has its origins in growth and aging', *J Bone Miner Res*, **18** (10), 1766–74.
3. Mayhew PM, Thomas CD, Clement JG, Loveridge N, Beck TJ, Bonfield W, Burgoyne CJ and Reeve J (2005). 'Relation between age, femoral neck cortical stability, and hip fracture risk', *Lancet*, **366** (9480), 129–35.
4. Mach DB, Rogers SD, Sabino MC, Luger NM, Schwei MJ, Pomonis JD, Keyser CP, Clohisy DR, Adams DJ, O'Leary P and Mantyh PW (2002). 'Origins of skeletal pain: sensory and sympathetic innervation of the mouse femur', *Neuroscience*, **113** (1), 155–66.
5. Ural A and Vashishth D (2006). 'Interactions between microstructural and geometrical adaptation in human cortical bone', J Orthop Res, **24** (7), 1489–98.
6. Cooper DM, Thomas CD, Clement JG, Turinsky AL, Sensen CW and Hallgrimsson B (2007). 'Age-dependent change in the 3D structure of cortical porosity at the human femoral midshaft', *Bone*, **40** (4), 957–65.
7. Gross TS, Damji AA, Judex S, Bray RC and Zernicke RF (1999). 'Bone hyperemia precedes disuse-induced intracortical bone resorption', *J Appl Physiol*, **86** (1), 230–5.
8. Bentolila V, Boyce TM, Fyhrie DP, Drumb R, Skerry TM and Schaffler MB (1998). 'Intracortical remodeling in adult rat long bones after fatigue loading', *Bone*, **23** (3), 275–81.
9. Burr DB, Hirano T, Turner CH, Hotchkiss C, Brommage R and Hock JM (2001). 'Intermittently administered human parathyroid hormone (1–34) treatment increases intracortical bone turnover and porosity without reducing bone strength in the humerus of ovariectomized cynomolgus monkeys', *J Bone Miner Res*, **16** (1), 157–65.
10. Roschger P, Rinnerthaler S, Yates J, Rodan GA, Fratzl P and Klaushofer K (2001). 'Alendronate increases degree and uniformity of mineralization in cancellous bone and decreases the porosity in cortical bone of osteoporotic women', *Bone*, **29** (2), 185–91.
11. Russo CR, Lauretani F, Seeman E, Bartali B, Bandinelli S, Di Iorio A, Guralnik J and Ferrucci L (2006). 'Structural adaptations to bone loss in aging men and women', *Bone*, **38** (1), 112–8.
12. Ural A and Vashishth D (2007). 'Effects of intracortical porosity on fracture toughness in aging human bone: a microCT-based cohesive finite element study', *J Biomech Eng*, **129** (5), 625–31.
13. Gurevitch O, Slavin S and Feldman AG (2007). 'Conversion of red bone marrow into yellow – Cause and mechanisms', *Med Hypotheses*, **69** (3), 531–6.

14. Waitches G, Zawin JK and Poznanski AK (1994). 'Sequence and rate of bone marrow conversion in the femora of children as seen on MR imaging: are accepted standards accurate'? *AJR Am J Roentgenol*, **162** (6), 1399–406.
15. Moore SG and Dawson KL (1990). 'Red and yellow marrow in the femur: age-related changes in appearance at MR imaging', *Radiology*, **175** (1), 219–23.
16. Mow VC, Ratcliffe A and Woo SL-Y (1990). *Biomechanics of Diarthrodial Joints*, Springer, New York.
17. Riggs BL, Melton LJ, Robb RA, Camp JJ, Atkinson EJ, McDaniel L, Amin S, Rouleau PA and Khosla S (2008). 'A population-based assessment of rates of bone loss at multiple skeletal sites: evidence for substantial trabecular bone loss in young adult women and men', *J Bone Miner Res*, **23** (2), 205–14.
18. Chavassieux P, Seeman E and Delmas PD (2007). 'Insights into material and structural basis of bone fragility from diseases associated with fractures: how determinants of the biomechanical properties of bone are compromised by disease', *Endocr Rev*, **28** (2), 151–64.
19. Silva MJ and Gibson LJ (1997). 'Modeling the mechanical behavior of vertebral trabecular bone: effects of age-related changes in microstructure', *Bone*, **21** (2), 191–9.
20. van der Linden JC, Homminga J, Verhaar JA and Weinans H (2001). 'Mechanical consequences of bone loss in cancellous bone', *J Bone Miner Res*, **16** (3), 457–65.
21. Weinstein RS and Hutson MS (1987). 'Decreased trabecular width and increased trabecular spacing contribute to bone loss with aging', *Bone*, **8** (3), 137–42.
22. Aaron JE, Shore PA, Shore RC, Beneton M and Kanis JA (2000). 'Trabecular architecture in women and men of similar bone mass with and without vertebral fracture: II. Three-dimensional histology', *Bone*, **27** (2), 277–82.
23. Jee WS (2001). 'Integrated bone tissue physiology: anatomy and physiology', In: *Bone Mechanics Handbook*, Cowin S (ed.) 2nd edition, CRC Press, Boca Raton, FL, 1–68.
24. Taylor JF (1992). 'The periosteum and bone growth', In: *Bone Growth VI*, Hall BK (ed.), CRC Press, Boca Raton, 21–52.
25. Hohmann EL, Elde RP, Rysavy JA, Einzig S and Gebhard RL (1986). 'Innervation of periosteum and bone by sympathetic vasoactive intestinal peptide-containing nerve fibers', *Science*, **232** (4752), 868–71.
26. Ito Y, Fitzsimmons JS, Sanyal A, Mello MA, Mukherjee N and O'Driscoll SW (2001). 'Localization of chondrocyte precursors in periosteum', *Osteoarthritis Cartilage*, **9** (3), 215–23.
27. Nakahara H, Bruder SP, Goldberg VM and Caplan AI (1990). '*In vivo* osteochondrogenic potential of cultured cells derived from the periosteum', *Clin Orthop Relat Res*, (259), 223–32.
28. Nakahara H, Bruder SP, Haynesworth SE, Holecek JJ, Baber MA, Goldberg VM and Caplan AI (1990). 'Bone and cartilage formation in diffusion chambers by subcultured cells derived from the periosteum', *Bone*, **11** (3), 181–8.
29. Allen MR, Hock JM and Burr DB (2004). 'Periosteum: biology, regulation, and response to osteoporosis therapies', *Bone*, **35** (5), 1003–12.
30. Islam A, Glomski C and Henderson ES (1990). 'Bone lining (endosteal) cells and hematopoiesis: a light microscopic study of normal and pathologic human bone marrow in plastic-embedded sections', *Anat Rec*, **227** (3), 300–6.
31. Taichman RS (2005). 'Blood and bone: two tissues whose fates are intertwined to create the hematopoietic stem-cell niche', *Blood*, **105** (7), 2631–9.

32. Adams GB and Scadden DT (2006). 'The hematopoietic stem cell in its place', *Nat Immunol*, **7** (4), 333–7.
33. Yin T and Li L (2006). 'The stem cell niches in bone', *J Clin Invest*, **116** (5), 1195–201.
34. Stout SD, Brunsden BS, Hildebolt CF, Commean PK, Smith KE and Tappen NC (1999). 'Computer-assisted 3D reconstruction of serial sections of cortical bone to determine the 3D structure of osteons', *Calcif Tissue Int*, **65**, 280–4.
35. Skedros JG, Holmes JL, Vajda EG and Bloebaum RD (2005). 'Cement lines of secondary osteons in human bone are not mineral-deficient: new data in a historical perspective', *Anat Rec A Discov Mol Cell Evol Biol*, **286** (1), 781–803.
36. Burr DB, Schaffler MB, Yang KH, Lukoschek M, Sivaneri N, Blaha JD and Radin EL (1989). 'Skeletal change in response to altered strain environments: is woven bone a response to elevated strain?' *Bone*, **10** (3), 223–33.
37. Kannus P, Haapasalo H, Sankelo M, Sievänen H, Pasanen M, Heinonen A, Oja P and Vuori I (1995). 'Effect of starting age of physical activity on bone mass in the dominant arm of tennis and squash players', *Ann Int Med*, **123**, 27–31.
38. Krane S (1977). 'Paget's disease of bone', *Clin Orthop Relat Res*, **127**, 24–36.
39. Krane SM (1980). 'Skeletal metabolism in Paget's disease of bone', *Arthritis Rheum*, **23** (10), 1087–94.
40. Silva MJ and Touhey DC (2007). 'Bone formation after damaging *in vivo* fatigue loading results in recovery of whole-bone monotonic strength and increased fatigue life', *J Orthop Res*, **25** (2), 252–61.
41. Uthgenannt BA, Kramer MH, Hwu JA, Wopenka B and Silva MJ (2007). 'Skeletal self-repair: stress fracture healing by rapid formation and densification of woven bone', *J Bone Miner Res*, **22** (10), 1548–56.
42. Currey JD (2003). 'The many adaptations of bone', *J Biomech*, **36** (10), 1487–95.
43. Buckwalter JA, Glimcher MJ, Cooper RR and Recker R (1996). 'Bone biology. I: Structure, blood supply, cells, matrix, and mineralization', *Instr Course Lect*, **45**, 371–86.
44. Brodsky B and Persikov AV (2005). 'Molecular structure of the collagen triple helix', *Adv Protein Chem*, **70**, 301–39.
45. Brodsky B and Ramshaw JA (1997). 'The collagen triple-helix structure', *Matrix Biol*, **15** (8–9), 545–54.
46. Knott L and Bailey AJ (1998). 'Collagen cross-links in mineralizing tissues: a review of their chemistry, function, and clinical relevance', *Bone*, **22** (3), 181–7.
47. Paschalis E (2007). 'Material properties: collagen', In: *The Bone Quality Book*, vol. 1. Dempster DW, Felsenberg D and Van Der Geest S (eds.), Excerpta Medica, Amsterdam, 42–8.
48. Seeman E and Delmas PD (2006). 'Bone quality–the material and structural basis of bone strength and fragility', *N Engl J Med*, **354** (21), 2250–61.
49. Martin E and Shapiro JR (2007). 'Osteogenesis imperfecta:epidemiology and pathophysiology', *Curr Osteoporos Rep*, **5** (3), 91–7.
50. Vashishth D, Gibson GJ, Khoury JI, Schaffler MB, Kimura J and Fyhrie DP (2001). 'Influence of nonenzymatic glycation on biomechanical properties of cortical bone', *Bone*, **28** (2), 195–201.
51. Gordon JA, Tye CE, Sampaio AV, Underhill TM, Hunter GK and Goldberg HA (2007). 'Bone sialoprotein expression enhances osteoblast differentiation and matrix mineralization *in vitro*', *Bone*, **41** (3), 462–73.

52. Roach HI (1994). 'Why does bone matrix contain non-collagenous proteins? The possible roles of osteocalcin, osteonectin, osteopontin and bone sialoprotein in bone mineralisation and resorption', *Cell Biol Int*, **18** (6), 617–28.
53. Young MF, Kerr JM, Ibaraki K, Heegaard AM and Robey PG (1992). 'Structure, expression, and regulation of the major noncollagenous matrix proteins of bone', *Clin Orthop Relat Res*, **281**, 275–94.
54. Chen J, McKee MD, Nanci A and Sodek J (1994). 'Bone sialoprotein mRNA expression and ultrastructural localization in fetal porcine calvarial bone: comparisons with osteopontin', *Histochem J*, **26** (1), 67–78.
55. Hunter GK and Goldberg HA (1993). 'Nucleation of hydroxyapatite by bone sialoprotein', *Proc Natl Acad Sci USA*, **90** (18), 8562–5.
56. Landis WJ, Hodgens KJ, Arena J, Song MJ and McEwen BF (1996) 'Structural relations between collagen and mineral in bone as determined by high voltage electron microscopic tomography', *Microsc Res Tech*, **33** (2), 192–202.
57. Landis WJ, Hodgens KJ, Song MJ, Arena J, Kiyonaga S, Marko M, Owen C and McEwen BF (1996). 'Mineralization of collagen may occur on fibril surfaces: evidence from conventional and high-voltage electron microscopy and three-dimensional imaging. *J Struct Biol*, **117** (1), 24–35.
58. Tondravi MM, McKercher SR, Anderson K, Erdmann JM, Quiroz M, Maki R and Teitelbaum SL (1997). 'Osteopetrosis in mice lacking haematopoietic transcription factor PU.1', *Nature*, **386** (6620), 81–4.
59. Yoshida H, Hayashi S, Kunisada T, Ogawa M, Nishikawa S, Okamura H, Sudo T and Shultz LD (1990). 'The murine mutation osteopetrosis is in the coding region of the macrophage colony stimulating factor gene', *Nature*, **345** (6274), 442–4.
60. Boyle WJ, Simonet WS and Lacey DL (2003). 'Osteoclast differentiation and activation', *Nature*, **423** (6937), 337–42.
61. Suda T, Takahashi N, Udagawa N, Jimi E, Gillespie MT and Martin TJ (1999). 'Modulation of osteoclast differentiation and function by the new members of the tumor necrosis factor receptor and ligand families', *Endocr Rev*, **20** (3), 345–57.
62. Teitelbaum SL and Ross FP (2003). 'Genetic regulation of osteoclast development and function', *Nat Rev Genet*, **4** (8), 638–49.
63. Matsuo K, Galson DL, Zhao C, Peng L, Laplace C, Wang KZ, Bachler MA, Amano H, Aburatani H, Ishikawa H and Wagner EF (2004). 'Nuclear factor of activated T-cells (NFAT) rescues osteoclastogenesis in precursors lacking c-Fos', *J Biol Chem*, **279** (25), 26475–80.
64. Wang ZQ, Ovitt C, Grigoriadis AE, Mohle-Steinlein U, Ruther U and Wagner EF (1992). 'Bone and haematopoietic defects in mice lacking c-fos', *Nature*, **360** (6406), 741–5.
65. Partington GA, Fuller K, Chambers TJ and Pondel M (2004). 'Mitf-PU.1 interactions with the tartrate-resistant acid phosphatase gene promoter during osteoclast differentiation, *Bone*, **34** (2), 237–45.
66. Takayanagi H, Kim S, Koga T, Nishina H, Isshiki M, Yoshida H, Saiura A, Isobe M, Yokochi T, Inoue J, Wagner EF, Mak TW, Kodama T and Taniguchi T (2002). 'Induction and activation of the transcription factor NFATc1 (NFAT2) integrate RANKL signaling in terminal differentiation of osteoclasts', *Dev Cell*, **3** (6), 889–901.
67. Rodan GA and Martin TJ (1981). 'Role of osteoblasts in hormonal control of bone resorption – a hypothesis', *Calcif Tissue Int*, **33** (4), 349–51.
68. Anderson DM, Maraskovsky E, Billingsley WL, Dougall WC, Tometsko ME, Roux

ER, Teepe MC, DuBose RF, Cosman D and Galibert L (1997). 'A homologue of the TNF receptor and its ligand enhance T-cell growth and dendritic-cell function', *Nature*, **390** (6656), 175–9.

69. Wani MR, Fuller K, Kim NS, Choi Y and Chambers T (1999). 'Prostaglandin E2 cooperates with TRANCE in osteoclast induction from hemopoietic precursors: synergistic activation of differentiation, cell spreading, and fusion', *Endocrinology*, **140** (4), 1927–35.
70. Jimi E, Nakamura I, Amano H, Taguchi Y, Tsurukai T, Tamura M, Takahashi N and Suda T (1996). 'Osteoclast function is activated by osteoblastic cells through a mechanism involving cell-to-cell contact', *Endocrinology*, **137** (8), 2187–90.
71. Takahashi N, Akatsu T, Udagawa N, Sasaki T, Yamaguchi A, Moseley JM, Martin TJ and Suda T (1988). 'Osteoblastic cells are involved in osteoclast formation', *Endocrinology*, **123** (5), 2600–2.
72. Yasuda H, Shima N, Nakagawa N, Mochizuki SI, Yano K, Fujise N, Sato Y, Goto M, Yamaguchi K, Kuriyama M, Kanno T, Murakami A, Tsuda E, Morinaga T and Higashio K (1998). 'Identity of osteoclastogenesis inhibitory factor (OCIF) and osteoprotegerin (OPG): a mechanism by which OPG/OCIF inhibits osteoclastogenesis *in vitro*', *Endocrinology*, **139** (3), 1329–37.
73. Simonet WS, Lacey DL, Dunstan CR, Kelley M, Chang MS, Luthy R, Nguyen HQ, Wooden S, Bennett L, Boone T, Shimamoto G, DeRose M, Elliott R, Colombero A, Tan HL, Trail G, Sullivan J, Davy E, Bucay N, Renshaw-Gegg L, Hughes TM, Hill D, Pattison W, Campbell P, Sander S, Van G, Tarpley J, Derby P, Lee R and Boyle WJ (1997). 'Osteoprotegerin: a novel secreted protein involved in the regulation of bone density', *Cell*, **89** (2), 309–19.
74. Yasuda H, Shima N, Nakagawa N, Yamaguchi K, Kinosaki M, Mochizuki S, Tomoyasu A, Yano K, Goto M, Murakami A, Tsuda E, Morinaga T, Higashio K, Udagawa N, Takahashi N and Suda T (1998). 'Osteoclast differentiation factor is a ligand for osteoprotegerin/osteoclastogenesis-inhibitory factor and is identical to TRANCE/RANKL', *Proc Natl Acad Sci USA*, **95** (7), 3597–602.
75. McHugh KP, Hodivala-Dilke K, Zheng MH, Namba N, Lam J, Novack D, Feng X, Ross FP, Hynes RO and Teitelbaum SL (2000). 'Mice lacking beta3 integrins are osteosclerotic because of dysfunctional osteoclasts', *J Clin Invest*, **105** (4), 433–40.
76. Teitelbaum SL (2000). 'Bone resorption by osteoclasts', *Science*, **289** (5484), 1504–8.
77. Bendall AJ and Abate-Shen C (2000). 'Roles for Msx and Dlx homeoproteins in vertebrate development', *Gene*, **247** (1–2), 17–31.
78. Ducy P (2000). 'Cbfa1: a molecular switch in osteoblast biology', *Dev Dyn*, **219** (4), 461–71.
79. Komori T, Yagi H, Nomura S, Yamaguchi A, Sasaki K, Deguchi K, Shimizu Y, Bronson RT, Gao YH, Inada M, Sato M, Okamoto R, Kitamura Y, Yoshiki S and Kishimoto T (1997). 'Targeted disruption of Cbfa1 results in a complete lack of bone formation owing to maturational arrest of osteoblasts', *Cell*, **89** (5), 755–64.
80. Otto F, Thornell AP, Crompton T, Denzel A, Gilmour KC, Rosewell IR, Stamp GW, Beddington RS, Mundlos S, Olsen BR, Selby PB and Owen MJ (1997). 'Cbfa1, a candidate gene for cleidocranial dysplasia syndrome, is essential for osteoblast differentiation and bone development', *Cell*, **89** (5), 765–71.
81. Robledo RF, Rajan L, Li X and Lufkin T (2002). 'The Dlx5 and Dlx6 homeobox genes are essential for craniofacial, axial, and appendicular skeletal development', *Genes Dev*, **16** (9), 1089–101.

82. Glass DA, 2nd, Bialek P, Ahn JD, Starbuck M, Patel MS, Clevers H, Taketo MM, Long F, McMahon AP, Lang RA and Karsenty G (2005). 'Canonical Wnt signaling in differentiated osteoblasts controls osteoclast differentiation', *Dev Cell*, **8** (5), 751–64.
83. Hu H, Hilton MJ, Tu X, Yu K, Ornitz DM and Long F (2005). 'Sequential roles of Hedgehog and Wnt signaling in osteoblast development', *Development*, **132** (1), 49–60.
84. Nakashima K, Zhou X, Kunkel G, Zhang Z, Deng JM, Behringer RR and de Crombrugghe B (2002). 'The novel zinc finger-containing transcription factor osterix is required for osteoblast differentiation and bone formation', *Cell*, **108** (1), 17–29.
85. Wetterwald A, Hoffstetter W, Cecchini MG, Lanske B, Wagner C, Fleisch H and Atkinson M (1996). 'Characterization and cloning of the E11 antigen, a marker expressed by rat osteoblasts and osteocytes', *Bone*, **18** (2), 125–32.
86. Feng JQ, Huang H, Lu Y, Ye L, Xie Y, Tsutsui TW, Kunieda T, Castranio T, Scott G, Bonewald LB and Mishina Y (2003). 'The Dentin matrix protein 1 (Dmp1) is specifically expressed in mineralized, but not soft, tissues during development', *J Dent Res*, **82** (10), 776–80.
87. Nampei A, Hashimoto J, Hayashida K, Tsuboi H, Shi K, Tsuji I, Miyashita H, Yamada T, Matsukawa N, Matsumoto M, Morimoto S, Ogihara T, Ochi T and Yoshikawa H (2004). 'Matrix extracellular phosphoglycoprotein (MEPE) is highly expressed in osteocytes in human bone', *J Bone Miner Metab*, **22** (3), 176–84.
88. Toyosawa S, Shintani S, Fujiwara T, Ooshima T, Sato A, Ijuhin N and Komori T (2001). 'Dentin matrix protein 1 is predominantly expressed in chicken and rat osteocytes but not in osteoblasts', *J Bone Miner Res*, **16** (11), 2017–26.
89. van Bezooijen RL, Roelen BA, Visser A, van der Wee-Pals L, de Wilt E, Karperien M, Hamersma H, Papapoulos SE, ten Dijke P and Lowik CW (2004). 'Sclerostin is an osteocyte-expressed negative regulator of bone formation, but not a classical BMP antagonist', *J Exp Med*, **199** (6), 805–14.
90. van Bezooijen RL, ten Dijke P, Papapoulos SE and Lowik CW (2005). 'SOST/sclerostin, an osteocyte-derived negative regulator of bone formation', *Cytokine Growth Factor Rev*, **16** (3), 319–27.
91. Hirose S, Li M, Kojima T, de Freitas PH, Ubaidus S, Oda K, Saito C and Amizuka N (2007). 'A histological assessment on the distribution of the osteocytic lacunar canalicular system using silver staining', *J Bone Miner Metab*, **25** (6), 374–82.
92. Plotkin LI, Manolagas SC and Bellido T (2002). 'Transduction of cell survival signals by connexin-43 hemichannels', *J Biol Chem*, **277** (10), 8648–57.
93. Yellowley CE, Li Z, Zhou Z, Jacobs CR and Donahue HJ (2000). 'Functional gap junctions between osteocytic and osteoblastic cells', *J Bone Miner Res*, **15** (2), 209–17.
94. Bonewald LF (2006). 'Mechanosensation and transduction in osteocytes', *Bonekey Osteovision*, **3** (10), 7–15.
95. Wang L, Wang Y, Han Y, Henderson SC, Majeska RJ, Weinbaum S and Schaffler MB (2005). 'In situ measurement of solute transport in the bone lacunar-canalicular system', *Proc Natl Acad Sci USA*, **102** (33), 11911–6.
96. Lanyon LE (1993). 'Osteocytes, strain detection, bone modeling and remodeling', *Calcif Tissue Int*, **53** (Suppl 1), S102–6; discussion S106–7.
97. Robling AG, Niziolek PJ, Baldridge LA, Condon KW, Allen MJ, Alam I, Mantila SM, Gluhak-Heinrich J, Bellido TM, Harris SE and Turner CH (2008). 'Mechanical

stimulation of bone *in vivo* reduces osteocyte expression of Sost/sclerostin', *J Biol Chem*, **283** (9), 5866–75.

98. Tatsumi S, Ishii K, Amizuka N, Li M, Kobayashi T, Kohno K, Ito M, Takeshita S and Ikeda K (2007). 'Targeted ablation of osteocytes induces osteoporosis with defective mechanotransduction, *Cell Metab*, **5** (6), 464–75.
99. Lane NE, Yao W, Balooch M, Nalla RK, Balooch G, Habelitz S, Kinney JH and Bonewald LF (2006). 'Glucocorticoid-treated mice have localized changes in trabecular bone material properties and osteocyte lacunar size that are not observed in placebo-treated or estrogen-deficient mice', *J Bone Miner Res*, **21** (3), 466–76.
100. Feng JQ, Ward LM, Liu S, Lu Y, Xie Y, Yuan B, Yu X, Rauch F, Davis SI, Zhang S, Rios H, Drezner MK, Quarles LD, Bonewald LF and White KE (2006). 'Loss of DMP1 causes rickets and osteomalacia and identifies a role for osteocytes in mineral metabolism', *Nat Genet*, **38** (11), 1310–5.
101. Frost HM (1991). 'Some ABC's of skeletal pathophysiology. 6. The growth/modeling/remodeling distinction', *Calcif Tissue Int*, **49** (5), 301–2.
102. Parfitt AM (1996). 'Skeletal heterogeneity and the purposes of bone remodeling: implications for the understanding of osteoporosis', In: *Osteoporosis*, Marcus R, Feldman D and Kelsey J (eds.), Academic Press, San Diego, CA, 315–29.
103. Hall BK and Miyake T (1992). 'The membranous skeleton: the role of cell condensations in vertebrate skeletogenesis', *Anat Embryol (Berlin)*, **186** (2), 107–24.
104. Kosher RA, Kulyk WM and Gay SW (1986). 'Collagen gene expression during limb cartilage differentiation', *J Cell Biol*, **102** (4), 1151–6.
105. Ornitz DM and Marie PJ (2002). 'FGF signaling pathways in endochondral and intramembranous bone development and human genetic disease', *Genes Dev*, **16** (12), 1446–65.
106. Vortkamp A, Lee K, Lanske B, Segre GV, Kronenberg HM and Tabin CJ (1996). 'Regulation of rate of cartilage differentiation by Indian hedgehog and PTH-related protein', *Science*, **273** (5275), 613–22.
107. Hartmann C (2007). 'Skeletal development: Wnts are in control', *Mol Cells*, **24** (2), 177–84.
108. Olsen BR (2006). 'Bone embryology', In: *Primer on the Metabolic Bone Diseases and Disorders of Mineral Metabolism*, 6th edition. Favus MJ (ed.), American Society for Bone and Mineral Research, Washington, DC, 2–6.
109. Akiyama H, Chaboissier MC, Martin JF, Schedl A, de Crombrugghe B (2002). 'The transcription factor Sox9 has essential roles in successive steps of the chondrocyte differentiation pathway and is required for expression of Sox5 and Sox6. *Genes Dev*, **16** (21), 2813–28.
110. Frost HM (1986). *Intermediary Organization of the Skeleton*, CRC Press, Boca Raton, FL.
111. Jee WS and Frost HM (1992). 'Skeletal adaptations during growth', *Sandoz J Med Sci*, **31**, 77–88.
112. Robling AG, Castillo AB and Turner CH (2006). 'Biomechanical and molecular regulation of bone remodeling', *Annu Rev Biomed Eng*, **8**, 455–98.
113. Hillam RA and Skerry TM (1995). 'Inhibition of bone resorption and stimulation of formation by mechanical loading of the modeling rat ulna *in vivo*. *J Bone Miner Res*, **10** (5), 683–9.
114. Parfitt AM (1984). 'The cellular basis of bone remodeling: the quantum concept reexamined in light of recent advances in the cell biology of bone', *Calcif Tissue Int*, **36** (Suppl 1), S37–45.

115. Adami S, Gatti D, Braga V, Bianchini D and Rossini M (1999). 'Site-specific effects of strength training on bone structure and geometry of ultradistal radius in postmenopausal women', *J Bone Miner Res*, **14** (1), 120–4.
116. Ahlborg HG, Johnell O, Turner CH, Rannevik G and Karlsson MK (2003). 'Bone loss and bone size after menopause', *N Engl J Med*, **349** (4), 327–34.
117. Hodsman AB and Steer BM (1993). 'Early histomorphometric changes in response to parathyroid hormone therapy in osteoporosis: evidence for de novo bone formation on quiescent cancellous surfaces', *Bone*, **14** (3), 523–7.
118. Jee WS, Li XJ and Schaffler MB (1991). 'Adaptation of diaphyseal structure with aging and increased mechanical usage in the adult rat: a histomorphometrical and biomechanical study', *Anat Rec*, **230** (3), 332–8.
119. Lindsay R, Cosman F, Zhou H, Bostrom MP, Shen VW, Cruz JD, Nieves JW and Dempster DW (2006). 'A novel tetracycline labeling schedule for longitudinal evaluation of the short-term effects of anabolic therapy with a single iliac crest bone biopsy: early actions of teriparatide', *J Bone Miner Res*, **21** (3), 366–73.
120. Uusi-Rasi K, Kannus P, Cheng S, Sievanen H, Pasanen M, Heinonen A, Nenonen A, Halleen J, Fuerst T, Genant H and Vuori I (2003). 'Effect of alendronate and exercise on bone and physical performance of postmenopausal women: a randomized controlled trial', *Bone*, **33** (1), 132–43.
121. Dempster D (2006). 'Bone modeling and remodeling', In: *The Bone Quality Book: A Guide to Factors Influencing Bone Strength*. Dempster D, Felsenberg D and van Der Geest S (eds.), Excerpta Medica, Amsterdam, Netherlands, 64–73.
122. Burr DB (2002). 'Targeted and nontargeted remodeling', *Bone*, **30** (1), 2–4.
123. Hert J, Fiala P and Petrtyl M (1994). 'Osteon orientation of the diaphysis of the long bones in man' *Bone*, **15** (3), 269–77.
124. Parfitt AM (1994). 'Osteonal and hemi-osteonal remodeling: the spatial and temporal framework for signal traffic in adult human bone', *J Cell Biochem*, **55** (3), 273–86.
125. Frost HM (1964). *Laws of Bone Structure*, Charles C. Thomas, Springfield, IL.
126. Parfitt AM (1983). The physiologic and clinical significance of bone histomorphometric data', In: *Bone Histomorphometry: Techniques and Interpretation*, Recker RR (ed.), CRC Press, Boca Raton, 143–223.
127. Parfitt AM (2000). The mechanism of coupling: a role for the vasculature', *Bone*, **26** (4), 319–23.
128. Hodsman AB, Bauer DC, Dempster DW, Dian L, Hanley DA, Harris ST, Kendler DL, McClung MR, Miller PD, Olszynski WP, Orwoll E and Yuen CK (2005). 'Parathyroid hormone and teriparatide for the treatment of osteoporosis: a review of the evidence and suggested guidelines for its use', *Endocr Rev*, **26** (5), 688–703.
129. Wolff J (1892). 'Das Gesetz der Transformation der Knochen,' A. Hirschwald, Berlin.
130. Cowin SC (1997). 'The false premise in Wolff's law', *Forma*, **12**, 247–62.
131. Pearson OM and Lieberman DE (2004). 'The aging of Wolff's 'law': ontogeny and responses to mechanical loading in cortical bone', *Am J Phys Anthropol*, Suppl 39, 63–99.
132. Rubin CT and Lanyon LE (1985). 'Regulation of bone mass by mechanical strain magnitude', *Calcif Tissue Int*, **37**, 411–17.
133. Turner CH, Forwood MR, Rho J-Y and Yoshikawa T (1994). 'Mechanical loading thresholds for lamellar and woven bone formation', *J Bone Miner Res*, **9**, 87–97.

134. Burr DB, Milgrom C, Fyhrie D, Forwood M, Nyska M, Finestone A, Hoshaw S, Saiag E and Simkin A (1996). '*In vivo* measurement of human tibial strains during vigourous activity', *Bone*, **18**, 405–410.
135. Frost HM (1987). 'Bone 'mass' and the 'mechanostat': a proposal', *Anatomical Record*, **219**, 1–9.
136. Frost HM (1990). 'Skeletal structural adaptations to mechanical usage (SATMU): 2. Redefining Wolff's law: the bone remodeling problem, *Anat Rec*, **226**, 414–22.
137. Hsieh YF, Robling AG, Ambrosius WT, Burr DB and Turner CH (2001). 'Mechanical loading of diaphyseal bone *in vivo*: the strain threshold for an osteogenic response varies with location', *J Bone Miner Res*, **16** (12), 2291–7.
138. Robling AG and Turner CH (2002). 'Mechanotransduction in bone: genetic effects on mechanosensitivity in mice', *Bone*, **31** (5), 562–9.
139. Rubin C, Judex S and Hadjiargyrou M (2002). 'Skeletal adaptation to mechanical stimuli in the absence of formation or resorption of bone', *J Musculoskelet Neuronal Interact*, **2** (3), 264–7.
140. Turner CH (1999). 'Toward a mathematical description of bone biology: the principal of cellular accommodation', *Calcif Tissue Int*, **65**, 466–71.
141. Turner CH (1998). Three rules for bone adaptation to mechanical stimuli', *Bone*, **23**, 399–407.
142. Hert J, Liskova M and Landrgot B (1969). 'Influence of the long-term, continuous bending on the bone. An experimental study on the tibia of the rabbit', *Folia Morphol*, **17**, 389–99.
143. Lanyon LE and Rubin CT (1984). 'Static vs dynamic loads as an influence on bone remodelling', *Journal of Biomechanics*, **17**, 897–905.
144. Robling AG, Duijvelaar KM, Geevers JV, Ohashi N and Turner CH (2001). 'Modulation of appositional and longitudinal bone growth in the rat ulna by applied static and dynamic force', *Bone*, **29** (2), 105–13.
145. Turner CH, Forwood MR and Otter MW (1994). 'Mechanotransduction in bone: do bone cells act as sensors of fluid flow?' *FASEB J*, **8** (11), 875–78.
146. Turner CH, Owan I and Takano Y (1995). 'Mechanotransduction in bone: role of strain rate', *Am J Physiol*, **269**, E438–E442.
147. Hsieh YF and Turner CH (2001). 'Effects of loading frequency on mechanically induced bone formation', *J Bone Miner Res*, **16** (5), 918–24.
148. Rubin C and McLeod KJ (1994). 'Promotion of bony ingrowth by frequency-specific, low-amplitude mechanical strain', *Clinl Orthopaed Rel Res*, **298**, 165–74.
149. Rubin C, Turner AS, Mallinckrodt C, Jerome C, McLeod K and Bain S (2002). 'Mechanical strain, induced noninvasively in the high-frequency domain, is anabolic to cancellous bone, but not cortical bone', *Bone*, **30** (3), 445–52.
150. Warden SJ and Turner CH (2004). 'Mechanotransduction in cortical bone is most efficient at loading frequencies of 5-10 Hz. *Bone*, **34**, 261–70.
151. Garman R, Gaudette G, Donahue LR, Rubin C and Judex S (2007). 'Low-level accelerations applied in the absence of weight bearing can enhance trabecular bone formation', *J Orthop Res*, **25** (6), 732–40.
152. Judex S, Lei X, Han D and Rubin C (2007). 'Low-magnitude mechanical signals that stimulate bone formation in the ovariectomized rat are dependent on the applied frequency but not on the strain magnitude', *J Biomech*, **40** (6), 1333–9.
153. Rubin C, Turner AS, Bain S, Mallinckrodt C and McLeod K (2001). 'Low mechanical signals strengthen long bones', *Nature*, **412**, 603–4.
154. Rubin CT and Lanyon LE (1984). 'Regulation of bone formation by applied dynamic loads', *J Bone Joint Surg Am*, **66** (3), 397–402.

155. Umemura Y, Ishiko T, Yamauchi T, Kurono M and Mashiko S (1997). 'Five jumps per day increase bone mass and breaking force in rats', *J Bone Miner Res*, **12** (9), 1480–5.
156. Robling AG, Burr DB and Turner CH (2001). 'Recovery periods restore mechanosensitivity to dynamically loaded bone', *J Exp Biol*, **204** (Pt 19), 3389–99.
157. Srinivasan S, Weimer DA, Agans SC, Bain SD and Gross TS (2002). 'Low-magnitude mechanical loading becomes osteogenic when rest is inserted between each load cycle', *J Bone Miner Res*, **17** (9), 1613–20.
158. Robling AG, Burr DB and Turner CH (2000). 'Partitioning a daily mechanical stimulus into discrete loading bouts improves the osteogenic response to loading', *J Bone Miner Res*, **15**, 1596–602.
159. Robling AG, Hinant FM, Burr DB and Turner CH (2002). 'Improved bone structure and strength after long-term mechanical loading is greatest if loading is separated into short bouts', *J Bone Miner Res*, **17** (8), 1545–54.
160. Robling AG, Hinant FM, Burr DB and Turner CH (2002). 'Shorter, more frequent mechanical loading sessions enhance bone mass', *Med Sci Sports Exerc*, **34** (2), 196–202.
161. Bass SL, Saxon L, Daly RM, Turner CH, Robling AG, Seeman E and Stuckey S (2002). 'The effect of mechanical loading on the size and shape of bone in pre-, peri-, and postpubertal girls: a study in tennis players', *J Bone Miner Res*, **17** (12), 2274–80.
162. Daly RM, Saxon L, Turner CH, Robling AG and Bass SL (2004). 'The relationship between muscle size and bone geometry during growth and in response to exercise', *Bone*, **34** (2), 281–7.
163. Kontulainen S, Sievanen H, Kannus P, Pasanen M and Vuori I (2003). 'Effect of long-term impact-loading on mass, size, and estimated strength of humerus and radius of female racquet-sports players: a peripheral quantitative computed tomography study between young and old starters and controls', *J Bone Miner Res*, **18** (2), 352–9.
164. Pavy-Le Traon A, Heer M, Narici MV, Rittweger J and Vernikos J (2007). 'From space to Earth: advances in human physiology from 20 years of bed rest studies (1986–2006)', *Eur J Appl Physiol*, **101** (2), 143–94.
165. LeBlanc AD, Spector ER, Evans HJ and Sibonga JD (2007). 'Skeletal responses to space flight and the bed rest analog: a review', *J Musculoskelet Neuronal Interact*, **7**(1), 33–47.
166. Jiang SD, Dai LY and Jiang LS (2006). 'Osteoporosis after spinal cord injury', *Osteoporos Int*, **17** (2), 180–92.
167. Myint PK, Poole KE and Warburton EA (2007). 'Hip fractures after stroke and their prevention', *QJM*, **100** (9), 539–45.
168. Jarvinen M and Kannus P (1997). 'Injury of an extremity as a risk factor for the development of osteoporosis', *J Bone Joint Surg Am*, **79** (2), 263–76.
169. Dietrick JE, Whedon GD, Shorr E, Toscani V and Davis VB (1948). 'Effect of immobilization on metabolic and physiologic functions of normal men', *Am J Med*, **4**, 3–35.
170. Frost HM (1960). 'Prescence of microscopic cracks *in vivo* in bone', *Henry Ford Hosp Med Bull*, **8**, 25–35.
171. Fazzalari NL, Forwood MR, Smith K, Manthey BA and Herreen P (1998). 'Assessment of cancellous bone quality in severe osteoarthrosis: bone mineral density, mechanics, and microdamage', *Bone*, **22** (4), 381–8.

172. Koszyca B, Fazzalari NL and Vernon-Roberts B (1989). 'Trabecular microfractures: nature and distribution in the proximal femur', *Clin Orthop Relat Res*, **244**, 208–16.
173. Taylor D, Hazenberg JG and Lee TC (2007). 'Living with cracks: damage and repair in human bone', *Nat Mater*, **6** (4), 263–8.
174. Martin RB (2003). 'Fatigue microdamage as an essential element of bone mechanics and biology', *Calcif Tissue Int*, **73** (2), 101–7.
175. Burr DB, Turner CH, Naick P, Forwood MR, Ambrosius W, Hasan MS and Pidaparti R (1998). 'Does microdamage accumulation affect the mechanical properties of bone?' *J Biomech*, **31**, 337–45.
176. Forwood MR and Parker AW (1989). 'Microdamage in response to repetitive torsional loading in the rat tibia', *Calcif Tissue Int*, **45**, 47–53.
177. Schaffler MB, Radin EL and Burr DB (1989). 'Mechanical and morphological effects of strain rate on fatigue of compact bone', *Bone*, **10**, 207–10.
178. Carter DR, Caler WE, Spengler DM and Frankel VH (1981). 'Fatigue behavior of adult cortical bone: the influence of mean strain and strain range', *Acta Orthop Scand*, **52** (5), 481–90.
179. Yerby SA and Carter DR (2001). 'Bone fatigue and stress fractures', In: *Musculoskeletal Fatigue and Stress Fractures*, Burr DB and Milgrom C (eds.), CRC Press, Bota Raton, Florida, USA, 85–103.
180. Boyce TM, Fyhrie DP, Glotkowski MC, Radin EL and Schaffler MB (1998). 'Damage type and strain mode associations in human compact bone bending fatigue', *J Orthop Res*, **16** (3), 322–9.
181. George WT and Vashishth D (2005). 'Damage mechanisms and failure modes of cortical bone under components of physiological loading', *J Orthop Res*, **23** (5), 1047–53.
182. Norman TL, Nivargikar SV and Burr DB (1996). 'Resistance to crack growth in human cortical bone is greater in shear than in tension', *J Biomech*, **29** (8), 1023–31.
183. Burr DB and Martin RB (1993). 'Calculating the probability that microcracks initiate resorption spaces', *J Biomech*, **26** (4–5), 613–6.
184. Burr DB, Martin RB, Schaffler MB and Radin EL (1985). 'Bone remodeling in response to *in vivo* fatigue microdamage', *J Biomech*, **18** (3), 189–200.
185. Allen MR, Iwata K, Phipps R and Burr DB (2006). 'Alterations in canine vertebral bone turnover, microdamage accumulation, and biomechanical properties following 1-year treatment with clinical treatment doses of risedronate or alendronate', *Bone*, **39** (4), 872–9.
186. Mashiba T, Hirano T, Turner CH, Forwood MR, Johnston CC and Burr DB (2000). 'Suppressed bone turnover by bisphosphonates increases microdamage accumulation and reduces some biomechanical properties in dog rib', *J Bone Miner Res*, **15** (4), 613–20.
187. Stepan JJ, Burr DB, Pavo I, Sipos A, Michalska D, Li J, Fahrleitner-Pammer A, Petto H, Westmore M, Michalsky D, Sato M and Dobnig H (2007). 'Low bone mineral density is associated with bone microdamage accumulation in postmenopausal women with osteoporosis', *Bone*, **41** (3), 378–85.
188. Noble BS, Peet N, Stevens HY, Brabbs A, Mosley JR, Reilly GC, Reeve J, Skerry TM and Lanyon LE (2003). 'Mechanical loading: biphasic osteocyte survival and targeting of osteoclasts for bone destruction in rat cortical bone', *Am J Physiol Cell Physiol*, **284** (4) C934–43.

189. Verborgt O, Gibson GJ and Schaffler MB (2000). 'Loss of osteocyte integrity in association with microdamage and bone remodeling after fatigue *in vivo*. *J Bone Miner Res*, **15** (1), 60–7.
190. Burr DB, Forwood MR, Fyhrie DP, Martin RB, Schaffler MB and Turner CH (1997). 'Bone microdamage and skeletal fragility in osteoporotic and stress fractures', *J Bone Miner Res*, **12** (1), 6–15.
191. Warden SJ, Burr DB and Brukner PD (2006). 'Stress fractures: pathophysiology, epidemiology, and risk factors', *Curr Osteoporos Rep*, **4** (3), 103–9.
192. Burr DB, Turner CH, Naick P, Forwood MR, Ambrosius W, Hasan MS and Pidaparti R (1998). 'Does microdamage accumulation affect the mechanical properties of bone?' *J Biomech*, **31** (4), 337–45.
193. Duncan RL and Turner CH (1995). 'Mechanotransduction and the functional response of bone to mechanical strain', *Calcif Tissue Int*, **57** (5), 344–58.
194. Cowin SC, Moss-Salentijn L and Moss ML (1991). 'Candidates for the mechanosensory system in bone', *J Biomech Eng*, **113** (2) 191–7.
195. Weinbaum S, Cowin SC and Zeng Y (1994). 'A model for the excitation of osteocytes by mechanical loading-induced bone fluid shear stresses', *J Biomech*, **27** (3), 339–60.
196. Hung CT, Allen FD, Pollack SR and Brighton CT (1996). 'What is the role of the convective current density in the real-time calcium response of cultured bone cells to fluid flow?' *J Biomech*, **29** (11), 1403–9.
197. Malone AM, Anderson CT, Tummala P, Kwon RY, Johnston TR, Stearns T and Jacobs CR (2007). 'Primary cilia mediate mechanosensing in bone cells by a calcium-independent mechanism', *Proc Natl Acad Sci USA*, **104** (33), 13325–30.
198. Pavalko FM, Norvell SM, Burr DB, Turner CH, Duncan RL and Bidwell JP (2003). 'A model for mechanotransduction in bone cells: the load-bearing mechanosomes', *J Cell Biochem*, **88** (1), 104–12.
199. Hynes RO (1992). 'Integrins: versatility, modulation, and signaling in cell adhesion', *Cell*, **69** (1), 11–25.
200. Moss ML (1997). 'The functional matrix hypothesis revisited. 1. The role of mechanotransduction', *Am J Orthod Dentofacial Orthop*, **112** (1), 8–11.
201. Pavalko FM, Otey CA, Simon KO and Burridge K (1991). 'Alpha-actinin: a direct link between actin and integrins', *Biochem Soc Trans*, **19** (4), 1065–9.
202. Ingber DE (1993). 'Cellular tensegrity: defining new rules of biological design that govern the cytoskeleton', *J Cell Sci*, **104** (Pt 3), 613–27.
203. Ingber DE (1998). 'Cellular basis of mechanotransduction, *Biol Bull*, **194** (3), 323–5; discussion 325-7.
204. Weinbaum S, Guo P and You L (2001). 'A new view of mechanotransduction and strain amplification in cells with microvilli and cell processes, *Biorheology*, **38** (2–3), 119–42.
205. Hung CT, Allen FD, Pollack SR and Brighton CT (1996). 'Intracellular Ca^{2+} stores and extracellular Ca^{2+} are required in the real-time Ca^{2+} response of bone cells experiencing fluid flow', *J Biomech*, **29** (11), 1411–7.
206. Davidson RM, Tatakis DW and Auerbach AL (1990). Multiple forms of mechanosensitive ion channels in osteoblast-like cells', *Pflugers Arch*, **416** (6), 646–51.
207. Duncan R and Misler S (1989). 'Voltage-activated and stretch-activated Ba^{2+} conducting channels in an osteoblast-like cell line (UMR 106)', *FEBS Lett*, **251** (1–2), 17–21.

208. Ryder KD and Duncan RL (2001). 'Parathyroid hormone enhances fluid shear-induced [Ca^{2+}]i signaling in osteoblastic cells through activation of mechanosensitive and voltage-sensitive Ca^{2+} channels', *J Bone Miner Res*, **16** (2), 240–8.
209. Zhang J, Ryder KD, Bethel JA, Ramirez R and Duncan RL (2006). 'PTH-induced actin depolymerization increases mechanosensitive channel activity to enhance mechanically stimulated Ca^{2+} signaling in osteoblasts', *J Bone Miner Res*, **21** (11), 1729–37.
210. Miyauchi A, Notoya K, Mikuni-Takagaki Y, Takagi Y, Goto M, Miki Y, Takano-Yamamoto T, Jinnai K, Takahashi K, Kumegawa M, Chihara K and Fujita T (2000). 'Parathyroid hormone-activated volume-sensitive calcium influx pathways in mechanically loaded osteocytes', *J Biol Chem*, **275** (5), 3335–42.
211. Genetos DC, Geist DJ, Liu D, Donahue HJ and Duncan RL (2005). 'Fluid shear-induced ATP secretion mediates prostaglandin release in MC3T3-E1 osteoblasts', *J Bone Miner Res*, **20** (1), 41–9.
212. North RA (2002). 'Molecular physiology of P2X receptors', *Physiol Rev*, **82** (4), 1013–67.
213. Jorgensen NR, Geist ST, Civitelli R and Steinberg TH (1997). 'ATP- and gap junction-dependent intercellular calcium signaling in osteoblastic cells', *J Cell Biol*, **139** (2), 497–506.
214. You J, Jacobs CR, Steinberg TH and Donahue HJ (2002). 'P2Y purinoceptors are responsible for oscillatory fluid flow-induced intracellular calcium mobilization in osteoblastic cells', *J Biol Chem*, **277** (50), 48724–9.
215. Li J, Liu D, Ke HZ, Duncan RL and Turner CH (2005). 'The P2X7 nucleotide receptor mediates skeletal mechanotransduction', *J Biol Chem*, **280** (52), 42952–9.
216. Brambilla R and Abbracchio MP (2001). 'Modulation of cyclooxygenase-2 and brain reactive astrogliosis by purinergic P2 receptors', *Ann N Y Acad Sci*, **939**, 54–62.
217. Koolpe M, Pearson D and Benton HP (1999). 'Expression of both P1 and P2 purine receptor genes by human articular chondrocytes and profile of ligand-mediated prostaglandin E2 release', *Arthritis Rheum*, **42** (2), 258–67.
218. Suzuki A, Kotoyori J, Oiso Y and Kozawa O (1993). 'Prostaglandin E2 is a potential mediator of extracellular ATP action in osteoblast-like cells', *Cell Adhes Commun*, **1** (2), 113–8.
219. Kawaguchi H, Pilbeam CC, Harrison JR and Raisz LG (1995). 'The role of prostaglandins in the regulation of bone metabolism', *Clin Orthop Relat Res*, **313**, 36–46.
220. Bakker AD, Klein-Nulend J and Burger EH (2003). 'Mechanotransduction in bone cells proceeds via activation of COX-2, but not COX-1', *Biochem Biophys Res Commun*, **305** (3), 677–83.
221. Westbroek I, Ajubi NE, Alblas MJ, Semeins CM, Klein-Nulend J, Burger EH and Nijweide PJ (2000). 'Differential stimulation of prostaglandin G/H synthase-2 in osteocytes and other osteogenic cells by pulsating fluid flow', *Biochem Biophys Res Commun*, **268** (2), 414–9.
222. Forwood MR (1996). 'Inducible cyclo-oxygenase (COX-2) mediates the induction of bone formation by mechanical loading *in vivo*. *J Bone Miner Res*, **11** (11), 1688–93.
223. Li J, Burr DB and Turner CH (2002). 'Suppression of prostaglandin synthesis with NS-398 has different effects on endocortical and periosteal bone formation induced by mechanical loading', *Calcif Tissue Int*, **70** (4), 320–9.

224. Pead MJ, Skerry TM and Lanyon LE (1988). 'Direct transformation from quiescence to bone formation in the adult periosteum following a single brief period of bone loading', *J Bone Miner Res*, **3** (6), 647–56.
225. Pead MJ, Suswillo R, Skerry TM, Vedi S and Lanyon LE (1988). 'Increased 3H-uridine levels in osteocytes following a single short period of dynamic bone loading *in vivo*', *Calcif Tissue Int*, **43** (2), 92–6.
226. Forwood MR, Owan I, Takano Y and Turner CH (1996). 'Increased bone formation in rat tibiae after a single short period of dynamic loading *in vivo*', *Am J Physiol*, **270** (3 Pt 1), E419–23.
227. Forwood MR and Turner CH (1994). 'The response of rat tibiae to incremental bouts of mechanical loading: a quantum concept for bone formation, *Bone*, **15** (6), 603–9.
228. Boppart MD, Kimmel DB, Yee JA and Cullen DM (1998). 'Time course of osteoblast appearance after *in vivo* mechanical loading', *Bone*, **23** (5), 409–15.
229. Lakes R (1993). 'Materials with structural hierarchy', *Nature*, **361**, 511–15.
230. McKinley M and O'Loughlin VD (2008). *Human Anatomy*, 2nd edition,: McGraw-Hill Higher Education, New York, NY.
231. Roschger P, Paschalis EP, Fratzl P and Klaushofer K (2008). 'Bone mineralization density distribution in health and disease', *Bone*, **42**(3), 456–66.
232. Page-McCaw A, Ewald AJ and Werb Z (2007). 'Matrix metalloproteinases and the regulation of tissue remodeling', *Nat Rev Mol Cell Biol*, 2, **8** (3), 221–33.
233. Krishnan V, Bryant HU and Macdougald OA (2006). 'Regulation of bone mass by Wnt signaling', *J Clin Invest*, **116**, 1202–9.
234. Canalis E, Giustina A and Bilezikian JP (2007). 'Mechanisms of anabolic therapies for osteoporosis', *N Engl J Med*, **357** (9), 905–16.
235. Burr DB, Robling AG and Turner CH (2002). 'Effects of biomechanical stress on bones in animals', *Bone*, **30**, 781–6.
236. Fazzalari NL, Forwood MR, Smith K, Manthey BA and Hereen P (1998). 'Assessment of cancellous bone quality in severe osteoarthrosis: bone mineral density, mechanics, and microdamage', *Bone*, **22**, 381–8.

3
Bone repair and regeneration

N. BALDINI, E. CENNI, G. CIAPETTI, D. GRANCHI and L. SAVARINO, Istituto Ortopedico Rizzoli, Italy

Abstract: Bone tissue has remarkable repair capacity, and generally heals by regeneration. This unique potential, expressed during remodelling and bone fracture healing, is tuned by a complex interplay of active factors and responding cells, which resides on an informative extracellular matrix and acts under a strict genetic control and different mechanical stimuli. The coordinated interaction of these elements is increasingly understood thanks to progress in cellular and molecular biology. This chapter deals with the sequential events leading to bone repair, with special attention given to the role of mesenchymal stem cells in regenerating bone. The genetic control of bone healing, the pathways underlying such process and the regulation by a variety of growth factors and cytokines are outlined according to the recent literature. Understanding the key elements of bone regeneration and their cross-talk is not merely a theoretical advancement in the knowledge of the physiological turnover of bone tissue, but offers practical tools for increasing the efficacy of orthopaedic procedures, such as the delivery of pro-osteogenic growth factors or mesenchymal stem cells.

Key words: bone, bone marrow, bone morphogenetic proteins, bone repair, fracture, growth factor, mesenchymal stem cells, osteoblast, regeneration.

3.1 Introduction

Bone is a dynamic, vascular, living tissue that undergoes constant remodeling throughout life. Constant remodelling provides a mechanism for scar-free healing and regeneration of damaged bone tissue. This property applies not only to the sequence of events that are initiated in response to injury, such as fracture, but also to the healing of bone around and within endosseous implants. Notably, the molecular mechanisms that regulate skeletal tissue formation during embryological development are recapitulated during bone repair.[1] Multiple factors, including growth and differentiation factors, hormones, cytokines and extracellular matrix, interact with different cell types, including mesenchymal stem cells (MSCs), bone and cartilage forming cells, endothelial cells and bone resorbing cells that are recruited at the injury site. These factors regulate intracellular and extracellular molecular signalling for bone induction and conduction through various processes such as migration, proliferation, chemotaxis, differentiation and extracellular protein synthesis.[2]

The aim of this chapter is to describe the process of bone repair and regeneration under the new insights provided by cellular and molecular biology tools. First, the temporal and spatial sequence of events leading to bone healing is reported, based on histological findings from experimental implants and retrievals. In the second part, the role of stem cells, from the host or delivered using tissue engineering approaches, in the process of bone regeneration is described. The third part is an elucidation of the molecular events that determine precursor cells that form specific connective tissue, that is bone. The last part is focused on the complex system of different growth factors and cytokines which act as autocrine and/or paracrine effectors to regulate osteogenesis.

Ongoing research and further understanding of the bone healing process will aid the strategies for bone regenerative therapies.

3.2 Bone healing

The complex series of integrated cellular events that ultimately lead to bone healing has been extensively elucidated in experimental models.[3] Primary fracture healing is an artificial situation that occurs when rigid fixation devices (that is, screws and plates) are surgically applied so that the fracture surfaces are rigidly held in contact. In this process, there is little if any participation from the periosteum or external soft tissues, but a direct involvement of the cortex, the endosteum and the bone marrow. Osteoclasts on each side of the fracture undergo a tunnelling resorptive response whereby they re-establish new Haversian systems, therefore providing pathways for the penetration of blood vessels.[4] Most fractures, however, heal by conservative treatment (i.e. cast immobilization) or by elastic stabilization through external or intramedullary fixation devices, so that micromotion occurs between fracture surfaces. In secondary fracture healing, a large amount of reparative tissue (so called fracture callus) is generated by a combination of intramembranous and endochondral bone formation by the periosteum and the surrounding tissues, with a less important role for the bone marrow.[5]

The histological phases of bone healing can be summarized as: (1) an early inflammation phase (haematoma formation, inflammation, angiogenesis) with granulation tissue formation; (2) a reparative phase, with cartilaginous callus formation and replacement of callus by lamellar bone; and (3) a late bone remodelling phase in which the original bone shape is obtained.

3.2.1 Inflammation

Fracture trauma involves not only an interruption of skeletal integrity but also a disruption of normal vascular structures and nutrient flow at the fracture site, leading to a reduced oxygen tension and a disruption of marrow architecture. A blood clot (haematoma) is formed between the bone ends, acting as a source of signalling molecules (growth factors and cytokines) for monocyte–macrophages and osteo-chondroblast precursors.[6] Infiltrating macrophages and other inflammatory cells secrete fibroblast growth factor (FGF), tumor necrosis factor-α (TNF-α), PDGF and TGF-β, and also release a variety of cytokines, including interleukin-1 (IL-1) and interleukin-6 (IL-6). In turn, IL-1, IL-6 and TNF-α have a chemotactic effect on other inflammatory cells and osteoblast precursors.[7, 8] During this early phase, mesenchymal precursors proliferate and differentiate into the chondrogenic and osteogenic lineages[9] (Fig. 3.1). Newly formed blood vessels form by budding of pre-existing vessels through an enzymatic degradation of the basement membrane, followed by migration of endothelial cells toward the angiogenic stimulus, proliferation of endothelial cells, maturation of endothelial cells and organization into capillary tubes. This process is regulated by FGF, vascular endothelial growth factor (VEGF) and angiopoietin 1 and 2.[10]

3.2.2 Repair

Intramembranous ossification occurs within a few days after injury, whereas endochondral ossification occurs in tissues adjacent to the fracture site and spans a period of up to 28 days. The subperiosteal area and the soft tissues immediately surrounding the fracture form a so-called 'hard callus' and directly create bone. In this process, mesenchymal precursors recruited to the site of

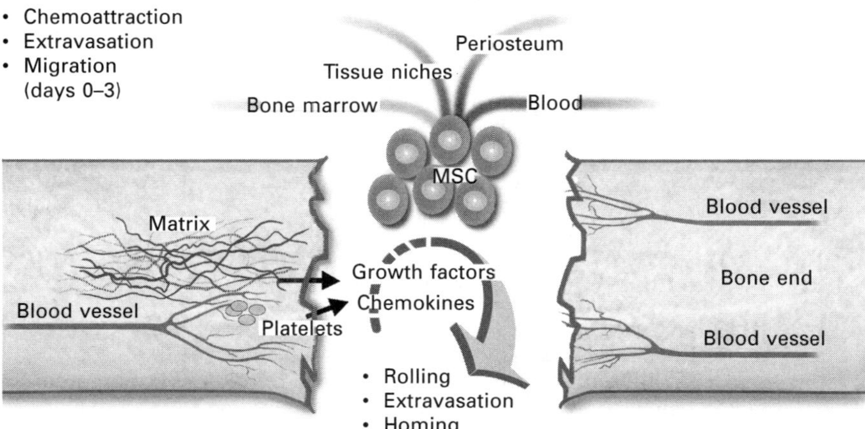

3.1 Mesenchymal stem cells (MSC) migrate from blood, periosteum, bone marrow and other tissue niches (perivascular) to the site of bone fracture. Growth factors, including TGF-β, FGF, PDGF, IGF-I and chemokines, including IL-1, IL-6 and TNF-α, are released from the extracellular matrix (ECM) and platelets to promote MSC recruitment, migration and proliferation, as well as homing to the healing site.

injury differentiate along the osteoblastic lineage and, eventually, produce both compact and trabecular bone in the absence of cartilage production. After 72 hours, osteoblasts from the cortex and committed osteoprogenitor cells from the periosteum proliferate and differentiate to form immature bone. Endochondral bone formation involves the recruitment, proliferation and differentiation of undifferentiated mesenchymal cells into cartilage. MSC proliferation can be detected as early as three days after fracture and is high for several days[11] (Fig. 3.2).

Chondrogenesis continues from day 7 to day 21, leading to the formation of a cartilaginous callus that bridges and stabilizes the fracture site. By nine days after fracture, the chondrocytes of the soft callus adjacent to the woven bone of the hard callus begin to elongate, portions of the chondrocyte membrane deliver calcium from the mitochondria into the extracellular matrix in packaged units (matrix vesicles) and cells express chondroblastic characteristics, as shown by the deposition of an extracellular matrix made of type II collagen and aggrecan.

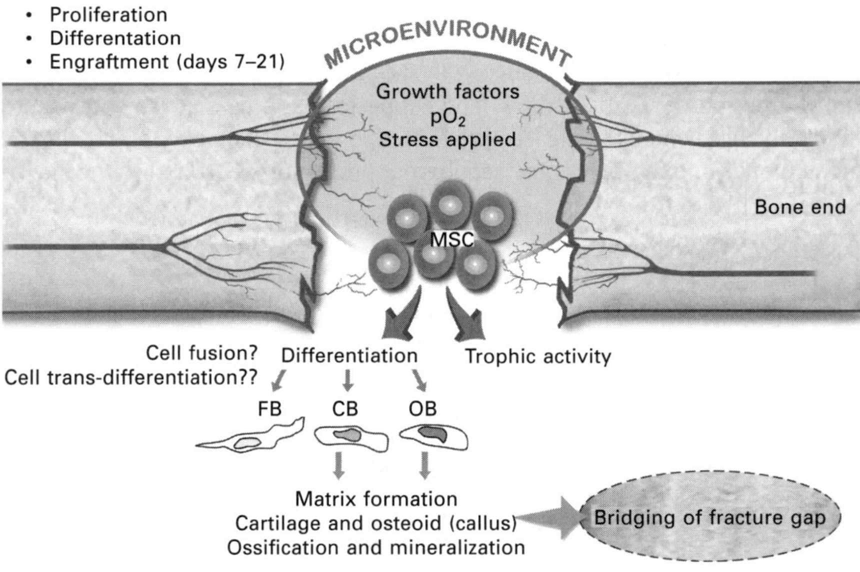

3.2 At the site of bone fracture mesenchymal stem cells (MSCs) undergo differentiation under the influence of microenvironmental factors, such as low oxygen tension, stress applied to the bone, including micromovements and several growth factors expressed at different time points during healing. Differentiation of MSCs to connective tissue lineages generates fibroblasts (FB), chondroblasts (CB) and osteoblasts (OB), which actively synthesize extracellular matrix to be calcified and converted to bone. Besides differentiating capacity, a relevant 'trophic activity' of MSCs has been recently hypothesized.[41]

After two weeks, these cells differentiate into hypertrophic chondrocytes that deposit type X collagen. Afterwards, this matrix is partially mineralized, resorbed and replaced by a matrix formed predominantly of type I collagen. To prepare the matrix for calcification, the chondrocytes release two types of enzymes, phosphatases and proteases.[12] Phosphatases provide phosphate ions that precipitate with the calcium delivered from the mitochondria to form calcified cartilage. Proteases degrade the proteoglycans that inhibit mineralization, allowing the chondrocytes to control the rate and physical chemistry of the mineralization process. After four or five weeks, the callus is mostly composed of calcified cartilage (hypertrophic chondrocyte mineralization of the matrix). This tissue becomes a target for chondroclasts, multinucleated cells that degrade the calcified cartilage matrix and, in doing so, send a signal that enables blood vessels to penetrate the tissue and bring perivascular mesenchymal stem cells that differentiate into osteoprogenitor cells and then into osteoblasts. Matrix metalloproteinase-expressing cells, including endothelial cells, facilitate vascular invasion, as well as removal of cartilaginous septa and any remnants of chondrocytes.[13]

Tissues derived from intramembranous and endochondral ossification grow in size until they unite. After about six to seven weeks, there is a combination of calcified cartilage and newly formed woven bone. The transition from cartilage to bone involves a highly programmed series of events for cell removal and matrix modification. During endochondral fracture healing, chondrocytes undergo a process of programmed cell death (apoptosis).[14] Calcification of cartilage starts at the interface between the maturing cartilage and newly formed woven bone. Once the cartilage component of the callus has been resorbed, there are two new surfaces of bone: an inner surface that has grown over the original cortex and an outer thinner layer that has encapsulated the callus and forms the new interface with the periosteum. Thus, a trabecular structure is seen bridging these surfaces in the space that was previously occupied by cartilage.

Since the outer shell is located far from the geometric center of the bone, it will be responsible for the majority of weight bearing.[15] This outer shell is connected to the original cortex via trabecular-like structures that provide sufficient support in order to stabilize the fracture. This represents an efficient mechanism, using minimal material, to restore rapidly biomechanical stiffness and strength and allow for remodeling on internal surfaces. The exact role of osteoclasts in fracture repair is still uncertain,[16] even though they probably contribute to vascular invasion and early endochondral ossification. Lamellar bone starts forming soon after the collagen matrix of either tissue becomes mineralized. At this point, vascular channels with accompanying osteogenic precursors penetrate the mineralized matrix and osteoblasts form new lamellar bone upon the recently exposed surface of the mineralized matrix.

3.2.3 Remodelling

Eventually, fracture healing is completed during the remodelling phase, in which cooperation between osteoblasts and osteoclasts occurs, progressively converting the fracture callus to a bony structure capable of supporting physiological mechanical loads. Unlike long-bone expansion, in which there is a balance between periosteal appositional growth and bone resorption at the endosteal surface, remodelling of fracture callus occurs from the outer surface inward, balancing external removal with the addition of bone to internal surfaces.

Trabecular bone is first resorbed by osteoclasts, creating a shallow resorption pit known as Howship's lacunae. Each individual cell acidifies the local extracellular space and secretes active lysosomal enzymes which break down the bone matrix enzymatically. These enzymes include serine proteases, collagenases and tartrate-resistant acid phosphatase. The enzymatic destruction of bone matrix releases various proteins, including growth factors previously stored during bone formation. These, in addition to cytokines manufactured by osteoclasts and other cells, recruit adjacent osteoprogenitor cells to become osteoblasts. Osteoblasts enter the resorption pits created by the osteoclast and manufacture new bone matrix of either the woven or lamellar type. As the cells become entrapped within the bone matrix, they evolve to osteocytes.[17] Some osteoblasts eventually become flat surface cells lining the quiescent bone surfaces, that is, bone lining cells.

With load bearing, most forces across the diaphysis are axial, therefore the healing area is compressed while outside tension is created. Since compressive 'physiological' forces result in chondroblast development, whereas moderate tensile stress may stimulate bone formation, the fracture callus of a diaphyseal fracture healed by secondary bone union shows bone primarily on the outside of the callus, where tensile stress is applied, whereas in the callus centre mesenchymal precursors experience compressive forces with cartilage formation.

Angiogenesis is closely associated with bone resorption and bone formation. Angiogenic factors, such as vascular endothelial growth factor and endothelin, are regulators of osteoclast and osteoblast activity, but the formation of blood vessels also serves as a way of transporting circulating osteoblast and osteoclast precursors to sites undergoing active remodelling. The close association between bone and vessels plays a pivotal role in the regulation of bone remodelling and fracture repair. The interface between bone forming surfaces and bone marrow is lined by vascular structures, the paratrabecular sinusoidal capillaries. An osteoblastic layer makes up the osseous wall of the capillary, the opposite wall being formed by endothelial cells.

Bone remodelling is also related to the existence of an increased flow through microvessels that conform closely to the contour of the cancellous bone surface.[18] A specialized vascular structure, the bone remodelling compartment (BRC), has been characterized[19] and shown to be composed of flattened cells with all the characteristics of bone lining cells. Immunoreactivity for all major osteotropic growth factors and cytokines has been shown in the cells lining the BRC, which makes it a candidate structure for resorption and formation coupling. The secretion of these factors inside a confined space separated from the bone marrow would facilitate local regulation of the remodelling process without interference from growth factors secreted by blood cells in the marrow space. The BRC could constitute an environment where cells inside the structure are exposed to denuded bone and where osteoclast/ osteoblast activity could be directly regulated by integrins and other matrix factors.

As clearly pointed out by Davies,[20] when considering bone healing and regeneration around endosseous implants, one has to take into account both the texture of the implant surface and the type of bone macroarchitecture. In fact, the relatively slow regeneration of peri-implant cortical bone relies exclusively on lamellar remodelling, whereas the generation of peri-implant trabecular bone may involve, not only remodelling of existing lamellar trabeculae, but can also include the rapid formation of new trabeculae by the recruitment of new populations of osteogenic cells within the healing compartment. In fact, cancellous bone has a very high surface area which is contiguous with the marrow compartment.

Since marrow contains not only mesenchymal osteoprogenitor cells but also a rich vasculature that can supply both the circulating mononuclear precursors to osteoclasts and the endothelial population needed for angiogenesis, it is not surprising that trabecular bone can remodel far more quickly than cortical bone. Around endosseous implants, osteoblasts may lay down bone on the old bone surface or on the implant itself.[21] The first occurs in cortical bone as a result of osteogenic activity that does not create bone on the implant, but around it, starting from damaged tissue toward the implant. In contrast, in contact osteogenesis, new bone forms first on the implant surface that is colonized by bone cells before bone matrix formation begins, in a very similar way as at sites of remodelling where a resorption surface of old bone is populated by osteogenic cells that are separated from the old bone by a proteoglycan-rich collagen-free cement line matrix (Fig. 3.3).[22] In fact, in this process of *de novo* bone formation, the collagen compartment of bone is also separated from the underlying substratum by a collagen-free layer containing proteoglycans and non-collagenous bone proteins (osteopontin and bone sialoprotein).[23]

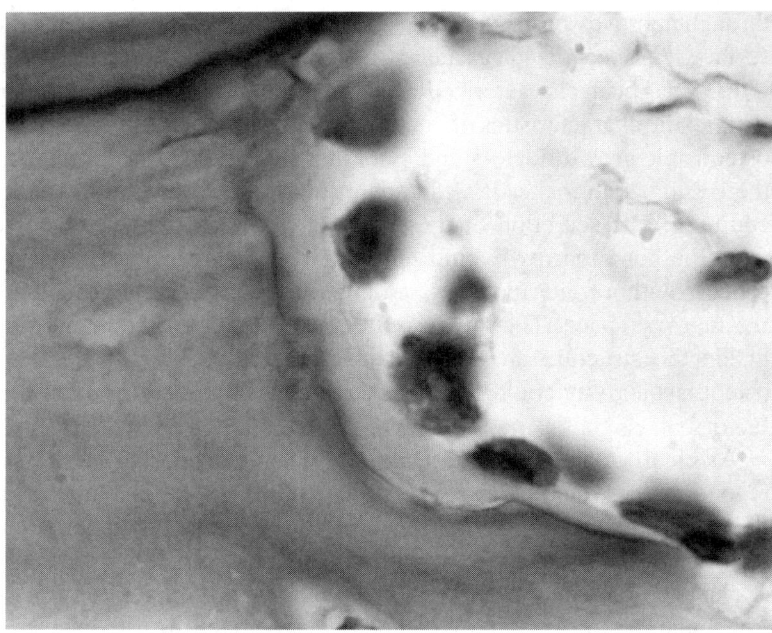

3.3 At sites of remodelling, a resorption surface of old bone is populated by osteogenic cells that are separated from the old bone by a proteoglycan-rich collagen-free cement line matrix (HE, × 60).

3.3 Role of stem cells in bone repair

As previously summarized, skeletal integrity after bone fracture is usually restored by the natural healing mechanisms of bone repair, sometimes with the help of proper orthopaedic tools to optimize mechanical stability. But when bone loss is too large, as a consequence of trauma, spinal fusion, tumour resection, arthrodesis, metabolic diseases, non- or delayed union, implant failure, as well as old age or poor bone quality, additional strategies are needed to potentiate secondary bone union, and bone regeneration or bone engineering is advocated.[24]

In the original work by Friedenstein *et al.*,[25] clonogenic, multipotential precursors in the bone marrow stroma were first described, and these cells were termed 'colony forming unit fibroblasts' (CFU-Fs). The current term 'stem cell' means elements capable of proliferation, self-renewal, conversion to differentiated cells and *in vivo* regeneration of tissues. There are two types of stem cells, embryonic and non-embryonic or adult stem cells. Embryonic stem cells (ESC) are derived from the inner cells of the blastocyst a few days after egg fertilization and can be converted into cells of any lineage. In contrast, stem cells from adult bone marrow have been characterized and extensively used for the treatment of blood disorders. Although the stemness of such cells has not been definitely demonstrated yet, the popular acronym MSC stays for 'multipotent mesenchymal stromal cells', encompassing plastic-adherent, non-haemopoietic (CD34$^-$), stroma-derived cells that are able to differentiate into osteoblasts, adipocytes, or chondroblasts *in vitro*.[26, 27]

Concerning clinical applications, the use of ESC, which have to be fully differentiated prior to transplantation to avoid teratoma formation, is not presently allowed, whereas autologous MSC are currently used in clinical trials for the treatment of ischaemic heart disease, vascular diseases, spinal cord lesions, non-union of bone, osteogenesis imperfecta, neurological diseases, Parkinson disease, Huntington disease and type I diabetes.[28]

Adult stem cell research does not inspire the controversy that surrounds ESC research because it does not require the destruction of an embryo. MSC have been isolated from bone marrow, the cambium layer of the periosteum, fat, muscle, synovium, dental pulp and amniotic fluid, as well as from foetal tissues, such as umbilical cord blood and others, but their *in vivo* incidence, activities and repositories are still partially understood. Unfortunately, no unique surface antigen is expressed by MSC and this hampers MSC enrichment from heterogeneous populations. STRO-1 antigen, which is present on fibroblast colony-forming unit (CFU-F) cells in adult human bone marrow cells and potentially defines a MSC precursor subpopulation, is common to erythroid precursors. The Oct-4 transcription factor, which is expressed in totipotent ESC and has a unique role in determining pluripotency and stemness, has been detected in human peripheral blood mononuclear cells.[29] Recently, the stage-specific embryonic antigen-4 (SSEA-4), previously thought to be exclusively present on ESC, erythrocytes and some neural cells, has been described as a marker for MSC.[30]

MSC are positive for a number of antigens, including CD105, CD90, CD73, LNGFR, D7-Fib and CD45, but some of them are lost during *in vitro* expansion,[31] therefore MSC are identified through a combination of physical, morphological and functional assays. Owing to the lack of pure, reliable markers for MSC, their tracking from repositories to sites of activity, such as bone or fracture site, is challenging, and most of our knowledge about MSC biology has been attained using culture-manipulated cells.

The bone marrow (BM) is filled with a network of stromal cells and haematopoietic cells, with the first group made of both committed cells, such as adipocytes and osteoblasts, and multipotent precursor cells. The frequency of MSC in the BM is very low (0.001–0.01%). Adipose tissue (AT) also contains stem cells similar to BM-derived MSC. These cells, termed AT-derived stem cells, can be isolated in large numbers from cosmetic liposuction and show multilineage differentiation. The frequency of colony-forming fibroblasts, the actual *in vitro* osteogenic precursor component in the MSC population, has been found to be 1:100 in purified AT-derived cells, that is, some 500-fold more than that found in BM.[32]

The presence of bone precursors in the circulating blood is contentious. Isolation of mesenchymal precursor cells has been obtained with or without prior growth factor mobilization, but the yield is very low and dependent on the isolation method.[33] The number of such precursors may be underestimated owing to the technique of isolation through plastic adherence. Interestingly, their frequency increases after bone fractures, acute burns and myocardial infarction.[34, 35] As previously mentioned, subendothelial pericytes, which provide mechanical support, stability, and contractility to small and large vessels, are claimed to be MSC precursors, as they originate osteoblasts, chondroblasts and adipocytes.[36]

MSC can also be grown from adult human liver and heart. Similarly to adult BM derived cells, a population of multipotent, clonogenic, telomerase-positive cells, able to differentiate into cell types morphologically and functionally corresponding to derivatives of the three germ layers, was produced in culture.[37] This population is likely to correspond to the 'multipotent adult progenitor cells' described below.

Despite a body of literature describing the putative adult MSC, evidence that multipotent MSC actually exist *in vivo* is still lacking. A potential equivalent of ESC has been identified within the MSC adult heterogeneous population and termed multipotent adult progenitor cells (MAPC). MAPC show some features of ESC, including differentiation potential for multilineages, extensive proliferation and, when injected into an early blastocyst, contribution to most somatic cell types.[38] In summary, these cells, similar to ESC, fully gratify the stem cell definition, but in contrast to ESC, can be selected from autologous BM and used undifferentiated without the risk of teratoma formation, or, after genetic manipulation, in local and systemic therapies.

It is hard to develop a consensus opinion about MSC plasticity, since the differences in experimental protocols result in different MSC populations being isolated and assayed. MSC can repair injured tissue by differentiating into the phenotype of damaged cells, by releasing cytokines and growth factors and by undergoing cell fusion. The ability of MSC to differentiate into committed cells, that is, adipocytes or chondrocytes, to be followed by their 'regression' to an intermediate step (de-differentiation) and progression along the osteoblastic lineage, as well as an epithelial-to-mesenchymal transition process, termed 'transdifferentiation', have been referred to as evidences of their *in vivo* plasticity. However, according to some authors, cell fusion, instead of transdifferentiation or de-differentiation, is the process underlining the change of MSC from a phenotype to another and the plasticity of MSC might be simply related to population heterogeneity.[39]

The matrix compliance may initially guide MSC into a development lineage, even if is not sufficient to complete terminal differentiation.[40] On soft substrates (0.1–1 kPa) mimicking the compliance of brain tissue, MSC show a neuronal phenotype; on substrates of intermediate stiffness (8–17 kPa), resembling muscle, they differentiate into myoblasts; on stiff substrates (25–40 kPa), resembling osteoid, MSC differentiate into osteoblasts. It should be noted that if this 'physical' commitment is prolonged for a few weeks, the differentiation to a lineage is not reversed by the addition of soluble factors specific for another lineage, consistent with the relative insensitivity of differentiated cells to elasticity. This underlines the role of the microenvironment, and specifically of the mechanical properties, in determining the fate of undifferentiated cells and may be suggested as an additional mechanism for MSC homing (Fig. 3.4).

Multipotent MSC are attractive for tissue engineering approaches. In fact (1) they are a population of adult undifferentiated cells that can be obtained without previous mobilization; (2) they can be easily isolated from the BM through simple mechanical disruption; (3) they are able to escape recognition by immune cells and exhibit immunosuppressive effects; and (4) under optimal conditions, they can undergo 25–40 passages *in vitro*, demonstrating a good capacity for self replication.

Three different modes of delivering MSC in scaffolds at the implant site are currently being investigated: MSC loaded into scaffolds *in vitro* and, after a short incubation, implantation of the cell-loaded scaffold; cell-scaffold composite incubated in differentiation medium to stimulate MSC progression into a specific lineage; and implantation of scaffold with specific sites for cell anchorage or factors recruiting cells (chemotaxis). These approaches have been used in animal models but rarely in humans.

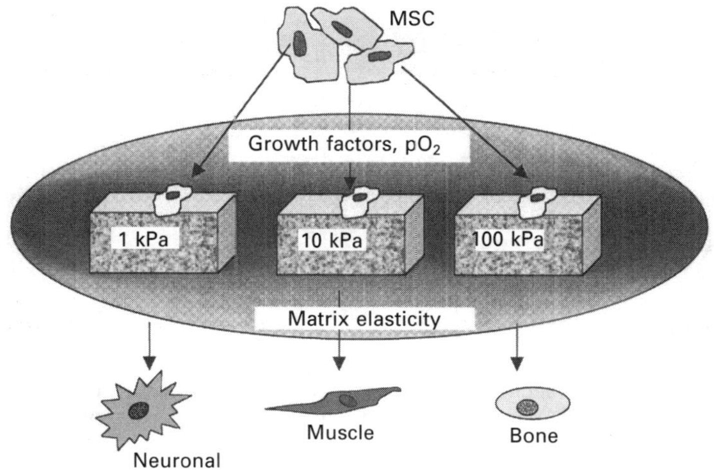

3.4 The differentiation of MSCs to cell lineages is influenced by the compliance of the surrounding extracellular matrix, too, which gives a mechanical signal to the cells. As described by Engler *et al.*,[40] a soft substrate (1 kPa) may induce MSCs to a neuronal type; an intermediate (10 kPa) to myoblastic cell, and a rigid one (100 kPa) turns MSCs to osteoblasts.

There is increasing evidence that although MSC are able to differentiate into lineage-specific cells under the microenvironment into which they are transplanted, the therapeutic effect of MSC proceeds in a different way. In fact, after MSC engraftment into damaged tissue, only a relatively small number of MSC differentiate. Therefore, improvement in tissue healing following MSC engraftment could be due to anti-inflammatory cytokine production, growth factors upregulation and immunomodulatory properties of MSC. This 'trophic' activity of MSC results in inhibition of scarring and of apoptosis, stimulation of angiogenesis and induction of proliferation for resident progenitor cells[41] (Fig. 3.5).

BM has long been a source of adult stem cells for tissue engineering. A more recently described source of multipotent cells are processed lipoaspirate cells (PLA cells) from AT. Some differences between AT and BM-derived multipotent cells have been highlighted. Some surface markers associated with haematopoiesis and migration, as well as some adhesion molecules, are differently expressed in BM- and AT-MSC. BM stromal cells (BMSC) exhibit greater expression of vascular cell adhesion molecule-1 and less expression of α4 integrin and intercellular adhesion molecule-1 than those from AT. These adhesion molecules have been implicated in stem cell mobilization and homing, suggesting that AT and BM-derived multipotent cells may have

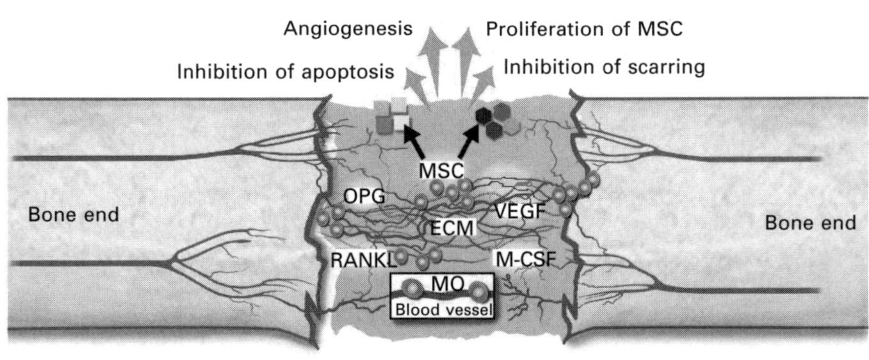

3.5 Trophic activity of MSCs. At the site of healing, a number of factors are secreted by monocytes (MO) and hosted by extracellular matrix (ECM). In addition to their differentiation ability between tissue specific lineages at the site of regeneration, MSCs secrete an array of bioactive factors that inhibit scarring, inhibit apoptosis (narrow or contain the field of injury), stimulate angiogenesis and stimulate the mitosis of tissue-intrinsic stem or progenitor cells. This capacity has been recently described as 'trophic activity' by Caplan.[41] OPG: osteoprotegerin; RANKL: receptor activator for nuclear factor kappaB-ligand; M-CSF: macrophage colony-stimulating factor; VEGF: vascular endothelial growth factor.

different homing properties at distant sites. Aspirates from either source can be harvested during routine elective medical procedures and, because of their mesenchymal origin, have been used to engineer such tissues as cartilage, bone, adipose tissue and blood vessels.[42]

Based on the assumption that the default pathway of human MSC is osteogenic, the achievement of an appreciable new bone formation using BMSC seems a relatively easy task. However, a variety of limiting factors account for such paucity of human applications, including the large numbers of cells that are needed to generate relatively small amounts of tissue, the low proportion of non-haemopoietic stromal cells in BM, the low frequency of CFU-forming fibroblasts or MAPC in adult tissues, the difficulty of a wide expansion of MSC without decreasing the proliferation ability and the risk of bacterial contamination during prolonged *ex vivo* manipulation. At the time of implantation, MSC should also resist the impact of transplantation and the relatively hostile environment of the injured site, including ischaemia and inflammation.

3.4 Molecular events of bone repair and regeneration

Cells activities in the sequential phases of bone healing are regulated by transcriptional programmes involving hundreds of genes. The development of microarray technology has allowed a large-scale analysis of the 'fracture healing transcriptome' to be performed, also distinguishing the different stages of bone repair.[43] Li *et al.* have identified genes that are differentially expressed during the early stages of bone repair by comparing the gene expression profile of non-fractured with post-fractured rat femurs.[44] More recently, the same authors analyzed the 'fracture healing proteoma' in order to dissect and characterize functionally proteins that are differentially expressed during bone repair.[45]

Genes with energy derivation, transport and binding activities are significantly up-regulated on day 1 after fracture. The proteomic functional analysis has revealed that preparation for fracture healing includes both cell-cycle regulation and cell-to-cell signalling. The first provides a molecular basis for the observation that cell division peaks on the first day after fracture and the second confirms that cell communication is essential to initiate bone repair.[46] Insulin-like growth factor I (IGF-I), platelet derived growth factor (PDGF) and the mitogen-activated protein kinase (ERK/MAPK) signalling pathway are significantly expressed during the inflammation phase. On day 4 after fracture, the haematoma is invaded by undifferentiated cells and vascularized connective tissue, while macrophages remove debris and neutrophils decrease.

Gene expression profiling shows that some genes continue to rise from days 1 to 4, while others are constantly up-regulated. Genes of the first group are functionally associated with the repair process including IGF-I, PDGF, fibroblast growth factor receptor (FGFR), fibronectin, matrix metalloproteinases, glypican, byglican, osteomodulin, osteonectin, tenascin C, cartilage collagen (type VI and XI) and bone collagen (type I, V, VI, and XII). In contrast, many of the constantly up-regulated genes control cell growth and survival, and they fall into activity groups with a general function such as binding, transport and catalytic activity.

On day 4, osteoblast progenitors differentiate and synthesize immature osteoid. From the molecular point of view, direct ossification is a relatively quiet stage and the essential molecular activity is the regulation of cell death. Proteomic analysis reveals that proteins, differentially expressed, belong to a single interacting network associated with cell death, immune response and cell signalling, and IL6 is strongly expressed and plays a pivotal role in coordinating the three functional groups.

On day 7, a number of molecular events testify the start of endochondral ossification that is observed histologically later.[47] Chondrogenesis represents the most active molecular event. Several molecular pathways are active, including PDGF, vascular endothelial growth factor (VEGF) and peroxisome proliferator-activated receptor alpha (PPAR). In the downstream of the above-mentioned pathways, the proteins related to PI3K/AKT, a cell survival signalling, are the most significantly expressed.

On day 14, hypertrophic chondrocytes are the dominant cell type. In the hard callus, BM is evident and osteoclast-like cells remove cartilage and create a space where osteoblasts are able to form woven bone. Proteins significantly expressed in this phase suggest that at least six pathways are potentially active; of these, PPAR is involved also at the chondrogenesis stage, while apoptosis and p38/MAPK signalling are uniquely significant during endochondral ossification. When endochondral ossification comes to an end (day 28), bone repair enters the remodelling phase. P13K/AKT, IGF-I, MAPK/ERK and integrins are some of the pathways involved.

Among the variety of cells and signalling pathways that regulate bone repair and regeneration, a central role is the ability of MSC to differentiate into bone forming cells. By using microarray technology, we have studied the gene expression profile of human MSC cultured *in vitro* and undergoing osteogenic induction. The analysis was performed at different time points until MSC were able to form mineral nodules *in vitro*.[48] We focused on up-regulated genes with a biological function relevant to osteogenesis, such as cell communication, morphogenesis and skeletal development, Wnt signaling, TGFβ signalling, angiogenesis, cell cycle and apoptosis. In the early stage of differentiation, we observed genes involved in cell cycle, while in further stages the expression of growth factor signalling pathways, bone-related genes and adhesion molecules gradually increased. Genes typical of angiogenesis and morphogenesis were up-regulated in the final steps of mineralization, suggesting that mature osteoblast induces the growth of other tissues involved in bone development. A list of bone-related genes which might be useful to monitor the functional status and activity of cultured MSC is shown in Table 3.1.

Several signalling systems are known to play important roles in driving the differentiation of MSC in bone forming cells.[49]

Table 3.1 'Bone related genes' significantly up-regulated during MSC differentiation with a relative difference greater than 3 in comparison to undifferentiated MSCs. Differentiation status has been defined as 'early', which includes the phases before the first confluence of MSC, 'intermediate', which means MSC able to produce alkaline phosphatase and generate 'colony forming units', and 'late', in which differentiated MSC acquire the competence to deposit mineral nodules *in vitro*

Differentiation status	Gene title	Gene symbol
Early, intermediate	Bone morphogenetic protein 1	BMP1
	Cadherin 11, type 2, OB-cadherin (osteoblast)	CDH11
	Collagen, type X, alpha 1 (Schmid metaphyseal chondrodysplasia)	COL10A1
	Collagen, type XII, alpha 1	COL12A1
	Fibrillin 1	FBN1
	Insulin-like growth factor 2 (somatomedin A)	IGF2
	Integrin-binding sialoprotein (bone sialoprotein, bone sialoprotein II)	IBSP
	PDZ and LIM domain 7 (enigma)	PDLIM7
	Periostin, osteoblast specific factor	POSTN
	Secreted protein, acidic, cysteine-rich (osteonectin)	SPARC
Intermediate	Alkaline phosphatase, liver/bone/kidney	ALPL
	C-type lectin domain family 3, member B (tetranectin)	CLEC3B
	Epidermal growth factor receptor (erythroblastic leukemia viral (v-erb-b) oncogene homolog, avian)	EGFR
	Proline/arginine-rich end leucine-rich repeat protein	PRELP
	Tumour necrosis factor receptor superfamily, member 11b (osteoprotegerin)	TNFRSF11B
Early, intermediate, late	Cartilage oligomeric matrix protein	COMP
	T-box 3 (ulnar mammary syndrome)	TBX3
Intermediate, late	Ankylosis, progressive homolog (mouse)	ANKH
	SRY (sex determining region Y)-box 9	SOX9

3.4.1 Wnt signalling pathway

Wnts, a family of secreted glycoproteins with multiple inhibitors, are ligands of the family of membrane-spanning frizzled (FZD) receptors involved in various aspects of cellular biology. Wnt proteins activate two different pathways, namely 'canonical' and 'non-canonical' Wnt signalling. The first one involves the formation of a complex between Wnt proteins, FZD and low density lipoprotein receptor-related protein 5 (LRP5) or LRP6 receptors. In 'non-canonical' Wnt signaling, Wnt5a binds FZD proteins, activates heterotrimeric G proteins and increases intracellular calcium via protein kinase C-dependent mechanisms or induces Rho- or c-Jun N-terminal kinase (JNK)-dependent changes in the actin cytoskeleton.[50] Wnt proteins regulate cell growth, differentiation, function and death, and the canonical pathway appears to be particularly important for bone biology.[51]

The binding of Wnt proteins to the FZD/LRP5/6 complex generates a signal through the proteins Dishevelled, Axin and Frat-1, which inhibit the activity of glycogen synthase kinase 3 (GSK3). GSK3 inactivity blocks the phosphorylation of ß-catenin and prevents its degradation in the cytoplasm by the ubiquitin-pathway, leading to translocation of β-catenin to the cell nucleus where it cooperates with transcription factors of the T-cell factor/lymphoid enhancer factor (TCF/LEF) family in regulating target gene expression.[52]

Wnt signalling may be affected by extracellular antagonists, including the secreted FZD related protein (sFRP) family, Wnt inhibitory factor 1 (WIF-1), while LRP5/6 coreceptor activity is inhibited by members of the SOST (Sclerosteosis gene product) and Dickkopf (Dkk) families. There is considerable *in vitro* evidence indicating that the Wnt 'canonical' pathway plays a critical role in bone formation resulting in the expression of osteoblast-specific markers.[53] It is likely that β-catenin activity is required in a bipotential precursor of the osteoblast lineage, the so-called osteochondroprogenitor, and indeed its absence steers the fate of mesenchymal precursors toward chondrogenesis.[54] The osteoblast differentiation is regulated by the effect β-catenin on transcription factors. β-catenin/TCF1 complex enhances expression and promoter activity of Runx2, while low levels of β-catenin seem to address the differentiation into the chondrocyte lineage.

3.4.2 Signalling TGFβ

Several members of the transforming growth factor β (TGFß) superfamily, such as the bone morphogenetic proteins (BMP), have potent osteogenic effects. The activity of BMP was first identified in the 1960s,[55] but proteins responsible for osteogenesis remained unknown until the purification and sequencing of bovine BMP3 (osteogenin) and cloning of human BMP2 and 4 in the late 1980s.[56]

The BMP/TGFβ superfamily signalling is transduced through two types of serine/threonine kinase receptors. Three type I receptors have been shown, namely type IA and IB BMP receptors (BMPR-IA or ALK-3, and BMPR-IB or ALK-6) and type IA activin receptor (ActR-IA or ALK-2). Three type II receptors for BMP have also been identified, including type II BMP receptor (BMPR-II) and type II and IIB activin receptors (ActR-II and ActR-IIB). Whereas BMPR-IA, IB and II are specific to BMPs, ActR-IA, II and IIB are also signalling receptors for activins.[57] The BMPR-IB activity is necessary for the initial steps of chondrogenesis, while BMPR-IA regulates the induction of chondrocyte hypertrophy.

BMPs transmit signals through Smad-dependent and Smad-independent pathways, including ERK, JNK and p38/MAPK pathways. There are three classes of Smads: (1) receptor-regulated Smads (R-Smads) which can be activated by BMP (BMPR-Smad), such as Smad 1, 5 and 8, or TGFß (TGFR-Smad), such as Smad 2 and 3; (2) common partner BMP and TGFß mediator Smads (Co-Smads), such as Smad 4; (3) inhibitory Smads, such as Smad 6 and 7.[58] Phosphorylated R-Smads bind to the common partner Smad-4. These complexes translocate into the nucleus and regulate transcription of target genes by interacting with various transcription factors and transcriptional co-activators or co-repressors. BMPR-Smads facilitate expression of Distal-less homeobox 5 (Dlx5) in osteoblasts, which induces expression of Runx2 and Osterix (Osx) in osteoprogenitor cells. The inhibitory Smads negatively regulate signalling by the R-Smads and Co-Smads.[59] Although the Smads are critical mediators in the TGFß signalling pathway, BMP2 can activate Smad-independent pathways, including MAP kinases (ERK, JNK and p38) which have distinct roles in regulating alkaline phosphatase and osteocalcin expression in osteoblastic cells.[60]

3.4.3 Hedgehog signalling

Indian hedgehog (Ihh) is produced by pre-hypertrophic chondrocytes and its signalling appears to act directly on osteoblast progenitors located in the perichondrium.[61, 62] Ihh signalling plays a crucial role in regulating the temporal and spatial programme of early osteoblast commitment, but its role is limited to this stage. In fact, when Smo (smoothened homolog) activity, which encodes an obligatory component of the Hh signaling pathway, is removed in Osx+ osteoblast precursors, normal bone osteoblasts are generated and the endochondral skeleton at birth is indistinguishable from the wild type.[63]

3.4.4 Fibroblast growth factor (FGF) signalling

The FGF-family polypeptides play a critical role in regulating endochondral and intramembranous ossification through four related tyrosine kinase receptors (Fgfr1-Fgfr4). Fgfr1 is expressed in hypertrophic chondrocytes and Fgfr1 signalling has stage-specific effects on osteoblast maturation: it acts to stimulate differentiation in osteoprogenitor cells, whereas it functions to arrest the maturation of differentiated osteoblasts.[64] FGFs 2, 9 and 18 probably bind Fgfr1 in osteoblasts. Although FGFs 9 and 18 represent the predominant signals during embryo development, FGF2 seems to be the most relevant in postnatal stages. In differentiated osteoblast, FGF2 activates Runx2 via MAPK pathway and plays an important role in the regulation of mineralization and bone formation. Fgf2r is expressed in reserve chondrocytes and appears to be downregulated in proliferating chondrocytes. Fgf2r shows tissue specific alternative splicing, resulting in epithelial variants (b forms) and mesenchymal variants (c forms). Studies of the ligand binding demonstrate that FGF7 and 10, activate Fgfr2b, whereas FGF2, 4, 6, 8 and 9 activate Fgfr2c. FGF18 acts as a physiological ligand for Fgfr3, which regulates cell growth and differentiation of proliferating chondrocytes, while in differentiated osteoblasts it regulates bone density and cortical thickness.[65]

3.4.5 Ephrin signalling

Ephrins have a capacity for bidirectional signalling. Thus, when a cell expressing an ephrin receptor contacts a cell expressing an ephrin ligand, signals are transduced into both the cells by forward and reverse signalling, respectively. There are two classes of ephrins, the B class (B1 to B3) are ligands for EphB1-6 tyrosine kinase receptors, whereas class A ephrins (A1 to A5) are ligands for GPI-anchored EphA receptors (A1 to A10). In bone biology, ephrinB and its receptors control skeleton development.[66] A bidirectional signalling is also implicated in the communication between osteoblasts and osteoclasts: the ephrinB2 ligand in osteoclasts and EphB4 receptor in osteoblasts are responsible for a forward-reverse signalling which regulates osteoblast–osteoclast cooperation. The reverse signalling from EphB4 in osteoblasts to ephrinB2 in osteoclast progenitors leads to the inhibition of osteoclast differentiation, while the forward signalling through EphB4 induces osteogenic regulatory factors, such as Dlx5, Osx and Runx2.[67]

3.4.6 Mitogen-activated protein kinases (MAPK) signalling pathway

MAPKs are important signal transducing serine/threonine-specific protein kinases that are involved in many facets of cellular regulation. The MAPK pathway is activated by a variety of growth factors with a role in osteogenesis, including FGF, PDGF, TGFβ and IGFs. The extracellular stimuli lead to activation of a signalling cascade composed of MAP kinase, MAP kinase kinase (MKK or MAP2K) and MAP kinase kinase kinase (MKKK or MAP3K).

Recent studies have elucidated the physiological functions of these cascades in the control of gene expression, cell proliferation and programmed cell death. The MAPK cascade comprises distinct groups of protein kinases which have been characterized in mammals (Table 3.2).[68]

3.4.7 Transcription factors regulating osteoblast differentiation

Transcription factors address the commitment of MSCs to tissue-specific cell types, and Runx2 is considered to be a master regulatory switch which mediates the temporal activation and/or repression of genes differentiation which is essential for osteoblast differentiation.[69] Other genes are required to progress the differentiation programme, such as Osx, which encodes a transcription factor genetically 'downstream' of Runx2.[70] Runx2 is a member of the Runx (Runt-related factors) family of transcription factors. The family members, Runx1 and Runx3, are encoded by distinct unlinked genes but share a common DNA recognition motif and heterodimerize with the ubiquitous subunit Cbfß for stable DNA binding. Runx2 is abundantly expressed in calcified cartilage and bone. The peculiarity of Runx2 is the transactivation domain, rich in glutamine and alanine residues, which serves

Table 3.2 Families of mitogen-activated protein kinases

Family	Name	Function
Extracellular signal-regulated kinases	ERK1, ERK2	The ERKs (also known as classical MAPK) signalling pathways are activated in response to growth factors and regulate cell proliferation and cell differentiation.
	ERK5 (MAPK7)	Activated both by growth factors and by stress stimuli, it participates in cell proliferation.
	ERK3 (MAPK6) ERK4 (MAPK4)	Atypical MAPKs: ERK3/4 are mostly cytoplasmic protein which binds, translocates and activates the MK5 (PRAK, MAP2K5). ERK3 is known to be unstable unlike ERK4 which is relatively stable.
	ERK7/8. (MAPK15)	New members of MAPKs structurally related to ERK3/4.
c-Jun N-terminal kinases (JNKs)	MAPK8, MAPK9, MAPK10	Stress-activated protein kinases (SAPKs)
p38 isoforms	MAPK11, MAPK12 (ERK6), MAPK13, MAPK14	Both JNK and p38 signaling pathways are responsive to stress stimuli, such as cytokines, ultraviolet irradiation, heat shock and osmotic shock, and are involved in cell differentiation and apoptosis.

to activate osteocalcin and type I collagen α chain (Col1a1) genes. Targeted disruption of Runx2 results in the complete inhibition of bone formation, revealing that Runx2 is essential for both endochondral and membranous bone formation. Runx2 may be expressed in early osteoprogenitors, but is also required for osteoblast function beyond differentiation.

Many transcription factors involved in the regulation of osteoblast differentiation exert their action by interacting with Runx2. Some provide co-stimulatory signals, while others directly repress Runx2 function by affecting its DNA binding activity and/or transactivation potential (Table 3.3).

The second transcriptional regulator for the final stages of bone tissue formation is Osx. This contains a DNA-binding domain consisting of three C_2H_2-type zinc fingers and a proline- and serine-rich transactivation domain responsible for the activation of osteocalcin and Col1a1 genes. MSCs of Osx-null mutant mice express normal levels of Runx2, but they cannot differentiate into osteoblasts and deposit bone matrix. As a consequence, in Osx-null mice, no endochondral or intramembranous bone formation occurs. Interestingly, Osx-null osteoblast precursors in the periosteum of membranous bones express chondrocyte markers, such as Sox9 and Col2a1, suggesting that Runx2-expressing preosteoblasts are still bipotential cells and Osx acts downstream of Runx2 to induce osteoblastic differentiation of

Table 3.3 Transcription factors regulating Runx2 function

Upstream proteins	Msh homeobox 2 (*Msx2*), NK3 homeobox 2 (*Bapx1*), homeobox A2 (*Hoxa 2*), p53, twist homologs (*Twist 1-2*), DNA binding/transcription factor (*Shn3*)
Co-activators	Core-binding factor beta (*Cbfß*), Cbp/p300-interacting transactivator (*Cited2*), monocytic leukemia zinc finger protein (*MOZ, MYST3*), MOZ related factor (*MORF, MYST4*), retinoblastoma protein (*pRb*), transcriptional coactivator with PDZ-binding motif (*TAZ*)
Co-repressors	Histone deacetylases (*HDACs*), Groucho related genes/ transducin-like enhancer of split (*Grg/TLE*), yes-associated protein (*YAP*), SMAD specific E3 ubiquitin protein ligase 1 (*Smurf1*)
Transcription factor partners with positive effect	Activator-protein 1 (*AP-1*) (*c-Fos* and *c-Jun*), BMP responsive Smads (*Smad1* and *Smad5*), v-ets erythroblastosis virus E26 oncogene homolog 1 avian (*Ets1*), CCAAT/enhancer binding protein (*C/EBP*) β and δ, distal-less homeobox 5 (*Dlx5*), hairy and enhancer of split 1 (*Hes1*), product of the tumor suppressor gene *Men1* (*Menin*)
Transcription factor partners with inhibitory effect	Distal-less homeobox 3 (*Dlx3*), lymphoid enhancer-binding factor 1 (*Lef1*), Msh homeobox 2 (*Msx2*), peroxisome proliferator-activated receptor (*PPAR*), *Smad3*, hairy/ enhancer-of-split related with YRPW motif 1 (*Hey1*), signal transducer and activator of transcription 1 (*Stat1*)

osteochondroprogenitor cells. Osx may be induced by additional signalling pathways acting in parallel to, or independent of, Runx2. It has been shown that Runx2 is required but not sufficient for the BMP2-mediated Osx induction, since MAPK and protein kinase D (PKD) signalling pathways serve as points of convergence mediating the BMP2 effect on Osx expression in MSC, as well as other transcription factors downstream of BMP2. Cooperation between NFAT and Osx activates the Col1a1 and osteocalcin promoters and accelerates osteoblast differentiation and bone formation in a Runx2-independent manner.[71]

3.5 Role of growth factors in bone repair and regeneration

Growth factors (GF) are polypeptides that act locally as modulators of cellular functions. Their action may be autocrine (GF influences the cell of its origin or a cell with the same phenotype), paracrine (GF influences a neighbouring cell with a different phenotype) or endocrine (GF acts on a cell located at a remote anatomical site).[72] A single GF may have effects on multiple cell types and may induce different functions. GF bind to target cell receptors and induce an intracellular signal transduction that reaches the nucleus and determines the biological response. This system is redundant, a single GF may bind to different receptors.

The most important GF acting on bone are bone morphogenetic proteins (BMP), transforming growth factor-β (TGF-β), fibroblast growth factor (FGF), platelet-derived growth factor (PDGF), vascular endothelial growth factor (VEGF) and insulin-like growth factors (IGFs) (Table 3.4). As previously mentioned, during bone repair and regeneration, GF are produced by the cells of the microenvironment, such as inflammatory cells, fibroblasts, endothelial cells, BMSC and osteoblasts. GF play a role during all the phases of bone repair. In the inflammation phase, the major contributors are the GF released by platelet α-granules (TGF-β, PDGF, VEGF and IGF), whereas macrophages and other inflammatory cells secrete FGF, PDGF and TGF-β. Migration of osteoprogenitors is enhanced by BMP, PDGF, FGF and VEGF. PDGF and FGF also stimulate the proliferation of periosteum-derived cells and may contribute to the mitogenic response of the periosteum in the early stages of bone repair.[73] Proliferation and differentiation of osteoprogenitor cells are modulated by TGF-β, IGF, BMP-6, BMP-2 and BMP-7, and the vascular ingrowth into the repairing bone is regulated by VEGF and FGF-2. The temporal response of GF in fracture repair has been investigated in mice.[74]

TGF-β and PDGF increase in the first two days from the seeding of bone marrow cells in osteogenic medium, then decrease but increase again at day 7, with a second peak at day 14. VEGF peaks at day 4 and returns

Table 3.4 Growth factors and their role in bone repair

Growth factor	Physiological source	Receptor class	General function	Action on bone
Bone morphogenetic proteins (BMP)	Osteoprogenitor cell, osteoblast, chondrocyte, endothelial cell (BMP-2)	Serine threonine sulphate	Chondro-osteogenesis. BMP -2 through -7 and BMP-9 are osteoinductive	Precursor chemotaxis, induction of proliferation, differentiation and matrix synthesis, contribute to angiogenesis
Transforming growth factor β (TGF-β)	Platelet, bone marrow stromal cell, osteoblast, chondrocyte, endothelial cell, fibroblast, macrophage	Serine threonine sulphate	Immunosuppressor; proangiogenic; stimulation of cell growth, differentiation and extracellular matrix synthesis	Stimulation of undifferentiated mesenchymal cell proliferation; osteoblast precursor recruiting; osteoblast and chondrocyte differentiation (but inhibition of terminal differentiation); bone matrix production; recruitment of osteoclast precursors
Fibroblast growth factor (FGF)	Macrophage, monocyte, bone marrow stromal cell, chondrocyte, osteoblast, endothelial cell	Tyrosine kinase	Proangiogenic; mitogenic for fibroblast and smooth muscle cells of the vascular wall	FGF-1 induces chondrocyte maturation; FGF-2 induces osteoblast proliferation and differentiation, inhibits apoptosis of immature osteoblasts while stimulating apoptosis of mature

				osteocytes, stimulates bone resorption
Platelet-derived growth factor (PDGF)	Platelet, osteoblast, endothelial cell, monocyte, macrophage	Tyrosine kinase	Mitogen for connective tissue cells, chemotactic for monocytes, macrophages and smooth muscle cells; proangiogenic	Stimulates osteoprogenitor proliferation and differentiation
Vascular endothelial growth factor (VEGF)	Endothelial cell, osteoblast, platelet	Tyrosine kinase	Proangiogenic; chemotactic for endothelial cell	Conversion of cartilage into bone; osteoblast proliferation and differentiation; induces RANK expression in osteoclast precursors
Insulin-like growth factor (IGF)	Osteoblasts, chondrocyte, hepatocyte, endothelial cell	Tyrosine kinase	Regulation of growth hormone biological activity	Stimulates osteoblast proliferation and bone matrix synthesis; bone resorption

to baseline levels at 1 week. IGF-1 is high during the first four days, then decreases at day 8 and increases later on. FGF-2 and BMP-2 peak at day 14, then decrease. A strong correlation has been demonstrated between VEGF, TGF-β and IGF-1, suggesting that they act coordinately in osteoprogenitor cell growth. A similar correlation is evident among BMP-2, PDGF and FGF-2, and between TGF-β and PDGF.

3.5.1 Bone morphogenetic proteins (BMP)

These belong to the TGF-β superfamily, which includes the BMP (except BMP-1), TGF-β, growth differentiation factors (GDF), activins, inhibins and the Müllerian substance. BMP are stored in the bone extracellular matrix and are mainly produced by osteoprogenitor cells, osteoblasts and chondrocytes.[75] Other cell types can also synthesize BMP, such as endothelial cells, which produce BMP-2.[76] Mature osteoblasts and chondrocytes do not express significant levels of BMP, but both have increased BMP expression in fracture repair.[77] BMP expression is induced by stimuli such as mechanical stress at regions undergoing bone tissue formation.[78]

Even if BMP are structurally and functionally related, each type has a unique role as well as a distinct temporal expression pattern during the bone repair process.[79] BMP-2 and -4 are expressed early by MSC, then are expressed throughout the bone healing process. BMP-7 (also known as osteogenic protein-1 or OP-1) is expressed from day 7 and peaks at 2–4 weeks.

BMP induce a cascade of events for chondro-osteogenesis, including chemotaxis, mesenchymal and osteoprogenitor cell proliferation and differentiation, angiogenesis and synthesis of extracellular matrix. BMP-2 and -4 are chemoattractive proteins for mesenchymal progenitor cells (MPC), suggesting a functional role for the recruitment of MPC during bone development and remodelling, as well as in fracture healing. BMP-4 works together with VEGF to recruit osteoblast precursors.[80] BMP-2, -6 and -9 stimulate the differentiation of pluripotent MSC into osteoprogenitor cells and BMP-2, -4, -7 and -9 further differentiate them to become osteoblasts. BMP-2 upregulates runx-2 and osterix expression.[81] BMP-2, -4, -6, -7 and -9 increase alkaline phosphatase and osteocalcin and lead to calcium deposition.

Most BMP are able to differentiate osteoblasts into osteocytes. BMP-13 stimulates the proliferation and differentiation of chondrocytes.[82] BMP-14, also known as the growth differentiation factor-5, promotes the chondrogenic differentiation and influences endochondral bone growth.[83] BMP-2 through -7 and BMP-9 are able to induce *de novo* bone formation after ectopic implantation.[84] The osteoinductive activity of BMP-3 depends on the experimental conditions and the stage of differentiation; it may have an inhibitory effect in the presence of BMP-2 and BMP-7.[85] BMP stimulate the synthesis of other GF, such as IGF and VEGF.[86] BMP also initiate the release of factors that promote osteoclast generation. Therefore, large doses of BMP may lead to resorption that precedes the appearance and the effects of osteoblasts.[87]

Five isoforms of transforming growth factor-β (TGF-β1 through TGF-β5) have been identified so far. TGF-β1 and TGF-β2 are stored in the bone extracellular matrix and in the blood as a latent form linked to TGF-β-binding protein-1. TGF-β1 has been detected in bone, cartilage and platelet α-granules, but it is produced by many cell types, including fibroblasts, macrophages and endothelial cells, whereas TGF-β2 is produced by osteoblasts and endothelial cells. In bone healing, TGF-β plays a role during chondrogenesis and endochondral bone formation.[88] TGF-β1 initiates signalling for BMP synthesis by osteoprogenitor cells, recruits osteoblast precursors, stimulates MSC to differentiate and produce matrix and alkaline phosphatase and stimulates the formation of osteoid and extracellular proteins such as collagen, proteoglycans, osteopontin, osteonectin and alkaline phosphatase.[89] However, TGF-β1 blocks terminal differentiation and suppresses mineralization, therefore it has a positive function in the early phases of bone repair but an inhibitory effect on differentiation in the terminal stage.[90] In addition, TGF-β1 has a limited osteoinductive potential.[91] It acts as a 'coupling factor' between osteoblasts and osteoclasts[92] since it favours the recruitment of hematopoietic precursors of osteoclasts.[93] However, TGF-β1 inhibits osteoclastic bone resorption and stimulates osteoprotegerin production.[94]

3.5.2 Fibroblast growth factors (FGF)

These are a family of 24 structurally related polypeptides that stimulate the proliferation of bone marrow cells, osteoblasts, chondrocytes, fibroblasts, myocytes and endothelial cells. The most abundant FGF are FGF-1 and FGF-2. Both have been identified in the early phases of bone healing and are associated with chondrocyte and osteoblast functions. In particular, FGF-1 is important for chondrocyte maturation.[95] FGF-2 is synthesized by osteoblasts and stored in the extracellular matrix; it induces osteoblast proliferation and differentiation, upregulates runx-2[96] and osteocalcin,[97] and favours bone nodule formation.[98] FGF-2 inhibits apoptosis of immature osteoblasts while stimulating apoptosis of mature osteocytes.[99, 100] FGF-2 also regulates osteoclastogenesis both indirectly by osteoblast-mediated mechanisms and directly by stimulation of bone pit resorption, via signal transduction pathways involving RANK-L, cyclo-oxygenase-2 and p42/p44 MAPK activation.[101] In addition, the proangiogenic effect of FGF-2 may be useful in bone repair, where an adequate vascular contribution is required. Angiogenesis elicited by FGF-2 is also accompanied by increased osteoclast formation and bone pit resorption.[102]

3.5.3 Platelet derived growth factor (PDGF)

This is secreted in the form of dimer with different combinations of A, B, C and D chains. It is present in platelet α-granules, monocytes, macrophages, endothelial cells and osteoblasts.[103] PDGF acts both in the first phase of bone repair, stimulating the proliferation of osteoprogenitors, and during the differentiation stage. PDGF is released by platelet α-granules during the early phases of fracture healing[104] and afterwards by the cells of the bone repair site. PDGF-BB is generally considered more effective than PDGF-AA in stimulating mitogenic activity on the skeleton,[105] but PDGF-AA also influences bone healing, together with BMP-2 and TGF-β.[106]

3.5.4 Vascular endothelial growth factor (VEGF)

This is produced by endothelial cells and osteoblasts. In the early stages of bone repair, VEGF is also released by platelet α-granules. Even if angiogenesis is the most known effect of VEGF, it is also required for osteoblast proliferation and differentiation.[107] VEGF is involved in the conversion of cartilage to bone callus during fracture repair[108] and increases the number of osteoblasts.[109] VEGF also favours osteoclastogenesis inducing RANK expression in osteoclast precursors.[110]

3.5.5 Insulin-like growth factors (IGF)

Two insulin-like growth factors (IGF) have been identified (IGF-I or somatomedin C and IGF-II). The serum concentration of IGF-I is mainly regulated by the growth hormone (GH) and the biological actions of IGF are modulated in a cell-specific manner by IGF-binding proteins.

IGF-I is primarily produced by liver cells in response to GH. Other sources are the bone matrix, endothelial cells, osteoblasts and chondrocytes. The target tissue of IGF-I are muscle, cartilage, bone, liver, kidney, nerves, skin and lungs. IGF-I is more potent than IGF-II and has been localized in healing fractures,[111] even if IGF-II is the most abundant growth factor in bone. In the first phases of bone repair, IGF-I stimulates osteoblast proliferation[112] and promotes bone matrix formation by fully differentiated osteblasts.[113] IGF-II acts at a later stage of endochondral bone formation and stimulates type I collagen production, cartilage matrix synthesis and cell proliferation.[114] IGF is regarded as a link between bone formation and bone resorption.[115]

3.5.6 Protein therapy with recombinant growth factors

The rationale for the therapeutic use of GF to stimulate bone healing is based on the hypothesis that the selection of an appropriate signalling GF may be sufficient to induce or accelerate the entire healing process.[116] The possible clinical applications for GF in bone repair and regeneration include acceleration of fracture healing, treatment of non-unions and pseudoarthrosis, enhancement of primary spinal fusion and, in general, treatment of bone defects and large bone loss. GF administration has been attempted, either through protein therapy, in which a recombinant (rh) GF is directly delivered to the regeneration site with or without a carrier matrix, or gene therapy, in which a GF is delivered indirectly by the transfection of its encoding gene. A special type of protein therapy is the use of autologous or homologous platelet rich plasma as a source of GF, or of demineralized bone matrix.

BMP-2 and BMP-7 are commercially available through the use of recombinant DNA technology. They may be administered by a buffer delivery system or combined with a carrier, in order to prevent rapid diffusion of the GF away from the healing site and to provide sustained release. In fact, using a buffer delivery system, less than 5% of the BMP dose remains at the application site, whereas combinations of BMP with a carrier increases the retention up to 55%.[117] The carrier used for the delivery of rhBMP may also be a scaffold for the newly formed bone.

Preclinical studies have provided evidence of the efficacy of rhBMP in the healing of critical-sized bone defects.[118] The first feasibility clinical trial on the application of rhBMP bound to an absorbable collagen sponge was performed in patients with a fresh open tibial fracture and demonstrated that the application of rhBMP was feasible and safe and favoured primary healing.[119] Several clinical studies have been published on the effects of rhBMP-7 or rhBMP-2 in bone healing or in delayed unions/non-unions. A randomized study has evaluated the use of rhBMP-2 absorbed to a collagen sponge in open tibial fractures, showing a significant reduction in healing time, number of additional procedures and infection.[120] BMP-7 was investigated in a variety of orthopaedic conditions, including non-unions, periprosthetic fractures, osteotomy, enhancement of bone stock, distraction osteogenesis, free fibular graft and arthrodesis.[121–123] Treatment with rhBMP also stimulates angiogenesis and reduces the rate of infection. A prerequisite for BMP to have a positive effect seems to be the presence of mesenchymal stem cells. As BMP are required not only to stimulate the proliferation and differentiation of BMSC, but also to maintain the osteoblastic phenotype, a successful treatment requires a high dose and a long exposure time.[124]

TGF-β has been used to enhance bone growth in experimental animals,[125] but its therapeutic potential seems limited owing to its unforeseen side effects.[126] rhFGF-2 accelerates bone repair in experimental animals,[127] but this effect is present only if FGF-2 is administered within 24 hours after fracture,[128] suggesting that the window for anabolic effects of exogenous FGF is limited to the early phase of the healing process. PDGF increases callus density in tibial osteotomies of rats,[129] but at present its therapeutical potential is unclear.[126] Animal studies have demonstrated that IGF may be administered systemically to increase bone formation. IGF-I effects were age-dependent, being absent in young, rapidly growing animals.[130] In a rat tibia model, the local administration of IGF-I had a greater stimulating effect on fracture healing than TGF-β; the application of both GF resulted in a significantly higher maximum load and torsional stiffness.[131]

Although recombinant GF may be used for specific clinical applications, there is concern that a single dose of exogenous protein will not induce an adequate biological response in patients, particularly in situations in which the viability of the host bone and surrounding soft tissues is compromised. A better strategy for protein delivery might be gene therapy, which involves the transfer of genetic information to cells. There are two ways to deliver the required GF gene to the regeneration site: it can be delivered directly to the tissue so that host cells are transfected and express the protein (*in vivo* transduction) or the gene can be delivered through transfection of cultured cells, which are implanted at the regeneration site (*in vitro* transduction). In general, the duration of protein synthesis after gene therapy depends on the technique used to deliver the gene to the cell. Both short-term and long-term expression are possible. The treatment of the bone repair defects usually requires short-term protein production, while long-term expression is useful in chronic diseases such as osteoporosis. MSC, genetically engineered to express BMP-2,[132] have been shown to stimulate osteogenesis and angiogenesis. Before the clinical application of the gene therapy, however, questions concerning the safety of viral vectors and the immunological reactions to viral proteins need to be addressed.

Autologous or homologous platelet rich plasma (PRP) is used to accelerate bone repair through the osteogenic GF released from platelet α-granules during activation.[133] The advantages of PRP lie in its mimicking the GF effects of the physiological wound healing and regenerative tissue processes. Moreover, if autologous PRP is used, immunological reactions are avoided. The drawbacks consist in the unpredictability of GF concentrations in different preparations, owing both to individual factors and to different preparation methods. The efficiency of PRP in improving bone regeneration is increased by its combination with bone allografts.[134] A recent prospective, randomized, controlled clinical study has demonstrated that PRP alone or combined with bone marrow stromal cells increases the osteogenetic potential of lyophilized bone chips.[135]

3.5.7 Demineralized bone matrix

DBM is the product of acid extraction of allograft bone, resulting in the loss of most of the mineralized component. It contains type I collagen, non-collagenous proteins and osteoinductive GF (BMP, GDF, TGF-β1, -2 and -3). The osteoinductive properties of DBM depend on the type of bone, the sterilization process, the formulation, the amount and the ratios of different BMP present.[136]

The therapeutic use of rhGF has some drawbacks. There are possible adverse effects of GF, such as immunological reactions. The long-term effects and possible genetic alterations in humans remain unknown. Excessive bone formation has been observed, although only after large doses. Pregnancy is a contraindication to the use of rhGF and applications in children must be carefully considered. The ideal timing of administration and the most effective dose to be administered, which could influence the effects on fracture healing,[137] have not been investigated in depth. Further research and controlled clinical studies are necessary to address the differences in bone repair mechanisms between specific conditions and to provide evidence-based guidelines for an appropriate GF therapy to optimize bone healing.[138]

3.6 References

1. Ferguson C, Alpern E, Miclau T and Helms JA. 'Does adult fracture repair recapitulate embryonic skeletal formation?' *Mech Dev*, 1999, **87**, 57–66.
2. Dimitriou R, Tsiridis E and Giannoudis PV. 'Current concepts of molecular aspects of bone healing', *Injury*, 2005, **36**, 1392–404.
3. Einhorn TA. 'The cell and molecular biology of fracture healing', *Clin Orthop*, 1998, **355S**, 7–21.
4. Einhorn TA. 'The science of fracture healing', *J Orthop Trauma*, 2005, **19**(Suppl), S4–S6.
5. McKibbin B. 'The biology of fracture healing in long bone', *J Bone Joint Surg*, 1978, **60B**, 150–62.
6. Brighton CT and Hunt RM. 'Early histological and ultra-structural changes in medullary fracture callus', *J Bone Joint Surg*, 1991, **73A**, 832–47.
7. Kon T, Cho T, Aizawa T, Yamazaki M, Nooh N, Graves D, Gerstenfeld LC and Einhorn TA. 'Expression of osteoprotegerin, receptor activator of NF-κB ligand (osteoprotegerin ligand) and related proinflammatory cytokines during fracture healing', *J Bone Miner Res*, 2001, **16**, 1004–14.
8. Einhorn TA, Majeska RJ, Rush EB, Levine PM and Horowitz MC. 'The expression of cytokine activity by fracture callus', *J Bone Miner Res*, 1995, **10**, 1272–81.
9. Shea CM, Edgar CM, Einhorn TA and Gerstenfeld L. 'BMP treatment of C3H10T1/2 mesenchymal stem cells induces both chondrogenesis and osteogenesis', *J Cell Biochem*, 2003, **90**, 1112–27.
10. Gerstenfeld LC, Cullinane DM, Barnes GL, Graves DT and Einhorn TA. 'Fracture healing as a post-natal developmental process: molecular, spatial, and temporal aspects of its regulation', *J Cell Biochem*, 2003, **88**, 873–4.
11. Iwaki A, Jingushi S, Oda Y, Izumi T, Shida JI, Tsuneyoshi M and Sugioka Y. 'Localization and quantification of proliferating cells during rat fracture repair. Detection of proliferating cell nuclear antigen by immunohistochemistry', *J Bone Miner Res*, 1997, **12**, 96–102.
12. Nakagawa Y, Shimizu K, Hamamoto T, Suzuki K, Ueda R and Yamamuro T.

'Calcium-dependent neutral protease (Calpain) in fracture healing in rats', *J Orthop Res*, 1994, **12**, 58–69.

13. Deckers MM, Van Beek ER, Van Der Pluijm G, Wetterwald A, Van Der Wee-Pals L, Cecchini MG, Papapoulos SE and Löwik CW. 'Dissociation of angiogenesis and osteoclastogenesis during endochondral bone formation in neonatal mice', *J Bone Miner Res*, 2002, **17**, 998–1007.
14. Lee FY, Choi YW, Behrens FF, DeFouw DO and Einhorn TA. 'Programmed removal of chondrocytes during endochondral fracture healing', *J Orthop Res*, 1998, **16**, 144–50.
15. van der Meulen MC, Jepsen KJ and Mikic B. 'Understanding bone strength: size isn't everything', *Bone*, 2000, **29**, 101–4.
16. McDonald MM, Dulai SK, Godfrey C, Sztynda T and Little DG. 'Single dose zoledronic acid treatment is superior to continuous treatment in enhancing hard callus formation and strength without delaying remodelling', *Bone*, 2006, **38**, (Suppl 3): 57.
17. Gerstenfeld LC, Alkhiary YM, Krall EA, Nicholls FH, Stapleton SN, Fitch JL, Bauer M, Kayal R, Graves DT, Jepsen KJ and Einhorn TA. 'Three-dimensional reconstruction of fracture callus morphogenesis', *J Histochem Cytochem*, 2006, **54**, 1215–28.
18. Eriksen EF, Eghbali-Fatourechi GZ and Khosla S. 'Remodeling and vascular spaces in bone', *J Bone Miner Res*, 2007, **22**, 1–6.
19. Hauge EM, Qvesel D, Eriksen EF, Mosekilde L and Melsen F. 'Cancellous bone remodeling occurs in specialized compartments lined by cells expressing osteoblastic markers', *J Bone Miner Res*, 2001, **16**, 1575–82.
20. Davies JE. 'Understanding peri-implant endosseous healing', *J Dental Edu*, 2003, **67**, 932–49.
21. Osborn JF and Newesely H. 'Dynamic aspects of the implant-bone interface', In *Dental Implants: Materials and Systems*, Heimke G (ed.) Carl Hanser Verlag München, 1980, 111–23.
22. Davies JE. '*In vitro* modeling of the bone/implant interface', *Anat Rec*, 1996, **245**, 426–45.
23. Hosseini MM, Sodek J, Francke R-P and Davies JE. 'The structure and composition of the bone-implant interface', In: *Bone Engineering*, Davies JE (ed.) em squared Inc, Toronto, 2000, 296–304.
24. Kraus K and Kirker-Head C. 'Mesenchymal stem cells and bone regeneration', *Vet Surg*, 2006, **35**, 232–42.
25. Friedenstein AY, Chailakhyan RK and Lalykina KS. 'The development of fibroblast colonies in monolayer cultures of guinea pig bone marrow and spleen cells', *Cell Tissue Kinetics*, 1970, **3**, 392–403.
26. Horwitz EM, Le Blanc K, Dominici M, Mueller I, Slaper-Cortenbach I, Marini FC, Deans RJ, Krause DS and Keating A. 'Clarification of nomenclature for MSC: The International Society for Cellular Therapy position statement', *Cytotherapy*, 2005, **5**, 393–5.
27. Dominici M, Le Blanc K, Mueller I, Slaper-Cortenbach I, Marini F, Krause D, Deans R, Keating A, Prockop D and Horwitz E. Minimal criteria for defining multipotent mesenchymal stromal cells. 'The International Society for Cellular Therapy position statement', *Cytotherapy*, 2006, **8**, 315–7.
28. Giordano A, Galderisi U and Marino I. 'From the laboratory bench to the patient's bedside: an update on clinical trials with mesenchymal stem cells', *J Cell Physiol*, 2007, **211**, 27–35.

29. Zangrossi S, Marabese M, Broggini M, Giordano R, D'Erasmo M, Montelatici E, Intini D, Neri A, Pesce M, Rebulla P and Lazzari L. 'Oct-4 expression in adult human differentiated cells challenges its role as a pure stem cell marker', *Stem Cells*, 2007, **25**, 1675–82.
30. Gang EJ, Bosnakiovski D, Figueiredo CA, Visser JW and Erlingeiro RC. 'SSEA-4 identifies mesenchymal stem cells from bone marrow', *Blood*, 2007, **109**, 1743–51.
31. Bielby R, Joens E and McGonagle D. 'The role of mesenchymal stem cells in maintenance and repair of bone', *Injury*, 2007, **3851**, S26–S32.
32. Fraser JK, Wulur I, Alfonso Z and Hedrick MH. 'Fat tissue: an underappreciated source of stem cells for biotechnology', *Trends Biotechnol*, 2006, **24**, 150–4.
33. Roufosse CA, Direkze NC, Otto WR and Wright NA. 'Circulating mesenchymal stem cells', *Int J Biochem Cell Biol*, 2004, **36**, 585–97.
34. Eghbali-Fatourechi GZ, Lamsam J, Fraser D, Nagel D, Riggs BL and Khosla S. 'Circulating osteoblast-lineage cells in humans', *New Engl J Med*, 2005, **352**, 1959–66.
35. Fox JM, Chamberlain G, Ashton BA and Middleton J. 'Recent advances into the understanding of mesenchymal stem cell trafficking', *Br J Haematol*, 2007, **137**, 491–502.
36. Collett GDM and Calfield AE. 'Angiogenesis and pericytes in the initiation of ectopic calcification', *Circ Res*, 2005, **96**, 930–8.
37. Beltrami AP, Cesselli D, Bergamin N, Mercon P, Rigo S, Puppato E, D'Aurizio F, Verardo R, Piazza S, Pignatelli A, Poz A, Baccarani U, Damiani D, Fanin R, Mariuzzi L, Finato N, Masolini P, Burelli S, Belluzzi O, Schneider C and Beltrami CA. 'Multipotent cells can be generated *in vitro* from several adult human organs (heart, liver, and bone marrow)', *Blood*, 2007, **110**, 3438–46.
38. Jiang Y, Jahargidar BN, Reinhardt RL, Schwartz RE, Keene CD, Ortiz-Gonzalez XR, Reyes M, Lenvik T, Lund T, Blackstad M, Du J, Aldrich S, Lisberg A, Low WC, Largaespada DA and Verfaillie CM. 'Pluripotency of mesenchymal stem cells derived from adult marrow', *Nature*, 2002, **418**, 41–9.
39. Popp FC, Piso P, Schlitt HJ and Dahlke MH. 'Therapeutic potential of bone marrow cells for liver diseases', *Curr Stem Cell Res Ther*, 2006, **1**, 411–8.
40. Engler AJ, Sen S, Sweeney HL and Discher DE. 'Matrix elasticity directs stem cell lineage specification', *Cell*, 2006, **126**, 677–89.
41. Caplan I. 'Adult mesenchymal stem cells for tissue engineering versus regenerative medicine', *J Cell Pysiol*, 2007, **213**, 341–7.
42. Barrilleaux B, Phinney DG, Prockop DJ and O'Connor KC. 'Review: Ex vivo engineering of living tissues with adult stem cells', *Tissue Eng*, 2006, **12**, 3007–19.
43. Hadjiargyrou M, Lombardo F, Zhao S, Ahrens W, Joo J, Ahn H, Jurman M, White DW and Rubin CT. 'Transcriptional profiling of bone regeneration', Insight into the molecular complexity of wound repair', *J Biol Chem*, 2002, **277**, 30177–82.
44. Li X, Quigg RJ, Zhou J, Ryaby JT and Wang H. 'Early signals for fracture healing', *J Cell Biochem*, 2005, **95**, 189–205.
45. Li X, Wang H, Touma E, Rousseau E, Quigg RJ and Ryaby JT. 'Genetic network and pathway analysis of differentially expressed proteins during critical cellular events in fracture repair', *J Cell Biochem*, 2007, **100**, 527–43.
46. Kalfas IH. 'Principles of bone healing', *Neurosurg Focus*, 2001, **10**, E1.
47. Jingushi S, Joyce ME and Bolander ME. 'Genetic expression of extracellular

matrix proteins correlates with histologic changes during fracture repair', *J Bone Miner Res*, 1992, **7**, 1045–55.
48. Leonardi E, Ochoa-Garay J, Granchi D, Devescovi V, Pagani S, Ciapetti G and Baldini N. 'Genetic control on osteoblast differentiation: a gene expression analysis', *9th International Conference on Tooth Morphogenesis and Differentiation*, Zurich, September 4–8, 2007, Zurich, Switzerland. Abstract Book, 105.
49. Huang W, Yang S, Shao J and Li YP. 'Signaling and transcriptional regulation in osteoblast commitment and differentiation', *Front Biosci*, 2007, **12**, 3068–92.
50. Veeman MT, Axelrod JD and Moon RT. 'A second canon. Functions and mechanisms of beta-catenin independent Wnt signaling', *Dev Cell*, 2003, **5**, 367–77.
51. Westendorf JJ, Kahler RA and Schroeder TM. 'Wnt signaling in osteoblasts and bone diseases', *Gene*, 2004, **341**, 19–39.
52. Fujita K and Janz S. 'Attenuation of WNT signaling by DKK-1 and -2 regulates BMP2-induced osteoblast differentiation and expression of OPG, RANKL and M-CSF', *Mol Cancer*, 2007, **6**, 71–83.
53. Jackson A, Vayssiere B, Garcia T. Newell W, Baron R, Roman-Roman S and Rawadi G. 'Gene array analysis of Wnt-regulated genes in C3H10T1/2 cells', *Bone*, 2005, **36**, 585–98.
54. Day TF, Guo X, Garrett-Beal L and Yang Y. 'Wnt/beta-catenin signaling in mesenchymal progenitors controls osteoblast and chondrocyte differentiation during vertebrate skeletogenesis', *Dev Cell*, 2005, **8**, 739–50.
55. Urist MR. 'Bone formation by autoinduction', *Science*, 1965, **150**, 893–9.
56. Wozney JM. 'The bone morphogenetic protein family and osteogenesis', *Mol Reprod Dev*, 1992, **32**, 160–7.
57. Chen D, Zhao M and Mundy GR. 'Bone morphogenetic proteins', *Growth Factors*, 2004, **22**, 233–41.
58. Wan M and Cao X. 'BMP signaling in skeletal development' *Biochem Biophys Res Commun*, 2005, **328**, 651–7.
59. Lee MH, Kwon TG, Park HS, Wozney JM and Ryoo HM. 'BMP-2-induced Osterix expression is mediated by Dlx5 but is independent of Runx2', *Biochem Biophys Res Commun*, 2003, **309**, 689–94.
60. Lai CF and Cheng SL. 'Signal transductions induced by bone morphogenetic protein-2 and transforming growth factor-beta in normal human osteoblastic cells', *J Biol Chem*, 2002, **277**, 15514–22.
61. Chung UI, Schipani E, McMahon AP and Kronenberg HM. 'Indian hedgehog couples chondrogenesis to osteogenesis in endochondral bone development', *J Clin Invest*, 2001, **107**, 295–304.
62. Long F, Chung UI, Ohba S, McMahon J, Kronenberg HM and McMahon AP. 'Ihh signaling is directly required for the osteoblast lineage in the endochondral skeleton', *Development*, 2004, **131**, 1309–18.
63. Rodda SJ and McMahon AP. 'Distinct roles for Hedgehog and canonical Wnt signaling in specification, differentiation and maintenance of osteoblast progenitors', *Development*, 2006, **133**, 3231–44.
64. Jacob AL, Smith C, Partanen J and Ornitz DM. 'Fibroblast growth factor receptor 1 signaling in the osteochondrogenic cell lineage regulates sequential steps of osteoblast maturation', *Dev Biol*, 2006, **296**, 315–28.
65. Ornitz DM. 'FGF signaling in the developing endochondral skeleton', *Cytokine Growth Factor Rev*, 2005, **16**, 205–13.
66. Mundy GR and Elefteriou F. 'Boning up on ephrin signaling', *Cell*, 2006, **126**, 441–3.

67. Zhao C, Irie N, Takada Y, Shimoda K, Miyamoto T, Nishiwaki, Suda T and Matsuo K. 'Bidirectional ephrinB2-EphB4 signaling controls bone homeostasis', *Cell Metab*, 2006, **4**, 111–21.
68. Chang L and Karin M. 'Mammalian MAP kinase signalling cascades', *Nature*, 2001, **410**, 37–40.
69. Lian JB, Javed A, Zaidi SK, Lengner C, Montecino M, van Wijnen AJ, Stein JL and Stein GS. 'Regulatory controls for osteoblast growth and differentiation: role of Runx/Cbfa/AML factors', *Crit Rev Eukaryot Gene Expr*, 2004, **14**, 1–41.
70. Nakashima K, Zhou X, Kunkel G, Zhang Z, Deng JM, Behringer RR and de Crombrugghe B. 'The novel zinc finger-containing transcription factor osterix is required for osteoblast differentiation and bone formation', *Cell*, 2002, **108**, 7–29.
71. Koga T, Matsui Y, Asagiri M, Kodama T, de Crombrugghe B, Nakashima K, Takayanagi H. 'NFAT and Osterix cooperatively regulate bone formation', *Nat Med*, 2005, **11**, 880–5.
72. Lieberman JR, Daluilski A and Einhorn TA. 'The role of growth factors in the repair of bone. Biology and clinical applications', *J Bone Joint Surg Am*, 2002, **84-A**: 1032–44.
73. Malizos KM and Papatheodorou LK. 'The healing potential of the periosteum. Molecular aspects', *Injury*, 2005, **36S**, S13–S19.
74. Einhorn TA. 'The cell and molecular biology of fracture healing', *Clin Orthop*, 1998; 355S, S7–S21.
75. Chubinskaya S, Merrihew C, Cs-Szabo G, Mollenhauer J, McCartney J, Rueger DC and Kuettner KE. 'Human articular chondrocytes express osteogenic protein-1', *J Histochem Cytochem*, 2000, **48**, 239–50.
76. Bouletreau PJ, Warren SM, Spector JA, Peled ZM, Gerrets RP, Greenwald JA and Longaker MT. 'Hypoxia and VEGF up-regulate BMP-2 mRNA and protein expression in microvascular endothelial cells: implications for fracture healing', *Plast Reconstr Surg*, 2002, **109**, 2384–97.
77. Bostrom MP. 'Expression of bone morphogenetic proteins in fracture healing', *Clin Orthop*, 1998, **335** (Suppl): S116–S123.
78. Nakase T and Yoshikawa H. 'Potential role of bone morphogenetic proteins (BMPs) in skeletal repair and regeneration', *J Bone Miner Metab*, 2006, **24**, 425–33.
79. Cho TJ, Gerstenfeld LC and Einhorn TA. 'Differential temporal expression of members of the transforming growth factor beta superfamily during murine fracture healing', *J Bone Miner Res*, 2002, **17**, 513–20.
80. Peng H, Wright V, Usas A, Gearhart B, Shen HC, Cummins J and Huard J. 'Synergistic enhancement of bone formation and healing by stem cell-expressed VEGF and bone morphogenetic protein-4', *J Clin Invest*, 2002, **110**, 751–9.
81. Lee MH, Kim YJ, Kim HJ, Park HD, Kang AR, Kyung HM, Sung JH, Wozney JM, Kim HJ and Ryoo HM. 'BMP-2-induced Runx2 expression is mediated by Dlx5, and TGF-beta 1 opposes the BMP-2-induced osteoblast differentiation by suppression of Dlx5 expression', *J Biol Chem*, 2003, **278**, 34387–94.
82. Cheng H, Jiang W, Phillips FM, Haydon RC, Peng Y, Zhou L, Luu HH, An N, Breyer B, Vanichakarn P, Szatkowski JP, Park JY and He TC. 'Osteogenic activity of the fourteen types of human bone morphogenetic proteins (BMPs)', *J Bone Joint Surg*, 2003, **85-A**: 1544–52.
83. Chhabra A, Zijerdi D, Zhang J, Kline A, Balian G and Hurwitz S. 'BMP-14 deficiency inhibits long bone fracture healing: a biochemical, histologic, and radiographic assessment', *J Orthop Trauma*, 2005, **19**, 629–34.

84. Wang EA, Rosen V, D'Alessandro JS, Bauduy M, Cordes P, Harada T, Israel DI, Hewick RM, Kerns KM, LaPan P, Luxenberg DP, McQuaid D, Moutsatsos IK, Nove J and Wozney JM. 'Recombinant human bone morphogenetic protein induces bone formation', *Proc Natl Acad Sci USA*, 1990, **87**, 2220–4.
85. Kan L, Hu M, Gomes WA and Kessler JA. 'Transgenic mice overexpressing BMP4 develop a fibrodysplasia ossificans progressive (FOP)-like phenotype', *Am J Pathol*, 2004, **165**, 1107–15.
86. Deckers MM, van Bezooijen RL, van der Horst G, Hoogendam J, van Der Bent C, Papapoulos SE and Löwik CW. 'Bone morphogenetic proteins stimulate angiogenesis through osteoblast-derived vascular endothelial growth factor A', *Endocrinology*, 2002; **143**, 1545–53.
87. Kanatani M, Sugimotu T, Kaji H, Kobayashi T, Nishiyama K, Fukase M, Kumegawa M and Chihara K. 'Stimulatory effect of bone morphogenetic protein-2 on ostoeblast-like cell formation and bone-resorbing activity', *J Bone Miner Res*, 1995, **10**, 1681–90.
88. Barnes GL, Kostenuik LC, Gerstenfeld LC and Einhorn TA. 'Growth factor regulation of fracture repair', *J Bone Miner Res*, 1999, **14**, 1805–15.
89. Sandberg MM, Hannu TA and Vuorio EI. 'Gene expression during bone repair', *Clin Orthop*, 1993, **289**, 292–312.
90. Spinella-Jaegle S, Roman-Roman S, Faucheu C, Dunn FW, Kawai S, Galléa S, Stiot V, Blanchet AM, Courtois B, Baron R and Rawadi G. 'Opposite effects of bone morphogenetic protein-2 and transforming growth factor-beta1 on osteoblast differentiation', *Bone*, 2001, **29**, 323–30.
91. Tsiridis E, Upadhyay N and P Giannoudis. 'Molecular aspects of fracture healing: which are the important molecules?' *Injury*, 2007, **38S**, S11–S25.
92. Erlebacher A, Filvaroff EH, Ye JQ and Derinck R. 'Osteoblastic responses to TGF-β during bone remodeling', *Mol Biol Cell*, 1998, **9**, 1903–18.
93. Quinn JMW, Itoh K, Udagawa N, Hausler K, Yasuda H, Shima N, Mizuno A, Higashio K, Takahashi N, Suda T, Martin T J and Gillespie MT. 'Transforming growth factor β affects osteoclast differentiation via direct and indirect actions', *J Bone Miner Res*, 2001, **16**, 1787–94.
94. Takai H, Kanematsu M, Yano K, Tsuda E, Higashio K, Ikeda K, Watanabe K and Yamada Y. 'Transforming growth factor-β stimulates the production of osteoprotegerin/osteoclastogenesis inhibitory factor by bone marrow stromal cells', *J Biol Chem*, 1998; **273**, 27091–6.
95. Jingushi S, Heydemann A, Kana SK, Macey LR and Bolander ME. 'Acidic fibroblast growth factor (aFGF) injection stimulates cartilage enlargement and inhibits cartilage gene expression in rat fracture healing', *J Orthop Res*, 1990, **8**, 364–71.
96. Zhang X, Sobue T and Hurley MM. 'FGF-2 increases colony formation, PTH receptor, and IGF-1 mRNA in mouse marrow stromal cells', *Biochem Biophys Res Commun*, 2002, **290**, 526–31.
97. Xiao G, Jiang D, Gopolakrishnan R and Franceschi RT. 'Fibroblast growth factor 2 induction of the osteocalcin gene requires MAPK activity and phosphorylation of the osteoblast transcription factor, Cbfa1/Runx2', *J Biol Chem*, 2002, **277**, 36181–7.
98. Pitaru S, Kotev-Emeth S, Noff D, Kaffuler S and Savion N. 'Effect of basic fibroblast growth factor on the growth and differentiation of adult stromal bone marrow cells: enhanced development of mineralized bone-like tissue in culture', *J Bone Miner Res*, 1993, **8**, 919–29.

99. Marie PJ. 'Fibroblast growth factor signaling controlling osteoblast differentiation', *Gene*, 2003, **316**, 23–32.
100. Mansukhani A, Bellosta P, Sahni M and Basilico C. 'Signaling by fibroblast growth factors (FGF) and fibroblast growth factor receptor 2 (FGFR2)-activating mutations blocks mineralization and induces apoptosis in osteoblasts', *J Cell Biol*, 2000, **149**, 1297–308.
101. Chikazu D, Hakeda Y, Ogata N, Nemoto K, Itabashi A, Takato T, Kumegawa M, Nakamura K and Kawaguchi H. 'Fibroblast growth factor (FGF)-2 directly stimulates mature osteoclast function through activation of FGF receptor 1 and p42 MAP kinase', *J Biol Chem*, 2000, **275**, 31444–50.
102. Collin-Osdoby P, Rothe L, Bekker S, Anderson F, Huang Y and Osdoby P. 'Basic fibroblast growth factor stimulates osteoclast recruitment, development, and bone pit resoption in association with angiogenesis *in vivo* on the chick chorioallantoic membrane and activates isolated avian osteoclast resorption *in vitro*', *J Bone Miner Res*, 2002, **17**, 1859–71.
103. Canalis E and Rydziel S. 'Platelet-derived growth factor and the skeleton', In: *Principles of Bone Biology*. JP Bilezikian, LG Raisz and GA Rodan (eds). Academic Press, San Diego, CA 1996, 619–26.
104. Gruber R, Varga F, Fischer MB and Watzek G. 'Platelets stimulate proliferation of bone cells: involvement of platelet-derived growth factor, microparticles and membranes', *Clin Oral Implants Res*, 2002, **13**, 529–35.
105. Mitlak BH, Finkelman RD, Hill EL, Li J, Martin B, Smith T, D'Andrea M, Antoniades HN and Lynch SE. 'The effect of systemically administered PDGF-BB on the rodent skeleton', *J Bone Miner Res*, 1996, **11**, 238–47.
106. Lalani Z, Wong M, Brey EM, Mikos AG and Duke PJ. 'Spatial and temporal localization of transforming growth factor-beta1, bone morphogenetic protein-2, and platelet-derived growth factor-A in healing tooth extraction sockets in a rabbit model', *J Oral Maxillofac Surg*, 2003, **61**, 1061–72.
107. Filvaroff EH. 'VEGF and bone', *J Musculoskel Neuron Interact*, 2003, **3**, 304–7.
108. Gerber HP, Vu TH, Ryan AM, Kowalski J, Werb Z and Ferrara N. 'VEGF couples hypertrophic cartilage remodelling, ossification and angiogenesis during endochondral bone formation', *Nat Med*, 1999, **5**, 623–8.
109. Hiltunen MO, Ruuskanen M, Huuskonen J, Mähönen AJ, Ahonen M, Rutanen J, Kosma VM, Mahonen A, Kröger H and Ylä-Herttuala S. 'Adenovirus-mediated VEGF-A gene transfer induces bone formation *in vivo*', *FASEB J*, 2003, **17**, 1147–9.
110. Yao S, Dawen L, Pan F and Wise GE. 'Effect of vascular endothelial growth factor on RANK gene expression in osteoclasts precursors and on osteoclastogenesis', *Arch Oral Biol*, 2006, **51**, 596–602.
111. Andrew JG, Hoyland J, Freemont AJ and Marsh D. 'Insulin-like growth factor gene expression in human fracture callus', *Calcif Tissue Int*, 1993, **53**, 97–102.
112. Manduca P, Palermo C, Caruso C, Brizzolara A, Sanguineti C, Filanti C and Zicca A. 'Rat tibial osteoblasts III: propagation in vitro is accompanied by enhancement of osteoblast phenotype', *Bone*, 1997, **21**, 31–9.
113. Mohan S, Nakao Y, Honda Y, Landale E, Leser U, Dony C, Lang K and Baylink DJ. 'Studies on the mechanism by which insulin like growth factor (IGF) binding protein-4 (IGFBP-4) and IGFBP-5 modulate IGF actions in bone cells', *J Biol Chem*, 1995, **270**, 20424–31.

114. Prisell PT, Edwall D, Lindblad JB, Levinovitz A and Norstedt G. 'Expression of insulin-like growth factors during bone induction in rat', *Calcif Tissue Int*, 1993, **53**, 201–5.
115. Rosen CJ. 'Insulin-like growth factor I and bone mineral density: experience from animal models and human observational studies', *Best Pract Res Clin Endocrinol Metab*, 2004, **18**, 423–35.
116. Tshamala M and van Bree H. 'Osteoinductive properties of the bone marrow. Myth or reality', *Vet Comp Orthop Traumatol*, 2006, **3**, 133–41.
117. Termaat MF, Den Boer FC, Bakker FC, Patka P and Haarman HJ. 'Bone morphogenetic proteins. Development and clinical efficacy in the treatment of fractures and bone defects', *J Bone Joint Surg Am*, 2005, **87**, 11367–78.
118. Johnson EE, Urist MR and Finerman GA. 'Resistant nonunions and partial or complete segmental defects of long bones', *Clin Orthop*, 1992, **277**, 229–37.
119. Riedel GE and Valentin-Opran A. 'Clinical evaluation of rhBMP-2/ACS in orthopaedic trauma: a progress report', *Orthopaedics*, 1999, **22**, 663–5.
120. Nordsletten L and Madsen JE. 'The effect of bone morphogenetic proteins in fracture healing', *Scand J Surg*, 2006, **95**, 91–4.
121. Giannoudis PV and Tzioupis C. 'Clinical applications of BMP-7. The UK perspective', *Injury*, 2005, **36S**, S47–S50.
122. Geesink RG, Hoefnagels NH and Bulstra SK. 'Osteogenic activity of OP-1 bone morphogenetic protein (BMP-7) in a human fibular defect', *J Bone Joint Surg Br*, 1999, **81**, 710–8.
123. Burkus JK, Dorchak JD and Sanders DL. 'Radiographic assessment of interbody fusion using rhBMP-2 with tapered interbody cages', *J Spinal Disord Tech*, 2002, **15**, 337–49.
124. ten Dijke P. 'Bone morphogenetic protein signal transduction in bone', *Curr Med Res Opinions*, 2006, **22**, S7–S11.
125. Lind M, Overgaard S, Ongpipattanakul B, Nguyen T, Bunger C and Soballe K. 'Transforming growth factor-β1 stimulates bone ongrowth to weight-loaded tricalcium phosphate coated implants: an experimental study in dogs', *J Bone Joint Surg Br*, 1996, **78**, 377–82.
126. Dimitriou R, Tsiridis E and Giannoudis PV. 'Current concepts of molecular aspects of bone healing', *Injury*, 2005, **36**, 1392–404.
127. Chen WJ, Jingushi S, Anzai J, Hirata G, Tamura M and Iwamoto Y. 'Effects of FGF-2 on metaphyseal fracture repair in rabbit tibiae', *J Bone Miner Metab*, 2004, **22**, 303–9.
128. Radomsky ML, Aufdemorte TB, Swain LD, Fox WC, Spin RC and Poser JW. 'A novel formulation of FGF-2 in a hyaluronan gel accelerates fracture healing in non-human primates', *J Orthop Res*, 1999, **17**, 607–14.
129. Nash TJ, Howlett CR, Martin C, Steele J, Johnson KA and Hicklin DJ. 'Effect of platelet-derived growth factor on tibial osteotomies in rabbits', *Bone*, 1994, **15**, 203–8.
130. Spencer EM, Liu CC, Si EC and Howard GA. '*In vivo* actions of insulin-like growth factor-I (IGF-I) on bone formation and resorption in rats', *Bone*, 1991, **12**, 21–6.
131. Schmidmaier G, Lucke M, Schwabe P, Raschke M, Haas NP and Wildemann B. 'Collective review: bioactive implants coated with poly(D,L-lactide) and growth factors IGF-I, TGF-beta1, or BMP-2 for stimulation of fracture healing', *J Long Term Effect Med Implants*, 2006, **16**, 61–9.

132. Musgrave DS, Pruchnic R, Bosch P, Ziran BH, Whalen J and Huard J. 'Human skeletal muscle cells in *ex vivo* gene therapy to deliver bone morphogenetic protein-2', *J Bone Joint Surg Br*, 2002, **84**,120–7.
133. Anitua E, Sànchez M, Nurden AT, Nurden P, Orive G and Andia I. 'New insights into and novel applications for platelet-rich fibrin therapies', *Trends Biotechnol*, 2006, **24**, 227–34.
134. Ilgenli T, Dundar N and Kal BI. 'Demineralized freeze-dried bone allograft and platelet-rich plasma vs. platelet-rich plasma alone in infrabony defects: a clinical and radiographic evaluation', *Clin Oral Investig*, 2007, **11**, 51–9.
135. Dallari D, Savarino L, Stagni C, Cenni E, Cenacchi A, Fornasari PM, Albisinni U, Rimondi E, Baldini N and Giunti A. 'Enhanced tibial osteotomy healing with use of bone grafts supplemented with platelet gel or platelet gel and bone marrow stromal cells', *J Bone Joint Surg Am*, 2007, **89**, 2413–20.
136. Bae HW, Zhao L, Kanim LE, Wong P, Delamarter RB and Dawson EG. 'Intervariability and intravariability of bone morphogenetic proteins in commercially available demineralised bone matrix products', *Spine*, 2006, **31**, 1299–1308.
137. Giannoudis P, Psarakis S and Kontakis G. 'Can we accelerate fracture healing? A critical analysis of the literature', *Injury*, 2007, **38S1**, S81–S89.
138. Veillette CJ and McKee MD. 'Growth factors – BMPs, DBMs, and buffy coat products: are there any proven differences amongs them?' *Injury*, 2007, **38S1**, S38–S48.

4
Biomechanical aspects of bone repair

D. LACROIX, Institute for Bioengineering of Catalonia (IBEC), Spain

Abstract: In this chapter some biomechanical aspects of bone repair are presented. The composition and structure of bone from a biomechanical point of view are first presented to highlight physical differences between cortical and trabecular bone. Then, the biomechanical properties of both types of bone are presented and discussed. The concept of poroelasticity is introduced to model bone and the effect of interstitial fluid flow on the overall mechanical response of bone is indicated. Finally bone repair and damage concepts are introduced. The remodelling of bone depending on the type of bone and its age is discussed. The damage present in the form of cracks in individual trabeculae and its effect on the overall mechanical response of bone are discussed.

Key words: biomechanics, bone, mechanical properties, remodelling, repair.

4.1 Bone composition and structure

4.1.1 Composition

Bone is a hard connective tissue that fulfils three main functions: (1) it gives support to the body structure, (2) it serves as a protection shield against external loadings and (3) it provides a framework that allows skeletal motion. Bone is made up of a mineral or inorganic phase (60–70% of the tissue), of water (5–8%) and of an organic matrix that makes up the remainder. Approximately 90% of the organic matrix is collagen and 10% are non-collagenous proteins. Bone strength is given mainly by its mineral phase made of non-stochiometric hydroxyapatite crystals ($Ca_{10}(PO_4)_6(OH)_2$) with carbonate ions (Hasegawa *et al.*, 1994). The small crystals are in the shape of needles, plates and rods located within and between collagen fibers. The plate-like crystals have dimensions of 20–80 nm long and 2–5 nm thick.

Bone contains four types of cells: (1) osteoprogenitor cells, (2) osteoblasts, (3) osteocytes and (4) osteoclasts, of which osteocytes are the most abundant. Bone contains a small number of mesenchymal cells called osteoprogenitor cells which have the ability to proliferate and differentiate into osteoblasts. The bone matrix is produced by the osteoblasts which differentiate into osteocytes when surrounded by bone matrix. Osteocytes are mature bone cells with extensive cell processes that project through the canaliculi. Through a network of cells, they establish contact and communication between adjacent osteocytes and the central canals of osteons via gap junctions (Donahue,

1998). The transmission of information is possible between osteocytes themselves and between osteocytes and osteoblasts on the bone surface through rapid fluxes of bone calcium across the gap junctions. In addition to the gap junctions, the interstitial fluid that surrounds the osteocytes and their processes provides an additional route for the diffusion of nutrients and waste products. This information network is also linked to the activity of osteoclasts, giant cells with 50 or more nuclei which have the function of removing bone matrix.

Bone can be viewed as a composite material made of solid and liquid phases. The solid phase is represented by the mineral phase whereas the liquid phase is represented by the interstitial fluid. The solid phase is made up of collagen type I produced by osteoblast bone cells. Apart from collagen type I, osteoblast produces a variety of non-collagenous proteins, including osteocalcin, osteopontin, osteonectin, and proteoglycans; regulatory factors, such as cytokines, growth factors and prostaglandins; and neutral proteases, alkaline phosphatase, and other enzymes that degrade the extracellular matrix and prepare it for calcification.

Bone collagen is constructed in the form of a triple helix of two identical $\alpha1$(I) chains and one unique $\alpha2$ chain stabilized by hydrogen bonding between hydroxyproline and other charged residues. This configuration gives a fairly rigid linear molecule of 300 nm long. Each molecule is aligned with the next in a parallel fashion in a quarter-staggered array to produce a collagen fibril. The collagen fibrils are then grouped in bundles to form the collagen fiber.

4.1.2 Bone structure

There are two types of bone: trabecular (spongy or cancellous) bone and cortical (dense or compact) bone (Fig. 4.1). Trabecular bone is found in the epiphysis and metaphysis of long bones and inside flat or small bones. Trabecular bone has an extensive network of small and interconnected plates and rods of individual trabeculae oriented according to the external loading. Cortical bone consists of layers with vascular channels surrounded by lamellar bone. This arrangement is called the osteon or Haversian system. The central canal of an osteon contains cells, vessels and nerves and the canals connecting osteons are called Volkmann's canals.

At the microscopic level, trabecular and cortical bones consist of two forms: woven and lamellar. Woven bone is considered to be immature bone or primitive bone and is found in the embryo, the newly born and in fracture healing. Woven bone has a matrix of interwoven coarse collagen fibers with osteocytes distributed more or less at random. It is less organized than lamellar bone. Woven bone is replaced by lamellar bone at age 2 or 3 years. Lamellar bone is a mature bone that results from the remodeling of

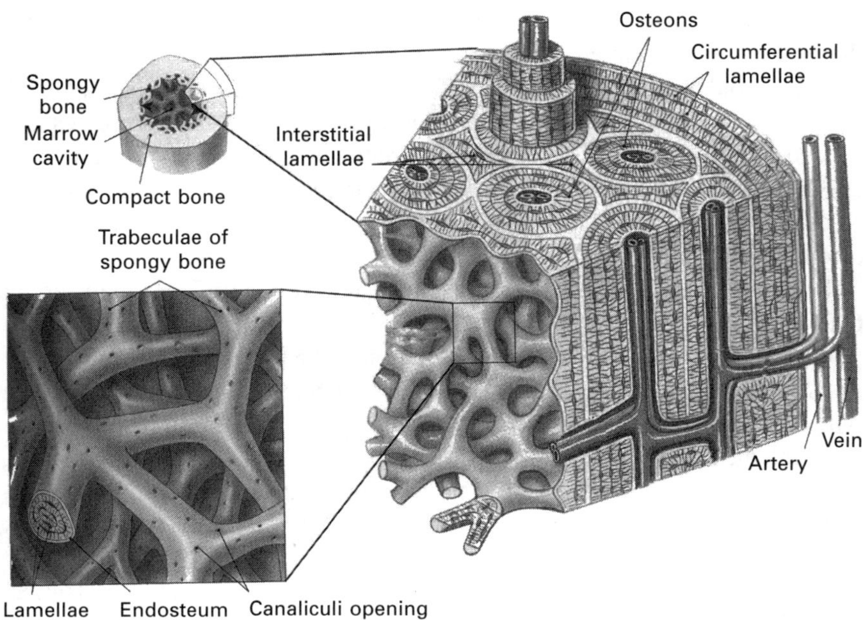

4.1 Structure of osseous tissue (adapted from Martini, 1989).

immature woven bone. Lamellar bone is highly organized; stress-oriented collagen of lamellar bone gives its anisotropic properties.

4.1.3 Bone physical properties

One of the fundamental differences between cortical and trabecular bone is its apparent porosity. Apparent porosity is the ratio of the mass bone tissue in a specimen to the bulk volume of the specimen. Typical apparent densities for cortical bone and trabecular bone are 1.85 g cm^{-3} and 0.30 g cm^{-3}, respectively with a much higher variability and standard deviation for trabecular bone. Physical properties vary from one bone to another depending on various parameters such as apparent density, ash density (total mineral content divided by bulk volume), histology (number of osteons, primary versus secondary bone), collagen composition and content, orientation of the collagen fibers and mineral, composition of the cement lines, bonding between the mineral and collagen phases, and accumulation of microcracks in the bone matrix and around osteons (Burstein *et al.*, 1975; Schaffler and Burr, 1988). Apparent density can be correlated to Young's modulus and ultimate strength using a power law with exponents for modulus ranging from 1.5 to 7.5. Volume fraction (proportional to apparent density) and mineral content (proportional to ash density) can also be correlated to Young's modulus and strength using a power law. Bone mineral content is the ratio between the mineral weight and the dry weight of the bone sample. The bone sample is burnt to determine its mineral content or the ash fraction. Water content is also important in the mechanical properties of cortical bone (Currey, 1988). Wet bone, as found *in situ*, is less stiff, less strong, and less brittle than fully dried bone.

4.2 Biomechanical properties of bone

Bone has a major advantage over engineering structural materials in that it is self-repairing and can alter its properties and geometry in response to changes in mechanical and metabolic demand. Bone properties also change from species to species. Bone physical properties differ from one person to another but also within one individual from one location to another. Owing to its different apparent porosity, mechanical properties of trabecular bone and cortical bone are clearly different (Ascenzi, 1988; Reilly *et al.*, 1974; Rho *et al.*, 1996).

4.2.1 Cortical bone

Cortical bone accounts for approximatively 80% of the skeletal mass. Cortical bone and relatively stiff trabecular bone have Young's moduli of about 17 GPa and 1 GPa, respectively (it also depends on the species and on the type of bone). Thus, most metals used in orthopedic applications are an order of magnitude stiffer than cortical bone. Human cortical bone is usually considered to be transversely isotropic with mechanical properties substantially different in the longitudinal direction (parallel to the axis of the osteons) than in the radial or circumferential directions but it has similar properties in the radial and circumferential directions. The modulus of cortical bone in the longitudinal direction is approximately 1.5 times its modulus in the transverse direction. The material properties measured can differ depending on the measuring techniques (Rho *et al.*, 1993). When ultrasound is employed, various velocities are measured from which the elastic coefficients are determined (Ashman *et al.*, 1987; Bonfield and Tully, 1982). The technical constants are then found by matrix inversion.

Cortical bone has a higher strength in compression than in tension and is stronger in the longitudinal direction than in the transverse direction. For longitudinal loading, cortical bone is a tough material because it can absorb substantial energy before fracture. Furthermore, cortical bone can be classified as a relatively ductile material for longitudinal loading since its ultimate strain for longitudinal loading is substantially larger than its yield strain. However, it is relatively brittle for transverse loading.

Cortical bone exhibits a viscoelastic behaviour, that is, it is sensitive both to strain rate and the duration of the applied loads (Carter and Hayes, 1976) (Fig. 4.2). Elastic modulus and strength have a power law correlation with strain rate with a coefficient of 0.06 approximately. The *in vivo* strain rate for bone can vary from of 0.001 to 0.01 per second in the course of daily activities. Thus, in this range of strain rate, the Young's modulus increases by approximately 15% whereas it is about 20% stronger (Fig. 4.3).

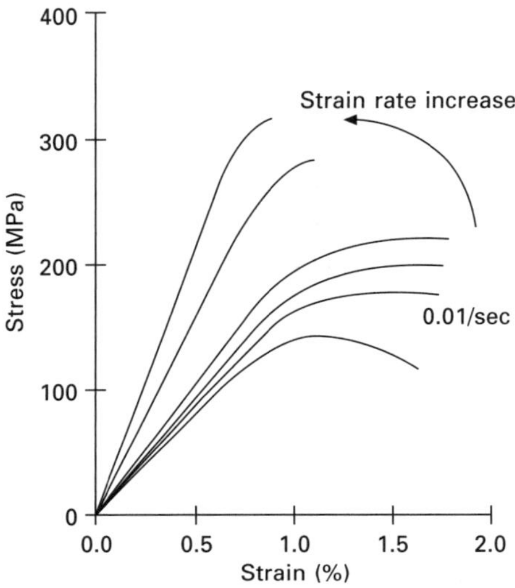

4.2 Strain rate dependence of cortical bone material behavior. Both modulus and strength increase for increased strain rates (adapted from McElhaney, 1966).

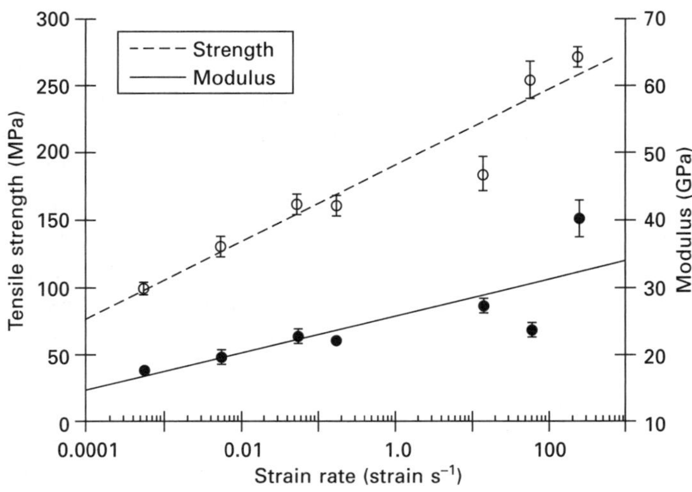

4.3 Dependence of modulus and ultimate tensile strength of human cortical bone for longitudinal loading as a function of strain rate (adapted from Wright and Hayes, 1976).

At very high strain rates representing high-impact trauma, cortical bone becomes more brittle. Thus, cortical bone exhibits a ductile to brittle transition as the strain rate increases (Schaffler *et al.*, 1989). The three characteristic stages of creep behavior as described in many conventional engineering materials are also observed in cortical bone (Fig. 4.4). The mechanical properties of cortical bone progressively deteriorate with aging for both men and women (Burr, 1997; Burstein *et al.*, 1976). During aging there is an embrittlement of cortical bone with a reduction in energy absorption (area under stress–strain curve) owing to a reduction in ultimate strain and therefore cortical bone becomes more brittle. As in any conventional engineering materials cortical bone is subject to fatigue failure (Burr *et al.*, 1985). However, owing to its ability to remodel, fatigue failure can be reduced significantly. Cracks that have been formed during strenuous activities can be closed and repaired through bone remodeling activity.

The fatigue mechanism for cortical bone can be described in three characteristic stages of fatigue fracture, corresponding to crack initiation, crack growth (propagation) and final fracture. In the primary stage, crack initiates owing to local stress concentration given by Haversian canals, lacunae or canaliculi. In the secondary stage, crack propagation results in a slow but steady further decrease in stiffness and strength. These microcracks propagate and tend to join together once they progress beyond the initiation stage. In the tertiary stage, fracture is preceded by a rapid decrease in the ability to support the load. The larger cracks run into weak material interfaces (cement lines) between the osteons and can lead to debonding of the osteons. However, imperfections in bone microstructure, such as the cement line, tend to stop the progression of cracks by changing the direction of crack

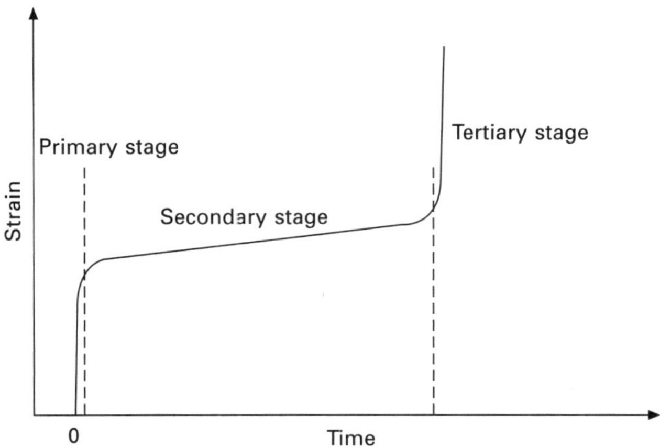

4.4 Schematic diagram showing the three stages of creep behavior of human cortical bone (adapted from Carter and Caler, 1985).

propagation from perpendicular to the loading direction to parallel to the loading direction. The final stage of fatigue fracture occurs because cracks coalesce and become so large that the weak interfaces can no longer absorb them. The cracks can thus cross the bone and induce bone failure.

4.2.2 Trabecular bone

Material properties of trabecular bone vary widely depending mainly on the anatomic location and age, for which the apparent density and the architecture can be markedly different (Ding *et al.*, 1997; Gibson, 1985) Trabecular bone is best described as an open-celled porous foam. Since trabecular bone is made up of a series of interconnecting trabeculae, it can be idealized as a combination of rod–rod, rod–plate, or plate–plate basic cellular structures where rods and plates represent thin and thick trabeculae, respectively. The mechanical properties can vary by a factor of ten depending on the type and orientation of these basic cellular structures (Fig. 4.5).

The architecture of trabecular bone depends on the thickness of individual trabeculae and the spacing between trabeculae. The architecture of trabecular bone results in anisotropic elastic properties found in elderly lumbar spine. However, in contrast to cortical bone, trabecular bone is nearly isotropic at some anatomic sites like the proximal humerus. For isotropic bones, the elastic modulus and the ultimate strength of trabecular bone in any direction are related to its apparent density ρ by a power-law relationship of the form:

$$E = a + b\rho^c$$

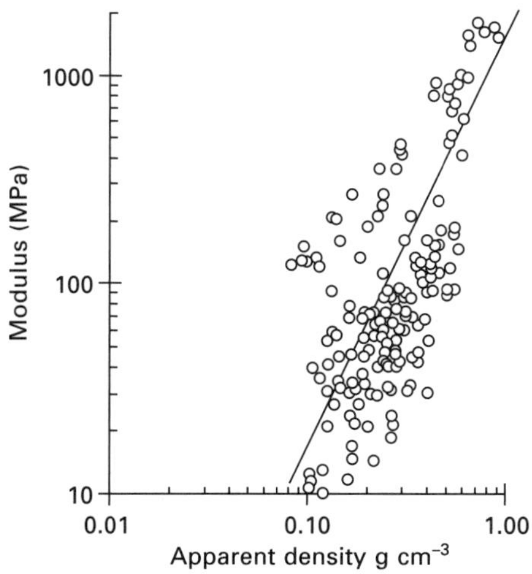

4.5 Compressive modulus as a function of apparent density for trabecular bone. (adapted from Keaveny and Hayes, 1993).

where a, b and c are constants that depend on the architecture of the tissue (Rice *et al.*, 1988). In general, the exponent c has a value of approximately 2.

Trabecular bone under compression has similar characteristics to porous foam materials such as wood. In the first stage, bone deforms in the linear elastic region, in which individual trabeculae bend and compress as the bulk tissue is compressed (Fig. 4.6). In the second stage, some trabeculae fail or buckle without an increase in loading (Turner, 1989). As more and more trabeculae fail, the strain increases until broken trabeculae begin to fill the pores, causing the specimen to stiffen. Thus, trabecular bone has a unique ability to resist large compressive load for a minimal mass. This energy absorption allows compressive strains of over 50% (Linde *et al.*, 1989). As in fiber-reinforced concrete, the tensile behavior of trabecular bone is poorer.

4.2.3 Bone poroelasticity

A poroelastic formulation can be used to describe the mechanical properties of bone. Fluid-filled porosities of bone can affect the mechanical response of the tissue, depending on the loading rate applied to the bone and the subsequent pressure that develops within the fluid. The interstitial fluid within bone has an important role in sustaining the load applied in the bone. Pore fluid pressure contributes to the total stress in the porous matrix medium and pore fluid pressure can also strain the porous matrix medium in addition to the strain developed from the loading. The presence of interstitial fluid is useful for transporting nutrients from the vasculature to the cells in the tissue and to transport waste products for removal. This fluid movement is created from the differences in pore fluid pressure developed by different pore volume strains associated with mechanical loading of the porous medium.

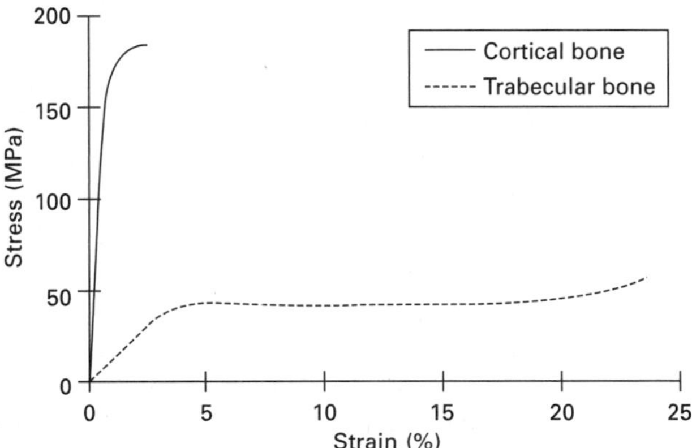

4.6 Example of typical compressive stress–strain behaviors of trabecular and cortical bone for different apparent densities (adapted from Keaveny and Hayes, 1993).

Two cases associated with the effects of fluid pressure are considered for the purpose of measuring the elastic constants in a poroelastic material: drained and undrained. In the drained case the fluid pressure in the pores is zero. This case can be achieved by removing the fluid from the pores before the test or doing the test so slowly that the pores will drain from a negligible fluid pressure. In the undrained case, the pores do not permit fluid to exit and therefore pressure builds in the bone pores when the tissue is loaded but the pressure cannot cause the fluid to move out of the specimen. The matrix elastic constants are the elastic constants of the non-porous material.

In the case of cortical bone, various levels of poroelasticy architecture can be defined to account correctly for the fluid effect within the cortical bone (Cowin, 1999). The porosity in the collagen-apatite is considered too small to play any role in the elastic constants, whereas the porosity of the inter-trabecular space is too large to have a physiological effect on the elastic stress–strain behavior since the fluid relaxes much faster than the loading rate. However, for the vascular porosity and the lacunar–canalicular porosity, the effect of fluid permeability and fluid pressure will depend greatly on loading rate. The permeability associated with the vascular porosity is much higher than the one from the lacunar–canalicular porosity (6.36×10^{-13} m^2 versus 1.47×10^{-20} m^2 respectively) (Zhang *et al.*, 1998). Bone tissue matrix has a bulk modulus of about 14 GPa whereas the bulk modulus of bone water is 2.3 GPa. Thus, solid bone matrix has a bulk modulus six times that of water. In the case of soft tissues, this ratio is about 1. Therefore, the incompressibility assumption of the fluid and solid phases, which is reasonable for soft tissue, is inappropriate for mineralized bone.

4.3 Bone damage and repair

4.3.1 Bone remodeling

Bone remodels throughout life to adapt its mechanical properties to the mechanical demands placed on it (Frost, 1987; Martin, 2000). Bone remodeling occurs on periosteal, endosteal, Haversian canal and trabecular surfaces. The metabolic turnover of trabecular bone is about eight times greater than that of cortical bone because of its greater surface area for cellular activity. Bone turnover is achieved through the joined activity of osteoclast (resorbing bone) and osteoblast (depositing bone) (Lanyon, 1993).

Osteoclast binds to the bone surface through cell attachment proteins called integrins and they resorb bone by isolating an area of bone under the region of cell attachment. The osteoclast then makes the local environment more acidic by production of hydrogen ions through the carbonic anhydrase system. The lowered pH increases the solubility of the apatite crystals and after the mineral is removed, the organic components of the matrix are hydrolyzed through acidic proteolytic digestion. Then osteoblasts produce bone matrix and osteoblasts become entrapped and differentiate into osteocytes.

With age, bone density diminishes and architecture changes. The reduction in density depends on a number of factors, including gender and anatomic site and is called osteoporosis (Fig. 4.7). In the lumbar spine, direct measurements have shown a decrease in trabecular bone density of approximately 50% from ages 20 to 80 years. With decreasing density, the number and thickness of the trabeculae decreases with preferential loss of vertical trabeculae, while the size of the intertrabecular spaces increases.

4.3.2 Bone failure

Damage and repair of individual trabeculae occurs in a physiological process throughout life and increase with age (Melvin, 1993). Small cracks within individual trabeculae (so called microfractures or microcracks) can be repaired by callus formation resulting in the formation of new woven bone or lamellar bone around the original crack. These microcracks are formed over time owing to the application of repetitive loading of low magnitude but whose number of cycles induces crack propagation failure of trabeculae. This damage process is particularly critical in osteoporotic bone where the remodeling process is much lower and can therefore lead more easily to rupture of individual trabeculae (Caler and Carter, 1989).

Four types of damage are found in bone: transverse cracks, shear bands, parallel cracks and complete fractures, of which the first two are dominant (Watchel and Keaveny, 1997). The formation of these small cracks induces local damage which could be seen as insignificant. However, this local damage

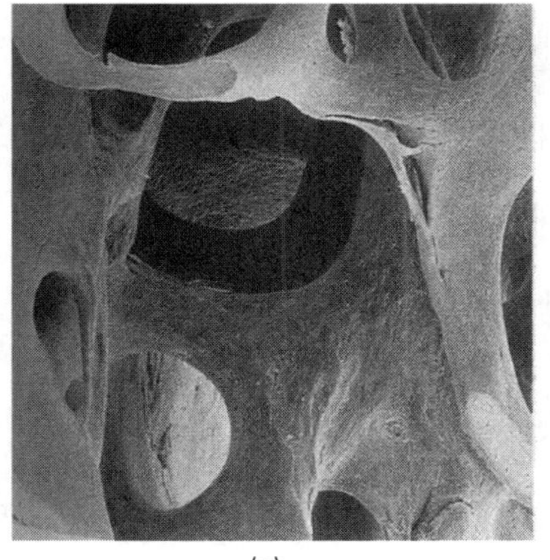
(a)

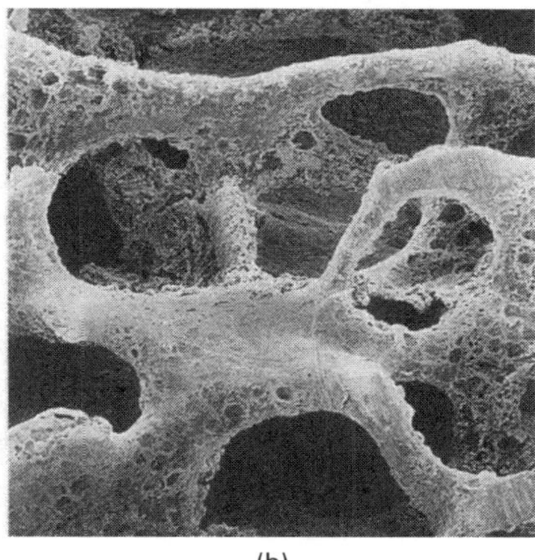
(b)

4.7 Scanning electron microscopy pictures of (a) a normal spongy bone and (b) a spongy bone with osteoporosis (from Martini, 1989).

can be so widespread that it can account for the large changes in mechanical properties of overloaded trabecular bone. Moreover, its detection in a clinical environment is more difficult owing to the fact that it can only be seen on a small scale. It is therefore difficult to evaluate the risk of fracture with this type of damage. Different factors can affect bone damage, such as strain rate or age. Loading at higher strain rates reduces the reduction in stress after the ultimate point is reached (Keaveny *et al.*, 1999). Elderly cortical bone, which is more brittle than younger bone, damages more easily than younger tissue when subjected to the same strain (Courtney *et al.*, 1996). Evidence in the literature on strain rate and age related effects led Keaveny (2001) to suggest that biomechanical effects of damage from a non-fracturing fall or overload may be most severe in elderly individuals who have brittle bone tissue and low bone density but who are subjected to loads at relatively low strain rates.

4.4 Conclusions

Bone is an intriguingly complex material with a very organized structure that confers it with anisotropic properties well adapted to the multiple loading present throughout human life. The mechanical properties are fundamentally anisotropic and can be described as a two phase material in which the interstitial fluid can play a determinant role in the mechanical response depending on the type of loading applied. Many factors can play a role in the mechanical properties of bone, in particular strain rate and age effects are very relevant for bone repair and its study with biomaterials.

4.5 Bibliography

Bilezikian, J.P., Raisz, L.G. and Rodan, G.A. (eds) (1996). *Principles of Bone Biology.* Academic Press, San Diego.

Buckwalter J.A., Einhorn, T.A. and Simon, S.R. (eds) (2000). *Orthopaedic Basic Science: Biology and Biomechanics of the Musculoskeletal System.* 2nd Edition, American Academy Orthopaedic Surgurgeons, Rosemont, Illinois.

Cowin, S.C. (ed) (2001). *Bone Mechanics Handbook.* 2nd Edition, CRC Press, Boca Raton.

Daniel D.M., Akeson W.H. and O'Connor J.J. (eds) (1990). *Knee Ligaments: Structure, Function, Injury, and Repair*. Raven Press, New York.

Fung Y.C. (ed) (1981). *Biomechanics: Mechanical Properties of Living Tissues*. Springer-Verlag, New York.

Martin, R.B. and Burr, D.B. (eds) (1989). *Structure, Function, and Adaptation of Compact Bone*. Raven Press, New York.

Mow V.C. and Hayes W.C. (eds) (1997). *Basic Orthopaedic Biomechanics*. 2nd edition, Lippincott-Raven, Philadelphia, PA.

Mow V.C. and Ratcliffe A. (eds) (1993). *Structure and Function of Articular Cartilage*. CRC Press, Boca Raton, FL.

Mow V.C., Ratcliffe A. and Woo S.L.-Y. (eds) (1990). *Biomechanics of Diarthrodial Joints*. Springer-Verlag, New York.

Odgaard, A. and Weinans, H. (eds) (1995). *Bone Structure and Remodeling*. World Scientific, Singapore.

4.6 References

Ascenzi, A. (1988). The micromechananics versus the macromechanics of cortical bone – a comprehensive presentation, *J Biomech Eng*, **8**, 143.

Ashman, R.B., Corin, J.D. and Turner, C.H. (1987). Elastic properties of cancellous bone: measurement by an ultrasonic technique, *J Biomech*, **20**, 979.

Bonfield, W. and Tully, A.E. (1982). Ultrasonic analysis of the Young's modulus of cortical bone, *J Biomed Eng*, **4**, 23–27.

Burr, D.B. (1997). Muscle strength, bone mass and age related bone loss, *J Bone Miner Res*, **12**, 1547.

Burr, D.B., Martin, R.B., Schaffler, M.B. and Radin, E.L. (1985). Bone remodeling in response to *in vivo* fatigue damage, *J Biomech*, **18**, 189.

Burstein, A.H., Zika, J.M., Heiple, K.G. and Klein, L. (1975). Contribution of collagen and mineral to the elastic-plastic properties of bone, *J Bone Joint Surg*, **A57**, 956.

Burstein, A.H., Reilly, D.T. and Martens, M. (1976). Aging of bone tissue: Mechanical properties, *J Bone Joint Surg*; **58B**: 82–86.

Caler, W.E. and Carter, D.R. (1989). Bone creep-fatigue damage accumulation, *J Biomech*, **22**, 625–635.

Carter, D.R. and Caler, W.E. (1985). A cumulative damage model for bone fracture, *J Orthop Res*; **3**: 84–90.

Carter, D.R. and Hayes, W.C. (1976). Bone compressive strength: the influence of density and strain rate, *Science*, **194**, 1174.

Courtney, A.C., Hayes, W.C. and Gibson, L.J. (1996). Age-related differences in post-yield damage in human cortical bone. Experiment and model, *J Biomech*, **29**, 1463–1471.

Cowin, S.C. (1999). Bone poroelasticity. *J Biomechanics*, **32**, 217–238.

Currey, J.D. (1988). The effects of drying and re-wetting on some mechanical properties of cortical bone, *J Biomech*, **21**, 439–441.

Ding, M., Dalstra, M., Danielsen, C.C., Kabel, J., Hvid, I. and Linde, F. (1997). Age variations in the properties of human tibial trabecular bone, *J Bone Joint Surg (Br)*, **79**, 995–1002.

Donahue, H.J. (1998). Gap junctional intercellular communication in bone: a cellular basis for bone mechanostat set point, *Calcif Tissue Int*, **62**, 85.

Frost, H.M. (1987). Bone 'mass' and the 'mechanostat', a proposal, *Anat Rec*, **219**, 1.

Gibson, L.J. (1985). The mechanical behaviour of cancellous bone, *J Biomech*, **18**, 317.

Hasegawa, K., Turner, C.H. and Burr, D.B. (1994). Contribution of collagen and mineral to the elastic anisotropy of bone, *Calcif Tissue Int*, **55**, 381.

Keaveny, T.M. (2001). Strength of trabecular bone. In *Bone Mechanics Handbook*. Cowin, S.C. (ed), 2nd edition, CRC Press, Boca Raton.

Keaveny, T.M. and Hayes, W.C. (1993). Mechanical properties of cortical and trabecular bone. In *Bone mechanics handbooks*, Hall, B.K. (ed), CRC Press, Boca Raton, FL, vol 7, pp 285–344

Keaveny, T.M., Wachtel, E.F. and Kopperdahl, D.L. (1999). Mechanical behaviour of human trabecular bone after overloading, *J Orthop Res*, **17**, 346–353.

Lanyon, L.E. (1993). Osteocytes, strain detection, bone modeling and remodeling, *Calcif Tissue Int*, **53** (sup), 102.

Linde, F., Hvid, I. and Pongsoipetch, B. (1989). Energy absorptive properties of human trabecular bone specimens during axial compression, *J Orthop Res*, **7**, 432–439.

Martin, R.B. (2000). Toward a unifying theory of bone remodeling, *Bone*, **26**, 1.

Martini, F.H. (1989). *Fundamentals of Anatomy and Physiology*. 4th edition, Prentice Hall International, New Jersey.

McElhaney, J.H. (1966). Dynamic response of bone and muscle tissue, *J Appl Physiol*, **21**, 1231–1236.

Melvin, J.W. (1993). Fracture mechanics of bone, *J Biomech Eng*, **115**, 549–554.

Reilly, D.T., Burstein, A.H. and Frankel, V.H. (1974). The elastic modulus for bone, *J. Biomech*, **7**, 271–275.

Rho, J.-Y., Ashman, R.B. and Turner, C.H. (1993). Young's modulus of trabecular and cortical bone material: ultrasonic and microtensile measurements, *J Biomech*, **26**, 111–119.

Rho, J.-Y., Tsui, T.Y. and Pharr, G.M. (1996). Elastic properties of human cortical and trabecular lamellar bone, *Bone*, **18**, 417–428.

Rice, J.C., Cowin, S.C. and Bowman, J.A. (1988). On the dependence of the elasticity and strength of cancellous bone on apparent density, *J Biomech*, **21**, 155–168.

Schaffler, M.B. and Burr, D.B. (1988). Stiffness of compact bone: effects of porosity and density, *J Biomech*, **21**, 13–16.

Schaffler, M.B., Radin, E.L. and Burr, D.B. (1989). Mechanical and morphological effects of strain rate on fatigue of compact bone, *Bone*, **10**, 207–214.

Turner, C.H. (1989). Yield behaviour of cancellous bone, *J Biomech Eng*, **111**, 1–5.

Watchel, E.F. and Keaveny, T.M. (1997). Dependence of trabecular damage on mechanical strain, *J Orthop Res*, **15**, 781–787.

Wright, T.M. and Hayes, W.C. (1976). Tensile testing of bone over a wide range of strain rates: Effect of strain rate, micro-structure and density. *Med Biol Eng*, **14**, 671–680.

Zhang, D., Weinbaum, S. and Cowin, S.C. (1998). Estimates of the peak pressures in the bone pore water, *J Biomech Eng*, **120**, 697–703.

Part II

Biomaterials

5 Properties and characterisation of bone repair materials

A. A. WHITE and S. M. BEST,
University of Cambridge, UK

Abstract: This chapter discusses material properties and characterisation, focusing on how to manipulate a material's properties through changes in chemistry, microstructure and processing; the relevant techniques to characterise the material thoroughly; and the interrelationship between different levels and types of material properties. The four main sections discuss (1) mechanical properties, (2) molecular and microstructural properties, (3) physiological effects and (4) the strengths and weakness of different material classes and their applications.

Key words: material characterisation, material properties, mechanical properties, microstructure, physiological effects.

5.1 Introduction

To perform successfully *in vivo*, an implant material must possess particular and well-controlled properties suited to each individual application. In major load-bearing situations, such as joint replacement, emphasis may be placed on the strength of the material and its ability to withstand repeated cycles of loading and unloading. The focus in repairing small bone defects, on the other hand, may lie on the chemical composition of the material and whether it is able to bond with surrounding bone tissue or trigger new growth.

While emphasis may be placed on one area, say strength, the situation is not so simple as to be able choose the strongest available material and implant it. We must first have an understanding of what microstructural properties influence that strength, and how to control them, and we must consider how susceptible that material's chemistry is to alterations in the body's environment. What, at first glance, may seem like the ideal material, could fail catastrophically when placed in the body. The better choice may be a weaker material that is inherently less susceptible to degradation *in vivo*, but whose microstructure can be altered to make it stronger and thus the more successful implant material for that application.

The important things to understand are (1) how to manipulate a material's characteristics through changes in chemistry, microstructure and processing; (2) the relevant techniques to characterise the material's properties thoroughly and (3) the interrelationship between different levels and types of material properties. Figure 5.1 illustrates this concept, showing how mechanical and microstructural and physiological effects interact with one another and come together to determine the *in vivo* success of the material. Indeed, examples can be given of relationships between any two of these property types and it is necessary to consider these associations as well as how all three interrelate and control the performance of an implant material.

This chapter is intended as an introduction to material properties and characterisation for non-materials specialists who seek to form a view of the most important material properties for an implant. It is divided into four main sections, one to discuss each of the three property categories listed above and displayed in Fig. 5.1 and one to compare the properties of the basic material classes. The mechanical properties section will define important mechanical characteristics and how they are evaluated. The following section, on microstructure and molecular properties, will focus on characteristics such as density, porosity, surface area, grain size and polymer structural and thermal attributes. The section on physiological effects examines attributes that come into play particularly when a material interacts with the local environment of the body. The final section brings together all of these property categories, comparing the relative performance of metals, ceramics and polymers, and how composites formed from different combinations of these materials might perform. Throughout reading this chapter, it may be helpful for the reader to refer to Table 5.1, which lists a wide range of material properties along with appropriate characterisation techniques.

5.2 Mechanical properties

When selecting a material for use as an implant, one of the major considerations is its required mechanical performance in the particular skeletal application.

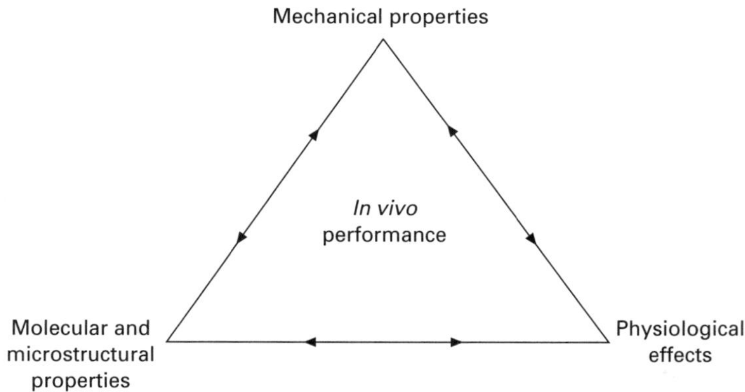

5.1 Interdependent relationship between different types of biomaterial properties and *in vivo* performance.

Table 5.1 Key material properties and relevant characterisation techniques

Property	Characterisation techniques	References
Mechanical		
Tensile strength	Tensile test	Dowling, 1998c
Compressive strength	Compression test	Dowling, 1998c
Flexural strength	3- and 4-point bend test	Wachtman, 1996a
Elastic (Young's) modulus	Calculation from stress–strain curve	–
Ductility	Calculation from strength test	–
Toughness	Single-edge notched beam Indirect measurement	Munz and Fett, 2001
Hardness	Indentation	Dowling, 1998b
Fatigue	Cyclic stress test	Dowling, 1998a
Creep	Constant stress test	Ferry, 1980
Microstructural and molecular		
Crystal structure	X-ray diffraction	Cullity and Stock, 2001
Composition	Rietveld analysis IR spectroscopy X-ray fluorescence spectroscopy	Will, 2006 Stuart, 2004 Buhrke *et al.*, 1997
Skeletal density	Pycnometry	Lowell *et al.*, 2006b
Porosity	Nitrogen adsorption – BJH	Barrett *et al.*, 1951
Surface area	Mercury porosimetry Nitrogen adsorption – BET	Lowell *et al.*, 2006c Braunauer *et al.*, 1938 Lowell *et al.*, 2006a
Grain size	Scanning electron microscopy Light microscopy	Bradon and Kaplan, 1999
Molecular weight	Gel permeation chromatography	Campbell *et al.*, 2000a
Thermal transition temperatures	Differential scanning calorimetry Thermo-mechanical analysis	Campbell *et al.*, 2000b
Environmental		
Wear	Hip joint wear simulator Multi-directional motion wear test	Lu and McKellop, 1997 Wang, 2001
Coefficient of friction	Dead load Inclined plane	Ludema, 1996
Corrosion potential	DC/AC/impedance electrochemistry	Lemons *et al.*, 1999
Dissolution/degradation rate	Absorption spectroscopy Emission spectroscopy	Williams and Bause, 1996
Surface composition	Auger electron spectroscopy X-ray photoelectron spectroscopy Fourier transform IR spectroscopy	Hayakawa *et al.*, 2008
Wettability	Contact angle measurement	Ratner, 2004
Surface roughness	Atomic force microscopy Scanning tunneling microscopy	Ratner, 2004

This section will define the most important mechanical criteria and how they are evaluated. Table 5.2 offers a comparison of mechanical data for several different types of replacement materials, along with those of bone.

5.2.1 The stress–strain curve

One of the most familiar diagrams to a materials scientist or engineer, a stress–strain graph provides several pieces of key mechanical data. Various strength tests can produce a stress–strain curve, the most common being uniaxial tension and compression tests (Dowling, 1998c). In these tests, the specimen is fitted between two plates and a load is applied either to squeeze the specimen together (compression) or to pull it apart (tension). Figure 5.2(a) shows a schematic of this procedure. As load is applied at a specified rate, the deformation of the specimen is measured, or vice versa. By dividing the load by the cross-sectional area of the specimen we get a value for stress (σ), while strain (ε) is calculated by dividing the change in length of the specimen by its original length. Using stress and strain values rather than load and deformation values normalises the data for a specimen's size and geometry.

By plotting stress against strain, we can get a good picture of the material's behaviour and work out some of its mechanical properties. Figure 5.3 shows a sample plot with examples of the shapes of curves for several different types of material behaviour. In the first region of a curve, between (1) and (2), the material's behaviour is elastic. Stress and strain are directly proportional to one another and deformation is recoverable, as atoms in the material's structure are displaced only slightly by the stretching of atomic bonds. The second, plastic region of a curve (if present) lies between (2) and (3). At a certain point, stress and strain are no longer proportional and permanent deformation occurs as whole arrays of atoms move to a new location in the crystal structure by breaking and reforming atomic bonds.

From the curves, we can obtain the following pieces of data:

- *Elastic (Young's) modulus, E.* Often referred to as the stiffness, it is the slope of the linear, elastic region of the stress–strain curve. The steeper the slope, the higher the Young's modulus and the higher the stiffness of a material. Some materials, mainly many polymers, do not have a linear elastic portion (see curve D). In this case either a tangent modulus is used, by drawing a line tangent to the curve at a specified stress and using its slope, or a secant modulus is taken from the slope of a line drawn from the origin to a specified point.
- *Yield strength*, σ_{ys}. This is the stress at the point when elastic deformation ends and plastic deformation begins (2). Many times the yield strength is cited as the 'strength' or 'tensile strength' of a material, since it represents

Table 5.2 Mechanical properties for common bone repair materials. (NB values for metal alloys are highly subjective to processing technique, which was not always specified in the data source. In general, one can expect that the lower values of strength and higher values of elongation correspond to annealed specimens, whereas the higher ranges of strength and lower ranges of elongation apply to cold-worked alloys.) Data compiled from various tables in Ratner *et al.*, 2004, pp 28, 69, 142, 157; Callister Jr., 2000a, pp 800-803; and Kokubo, 2008, pp 12, 79, 226, 288

Material	Tensile/bending strength (MPa)	Yield strength (MPa)	Compressive strength (MPa)	Elastic modulus (GPa)	Toughness ($MPa{\cdot}m^{1/2}$)	Elongation to fracture (%)
Bone (cortical)	50–150	30–70	160–250	4–30	2–12	0–8
Bone (cancellous)	10–20	–	23	0.2–0.5	–	–
Stainless steel	480–1000	200–800	–	190–210	20–95	20–55
Ti alloys	900–1200	830	450–1850	110–120	44–66	18
CoCr alloys	400–1900	450–1600	480–600	210–250	120–160	10
Hydroxyapatite	115–120	–	350–400	80–110	1.0	–
Glass-ceramic AW	220	–	1080	118	2.0	–
Alumina	280–600	–	4500	350	3–6	0
Zirconia	800–1500	–	1990	210–220	6.4–10.9	–
Polyethylene (incl. UHMWPE)	23–48	21–28	20	0.6–2.2	–	350–525
PMMA	35–80	54–73	80	2.2–4.8	0.7–1.6	0.5–6

UHMWPE = ultra high molecular weight polyethylene

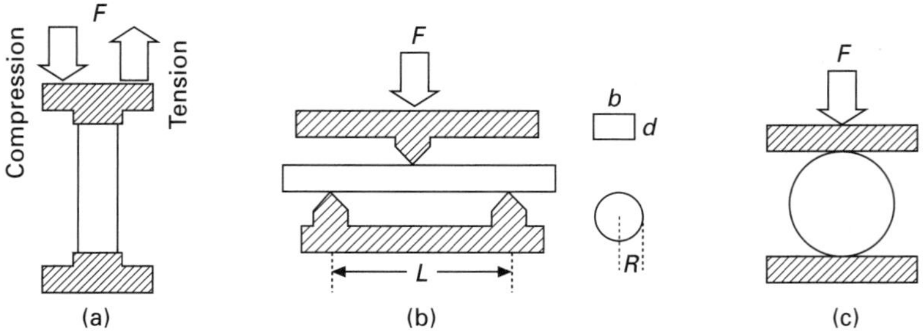

5.2 Schematics of strength tests. (a) Tensile and compression tests with a traditional dog-bone sample. (b) Flexural strength test. (c) Diametral compression test.

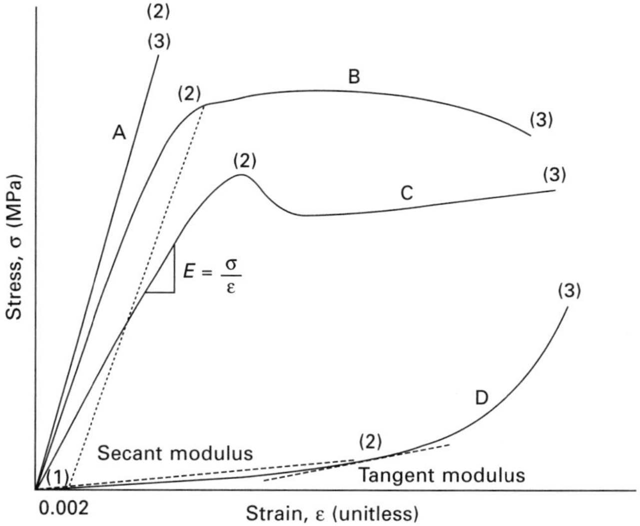

5.3 Stress–strain graph comparing tensile behaviour of different types of materials.

the highest practical strength of a material for many applications in which plastic deformation would render the material useless. When the yield point cannot be precisely identified, as is the case with many metals which undergo a gradual elastic to plastic transition, a line parallel to the elastic slope can be constructed at a specified strain (usually 0.002). The yield strength is then taken as the stress where the parallel line meets the curve.

- *Ultimate tensile strength,* σ_{UTS}. This is the highest stress a material experiences during a tensile test. It may or may not be the stress at which the material fails (compare curves A and D to B and C).

- *Failure Strength, σ_f.* This is the stress at catastrophic failure (3). It may or may not correspond to the ultimate tensile strength.
- *Work of fracture (toughness).* Taken as the area under the entire stress–strain curve, from origin to failure, this is a measure of the ability of a material to absorb energy up to fracture. Note that this is a slightly different concept from values most often cited as 'toughness', which are actually the fracture toughness and a measure of a material's ability to resist crack propagation (see Section 5.2.3).
- *Ductility, %EL or %RA.* Ductility is a measure of the amount of plastic deformation at fracture. Very generally, this can be seen by the shape of the stress–strain curve. Curve A undergoes extremely little plastic deformation, whereas Curves B, C and D display considerably more. Values of ductility can be given as percentage elongation (%EL) or percentage reduction (%RA) in area according to the following formulae:

$$\%EL = \frac{l_f - l_0}{l_0} \times 100\% \qquad [5.1]$$

$$\%RA = \frac{A_0 - A_f}{A_0} \times 100\% \qquad [5.2]$$

  where l_f and l_0 are the final and initial length, respectively and A_f and A_0 are the final and initial cross-sectional areas, respectively. A material with a low value of ductility (0–5%) is said to be brittle, whereas a material with a high value is said to be ductile.

The four different curves displayed in Fig. 5.3 are typical of different types of materials. Curve A displays the high modulus and brittle behaviour common to ceramics and bone cement. As no plastic deformation occurs in this case, points (2) and (3) are the same. Curve B shows a material with a moderate modulus, a fair degree of yielding, and the blurred elastic–plastic transition common to metals and alloys. The more distinct yield point and yielding behaviour of curve C is common of many polymers. Curve D displays the typical behaviour of elastic polymers, such as rubber. These are very general curve shapes and classifications, at best, but should give some idea of how varied material behaviour can be. Indeed the shape of a curve may differ considerably for the same material, depending on the processing conditions or testing environment.

5.2.2 Other strength tests

While tensile tests work well for most metals and polymers, ceramics pose more of a problem. First, it is difficult to prepare ceramic specimens with the right geometry (often a dog-bone shape) and their brittle nature makes it very hard to grip them properly. In some cases a compression test can provide the information needed. However, because materials can behave very differently in compression compared with tension, it is necessary to find another way to test the tensile properties of materials that cannot reliably undergo a uniaxial tensile test.

Flexural strength

A flexural or bend test can be performed on rod-shaped specimens with either rectangular or circular cross-sections. A schematic of the setup for a three-point bend test is shown in Fig. 5.2(b). This test can also be performed as a four-point bend test, wherein the load is applied at two contact points along the top, rather than just one, with a moderate distance between them. When the load is applied, the ends of the specimen bend upwards, forcing the mid-point lower. This places the top of the specimen in compression and the bottom in tension. Since the tensile strength of most brittle ceramics is approximately one-tenth that of the compressive strength, it can be assumed that the specimen fails due to tension and thus represents a good value for tensile strength. Care must be taken to ensure the specimen has broken as close to the centre as possible, and always between the contact points rather than towards the outside or at a contact point.

The formulae for calculating bending strength for a three-point bend are shown below, both for rectangular and circular cross-sections:

$$\sigma_{fs} = \frac{3FL}{2bd^2} \quad [5.3]$$

$$\sigma_{fs} = \frac{FL}{\pi R^3} \quad [5.4]$$

where F is the load, L is the distance between contact points, b and d are the width and depth of a rectangular cross-section specimen, respectively, and R is the radius of a circular cross-section specimen. The four-point bend test may be generally preferred over the three-point bend test for brittle ceramics. One cause for concern with the three-point test is that failure might be initiated prematurely on the top face by a flaw generated by the contact point at the centre of the specimen. As the centre is also where the peak load is, this is expected to be the failure location under normal conditions. In the case of the four-point bend test, the bending moment is constant between the top two contact points. In this case, however, premature failure caused by a test-induced flaw should be easily distinguishable from a correct result where the specimen breaks between the two contact points. It should be noted, as well, that four-point bend tests tend to give lower strength values for ceramics. Since the load is spread over a wide area, there is more of a probability of encountering failure-inducing flaws, such as micropores. A more detailed description of the procedure and calculations can be found in ASTM Standard C1161 and (Wachtman, 1996a).

Diametral compression

Another option for testing tensile strength is the diametral compression test, also known as the Brazilian disc test (Fell and Newton, 1970). This test is done on a round tablet or short, circular cross-section rod and can be particularly practical for brittle ceramics. In this test, a specimen is placed on its side so that its curved surface is touching the plates of a tensile tester (Fig. 5.2c). A compressive load is then applied, causing the specimen to crack vertically through its centre. Though the name and technique are misleading, this is actually a measure of tensile strength. A crack is initiated in the centre of the sample by a tensile load, which acts perpendicular to the applied load. The tensile strength is then calculated as shown:

$$\sigma = \frac{2F}{\pi D t} \quad [5.5]$$

where F is the applied load, D is the specimen diameter and t is its thickness. One of the advantages to this test is that the results are independent of the quality of the specimen surface.

With both the bend test and the diametral compression test, it must be noted that the results are size dependent. The larger the specimen used, the more volume is placed under stress, which means the probability of small cracks or flaws leading to catastrophic failure increases. Since brittle ceramics are particularly prone to problems to do with microcracks and pores (discussed more in Section 5.2.3 on toughness), the scatter in data is much higher than for other classes of material. Thus, statistical methods are important in order to make sensible use of data. Weibull statistics are the most useful for ceramic materials and are described in further detail by Wachtman (1996b).

5.2.3 Other mechanical properties

Hardness

Hardness tests are a measure of resistance to indentation and are notable for being fast, easy and non-destructive. A force is applied to an indenter, such as a steel ball or diamond pyramid, and the resulting size or depth of the indentation in the surface of the material is measured using a microscope. There are several different types of hardness tests, varying in the shape and material of the indenter and the scale of the load applied. Some of the more common tests are Brinell and Rockwell to measure macrohardness, Knoop to measure microhardness and Vickers to measure both macro- and microhardness. Nanoindentation can also be performed with a Berkovich test. Specific hardness formulae match each type of hardness test. Lower numbers indicate the material is easily scratched or dented, whereas higher numbers indicate more resistance to indentation. Hardness is often related to other properties, such as tensile strength. For steels, cast irons and brass, hardness and tensile strength have a linear relationship (Callister Jr., 2000b).

Shear and torsion

Sometimes a material may be subjected to transverse loads (shear) or twisting motions (torsion). For shear, imagine a cube, fixed at the bottom. A force is then applied across the top, parallel to the top face, distorting the cube into a parallelepiped. Shear stress may be calculated in a similar way to longitudinal stress, but with a modification for the angle. The shear stress, τ, is equal to the shear force divided by the initial area across which the shear force is applied. The shear strain, γ, is equal to the tangent of the angle through which the deformation occurs. Shear modulus, G, is then τ divided by γ. Like tensile deformation, shear deformation can also be elastic, in small quantities, or plastic in larger quantities.

Torsion involves a twisting motion about the long axis of a specimen. In this case, imagine a rod, fixed at the bottom, subjected to a torque around its top face. The top will be deformed by an angle φ relative to the bottom. Shear stress is then a function of the applied torque and shear modulus is a function of the angle of twist.

Poisson's ratio is a way of relating the deformation of a material along different axes. For example, a tensile specimen experiences an elongating strain along the z axis, reducing the cross-sectional area of the specimen proportionally and reducing the strain in the x and y directions. If the material is isotropic along the x–y face then $\varepsilon_x = \varepsilon_y$. Poisson's ratio, v, can then be represented as:

$$v = -\frac{\varepsilon_x}{\varepsilon_z} = -\frac{\varepsilon_y}{\varepsilon_z} \qquad [5.6]$$

The ratio can be useful for relating shear and elastic moduli by the equation:

$$E = 2G(1 + v) \qquad [5.7]$$

Fracture toughness

As mentioned previously, the general toughness of a material, in terms of its ability to absorb energy as it fractures, can be calculated by the area under a stress–strain curve. However, fracture toughness is a slightly different concept.

Materials can have many microscopic defects, such as microporosity, and macroscopic defects, such as cracks. At the edges of these defects or crack tips, any applied stress is concentrated, meaning the stress needed to break the material is lowered. If a material is tough, then it can deform plastically as the crack propagates, slowing or stopping the crack's motion, or it may have a second phase which hinders the crack's motion. However, if a material is brittle, then the concentrated stress causes the crack to propagate very quickly and catastrophically.

There are several ways to measure fracture toughness, one of the most common being the single-edge notched beam (Munz and Fett, 2001). This consists of a setup similar to the three-point bend test, wherein a notch as thin as possible is placed on the bottom face of the rod, where the specimen is in tension. If done properly, this notch will serve as a crack initiator and its propagation will cause the failure of the material. Fracture toughness, K_{Ic}, is calculated by:

$$K_{Ic} = Y\sigma\sqrt{\pi a} \quad [5.8]$$

where Y is a geometrical factor, σ is the stress at which catastrophic failure occurs and a is the crack length. (In the case of an internal crack, a represents the radius of the crack or one-half the crack length.) Toughness can also be measured indirectly, by indenting the sample with a hard enough load that cracks emanate from the corners of the indent. Measuring the length of the cracks enables an estimate of the toughness to be calculated.

Fatigue

When a material is placed under continuous cyclic stresses, it may fail by a mechanism called fatigue. Repetitive loading and unloading can create microscopic cracks that propagate little by little with each subsequent cycle. Because cracks and scratches concentrate stresses locally, it will take a much lower stress than the normal failure stress to propagate the crack and eventually cause failure. Thus the fatigue strength may be as little as one-quarter to one-third the material's tensile strength.

Fatigue is tested by a cyclic tension or bending test at different maximum stresses (Dowling, 1998a). The endurance limit is determined by the stress that causes little to no failure after 10^6 to 10^8 cycles. The fracture surface is normally perpendicular to the direction of the applied tensile stress. Because fatigue is due to the gradual formation and propagation of tiny cracks within the material, the failure mode is brittle, even with a normally ductile material.

The fatigue behaviour of a material is also sensitive to environment. Corrosion or other degradation of the material and the cycle rate will affect the endurance limit. In a phenomenon called corrosion fatigue, corrosion forms pits, which act as stress concentrators, causing cracks to initiate and propagate with each cycle. In some cases, processing conditions may also contribute to fatigue. Small scratches or grooves caused by machining can lower the endurance limit of a material, thus it is always best to have a smooth, polished specimen.

Viscoelastic creep

Many polymers, particularly amorphous polymers like plastics and rubber, are susceptible to a phenomenon called viscoelastic creep. (While metals and ceramics may also experience this phenomenon, they only do so at temperatures far exceeding body temperature.) 'Viscoelastic' refers to a type of behaviour in between elastic and viscous behaviour. With elastic behaviour, the material stretches immediately with applied load and immediately recovers upon removal of the load, like a rubber band. A viscoelastic material, on the other hand, like silly putty, has a delayed deformation upon application of stress. After removal of the stress, the material slowly recovers the strain, but never completely. The behaviour is also subject to the rate of strain. If the strain is fast, the material behaves more elastically; if slow, the material behaves more viscously. Viscoelastic creep, then, occurs when a constant load slowly deforms a material. This property can be significant for some polymers even at temperatures as low as body temperature and at modest stresses far below the yield stress. The higher the degree of crystallinity a polymer has, the less susceptible it is to creep. Creep is evaluated by applying an instantaneous load and measuring strain as a function of time (Ferry, 1980).

5.3 Molecular and microstructural properties

The microstructure of a material contributes a great deal to its overall properties. Atomic structure and chemical composition play a key role in determining the mechanical properties and the way in which the body interacts with the material. Pore size, grain characteristics (in the case of crystalline materials) and phase distribution also affect material properties. In the case of amorphous or semi-crystalline polymers, small changes in attributes like molecular weight, thermal transition temperatures and cross-linking can have a profound effect on the behaviour of a material.

5.3.1 Atomic structure

Atoms and molecules in a material can be oriented and packed in different ways. In the case of glasses and some types of polymers, the orientation is random and is referred to as amorphous. Metals and ceramics, on the other hand, are crystalline. This means that their atoms are linked together in an ordered, repeating fashion. Other polymers have some regions of order and are thus semi-crystalline. The crystal structure is made up of the repeating pattern of atoms overlaid on a lattice of repeating points in three dimensions. A unit cell can then be thought of as a box containing a significant enough portion of the crystal structure to describe the bulk arrangement of atoms. It may be one of several shapes, including cubic, tetragonal or hexagonal. The arrangement of atoms within the unit cell results in crystal structures such as face-centred cubic (named for atoms located at the centre of each cube face and the cube corners), body-centred cubic (atoms located on the cube corners and one at the centre) and hexagonal close packed. The packing efficiency of a structure depends on the amount of space taken up by atoms in the unit cell relative to empty space. For more detailed information on crystal structures, see Cullity and Stock (2001).

A crystalline material may consist of a single crystal or, more often, it may be polycrystalline, consisting of many crystals or grains. The orientation of the grains is typically random, although they can also have a preferred orientation. Amorphous and polycrystalline materials are normally isotropic, meaning their properties are the same in every direction. Anisotropy occurs in single crystals which have directionally dependent chemical bond strengths (in the case of polycrystalline materials, the crystals' random orientation evens out this effect) and in some composites, such as those reinforced with long, oriented fibres (see Section 5.5.4). As a composite material of long collagen fibrils intermixed with hydroxyapatite-like crystals, bone is anisotropic. In this case, mechanical properties will be better along the longitudinal fibre axis. Processing conditions can also create anisotropy in a material by orienting crystals. Polymers, for example, when drawn or extended in one direction, can have higher strength and stiffness in the drawing direction.

Despite what might seem like a perfect, infinitely repeating structure, all polycrystalline materials contain defects on several possible dimensional levels. On the 0-D level, crystal structures may contain vacancies, where an atom is missing, or interstitials, where smaller atoms force themselves in an empty space between larger atoms. On the 1-D level, an interruption in the normal alignment of atomic planes results in a dislocation. The 2-D level encompasses grain boundaries, where a mismatch occurs as two crystals meet. And finally, pores are an example of a 3-D defect.

Strengthening mechanisms

Manipulation of microstructural characteristics can alter the mechanical properties of materials. The effect of pores and grains will be discussed in following sections. Additionally, some materials can be strengthened by other mechanisms. Work hardening or cold working is a room-temperature process in which a metal is rolled or drawn. This produces more dislocations in the metal's crystal lattice, which, when they meet, form immovable jogs which stop dislocation motion. Solution hardening involves the addition of impurities or alloying to make it more difficult for dislocations to propagate. The different sized atoms of impurities or another metal in an alloy distort the original lattice, making dislocation motion more difficult. Semi-crystalline polymers can be strengthened by drawing or pulling a specimen uniaxially. This aligns the molecular chains in the structure, making the polymer stronger in the drawing direction.

Density

The term density can apply to a material on several levels. At the most basic level, density is related to the atomic weight of chemical elements in a structure and their tightness of packing. Skeletal density (also known as theoretical or true density), which can be measured by pycnometry, also includes second phases (an alloying phase or another phase of a composite) and crystallographic defects in its calculation. Pycnometry uses small gas molecules, such as He, to compare the volume of a reference container with one filled with a sample in order to give a value for skeletal density. Bulk density uses a volume calculated from the outer dimensions of a sample divided by its mass, thus accounting for micro- and macropores and giving a lower value of density than for skeletal density if any pores are present. For non-porous materials with complex geometries, their volume can be measured by the amount of liquid they displace, provided the material is not soluble in that liquid (Archimedes' principle). Relative density is then the percentage ratio of bulk to true density. Ceramics, for instance, are considered 'dense' if their relative density is at least 95%.

5.3.2 Phase composition

The chemical and crystallographic identities of the phases present in a material, along with their relative amounts, distribution and orientation, determine the material's intrinsic properties. Therefore it is very important to be able to identify these phases precisely. Phases may be distinguished in a number of different ways. If crystalline, the structure will have unique lattice parameters and an arrangement of atoms identifiable by X-ray diffraction (XRD). In the case of polycrystalline materials, Rietveld analysis applied to XRD data can determine the relative amounts of phases present in a specimen (Will, 2006). Infrared (IR) spectroscopy can identify the chemical bonds present in a material, their relative quantity, and any changes in the character or quantity of the bonds over time (Stuart, 2004). This technique is particularly useful for polymers, which are not crystalline.

The locations of different phases in a material can sometimes be determined by microscopy. Grains in metals can usually be seen in light microscopy and different phases in an alloy will reflect light differently. Scanning electron microscopy (SEM) is also useful, although sometimes phases might appear similar. In this case, an attached X-ray beam can be used for energy dispersive spectroscopy (EDS) to pinpoint an elemental analysis of a specific location in the specimen. This method is not as sensitive for determining elemental ratios as some other methods, however. When knowing the exact composition of a material is very important, such as in the case of calcium phosphates which have different dissolution behaviour depending on their Ca/P ratio, more sensitive methods like X-ray fluorescence (XRF) spectrometry are a better choice (Buhrke *et al.*, 1997).

5.3.3 Porosity

The porosity of a material contributes greatly to both its mechanical properties and the way in which it behaves *in vivo*. Pores in a material act as stress concentrators, decreasing mechanical properties, while increased surface area provides a greater means of environmental interaction. In some cases a material is made intentionally porous, namely in the case of scaffolds in which interconnected macropores of 100–400 μm in diameter are placed in the material to allow bone ingrowth (Fig. 5.4a). The increased surface area may then allow the degradable scaffold slowly to dissolve away as bone replaces it. Owing to inhibited mechanical properties, however, these scaffolds can only be used in non-major load-bearing situations.

Much smaller pores will also be detrimental to mechanical properties. A material may have microporosity as a result of incomplete densification during sintering of a ceramic powder (Fig. 5.4b) or defects remaining after casting a metal, for example. In this case, the micropores will decrease the mechanical properties of a material, limiting its use in load-bearing applications.

The size and distribution of pores can be measured by a variety of techniques. Mercury porosimetry characterises porosity by forcing mercury into the pores of a material. The pressure required to intrude mercury into the pores is inversely proportional to the size of the pores. Using this technique can give a complete set of information about pore size, distribution, and surface area and bulk and skeletal density (Lowell *et al.*, 2006c). However, it can only be used with stronger samples able to withstand the pressures involved in mercury intrusion.

In addition to knowing the surface area of a material that is evident to the naked eye, it is important to know the full surface area available for environmental interactions, such as aqueous dissolution. This includes the entire surface area of a geometrically complex implant like a scaffold, the surface area of a filler powder, or the sum of the external and 'internal'

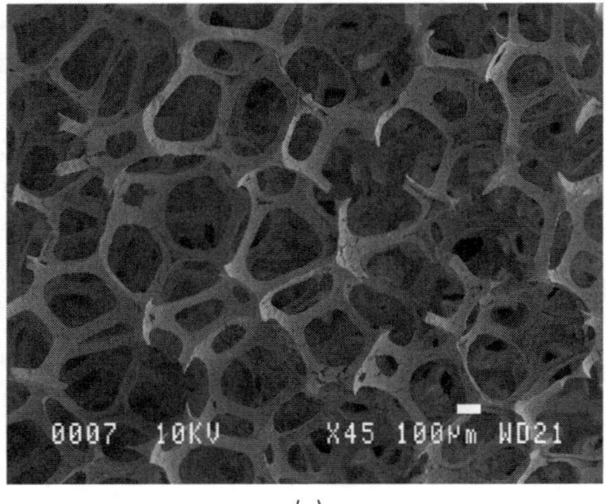

(a)

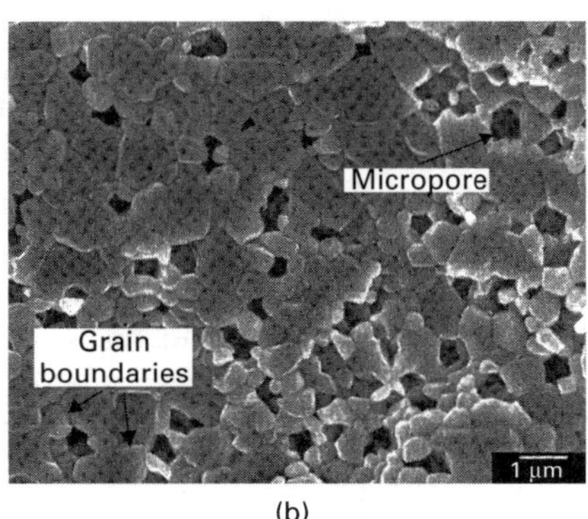

(b)

5.4 SEM micrographs of hydroxyapatite. (a) Macroporosity in a scaffold designed for bone ingrowth. Dip-coated hydroxyapatite scaffold made using the reticulated foam method. Courtesy J.H. Robinson, University of Cambridge. (b) Microporosity in sintered (densified) polycrystalline hydroxyapatite. Grains and grain boundaries are also evident.

surface areas of a material which may be riddled with micropores owing to incomplete densification during sintering. One of the standard techniques for doing this, as just mentioned, is mercury porosimetry. Another option, for more delicate materials, is nitrogen adsorption, in which gas molecules are physically adsorbed onto a solid surface. Using BET theory, one can use the data from nitrogen adsorption to calculate the specific surface area (Braunauer *et al.*, 1938), measured in units of m^2g^{-1}. A green (unsintered) ceramic powder may have a surface area of hundreds of square metres per gram, while a sintered powder may be in the low tens of square metres per gram. Pore size distributions can also be calculated from nitrogen adsorption data with BJH theory (Barrett *et al.*, 1951). Adsorption mechanisms are described in more detail in (Lowell *et al.*, 2006a).

5.3.4 Grain structure

As mentioned previously, the term 'grain' refers to a crystal in a polycrystalline material. Normally these grains are randomly oriented, but they can also have a preferred orientation, referred to as 'texture'. Where two grains meet, there is atomic mismatch, creating a grain boundary (Fig. 5.4b). Boundaries are areas of high energy, making them more chemically reactive than their surroundings. They also serve to improve mechanical properties by inhibiting dislocation motion. Heat treatments cause grains to grow in size, with the driving force being the reduction in boundary energy. However, mechanical properties are increased most when grains are smaller, as there are more grain boundaries to stop the propagation of dislocations. Additionally, fine-grained ceramics tend to have lower porosity since pores are removed by the easy vacancy transport that can occur along grain boundaries. Lower porosity, of course, means higher strength.

A smaller grain size improves many different mechanical properties. Surface wear has been found to improve in ceramics with fine grain size (Wang *et al.*, 2005) as well as strength and fracture toughness in ceramics and metals (DeWith *et al.*, 1981; Takaki *et al.*, 2001). The shape of grains also has an influence on the mechanical properties, as discussed in more detail by (Lee and Rainforth, 1994). At the same time, however, smaller grain size and increased grain boundary area has been found to increase corrosion of metal implant materials and increase dissolution of bioceramics *in vivo* (Placko *et al.*, 1998; Porter *et al.*, 2003).

Grain size can be measured from micrographs showing the grain structure. In some cases a sample may have to be etched with acid, which preferentially attacks grain boundaries, to reveal the grain structure. By drawing a line across the image and counting the number of times it intersects a grain boundary, the grain size can then be calculated by comparing this result with the scale bar.

5.3.5 Polymer structure and properties

Starting from the smallest structural level, characteristics like molecular weight, tacticity, chain configuration, degree of polymerisation and crosslinking can affect the behaviour of polymers. Properties such as crystallinity, melting temperature and glass-transition temperature are determined by these molecular-level characteristics. These, in turn, affect mechanical properties and *in vivo* response.

Molecular-level structural characteristics

During the polymerisation process, single, repeating units (mers) combine to form long chains of varying lengths. The molecular weight then represents the average total molar mass for one chain in a polymer. There are several ways in which to calculate molecular weight, including a number-average molecular weight and a weight-average molecular weight, the details of which can be found elsewhere (Campbell *et al.*, 2000a). The degree of polymerisation is a related concept and represents the number of mers in a polymer chain. During synthesis of a polymer, the degree of polymerisation can be followed over time using IR spectroscopy to measure the chemical bonds present and their relative quantity over time (Stuart, 2004). Molecular weight can be measured experimentally by osmotic pressure, gel permeation chromatography and light scattering, among other techniques (Campbell *et al.*, 2000a). The higher the molecular weight, the more rigid is the polymer. Soft waxes or resins have molecular weights on the order of 1000 g mol^{-1}, while solid, hard polymers have molecular weights on the order of 10 000–1 000 000 g mol^{-1}. One of the most widely used polymers in orthopaedic applications, ultra-high-molecular-weight polyethylene (UHMWPE), has a molecular weight of 4×10^6 g mol^{-1}.

Chains can arrange themselves in a variety of ways. Linear chains are simply long chains of monomers joined end-to-end. Branched chains, on the other hand occur when shorter chains grow off the longer chain. In an extreme example, a network polymer consists of many chains and many branches, bonded together at various points by crosslinks. Tacticity refers to the arrangement of side groups around a chain. An isotactic arrangement has all side groups on the same side, a syndiotactic alternates sides, whereas an atactic arrangement is completely random. When more than one type of monomer is present in the polymer structure, it is called a copolymer. The locations of the different monomers relative to one another results in different types of structures, including alternating (the monomers alternate back and forth), block (several monomers of each type join together and then alternate with a group of another monomer type) and random (completely random arrangement of monomer types).

The various components of the chemical structure of a polymer can be determined experimentally by a wide array of characterisation techniques. IR spectroscopy can identify the types of bonds present, while nuclear magnetic resonance can determine chemical groups. Wide-angle X-ray scattering determines the local structure of semi-crystalline polymers, while small-angle X-ray scattering can identify if a polymer is multi-phase, a copolymer, or an ionomer.

Degree of crystallinity

When polymer chains are arranged in a particularly compactable way, say a linear chain with small side groups in an isotactic configuration, they are better able to align and pack into an ordered structure. Secondary bonding can then occur between adjacent chain segments and regions of crystallinity can form. The complexity of the chain affects this, including the size of side groups, any branching, and the tacticity. While both isotactic and syndiotactic arrangements allow for crystallisation, atactic structures cannot crystallise. Owing to the size and complexity of all polymer chains, it is virtually impossible for them to be completely crystalline. Thus polymers are either amorphous or semi-crystalline.

The degree of crystallinity can be determined by the density of the material. The more crystalline, the more compact the structure is and thus the more dense the polymer is. In general, ductile semi-crystalline polymers have a crystallinity of about 50%, whereas very brittle ones are 90–95% crystalline. The degree of crystallinity can also be influenced by processing conditions. A slower cooling rate can allow for more crystallisation, as the chains have more time to arrange themselves in an orderly fashion. Along with the more ordered, dense structure comes an improvement in both tensile modulus and tensile strength.

Thermal transitions

Many polymers undergo two important thermal transitions – melting and glass transition. A melting temperature (T_m) is only present in semi-crystalline polymers. It occurs when the solid material with ordered, aligned chains turns into a randomly oriented viscous liquid. Owing to the range of molecular weights in the structure, it actually takes place over a range of a few degrees rather than at one, clearly-defined temperature. Like the degree of crystallinity, chain properties, like the size of side groups and ease of rotation, affect the melting temperature. It takes more energy to unpack a well-packed chain, resulting in a higher T_m. Branching, on the other hand, decreases T_m, as branching leads to defects in crystallinity. The rate at which the polymer is heated also affects the T_m; a higher rate results in a higher melting temperature.

The glass transition temperature (T_g) marks the point at which a polymer goes from rubbery behaviour to a rigid solid as it cools. As temperature decreases, the motion of large segments of polymer chains is reduced. All types of polymers experience a glass transition. The same molecular characteristics that affect T_m affect T_g in a similar way. The two temperatures are typically linked, as well; a change in one affects the other by the relationship T_g = 0.5–0.8T_m (Kelvin).

Several techniques can measure thermal transition temperatures in polymers. Differential scanning calorimetry (DSC) is perhaps the most widely used. DSC monitors heat flow to determine T_g and T_m (if present). Other techniques include thermomechanical analysis and dynamic mechanical analysis and are described in more detail elsewhere (Campbell *et al.*, 2000b).

Strengthening polymers

While polymers do not have a grain structure in the same way that metals and ceramics do, they can be strengthened in a number of different ways. As previously mentioned, increasing the crystallinity and molecular weight of a polymer will strengthen it. In the same way that grain boundaries impede dislocation motion, anything in a polymer's structure that will impede the slippage of segments of molecular chains will strengthen it. Crosslinking, mentioned briefly before, involves forming strong bonds between molecules previously only linked by weak Van der Waals forces. These strong bonds then stop chains from moving. Drawing, as mentioned before, strengthens semi-crystalline polymers in the drawing direction by aligning the molecular chains in the structure through uniaxial force.

5.4 Physiological effects

The way a material behaves in a standard room temperature atmosphere may vary substantially from its performance *in vivo*, where it must withstand a corrosive saline environment at 37°C, while negotiating interactions with other surrounding body fluids, tissues, biomolecules and cells. Some of the microstructural properties associated with *in vivo* behaviour have been described in the previous section, such as the effect of porosity on surface area and the consequential number of reaction sites with which body fluids may interact and the various structural properties of polymers. This section will discuss the properties that influence *in vivo* reactions such as corrosion, dissolution, degradation, inflammation and cell interaction with surfaces.

5.4.1 Metallic corrosion

The tendency to corrode is the primary problem facing metal implant use in the body. Corrosion degrades structural integrity and can create by-products that adversely affect biological functions. The ions, organic substances and dissolved oxygen contained in the body's environment make it electrochemically reactive to metals, leading to corrosion. Metals vary in their tendency to corrode, depending on electrode potential. This potential can be measured by AC, DC or impedance electrochemistry, as described by Lemons *et al.* (1999). Some metals, such as Au and Pt, are inert, whereas metals like Cr, Co, Al, Zn and Ti are quite reactive and easily corrode. Why, then, are the three main alloys in total joint replacement Ti alloys, Co alloys and stainless steel?

While aqueous corrosion in the body can be a hindrance, a similar electrochemical reaction with the oxygen in air, called dry corrosion, can be an advantage. Upon exposure to air, some metals immediately form an oxide layer on their surface, just a few nanometres thick. Since corrosion is a surface phenomenon, this oxide layer acts as a passivating layer, preventing the transport of metallic ions and electrons between the metal implant and body fluids. This serves to prevent both aqueous corrosion and leaching of any potentially irritating or toxic ions, such as Ni^{2+}, Cr^{3+} or Co^{2+}. Al, Cr and Ti are so reactive in air that they are almost always included as components in alloys to ensure an oxide layer will form. A nitric acid treatment on stainless steel is another common way to create this layer.

Once in the body, the passivating oxide layer does not always completely protect the metallic implant from corrosion. First, mechanical stresses may cause the oxide film to wear off. While it can reform, biological factors may affect its ability to do so. Biological macromolecules, such as proteins, cells and bacteria can upset the equilibria of corrosion reactions by altering the local pH, affecting electrode potential and affecting the amount of oxygen available to reform and maintain the layer. Weak points in the oxide layer can also cause what is known as pitting corrosion. This forms holes in the oxide layer that cannot be reformed. Fretting corrosion is a cyclic process in which the passive oxide layer is continuously removed and reformed, gradually wearing away at the surface of the implant. Finally, stress corrosion can occur in the presence of an applied load. It reacts by attacking the oxide layer at its weakest and forming small cracks that grow in length and depth over time, eventually leading to device failure.

5.4.2 Ceramic dissolution

Metals are made passive to aqueous corrosion in the body by first creating an oxide layer through dry corrosion. This is the reason why ceramics are not subject to corrosion. The Al_2O_3, ZrO_2, TiO_2, passivating layers that are formed are ceramic in structure and nature, and the strongly directional interatomic bonds in the structures mean that large amounts of energy are required for their disruption. Instead, ceramics may have a tendency to dissolve in aqueous environments, depending on their chemical composition and microstructure. In some cases this 'flaw' is turned into advantage by creating ceramic implants with a controlled dissolution rate.

Bioceramics (discussed in more detail in a later chapter) include Al_2O_3, ZrO_2, calcium phosphates, calcium carbonates and bioglasses, ranging on the scale of *in vivo* behaviour from bioinert (the body produces a fibrous capsule around the implant) to bioactive (the body directly bonds with the material) to bioresorbable (the body dissolves the material completely). Factors such as chemical composition (i.e. Ca/P ratio for calcium phosphates), porosity and even mechanical stress play a role in the rate and extent of degradation. The more chemically similar a material is to bone, the more likely the body is to recognise it and bond to it or interact with it in some way. Indeed, complete degradation of a ceramic is often planned and serves as a reservoir of useful ions (Ca^{2+}, CO_3^{2-}, Na^+, PO_3^{2-}) as the body rebuilds. Porous scaffolds are designed with the intention that bone will grow into their interconnected pores. However, it should be kept in mind that the larger surface area of the scaffold will make it more susceptible to dissolution and the nature of the structure will make it mechanically much weaker than an equivalent dense ceramic.

The dissolution rate of bioceramics can be predicted by immersing the material in an aqueous solution, like simulated body fluid, and monitoring its weight loss over time. More specific information about the dissolution products can be learned by performing spectroscopic analysis on the liquid as the material degrades (Williams and Bause, 1996). Care should be taken in selecting the specific technique to be used, however, as different techniques have different levels of sensitivities to specific elements. While this method can give a general idea of how the ceramic might perform in the body, a host of other factors, such as the presence of cells and proteins, local pH changes caused by inflammation and mechanical stresses, will play a role in the degree of dissolution that cannot be simulated.

5.4.3 Polymer degradation

Polymers degrade in the body through physiochemical processes. Hydrolysis is one type of degradation, wherein the polymer chains spread apart as biomolecules and water move into the structure. This process can cause the scission of any susceptible molecular functional groups. Polyethylene (PE), used in joint replacement prostheses, and polymethyl methacrylate (PMMA), used as bone cement, are not prone to this type of degradation. Material properties that combat this process are a high molecular weight and a high degree of crosslinking and crystallinity.

In some cases, the degradation process may be helpful to the material design. A small amount of swelling may be beneficial in locking a polymer into position. Additionally, a material may be designed to stay in the body only temporarily, completely degrading when its task is complete. As with ceramics, the potential for degradation can be evaluated by immersing the material in simulated body fluid and analysing the content of the liquid over time by spectroscopy (Williams and Bause, 1996).

In many cases, polymer degradation lowers the T_g, thus special care must be taken if using a polymer whose T_g is close to that of body temperature. If the T_g is lowered to less than 37°C, a strong polymer may become rubbery and weak. Other factors that can degrade polymer properties *in vivo* are adsorption of biomolecules, such as proteins, as well as calcification and other forms of mineralisation. Secondary effects of degradation should also be considered. Degradation products may cause a local alteration of pH and the degradation process can also leach low-molecular weight compounds from the polymer, such as plasticiser, which can weaken or embrittle the polymer and lead to faster dissolution.

Processing conditions and sterilisation procedures may also affect the properties of a polymer. Polymers particularly prone to hydrolysis, for instance, should be kept moisture-free during processing and storage to prevent any premature degradation. When considering a sterilisation technique, the advantages and disadvantages of each method should be taken into account. When using heat sterilisation, care must be taken to keep the temperature below T_g at all times to prevent changes in morphology. During chemical sterilisation procedures, on the other hand, a polymer may absorb the chemicals and later release them into the body. Additionally, irradiation can cause bond ruptures, which can lower the molecular weight, or can create new crosslinks, both of which will affect the mechanical properties. It can also generate free radicals that may interact with oxygen in the body to create unwanted by-products.

5.4.4 Tribological properties

Wear

When two materials in contact continuously rub against one another (most notably in joint replacements, in the case of orthopaedic applications), a gradual loss of matter will occur. Particulate debris contribute a great deal to orthopaedic device degradation and are the main factor limiting the long-term performance of joint replacement prostheses (Hallab *et al.*, 2004).

Wear may occur by abrasion, adhesion or fatigue. In the case of abrasion, a rougher or harder surface gradually wears away a softer surface. In the case of adhesion, a softer material may wear off and transfer onto the harder material, creating a film. Surface fatigue, on the other hand, gradually creates debris particles as changing cyclic stresses are repeatedly applied to the contact area. The wear particles may remain between the surfaces of the two interacting materials, they may be transferred from one surface to another, or they may be lost from the system. Generally it is the softer material which wears more quickly, a polymer in the case of a metal–polymer interface or the metal in the case of a metal–ceramic interface. Wear resistance can be improved by altering the microstructure and chemical structure of the material. For example, a higher molecular weight and degree of branching and crosslinking improve the wear of polymers, while a fine, narrowly distributed grain size gives better wear properties in ceramics.

The main problem with wear particles is not so much to do with decreased mechanical properties of the devices, but rather to do with the biological effects of the particle. Wear particles may be irritating to the body's tissues, causing an inflammatory reaction. In the case of hip prostheses, these wear particles can induce an inflammatory response which results in local bone loss around the implant (Jacobs *et al.*, 2001). Wear can be tested by several methods, including the hip joint wear simulator (Lu and McKellop, 1997), the multi-directional motion wear test (Wang, 2001) and the flat-on-ring wear test (Chiesa *et al.*, 2000).

Coefficient of friction

If two materials are in contact, the best way to avoid unnecessary wear is by having a low coefficient of friction between the two surfaces. The coefficient of friction is determined by measuring the ratio of the parallel force between the two surfaces in contact to the perpendicular force as the surfaces pass over one another. Several techniques have been developed to do this, the most simple of which are the dead load and inclined plane test, described in detail in Ludema's textbook on tribology (1996). He does recommend, however, seeking a published value for the coefficient for the two materials in question, in the first instance, as it can be very difficult to obtain consistent values of this property.

5.4.5 Surface properties

As the surface of a material is the first part of an implant the body's environment encounters, it drives the subsequent biological reactions. The body's response to surface characteristics and features is still not entirely understood, although some general trends in the types of properties that affect cell behaviour have emerged. Special methods must be employed to characterise surface properties, as the surface has a different reactivity compared with the bulk material. It also involves such a small amount of material that particularly sensitive equipment is needed and, additionally, the surface is easily contaminated by air or other substances. Ratner (2004) gives a good description of the important surface properties and the current technology involved in their characterisation. A review by Boyan *et al.* (1996) summarises typical cell behaviour towards different surface properties.

Surface composition

Perhaps the most obvious surface characteristic that influences the body's response to a material is the composition. The composition and chemical structure affect whether cells attach to the surrounding tissue, resorb the implant material or form a capsule around it. Bioceramics, particularly calcium phosphates, are noted for their chemical similarity to the inorganic constituent of bone. Thus, coatings of hydroxyapatite (HA) and tri-calcium phosphate

(TCP) have been shown to enhance *in vivo* response to implant materials (Jasty *et al.*, 1992). In addition to coatings, implanting ions favourable to the body within the surface of a material can change the binding behaviour of cells.

Fully characterising the surface composition of a material may be tricky, as traditional methods for determining composition, such as XRD, may penetrate too far into the material. The techniques recommended and described by Hayakawa *et al.* include Auger electron spectroscopy (AES), X-ray photoelectron spectroscopy (XPS) and Fourier transform infrared spectroscopy (FTIR) (Hayakawa *et al.*, 2008).

Wettability

Variation in surface charge has been shown to affect cellular spreading and affinity for the surface of a material (Hollinger and Schmitz, 1997). Charge makes a surface more conducive to tissue integration, with both a net positive or net negative charge shown to promote bone formation (Krukowski *et al.*, 1990; Hamamoto *et al.*, 1995). The surface energy and surface charge are directly related to wettability, which is the affinity of a surface for liquids. In a contact angle measurement (Ratner, 2004), a drop of water or other liquid is dropped onto the surface of the material and the angle the edge of the droplet makes with the surface is measured. If the droplet spreads out, the surface has good wettability and is said to be hydrophilic. If the droplet beads up, it has poor wettability and is hydrophobic. If a surface has a net negative or positive charge it will be hydrophilic, while if it has a neutral charge it will be hydrophobic. Thus, bone formation is increased on wettable, hydrophilic surfaces (Boyan *et al.*, 1996).

Surface roughness

According to research by Larsson *et al.* (1994), surface topology may influence the rate at which bone is formed next to the surface of an implant material more than oxide thickness or microstructure. Surface roughness can affect cellular adhesion, proliferation and phenotype (Burg *et al.*, 2000). Generally, porosity and roughness are more biologically favourable than smooth surfaces (Hanker and Giammara, 1988). A study by Boyan *et al.* (1996) found that virtually all parameters associated with cell proliferation, metabolism, matrix synthesis and differentiation were dependent on surface roughness.

A good overview of the surface roughness of a material can be obtained by SEM. However, techniques such as atomic force microscopy (AFM) and scanning tunnelling microscopy (STM) give a more sensitive, quantitative measurement. These techniques are described in detail by Ratner (2004).

5.5 Comparing material classes

The previous three sections have identified and discussed the mechanical and microstructural properties and physiological effects that are important to the *in vivo* performance of a material. We should now be prepared to compare material classes in terms of their overall performance and suitability for different bone repair requirements.

5.5.1 Metals

Metals possess a great many attributes which make them highly suitable for bone repair. Looking back to Table 5.2, we can compare the mechanical properties of metals used in biological applications to those of other material classes. First, metals possess excellent tensile strength which far outweighs any polymer and is markedly higher than any of the bioceramics, with the exception of zirconia. In compression, however, ceramics perform moderately better. Metals have a modulus on par with ceramics and are moderately ductile. More noticeable, however, is their toughness, which is about 20 times greater than that of ceramics. Although not listed in the table, metals are fairly hard, have a reasonable fatigue life compared with other materials and are easily machined. If selected properly, they also have good corrosion resistance and do not elicit adverse biological responses. Their ability to alloy also means their properties can be specifically tailored for a particular application.

However, metals are lacking in other aspects. First, while those used in biological applications are not toxic, they also do not interact with body tissue in a synergistic way, as calcium phosphates and biological glasses do. Also, while good mechanical properties can be beneficial, the strength and stiffness of metals actually considerably exceed those of bone. A theory referred to as Wolff's Law observes that bone tends to remodel itself according to the load under which it is placed. In other words, if an implant with superior mechanical properties is used in a major load-bearing orthopaedic application, the metal will then bear more of the stress than the bone, causing the bone to remodel itself accordingly.

5.5.2 Ceramics

Bioceramics are noted for their superior wear resistance, low coefficient of friction, high stiffness and resistance to oxidation. Looking at Table 5.2, we see that ceramics have very high compressive strengths, but comparatively much lower tensile strengths. Some ceramics (i.e. alumina) have high tensile strengths, greater than that of bone, while others (i.e. HA) have tensile strengths well below that of bone, which limits their use in major load-bearing applications. The low roughness of ceramics is also limiting. As mentioned in the previous section, the metals have, on average, a fracture toughness 20 times that of the ceramics. In particular the toughness of HA, the bioceramic most similar in composition to the inorganic component of bone, is far below that of cortical bone. Although bone contains a considerable amount of the inorganic 'ceramic' phase, the collagen fibrils which run longitudinally through it greatly improve its toughness, preventing the type of catastrophic failure that plagues biological glasses and calcium phosphates. The high stiffness of ceramics might also pose a problem in a load-bearing situation owing to modulus mismatch with surrounding bone tissue.

In compositional considerations and resulting *in vivo* behaviour, ceramics encompass a range of performances. Some, such as alumina and zirconia, are bioinert, having neither an adverse nor beneficial effect on the surrounding tissue. Others, like HA, are so similar in composition to the inorganic phase of bone that they can create a stable bond with it and are termed bioactive. Still others are bioresorbable, like TCP, dissolving over time as they donate their ions towards new bone growth. Bioactive glasses and glass ceramics, including Bioglass®, developed by Hench *et al.* (1971), and apatite-wollastonite (A-W) glass ceramic, encompass a wide range of biological behaviour, depending on the exact proportions of CaO, SiO_2, Na_2O and P_2O_5.

Were it not for their poor mechanical properties, the compositional similarity of some bioceramics to bone tissue would make them an ideal replacement material. With the current state of technology, materials like HA and bioactive glasses are limited to powders to fill in bony defects, non-major load-bearing applications, like middle ear implants and alveolar ridge reconstruction, and coatings on orthopaedic, dental and maxillofacial prosthetics. While the poor strength and toughness of HA and bioactive glasses limits their use, the significantly higher mechanical properties of glass ceramics enable their use in higher load-bearing situations in porous, granular and even bulk forms, mainly in the spinal area. Alumina and zirconia, on the other hand, with their superior mechanical properties compared with other bioceramics, can be used in situations requiring both strength and wear resistance, such as femoral heads and acetabular cups.

5.5.3 Polymers

The properties of polymers can vary considerably, depending on their degree of crystallinity and crosslinking and their molecular weight. Amorphous, rubbery polymers are soft and ductile, have a low modulus and can extend hundreds of times their original length. Semi-crystalline polymers, on the other hand, have much higher moduli and lower extensibilities. Common to many polymers is their high toughness. While some, such as PMMA, exhibit brittle behaviour, the vast majority used in biomedical applications exhibit yielding behaviour and thus are able to deform plastically to stop the propagation of microcracks, giving them a higher toughness. They must, however, have a sufficient yield strength to minimize plastic deformation, particularly in major load-bearing situations. If we compare the properties of PE in Table 5.2 to those of bone, they do not match well for any material property, except perhaps modulus for which PE is far closer to bone's modulus than are any of the other materials. We can also assume that the toughness value of PE will be higher than that of bone, considering the extent of elongation is drastically higher for PE than for bone. One should keep in mind, however, that PE represents the higher end of mechanical property values for polymers, so most polymers will be even less of a match for bone when it comes to strength and modulus.

Polymers must also be carefully selected based on glass transition temperature to ensure they resist creep at body temperatures. Additionally, if they are to be used in frictional settings, they should have sufficient crosslinking, molecular weight and other chemical properties to resist wear. UHMWPE is excellent in this regard, which is why it has been used commercially for over 30 years for load-bearing surfaces in total knee and hip replacements, such as acetabular cups in hip prostheses. Another benefit of polymers is the relative ease with which they are machined and the variety of products that can result, from sheets to films and coatings to fibres. Biologically speaking, polymers can be bioinert, resisting interaction with the body, or can be designed to be biodegradable, giving them a wide range of possible uses in the body. For the purpose of bone implant materials, biodegradable polymers, owing to their weak mechanical properties, are often combined with ceramic particulate reinforcements to create a scaffold material with a controllable degradation rate (see Section 5.5.4). PMMA, while an excellent bone cement material used to fix hip- and knee-joint prostheses, is limited in use owing to its brittleness.

5.5.4 Composites

A composite material consists of two or more phases, distinguishable on the macrostructural scale, whose constituents interact and result in a single material with unique properties. The synthesis of composite materials offers a way to combine properties of different material classes and to tailor the resulting properties for a specific application. Bone itself is a composite material consisting of a matrix of an HA-like inorganic phase reinforced with fibrils of collagen, suggesting that the best way to mimic its properties is with a composite material.

Several factors affect the overall properties of a composite, including the properties of the constituents, how well the phases are distributed and in what manner, and the loading of the two phases with respect to one another.

In some cases the properties of the composite material might be a weighted average of the properties of the constituents. But in other cases, perhaps owing to geometrical orientation or interfacial interactions, the phases might act synergistically and result in properties better than either of the constituent materials. Some requirements of a biocomposite are that it is biocompatible, has good strength and fatigue properties, good toughness and a modulus matching that of the material it is replacing.

Usually a reinforcing phase is either in the form of fibres (long or short) or particles. The aspect ratio distinguishes the two. If the ratio of the length to diameter of the phase is approximately the same, then it is a particle, whereas a large length to diameter ratio is representative of a fibre. Particle reinforcement provides isotropic properties, whereas aligned fibres result in anisotropic properties.

To describe fully a composite, the type of reinforcement, its loading, how well it is distributed throughout the matrix, its orientation (aligned or random) and its size with respect to the matrix should be specified. Smaller reinforcements offer more surface area with which to interact with the matrix. They also allow properties to be distributed throughout the material a bit better, if well dispersed.

Looking back at Table 5.2, let us try to determine two materials which might combine well to give us properties similar to bone. HA is a material with superb biological properties, but whose mechanical properties severely limit its *in vivo* use. Its modulus is higher than that of bone and its toughness is much lower. If we consider PE, with its much lower modulus and high toughness (explained in the previous section), it is not hard to imagine that a composite of these two materials would yield mechanical properties very similar to those of bone. Additionally, the HA would bring along its bioactivity to the normally inert PE. And indeed, in 1981 Bonfield *et al.* not only imagined this, but developed the composite into the promising bone repair material HAPEX™ (Bonfield *et al.*, 1981). This is an example of particulate reinforcement.

In some cases, one of the primary reasons for creating a composite biomaterial may be to control degradation. Rather than combine a particulate phase, like HA or TCP, with a nearly inert polymer, it instead can be combined with a biodegradable polymer, such as poly-L-lactide (PLLA), poly(lactic-*co*-glycolic acid) (PLGA) or polycaprolactone (PCL). By varying the loading of the reinforcing ceramic phase, the degradation rate of the polymer can be mediated. This arrangement has the mechanical advantages of the soft polymer countering the ceramic's brittleness and making it easier to shape, whereas the ceramic adds structural integrity to the polymer. This type of composite shows particular potential as a scaffold material.

The advantages in fibre reinforcement come mainly in toughness improvements and the opportunity to give anisotropic properties to the composite. If fibres are long and aligned, mechanical properties should be improved along the longitudinal direction. Unaligned long fibres or short fibres still offer a great deal of surface area with which to interact with the matrix while retaining isotropic properties. Fibres can improve toughness by bridging cracks or by fibre pull-out, wherein energy is absorbed by the frictional force required to pull the fibre out of place when fractured. In either case, the main goal of a fibre is to either stop crack propagation altogether or to elongate the path the crack has to take to propagate across the material.

If we return, briefly, to the original ideal goal of mimicking bone to achieve its properties, let us consider another scenario. Again, HA, as it is very similar to the inorganic component of bone, seems a good choice of matrix material. The main second phase of bone is collagen, in the form of bundled fibrils running longitudinally up and down the bone. If we remember that reinforcement size is an important factor, we know we need something on the scale of nanometres in diameter to simulate the reinforcing effect of the fibrils. Carbon nanotubes, with their nano-scale dimensions, high aspect ratio and excellent strength seem like a good possibility. This composite idea is discussed in more detail in the literature (White *et al.*, 2007).

A final consideration in forming composites is, of course, how they will react in the body and how the body will interact with them. It is important to consider the biological response to all constituent materials. In the case of carbon nanotube-reinforced HA, there is still a good deal of research that needs to be done to evaluate the biological impact of carbon nanotubes before the idea would be feasible *in vivo*.

5.6 Summary

This chapter broadly categorises material properties into three areas: mechanical properties, molecular and microstructural properties and physiological effects. Mechanical properties include, among others, strength, stiffness, toughness and fatigue. Molecular and microstructural properties contain density, porosity, surface area, grain size, composition, atomic structure, and polymer molecular weight and thermal transition temperatures. Properties such as wear, surface characteristics and tendencies toward corrosion, dissolution and degradation comprise the final category of physiological effects. Explanations of these properties and general characterisation advice are provided. The final section of the chapter seeks to compare material classes with respect to each of these property areas and suggests composites as a way to 'compromise' on properties and combine the best attributes of at least two separate materials.

One should take away two main points from this chapter. First, that material properties are controllable. At the same time, however, one must consider the second point, that material properties are all interrelated. Alterations in one property change another and, ultimately, all properties come together to determine *in vivo* behaviour. The key to success is to achieve an optimal balance of these properties.

5.7 References

Barrett E P, Joyner L G and Halenda P P (1951), 'The determination of pore volume and area distributions in porous substances: computations from nitrogen isotherms', *J Am Chem Soc*, **73**, 373–80.

Bonfield W, Grynpas M D, Tully A E, Bowman J and Abram J (1981), 'Hydroxyapatite reinforced polyethylene – a mechanically compatible implant material for bone replacement', *Biomaterials*, **2**, 185–6.

Boyan B D, Hummert T W, Dean D D and Schwartz Z (1996), 'Role of material surfaces in regulating bone and cartilage cell response', *Biomater*, **17**, 137–46.

Bradon D B and Kaplan W D (1999), 'Quantitative analysis of microstructure', in *Microstructural Characterization of Materials*, John Wiley & Sons, New York, 345–98.

Braunauer S, Emmett P H and Teller E (1938), 'Adsorption of gases in multimolecular layers', *J Am Chem Soc*, **60**, 309–19.

Buhrke V E, Jenkins R and Smith D K (1997), *A Practical Guide for the Preparation of Specimens for X-ray Fluorescence and X-ray Diffraction Analysis*, John Wiley & Sons, New York.

Burg K J L, Porter S and Kellam J F (2000), 'Biomaterial developments for bone tissue engineering', *Biomater*, **21**, 2347–59.

Callister Jr. W D (2000a), *Materials Science and Engineering: An Introduction*, John Wiley & Sons, New York.

Callister Jr. W D (2000b), 'Mechanical properties of metals', in *Materials Science and Engineering: An Introduction*, John Wiley & Sons, New York, 112–52.

Campbell D, Pethrick R A and White J R (2000a), 'Molecular mass determination', in *Polymer Characterization: Physical Techniques*, 2nd edition, Stanley Thornes, Cheltenham, UK, 15–50.

Campbell D, Pethrick R A and White J R (2000b), 'Thermal analysis', in *Polymer Characterization: Physical Techniques*, 2nd edition, Stanley Thornes, Cheltenham, UK, 362–407.

Chiesa R, Tanzi M C, Alfonsi S, Paracchini L, Moscatelli M and Cigada A (2000), 'Enhanced wear performance of highly crosslinked UHMWPE for artificial joints', *J Biomed Mater Res*, **50**, 381–7.

Cullity B D and Stock S R (2001), *Elements of X-ray Diffraction*, 3rd edition, Addison-Wesley, London.

DeWith G, Vandijk H J A, Hattu N and Prijs K (1981), 'Preparation, microstructure and mechanical properties of dense polycrystalline hydroxyapatite', *J Mater Sci*, **16**, 1592–8.

Dowling N E (1998a), 'Fatigue of materials: introduction and stress-based approach', in *Mechanical Behavior of Materials*, Prentice Hall, Upper Saddle River, NJ, 357–419.

Dowling N E (1998b), 'Hardness', in *Mechanical Behavior of Materials*, Prentice Hall, Upper Saddle River, NJ, 139–48.

Dowling N E (1998c), 'Mechanical testing: tension test and other basic tests', in *Mechanical Behavior of Materials*, Prentice Hall, Upper Saddle River, NJ, 102–65.

Fell J T and Newton J M (1970), 'Determination of tablet strength by the diametral-compression test', *J Pharm Sci*, **59**, 688–91.

Ferry J D (1980), *Viscoelastic Properties of Polymers,* 3rd edition, John Wiley & Sons, New York.

Hallab N J, Jacobs J J and Katz J L (2004), 'Application of materials in medicine, biology, and artificial organs: orthopedic applications', in Ratner B D, Hoffman A S, Schoen F J and Lemons J E (eds), *Biomaterials Science*, Elsevier, London, 527–55.

Hamamoto N, Hamamoto Y, Nakajima T and Ozawa H (1995), 'Histological, histocytochemical and ultrastructural study on the effects of surface charge on bone formation in the rabbit mandible', *Arch Oral Biol*, **40**, 97–106.

Hanker J S and Giammara B L (1988), 'Biomaterials and biomedical devices', *Science*, **242**, 885–92.

Hayakawa S, Tsuru K and Osaka A (2008), 'The microstructure of bioceramics and its analysis', in Kokubo T, *Bioceramics and their Clinical Applications*, Woodhead, Cambridge, UK, 53–77.

Hench L L, Splinter R J, Allen W C and Greenlee T K (1971), 'Bonding mechanisms at the interface of ceramic prosthetic materials', *J Biomed Mater Res*, **2**, 117–41.

Hollinger J O and Schmitz J P (1997), 'Macrophysiologic roles of a delivery system for vulnerary factors needed for bone regeneration', *Ann New York Acad Sci*, **831**, 427–37.

Jacobs J J, Roebuck K A, Archibeck M, Hallab N J and Glant T T (2001), 'Osteolysis: basic science', *Clin Orthop Rel Res*, **393**, 71–7.

Jasty M, Rubash H E and Paiement G D (1992), 'Porous-coated uncemented components in experimental total hip arthroplasty in dogs. Effect of plasma-sprayed calcium phosphate coatings on bone ingrowth', *Clin Orthop Rel Res*, **280**, 300–9.

Kokubo T, ed. (2008), *Bioceramics and Their Clinical Applications*, Woodhead, Cambridge, UK.

Krukowski M, Shively R A, Osdoby P and Eppley B L (1990), 'Stimulation of craniofacial and intramedullary bone formation by negatively charged beads', *J Oral Maxillofac Surg*, **48**, 468–75.

Larsson C, Thomsen P and Lausmaa J (1994), 'Bone response to surface modified titanium implants: studies on electropolished implants with different oxide thicknesses and morphology', *Biomater*, **15**, 1062–74.

Lee W E and Rainforth W M (1994), 'General influence of microstructure on ceramic properties', in *Ceramic Microstructures: Property Control by Processing*, Chapman & Hall, London, 67–123.

Lemons J E, Venugopalan R and Lucas L C (1999), 'Corrosion and biodegradation', in von Recum A F, *Handbook of Biomaterials Evaluation: Scientific, Technical and Clinical Testing of Implant Materials,* 2nd edition, Taylor & Francis, London, 155–70.

Lowell S, Shields J E, Thomas M A and Thommes M (2006a), 'Adsorption mechanisms', in *Characterization of Porous Solids and Powders: Surface Area, Pore Size and Density*, Springer, Dordrecht, Netherlands, 15–57.

Lowell S, Shields J E, Thomas M A and Thommes M (2006b), 'Density measurement', in *Characterization of Porous Solids and Powders: Surface Area, Pore Size and Density*, Springer, Dordrecht, Netherlands, 326–38.

Lowell S, Shields J E, Thomas M A and Thommes M (2006c), 'Pore size and surface characteristics of porous solids by mercury porosimetry', in *Characterization of Porous Solids and Powders: Surface Area, Pore Size and Density*, Springer, Dordrecht, Netherlands, 189–212.

Lu Z and McKellop H (1997), 'Frictional heating of bearing materials tested in a hip joint wear simulator', *Proc Inst Mech Eng Part H – J Eng in Med*, **211**, 101–8.

Ludema K C (1996), 'Friction', in *Friction Wear Lubrication: A Textbook in Tribology*, CRC Press, Boca Raton, FL, 69–110.

Munz D and Fett T (2001), 'Fracture Mechanics', in *Ceramics: Mechanical Properties, Failure Behaviour, Materials Selection*, Springer, New York, 19–52.

Placko H E, Brown S A and Payer J H (1998), 'Effects of microstructure on the corrosion behavior of CoCr porous coatings on orthopedic implants', *J Biomed Mater Res*, **39**, 292–9.

Porter A E, Patel N, Skepper J N, Best S M and Bonfield W (2003), 'Comparison of *in vivo* dissolution processes in hydroxyapatite and silicon-substituted hydroxyapatite bioceramics', *Biomater*, **24**, 4609–20.

Ratner B D (2004), 'Properties of materials: surface properties and surface characterization of materials', in Ratner B D, Hoffman A S, Schoen F J and Lemons J E (eds), *Biomaterials Science*, Elsevier, London, 40–59.

Ratner B D, Hoffman A S, Schoen F J and Lemons J E, eds. (2004), *Biomaterials Science*, 2nd edition, Elsevier, London.

Stuart B H (2004), *Infrared Spectroscopy: Fundamentals and Applications*, England, John Wiley & Sons, Chichester, UK.

Takaki S, Kawasaki K and Kimura Y (2001), 'Mechanical properties of ultra fine grained steels', *J Mater Proc Technol*, **117**, 359–63.

Wachtman J B (1996a), 'Measurements of elasticity, strength, and stress intensity factors', in *Mechanical Properties of Ceramics*, John Wiley & Sons, New York, 65–88.

Wachtman J B (1996b), 'Statistical treatment of strength', in *Mechanical Properties of Ceramics*, John Wiley & Sons, New York, 89–116.

Wang A (2001), 'A unified theory of wear for ultra-high molecular weight polyethylene in multi-directional sliding', *Wear*, **248**, 38–47.

Wang X T, Padture N P, Tanaka H and Ortiz A L (2005), 'Wear resistant ultra-fine-grained ceramics', *Acta Mater*, **53**, 271–7.

White A A, Best S M and Kinloch I A (2007), 'Hydroxyapatite-carbon nanotube composites for biomedical applications: a review', *Intl J Appl Ceram Technol*, **4**, 1–13.

Will G (2006), *Powder Diffraction: the Rietveld Method and the Two Stage Method to Determine and Refine Crystal Structures from Powder Diffraction Data*, Springer, Berlin.

Williams R T and Bause D E (1996), 'Elemental and chemical analysis', in Sibilia J P (ed), *A Guide to Materials Characterization and Chemical Analysis*, John Wiley & Sons, New York, 115–42.

6 Metals as bone repair materials

J. L. GONZÁLEZ-CARRASCO, Centro Nacional de Investigaciones Metalúrgicas (CENIM-CSIC) and CIBER-BBN, Spain

Abstract: Metals are the materials of choice for many structural implantable device applications and there is no reason to expect a change in the short or medium term. Processing-structure relations are described with special emphasis on Ti and Ti-base alloys, austenitic stainless steel and Co-based alloys, but other metallic materials in use are also presented. Mechanical properties and their relationship with the microstructure are summarized for static and dynamic loads. Chemical properties focus on corrosion behaviour, the nature of the passive films and the closely related ion release. Surface energy and surface charges, which are relevant for understanding the biological response, are also discussed. A detailed overview of the new family of Ti-base alloys with a lower Young's modulus, Ni-free Fe-based alloys, nanostructured alloys, biodegradable alloys and porous metals for the fabrication of scaffolds, is presented.

Key words: biodegradable alloys, Co-based alloys, corrosion behaviour, magnetic metallic materials, mechanical properties, metallic scaffolds, Ni-free alloys, shape memory alloys, stainless steels, Ti-base alloys, trends in metallic biomaterials.

6.1 Introduction

Materials in use within the body cover a wide spectrum, with examples of metals, ceramics, glasses, polymers and composites. Physical, chemical and mechanical characteristics make some materials more desirable than others.

The low Young's modulus and the viscoelastic nature of synthetic polymers often caused them to be excluded from load-bearing applications. Furthermore, it is very difficult to obtain medical grade polymers free of additives. The release of these additives under physiological constraints may lead to toxic or allergic processes.

Ceramics have been recognized as biomaterials particularly because of their good biocompatibility. Monolithic ceramics, however, are inherently brittle and fabrication is constricted, especially when considering recent improvements in prosthesis design. The inherent brittleness tends to limit their applications to devices where the loads are predominantly compressive in nature or as coatings.

Metals and their alloys are the biomaterials of choice as cyclic load-bearing implants because they combine a high mechanical strength with high fracture toughness.[1–3] Typical examples of highly loaded implants are hip and knee endoprosthesis, plates, screws, nails, and (Fig. 6.1). Besides orthopaedics, there are other markets, including oral and maxillofacial surgery. Metallic biomaterials are also used for unloaded components obviously not related to bone replacement/repair devices. The main limitation of metallic biomaterials is the release of toxic metallic elements, driven by corrosion that can lead to a variety of adverse tissue reactions and/or hypersensitivity reactions.

The objective of this chapter is to describe the composition, microstructure and properties of metallic biomaterials with a major emphasis on those widely used for bone replacement. Common metallic biomaterials used for loaded components are austenitic stainless steels, cobalt base alloys and titanium base alloys. The main advantages, disadvantages, and primary uses of these materials are listed in Table 6.1. In use since 1930, stainless steels still represent about 90% of osteosynthesis devices. They combine good mechanical properties with a reasonable biocompatibility. They are popular because they are easy to machine and less expensive than other metallic biomaterials. Cobalt base alloys are widely used for heavily loaded joints (wrought products) because of the excellent compromise between their various characteristics, such as intrinsic mechanical strength and wear resistance. Chromium is a major component (>18 wt%) that provides both austenitic steels and cobalt base alloys with a high stability against a variety of different forms of corrosion.

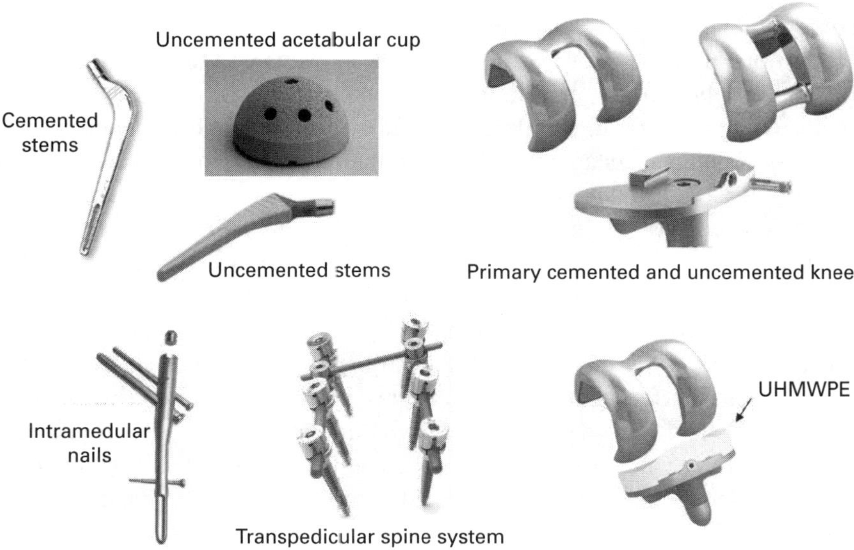

6.1 Photography showing different metallic prosthesis components (courtesy of Surgival SA, Spain). UHMWPE = ultra high molecular weight polyethylene.

Table 6.1 Main characteristics of orthopaedic metallic implant materials

	Advantages	Disadvantages	Primary uses
Stainless steels	Low cost; availability of processing	High modulus	Temporary devices (plates, screws) and hip stems
Co-base alloys	Wear resistance; corrosion; resistance; fatigue strength	High modulus; availability	Dentistry castings; hip and knee joints
Ti and Ti-base alloys	Biocompatibility; corrosion; fatigue strength; low modulus; low density	Wear resistance; low shear strength	Modular total hip replacement (THR) (stems); dental implants; maxillofacial and craniofacial implants; permanent devices (nails, pacemaker cases); fixation elements (screws, staples)

Titanium alloys were developed in the 1950s for aerospace applications but it was not until the 1960s they were used as surgical implant materials. Nowadays, about 2% of the total production of titanium tonnage is used for biomedical applications. Their attractiveness is primarily based on an excellent combination of corrosion resistance, biocompatibility, osseointegration and biofuntionality. Their low wear resistance, however, is the limiting factor for their application in articulating components.

The driving force in the development of new metallic biomaterials for surgical implants is an ageing population that demands implants with both a longer service life and greater reliability. The success of new designs depends upon knowledge of the properties that determine the interactions with living tissues, without the need for trial and error. Nowadays it is accepted that biocompatibility strongly depends on the interactions between the implant surface and physiological environment which can be extremely hostile and sensitive. Therefore, the physicochemical properties of the implant surface are relevant. Surface parameters that have been demonstrated to play an important role for *in vitro* and *in vivo* biocompatibility are frequently grouped in three categories: geometrical, chemical and electrical. Geometrical properties (roughness, topography) are related to the surface finishing or to surface modification techniques and, therefore, are out of the scope of this chapter. Electrical and chemical properties are related to properties of the passive films developed on the surface that obviously are linked to chemical composition of the bulk.

6.2 Common metallic biomaterials

6.2.1 Austenitic stainless steels

The first stainless steel utilized for fabrication of implants was developed in 1926 by Krupp (Essen-Germany). It contained 18% chromium and 8% nickel and became popular as 18-8 (type 302 in modern classification). The key function of chromium is to allow the formation of a protective Cr-rich passive film on the surface. Later some molybdenum was added to improve the pitting corrosion resistance. It was called 18-8Mo and became later type 316 stainless steel. With the introduction of vacuum technology in 1950, it was possible to reduce the carbon content from 0.08 to about 0.03 wt% maximum, yielding an increase in the corrosion resistance. The main rationale for addition of nickel, in the range 9–15 wt%, is to ensure an austenitic state at room temperature for the high chromium content used. Compositions of this and other alloys are listed in Table 6.2.

Nowadays, about 1% of the total production of stainless steel is used for biomedical applications. Surgical and dental instruments are manufactured from commercial-grade stainless steel. However, for implant-grade stainless steels, special production routes such as vacuum melting (VM), vacuum arc remelting (VAR) or electroslag refining (ESR) are used to increase the resistance to pitting and crevice corrosion, as well as to decrease quantity and size of the non-metallic inclusions. Austenitic stainless steels constitute the largest stainless steel family in terms of number of alloys and use. They are popular because are relatively inexpensive, easy to machine using common techniques and their mechanical properties can be controlled over a wide range for optimal strength and ductility.

Vacuum melted 316L stainless steel remains the most widely used stainless steel for implant devices. They find applications mostly as bone screws, bone plates, intramedullary nails and rods and other temporary fixation devices. The microstructure consists of austenite with a single face-centered cubic (fcc) structure called the γ phase. The ferrite, α phase with a body-centered cubic (bcc) structure, should not be present, not only from the standpoint of its corrosion resistance but also because of its ferromagnetic behaviour. Sulphide inclusions predispose the steel to pitting-type corrosion at the metal–inclusion interface and, therefore, their presence must be also avoided. Passivation treatments applied at the last moment of the fabrication of the components are used to remove inclusions emerging at the surface. The recommended grain size is ASTM No. 6 (< 100 μm) or finer. Another feature of the microstructure is the texture as the result of a preferred orientation of deformed grains. Figure 6.2 shows a typical micrograph of the 316 LVM steel in the cold worked and aged condition. Within the grains, thermal twins that developed during ageing are observed.

The austenitic stainless steels work-harden very rapidly and therefore

Table 6.2 Chemical compositions of common metallic biomaterials used for implantable devices

	ASTM designation	Cr	Ni	Mo	Al	V	W	Mn	C	0	N	Fe	Co	Ti
316L	F138	17–19	13–15	2.2–3				2	0.03		0.10	Bal.		
CoCr (as cast)	F 75	27–30	1	5–7			–		0.35				Bal.	–
	F90	19–21	9–11				14–16	1–2	0.05–0.15			3	Bal.	
CoCr (as wrought)	F562	19–21	33–37	9–10.5			–	0.15	0.025			1	Bal.	1
Cp-Ti	F67	–	–	–			–	–	0.08	0.2–0.4	0.03–0.05	0.2–0.5		Bal.
Ti-6Al-4V	F136	–	–	–	5.5–6.5	3.5–4.5			0.08	0.13	0.05	0.25		Bal.

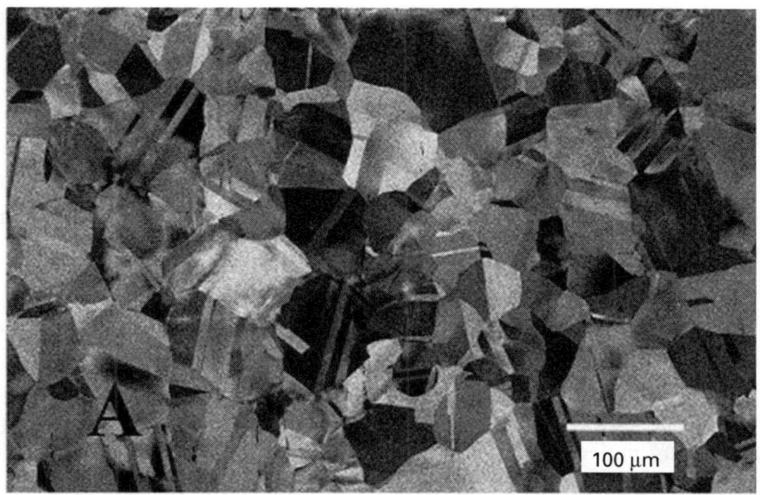

6.2 Backscattered electron image revealing the grain size of a non etched section of 316 L (courtesy of M. Multigner, CENIM).

cannot be cold worked without intermediate heat treatments. However, such heat treatments should not induce the formation of chromium carbide at the grain boundaries which may decrease the corrosion resistance.

6.2.2 Co-based alloys

There are two types of CoCr alloys extensively used in implant fabrications such as the knee and hip. The castable CoCrMo alloy known as 'Vitallium' was formerly introduced by Venable and Stucke in 1936.[4] This alloy has been used for many decades in dentistry too. The second group of alloys is processed by hot forging (wrought alloys) and contains tungsten and a higher nickel content. The two basic elements of the CoCr alloys form a solid solution of up to 65% Co. Although a number of specifications exist for cobalt-base alloys, the main alloys used are Co-28Cr-6Mo cast alloy (ASTM F 75), Co-20Cr-15W-10Ni wrought alloy (ASTM F 90) and Co-35Ni-20Cr-10Mo (ASTM F562).

The cast alloys contain up to 0.5 wt% carbon to improve the castability by lowering the melting temperature to ~1350°C. The normal fabrication involves a lost wax method by using a wax pattern of the desired component. The chromium enhances the corrosion resistance as well as the strength of the alloy. The molybdenum is added to produce finer grains, which results in higher strengths for both cast and wrought components. The microstructure of the cast products consist of a cobalt-rich matrix (α phase) with an fcc structure. Strengthening is produced by a solid solution of alloying elements and precipitation of carbides ($M_{23}C_6$, M_7C_3, M_6C, where M= Co, Cr or Mo). There can also be interdendritic Co- and Mo-rich sigma intermetallics. Overall, the volume fractions of alpha and carbide phases are about 85% and 15%, respectively. In the as-cast products, however, segregation during cooling and a coarse grain size (~ 4 mm) structure that can strongly influence implant properties, often negatively, cannot be avoided. Powder metallurgical techniques, such as hot isostatic pressing (HIP), are used to enhance the mechanical properties by improving the microstructure of the alloy (grain size of about ~ 8 μm). The associated finer distribution of carbides has a hardening effect as well.

Wrought alloys have a lower Cr content (19–21 wt%) and higher levels of Ni, Fe or Mn to stabilize the fcc phase in the annealed condition. Further mechanical deformation (about 50% cold working) causes the transformation to a hexagonal close-packed (hcp) phase that forms via a shear-induced martensitic-type transformation. In this condition the microstructure consists of a fcc matrix with fine hcp platelets, which causes an improvement in the mechanical properties. Additional hardening may be obtained by precipitation of Co_3Mo carbides on the hcp platelets during ageing between 500 and 600°C. The superior mechanical properties of the wrought CoNiCrMo alloy make it suitable for the fabrication of stems for hip joint prostheses.

6.2.3 Ti and Ti-base alloys

Attempts to use titanium for implant fabrication date back to the late 1930s. Titanium has a low density (4.5 g cm^{-3}) and can be greatly strengthened by alloying and thermomechanical processing techniques. Owing to their high reactivity in the presence of oxygen, an inert atmosphere or vacuum is required during high temperature processing. Commercially pure titanium (CP-Ti) is essentially α titanium (hcp crystal structure) and is available in four grades. The primary difference between grades is the oxygen and iron content. Oxygen in particular has a great influence on ductility and strength. These materials also contain hydrogen (0.015 wt%) and carbon (0.08 wt%). CP-Ti is selected for its excellent corrosion resistance, especially in applications where high strength is not required. Depending on the cold working conditions, grain diameters in the range 10–150 μm are obtained.

Pure titanium undergoes a phase transformation, changing with increasing temperature from an hexagonal close packed (hcp) structure, called the α phase, to a body-centered cubic (bcc) structure, referred to as the β phase. The transition temperature takes place at around 885°C. Below the β-transus temperature, diffusion processes are substantially slower. The completion of transformation on heating to β is strongly influenced by elements stabilizing the α phase (like O, Al, N, C), raising the transition temperature, or the β phase (like V, Nb, Mo, Ta), lowering the transition temperature. At high cooling rates from temperatures above the martensite start (Ms) temperature, the β phase transforms into the α phase by a diffusionless transformation mechanism, leaving behind a metastable microstructure. The martensite can be further split into hexagonal α′-martensite and orthorhombic α″-martensite if quenching takes place below about 900°C. The existence of these phase transformations and their dependence on the alloy composition form the basis for the classification of the Ti-base alloys, as schematically illustrated in Fig. 6.3. Depending on their microstructure, commercial titanium alloys are classified into three groups: α, α+β and β alloys. There is further subdivision into near-α, which have a minor fraction of β-stabilizing elements, and metastable β alloys, for which β no longer transforms to martensite upon fast quenching. The α+β alloys, the most widely used alloy group, have a β volume fraction at room temperature in the range of 5–40%.

The continuous increase in the use of pure titanium and Ti-6Al-4V (α+β), particularly the extra-low interstitial variant (ELI), when compared to conventional stainless steels and cobalt base alloys results from their lower modulus, superior biocompatibility and enhanced corrosion resistance. Ti-6Al-7Nb and Ti-5Al-2.5Fe are metallurgically quite similar to Ti-6Al-4V. They were the first alloys specifically developed for the biomaterials field eliminating the vanadium, which is considered a toxic element in terms of its biocompatibility.

Ti-6Al-4V is a biphasic (α+β) alloy available in wrought, cast and powder metallurgy (PM) forms. The processing history (heat treatments, mechanical

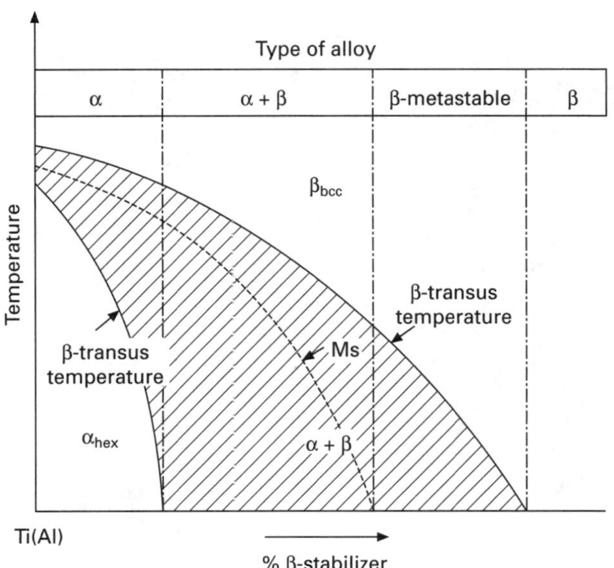

6.3 Schematic phase diagram for Ti alloys showing their classification.

working) and the interstitial (primarily oxygen) content determine the volume fractions of the α and β phases. The β phase is stable at room temperature only if the vanadium content is greater than 15%. When slowly cooled, the alloy may contain up to about 90 vol% of the α phase. This phase precipitates as plates or needles which have a specific crystallographic orientation within grains of the β matrix. Depending on the phase morphology, the microstructures are classified into three categories: lamellar, equiaxed or bimodal (a mixture of both).

Lamellar structures are obtained by heat treatments. Slow cooling at the furnace from the β phase field allows precipitation of the α phase at the β-grain boundaries forming plates that grow towards the grain interior, as can be seen in Fig. 6.4. The resulting lamellar structure is fairly coarse. Higher cooling rates, for instance in air, give rise to a microstructure consisting of a fine needle-like α phase referred to as acicular. At intermediate cooling rates, Widmanstätten structures are obtained. Finer lamellar structures can be obtained by water quenching the alloy from the β-transus temperature followed by annealing at intermediate temperatures in the biphasic region. Quenching from temperatures higher than 900°C results in an acicular or sometimes fine-lamellar hcp martensite (α′), while quenching from the 750–900°C temperature range produces an orthorhombic martensite (α″) that is a rather soft martensite. This phase can also form as a stress-induced product by straining metastable β.

Equiaxed microstructures are obtained by applying a severe deformation (>75% reduction) to the alloy in the biphasic condition and subsequent

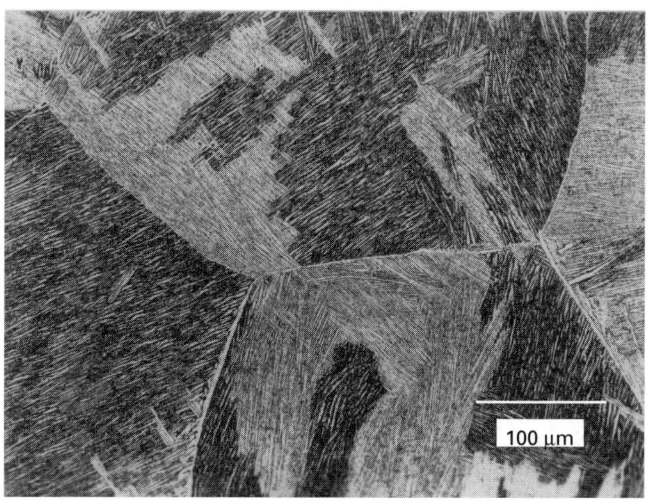

6.4 Optical micrograph showing the microstructure of the Ti-6Al-4V alloy annealed at 1100°C for 2 hours, then slowly cooled within the furnace (courtesy of J. Chao, CENIM).

annealing below the β transus temperature between 480 and 650°C. The resulting microstructure, so-called mild annealed, strongly depends upon the previous working. Figure 6.5 illustrates the typical biphasic microstructure consisting of bright (β phase) and dark (α phase) zones.

Bimodal microstructure consists of isolated primary α grains in a transformed β matrix. This microstructure may be developed by solution treatment below the β transus, typically between 900 and 950°C, followed by air cooling and ageing below 700°C.

6.3 Other metallic materials

6.3.1 NiTi shape memory alloys

In recent years the largest commercial successes of shape memory alloys are linked to medical applications owing to their good corrosion resistance and unique capacity to return to a previous shape when subjected to an appropriate thermal procedure.[5,6] A widely known NiTi alloy is Nitinol (an acronym for NiTi Naval Ordnance Laboratory) that contains about 50 at% Ni and small amounts of Co, Cr, Mn and Fe. The shape memory effect is related to the diffusionless reversible martensitic transformation induced by changes in the temperature, as illustrated in Fig. 6.6. It is characterized by its transition temperatures M_s and M_f which refer to the start and finish of the formation and growth of the low-temperature phase martensite on cooling, and A_s and A_f, which refer to the start and finish of the formation and growth of the high-temperature phase austenite on heating. The overall

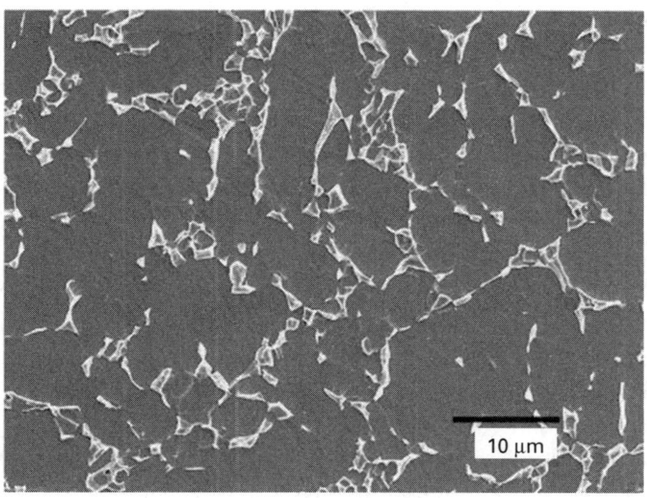

6.5 Secondary electron image revealing the biphasic microstructure in an etched section of Ti-6Al-4V.

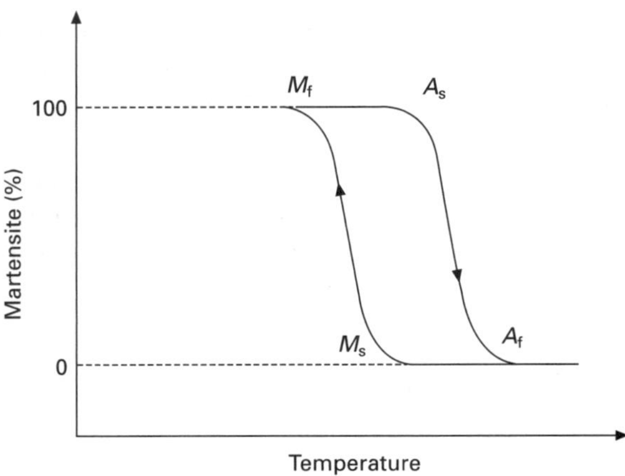

6.6 Schematic representation of the martensite transformed during cooling and heating periods under constant stress.

transformation describes a hysteresis of the order of 10–50°C, although the beginning and end of the transformation during heating and cooling extends over a much larger temperature range.[6] The transformation temperature strongly depends on the Ni content which provides the ability to tailor the properties to a specific application.[7]

Titanium–nickel alloys show unusual properties, that is, if they are deformed below the transformation temperature, they revert back to their original shape as the temperature is raised. The great advantage is that the device can be implanted in an optimal shape and after surgery the desired functional shape is obtained *in situ* by the action of body heat.

A second important property is the ability of the material to recover an apparently plastic strain on loading at a temperature above A_f, as illustrated in Fig. 6.7. The amount of this reversible deformation is much greater (~ 8–10%) than the conventional elastic strain (< 0.2 %). If deformed above M_s but below A_f, some strain-induced martensite will remain stable, leading to an incomplete shape restoration. This pseudoelasticity or superelasticity is also closely related to the martensitic phase transformation, which is also thermoelastic in nature. It is worth remarking that once the critical stress is reached, the sample will start to transform to martensite. During further straining, the stress is almost constant until the austenite is fully transformed. The temperature dependent character of the superelastic effect is of less importance because of the stable temperature of the human body.

The martensitic transformation in Nitinol causes an abrupt change in the Young's modulus E and yield stress (see Table 6.4). When changing shape, the alloys can recover substantial amounts of strain or generate a force as a consequence of variations in the body temperature, which has triggered a number of commercial applications. In the field of orthopaedics, applications

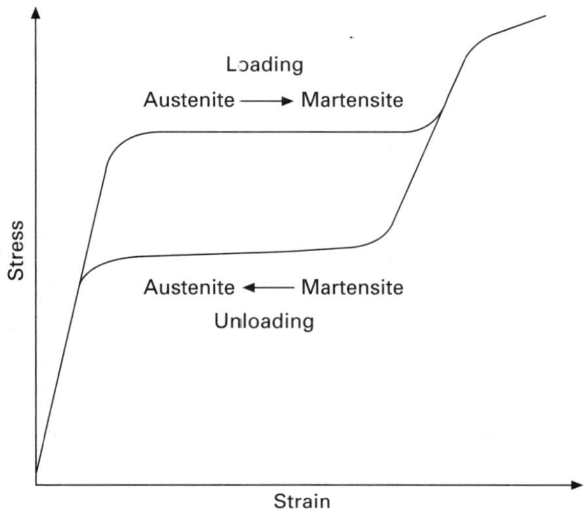

6.7 Schematic representation of stress induced martensite transformation at constant temperature.

extend from bone anchors to a variety of devices for osteosynthesis bone staples.

The potential release of Ni has been the driving force for great activity in its surface modification. Thermal oxidation of the alloy, performed under low oxygen partial pressure, leads to the formation of a pure stochiometric TiO_2 on the surface.[8] This layer improves the electrochemical corrosion resistance of the alloy by increasing the breakdown potential and decreasing the maximum current density and Ni ion release and, therefore, may avoid toxic reactions associated with Ni.[9] A critical overview of Nitinol surfaces and their modifications for medical applications has been recently published.[10]

6.3.2 Zirconium alloys

Zr-2.5% Nb is a biocompatible, high-strength alloy that possesses an elastic modulus of 100 GPa. Thermal oxidation of the alloy under dry oxygen flow at temperatures near the eutectoid temperature (590–700°C) for a few hours gives rise to the formation of an outer zirconia layer of about 5 μm in thickness. The resulting monoclinic zirconia surface contains grains that are 40 nm wide and 200 nm long, arranged in a brick work pattern that is resistant to grain pull out and lateral fracture.[11] The oxidized alloy material, which combines the abrasion resistance of ceramics with the toughness of metals, was recently introduced commercially for knee arthroplasty components.[12] The thermally oxidized alloy is burnished to create a smooth bearing surface. In this condition the material shows excellent wear behaviour against polyethylene components, with reduced wear particle generation.[13]

The UHMWPE cups articulating with smooth OxZr heads showed a 45% wear reduction in comparison with CoCr heads under identical conditions. Moreover, particle analysis of UHMWPE wear debris showed significantly fewer particles.

6.3.3 Tantalum

Tantalum has an excellent corrosion resistance,[14] being among the most biocompatible metals used for implantable devices.[15] The high density (16.6 g cm^{-3}) and its poor mechanical properties preclude its use for the fabrication of large components, however, it provides excellent fluoroscopic visibility. Tantalum has been used successfully in sheets and plates for cranioplasty and reconstructive surgery. Recently, tantalum has gained interest for the fabrication of scaffolds for bone ingrowth.

6.3.4 Magnetic materials

The magnetic field application in orthopaedics attracts the interest of scientists and clinicians. Both static magnetic fields and pulsed electromagnetic fields are used in combination with or without metallic magnetic materials implanted into the body. In this sense, many medical applications range from their simple use for retention, through maxillofacial, orthopaedics and fracture healing, helping to maintain stability of joints like the elbow or shoulder.

A ferromagnetic material may be either hard, which means that once magnetized it retains its magnetization even in the absence of magnetic fields, that is a permanent magnet, or soft, meaning it is easy to magnetize or demagnetize. An overview of their applications in medicine can be found elsewhere.[16] Among hard magnetic materials are the modern permanent magnets based on intermetallic compounds of rare earths and 3*d* transition metals with very high magnetocrystalline anisotropy, such as $Nd_2Fe_{14}B$ and $SmCo_5$. Typical examples of soft ferromagnetic materials are ferritic stainless steels and Fe–Pt alloys. However, Fe–Pt alloys have both soft (< 39.5 at% Pt) and hard (> 39.5 at% Pt) magnetic properties and can be used for the fabrication of castable devices. In this system, the relatively large Pt content makes them corrosion resistant.[17]

One of the main advantages of magnetic materials is that they allow the application of forces *in situ* without physical contact. With regard to bone growth, it is worth mentioning the use of magnetic materials in distraction devices which are implanted in young patients diagnosed with bone tumour, who have not completed their growth at the time of surgery. When the patient grows, the implant is extended by activating a magnetic force. The lengthening procedures, which do not require additional surgery, enable the patient to reach skeletal maturity with no or very minimal leg length discrepancy

(Stanmore Implants Worldwide Limited and Birmag prosthesis). Figure 6.8 shows the growth module of the Stanmore Implants Worldwide Limited JTS® prosthesis. An external rotating magnetic field interacts with a powerful magnet mounted inside the prosthesis, causing it to rotate in synchronization. This generates a very small torque. The torque is then amplified through a gearbox driving a power screw and telescoping the prosthesis at a rate of 1 mm in 4 minutes. During extending procedures, the patients reported no discomfort, no sensation and no noise. These devices eliminated the risk of infection of traditional devices caused by the pins connecting the bone with the external pieces.

Another common use of magnetic materials is in dentistry for prosthodontic and orthodontic applications.[18] A common application is the retention of implant-supported overdentures or maxillofacial prostheses. Magnetic attachments investigated for dental appliances consist of a magnet combined with a yoke cap and its keeper.[17, 19] The magnetic force would be proportional to the magnetic field of the magnet and the saturation magnetization of the soft ferromagnetic material. Not only excellent magnets but also soft magnetic stainless steel with high corrosion resistance could be developed for such magnetic attachments. In high-purity ferritic stainless steels, chromium added to improve the corrosion resistance decreases the saturation magnetization. According to Takada and Okuno[20] chromium contents below 17% might limit their use in dental magnetic attachments. PM2000, namely (wt%) 20Cr-5Al-0.5Y_2O_3 balance Fe is a ferritic commercial alloy obtained by powder metallurgy that has being investigated for potential applications as a biomaterial.[21] It has been shown that PM2000 is a soft magnetic material with a saturation magnetization of about 135 emu g^{-1}. The higher iron content of the alloy does not compromise the good corrosion behaviour, especially when coated with alumina by thermal oxidation for which a superior *in vitro* corrosion resistance has been reported.[22]

The ferromagnetic character will obviously prohibit the use of medical control techniques based on strong magnetic fields,[23] primarily because of the risks associated with their movement or dislodgment, as happens with patients wearing, for instance, cardiac pacemakers, electrical implants, prosthetic cardiac valves, aneurysm clips or simply rejected by discomfort.

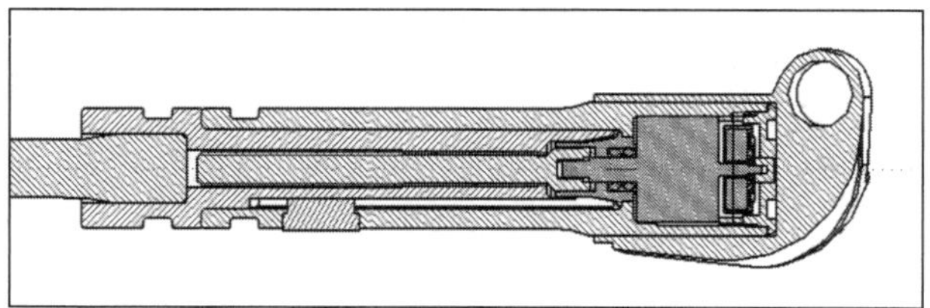

6.8 Growth module of Stanmore prosthesis (courtesy of Stanmore Implants Worldwide Limited JTS).

6.4 Properties

6.4.1 Mechanical properties

The mechanical properties of the alloy will determine its capability for use in the fabrication of load-bearing components. In addition to the chemical composition and impurities of the alloy, mechanical properties are strongly dependent on its microstructure (grain size, texture, amount and distribution of phases). Variations in the processing conditions (thermal treatments, thermomechanical processing, surface treatments) may lead to differences in the microstructure that are also manifested in the mechanical properties of the bulk.[24] Therefore, properties can vary from one product to another and often mechanical properties are only valid for a certain range of products and dimensions. Table 6.3 summarizes the microstructural features of common metallic alloys that are relevant for their mechanical properties. The relevance of a fine grain size is explained by the relationship between yield stress and grain diameter given by the Hall–Petch expression.[25,26] From this expression it follows that for a given composition higher yield stresses may be achieved by a metal with a smaller grain diameter. The preferred orientation of deformed grains, that is the crystallographic texture, may also be a notable feature influencing the mechanical properties. A summary of the relevant mechanical properties is provided in Table 6.4.[1–3, 27–29] For comparative purposes values for cortical bone are also included. From the above considerations it follows that the table should only be taken as a general guide.

Mechanical properties of austenitic stainless steels are strongly dependent on the cold work applied during processing, it being possible to harden the alloy by applying up to about 60% of cold deformation. For instance, the 30% cold worked steel may present a twofold increase in the yield strength relative to the annealed state. The presence of ferrite and carbides are considered to be defects.

Table 6.3 Microstructural features of common metallic alloys relevant to their mechanical properties

	Major phases and crystalline structure	Other possible phases	Average grain size
316LVM	γ (fcc)	Ferrite and carbides	< 100 mm
CoCr cast alloy	fcc	Carbides (~ 15%)	~ 4 mm
CoCr wrought	fcc + hcp	Carbides	< 0.1 mm
Ti-6Al-4V	α (hcp) and up to 10% β (bcc)		15–20 mm

Table 6.4 Characteristic mechanical properties of various metallic biomaterials compiled from different sources. na = data is not available

	Density (g cm^{-3})	$\sigma_{C.2}$ (MPa)	σ (MPa)	Young's modulus E (GPa)	Fatigue limit	Toughness (MPa$\sqrt{m}$)
Ta	16.6	138–345	205–515	185–190	na	na
316 L	7.9	172–690	485–860	190–200	241–820	100
CoCrMo	8.4	450–648	655–860	210–230	207–310	100
CoNiCrMo	9.2	240–1585	793–1793		586–793	
Ti	4.5	170–485	240–760	105	300–430	na
Ti-6Al-4V	4.4	760–895	900–970	110	500–689	80
β Ti-alloys		530–1060	590–1310	55–100	na	na
NiTi austenitic	6.7	100–800	800–1500	70–110	350	na
NiTi martensitic		50–300	100–1100	21–69		na
Mg alloys	1.7–2	100–200	220–290	45	na	28
Al_2O_3		–	280–550	380	na	4.2–5.9
Cortical bone	1.8–2.1	–	50–150	7–30	na	2–12

Cast Co-base alloys usually have large grain sizes (~ 4 mm) and undesirable defects like inclusions and micropores that impair their mechanical properties. Wrought Co-base alloys are multiphasic and hardening derives from the combination of cold working, grain size refinement (~ 8 μm), solid solution hardening and carbide precipitation (up to 15%). The resulting mechanical properties make the alloys among the strongest available for implant applications.

Commercially pure titanium has a relative low strength and high ductility. Cold working (around 30 %) is used to enhance mechanical properties. Differences in yield strength between the different grades result from variations in the interstitial and impurity level. Similarly, for a given grain size, fatigue strengths are also increased with higher levels of oxygen.[30]

Mechanical properties of Ti-6Al-4V are affected by the processing and oxygen content. Solution treatments and further ageing can increase the strength of α+β alloys by 30–50% over the annealed condition. Equiaxed microstructures provide high strength and ductility and relatively low fracture toughness, whereas a lamellar structure provides good fracture toughness but with some compromise on strength and ductility.[31] With regard to the high cycle fatigue, the bimodal microstructure provides the highest value followed by the equiaxed structure, with the lamellar structure having the lowest fatigue resistance. In addition, for a given microstructure, finer microstructures result in higher cycle fatigue strength.[32] With regard to their biofunctionality value, which is given by the ratio of the fatigue strength over the Young's modulus, titanium and its alloys demonstrate their superiority.

One of the major problems in orthopaedic surgery is the large mismatch of the Young's modulus between the bone and the metallic implant. Assuming that the system bone/metal is rigid and has an isoelastic behaviour, for a given strain, the amount of stress carried out by the bone will be lower, as illustrated in Fig. 6.9. This phenomenon, so-called 'stress shielding', affects the bone remodelling and healing process, leading to bone resorption and eventual aseptic loosening. This is particularly a problem with young and more active patients. As deduced from Table 6.4, the stress shielding effect would be more pronounced with austenitic stainless steels and cobalt alloys.

Overall, the mechanical properties of metallic alloys are well above those of natural bone. Here it is worth remarking that bone is a living tissue that has the capability to self repair microdefects generated during the daily activity. Metallic implants, however, have to be over designed since, although loads are rather low, they are cyclic and occasionally very high. Moreover, these stresses fluctuate depending on the daily activity. For instance, during movement, the main load on a femoral head is about twice the body weight. The load varies with the position in the walking cycle and reaches a peak of about four times the body weight at the hip and three times the weight at the knee. Peak loads during jumping can be as high as 10 times body weight. The frequency of loading and load cycles are also important. Typically a person may take one to two million steps per year.[33] Thus, it is not strange that most of the mechanical failures of orthopaedic implants are due to a fatigue mechanism. Often the fatigue failure is associated with design-induced stress concentration.[34] Therefore, fatigue strength becomes relevant for most load-bearing components.

In this sense it is important to note that the presence of defects at the surface produced during machining or at the moment of the surgery may impair fatigue strength, irrespectively of the alloy microstructure. In Fig.

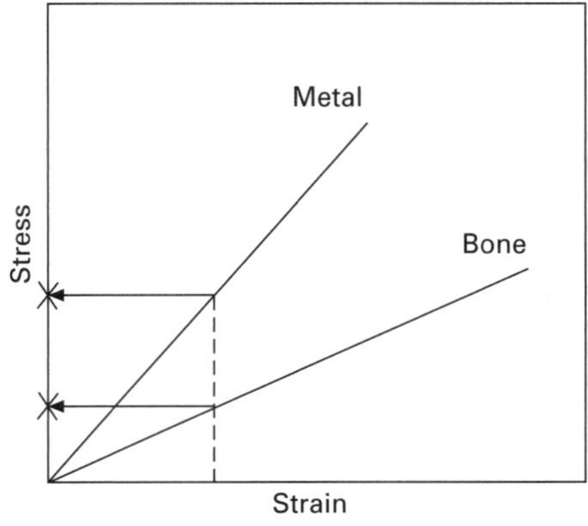

6.9 Schematic representation of the dependence of the stress and elastic strain of a metallic biomaterial and the natural bone.

6.10, it can be seen that the fatigue strength of fine- and coarse-grained Ti-6Al-4V significantly decreases when a notch is present.[34] This decrease is even greater than expected, considering the magnitude (1.95) of the stress concentration factor. The fatigue strength under the notch of the fine grained material is only slightly higher than that of the coarse grained material, which suggests (taking into account the difference in the fatigue limit of unnotched specimens of both microstructures) that the effect of the as-machined notch is more severe in the fine grained material. Viceconti *et al.*, studying a group of hip prostheses with a small systematic machining defect that produced a stress concentration factor of 1.13, which is equivalent to that produced by the notch (1.95), reported a fatigue limit reduction factor of 1.4.[35]

A further consideration concerns the effect of surface treatments on the mechanical properties of the bulk. For instance, efforts to improve the osteointegration, fixation and stability of Ti implants have been addressed by creating a rough surface that increases the surface area available for bone/implant apposition. Particularly important has been the activity for the production of randomly rough surfaces by sandblasting, which is mechanical abrasion of the surface by using oxide particles (mostly SiO_2, ZrO_2, or Al_2O_3) with angular shapes that are shot against the implant. The treatment yields a severe plastic deformation of the surface which causes a roughness increase, whose magnitude depends on size, shape and the kinetic energy of the particles reaching the surface. In addition, the treatment leaves compressive residual stresses with a maximum value close to the surface.[36] This compressive stress state is known to delay crack initiation and/or slow

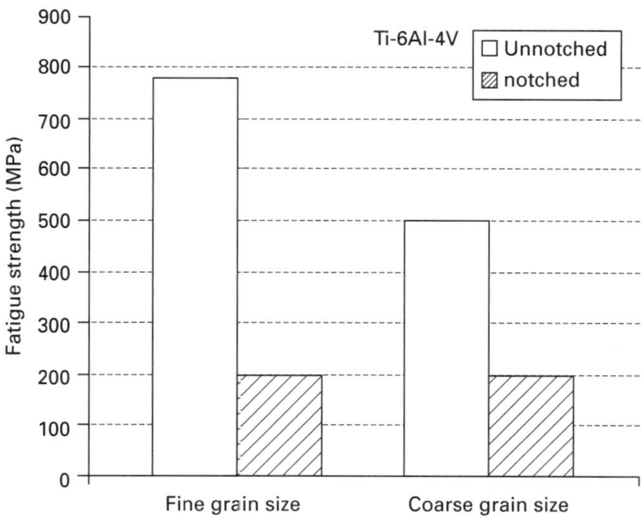

6.10 Fatigue strength of unnotched and notched specimens as a function of microstructure (adapted from Chao and López[34]).

down crack propagation, resulting in an increased fatigue resistance. However, blasting of the Ti-6Al-4V alloy leads to a pronounced decrease in the fatigue strength during either axial or bending fatigue tests, as can be seen in Fig. 6.11.[37] The fatigue limit decreases with increasing roughness, about a 20% decrease for fine blasting (*Ra* ~ 2 μm) and up to about 40% for samples with coarse blasting (*Ra* ~ 7 μm), where *Ra* is the roughness parameter.[38] This fatigue behaviour of sandblasted Ti-6Al-4V is somewhat puzzling since blasting of cp-Ti, causing similar microstructural damage, enhances the fatigue properties.[39]

6.4.2 Chemical properties

Corrosion of metallic biomaterials is undesirable because it may reduce the structural integrity of the implant or it may release products that may be potentially toxic to the host. Additionally, corrosion may interact with other mechanical processes (e.g. fatigue, fretting, wear) causing premature structural failure or accelerating metal ion release. Therefore, the need to ensure minimal corrosion has been a major determining factor in the selection of materials for use in the body environment.

Corrosion is the result of an electrochemical reaction with biological fluids that are very aggressive owing to the presence of chloride ions, although it has recently become apparent that proteins present in extracellular fluids are able to influence the corrosion.[40] Moreover, temporary variations in the normal pH of the body fluids (~7.4 at 37°C) in surgery caused by hematoma (pH ~ 4) or infections (pH ~ 9) make the environment much more aggressive for metals.

Metallic biomaterials are normally considered to be highly corrosion

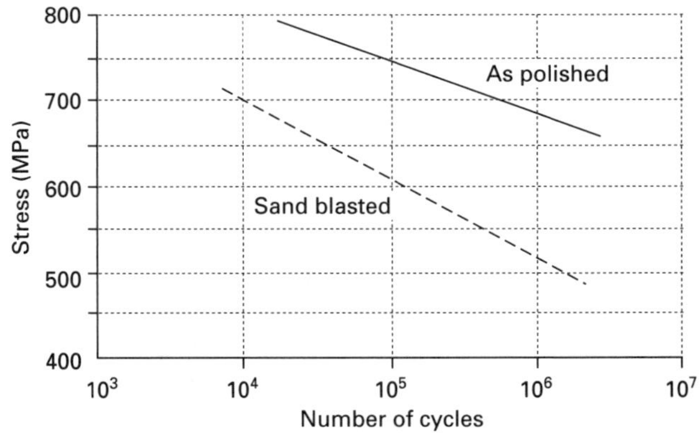

6.11 Stress versus number of cycles for polished and sand blasted Ti-6Al-4V during axial loading in Ringer's solution (adapted from Leinenbach and Eifler[37]).

resistant owing to the presence of an extremely thin passive oxide film (< 7 nm) which spontaneously forms on their surfaces, even in solutions with low oxygen contents, and which serves as a physical barrier against the action of the aggressive fluids. According to Marcus[41] the role of alloying elements in the passivation of alloys is based on the metal–oxygen and the metal–metal bond strengths. Alloying elements with a high energy of adsorption of oxygen and low metal–metal bond energy are predicted to enhance passivity. For instance, the relatively high energy of adsorption of oxygen ($\Delta H_{ads} = 737$ kJ mol^{-1}) and the low Cr–Cr bond strength ($\Delta H_B = 99.1$ kJ mol^{-1}) allow the easy breaking of the metal–metal bond, favouring oxide nucleation. Alloying elements that have a high metal–metal bond strength cause a lowering of the dissolution rate by increasing the activation energy barrier for the disruption of the metal–metal bonds in the alloy surface, thus they are so-called dissolution blockers.

Once the oxide passive film is formed, the corrosion behaviour depends to a large extent on its structure and chemistry, which are themselves dependent on the thermal, mechanical and electrochemical history. Passivation of stainless steel and Co-base alloys lie in the formation of Cr-rich oxide films, whereas Ti-base alloys yield to the formation of outer Ti-rich oxide films. In recent years there has been increasing interest in the nature of the oxide developed on the surface of Ti and Ti-based alloys and its biological significance. It has been shown by Scanning Auger Microscopy that composition of the passive film on the Ti-6Al-7Nb is heterogeneous and reflects the underlying $\alpha+\beta$ microstructure of the substrate.[42] The oxide layer developed on the α phase is enriched in Al by a factor of two, while the oxide above the β phase has a sixfold higher Nb content. These compositional differences were found to point to small variations in surface charges.

The most corrosion-resistant materials are titanium and its alloys, followed by wrought and cast cobalt base alloys. Type 316L is the least corrosion resistant of the implant metals.[43] Passivating steel in a 20–40 vol% nitric acid solution at 60°C for 30 minutes removes surface defects which could serve as pit sites and improves their corrosion behaviour. The same ranking can be observed during the measurement of polarization resistance. Corrosion takes place by several mechanisms that may occur alone (pitting, crevice, galvanic, intergranular) or be assisted by external loads (stress-corrosion cracking, corrosion fatigue and fretting corrosion).[44]

Pitting corrosion refers to a severe form of localized attack that results in the release of significant amounts of metal ions. It is manifested by the presence of cavities at the surface. Pits may be initiated at surface defects in the material or passive film. Their formation is attributed to the interaction of aggressive ions, such as Cl^-, with the passive film. Once the passive film is broken, the forming pit becomes covered by precipitates that restrict the entry of the solution and oxygen into the pit, making repassivation impossible.

To increase the pitting corrosion resistance in a saline environment it is important to keep the inclusion content at the surface to a minimum level.

Crevice corrosion is a form of corrosion related to metal surfaces that are partially shielded from the body fluids. This situation occurs, for instance, at interfaces between different parts of a device (plate and screw) or in the presence of a crevice – a narrow, deep crack. This form of corrosion is particularly important for the type 316 L stainless steel. The problem can often be eliminated by an appropriate design.

Galvanic corrosion takes place when two different metals are in physical contact in the presence of an ionic medium. This situation may occur when the plate and the screw are made of dissimilar alloys. This form of corrosion depends on a large number of factors including the relative areas of contact and the actual metal couple involved.

Intergranular corrosion occurs when the grain boundary becomes anodic or cathodic to the rest of the grains. Microstructural features at grain boundaries that account for this mechanism are the presence of impurities or precipitates that cause near the grain boundaries depletions of elements forming the passive layer.

Stress corrosion is observed when a metal is subjected to a tensile stress in the presence of an aggressive environment. Several mechanisms, including plastic properties of the alloy and selective adsorption of ion species at strained areas, have been shown to be important in this complex interaction.

Corrosion fatigue results from the simultaneous interaction of electrochemical reactions and cyclic loading. The corrosive attack may accentuate imperfections at the surface leading to a decrease in the fatigue strength.

Fretting corrosion occurs when two opposing surfaces rub against each other in the body environment under small amplitude motion. Depending on the intensity of the movement between the contacting surfaces, it may give rise to a large amount of corrosion products that accumulate at the adjacent tissues. The weight loss of the implant is proportional to the load, the number of cycles and the amplitude of stresses, and inversely proportional to the hardness of the material. The repassivation capability of the passive film in case of its damage during surgery or by fretting metal against metal during service (plate/screw system) is also a very important factor. The growth of the passive layer in saline mediums is known to be superior for Ti and its alloys as compared to that of other materials. Nevertheless, for the articulating surfaces of the implants, a coating of hard layers of non-abrasive materials is recommended.

The corrosion process may have a significant influence in the implant/body interaction through the slow flow of ions that could cause an accumulation of metal in the surrounding tissues.[45] Other sources of metal ions may result from mechanical effects under frictional conditions or as a result of electrochemical equilibrium with body fluids. For instance, while the oxides of Al, Cr, Nb, Ta, Ti and V are stable owing to a more negative heat of formation than that of water, the oxides of Co and Ni are unstable because of a less negative heat of formation.[46] The interaction between the oxides forming the passive layer and the body fluid increases with increasing heat of formation of the oxide, resulting in a higher solubility. Consistently, Co-, Fe- and Ni-oxides have a considerable solubility, whereas Ti-oxide is practically insoluble. Experimental determination of the rate of nickel release from the CoNiCrMo alloy and 316L stainless steel in the Ringer's solution reveals that although the cobalt alloy has a greater initial release of nickel ions, the rate of release was about the same (3×10^{-10} g/cm^2/day) for both alloys despite the nickel content for the former alloy being about three times that of austenitic steel.[47]

Recently, it has been reported that austenitic stainless steels show a higher sensitivity to corrosion in cross-sectional specimens (transversal cuts with respect to the rolling direction) and compared to longitudinal sections they release nickel ions at rates 10–100 times higher.[48] The effect is less intense for medical grade steels (ASTM-138) for which a remelting process is added to the standard metallurgical process in order to reduce the inclusion content and notably the sulphur concentration. Its nickel release rate is very low and increases from 0.2 to 0.25 μg cm^{-2} week^{-1} when going from an S_{trans}/S_{long} ratio of 0.2 to 0.25, where S refers to section. The release of nickel increases with cold working (23%), except for the medical grade steels.

6.4.3 Physical surface properties

Because the interactions between cells and tissues with biomaterials at the tissue implant interface are almost exclusively surface phenomena, the surface properties of implant materials are of great importance.[49] Surface parameters are frequently grouped in three categories: geometrical, chemical and physical. Next we will describe the physical properties (surface charge and surface energy) that have been demonstrated to play an important role in *in vitro* biocompatibility.

Surface charges

The first event that takes place soon after implantation of a biomaterial is the adsorption of a monolayer of soluble proteins from physiological fluids that cover the implant. The protein adsorption is selective and depends on the biophysical and biochemical characteristics of the surface, particularly the electrical charges. This protein layer transforms the implant in a biologically recognizable surface through specific receptors located in the cell membrane. The composition of the adsorbed protein layer influences the later cellular behaviour. Thus, if the proteins required for cellular adhesion adsorb on the surface of the implant in a proper conformation, osseointegration will be favoured. In constrast, if the proteins are adsorbed in a state that cannot be recognized by the cells, the implants may be identified as a foreign material and trigger an immune response.[50] The cells attach to positively or negatively charged surfaces but the morphology of the cells can vary depending on the electrical charge.[51]

Surface charges are relevant for anchorage-dependent cells such as osteoblasts. The attachment and spreading of osteoblasts is strong on very positively charged surfaces, with intimate contact between the ventral cell membrane and the biomaterials surface.[52] On negatively charged surfaces, however, osteoblasts tend to show a stand-off morphology with localized attachment points.[53]

As a quantitative measure, the isoelectric point (IEP), or the pH at which its zeta potential is equal to zero, is often used to investigate the surface charges. The surface tends to be more negative when IEP is inferior to the physiological pH (7.4) and more positive when it is superior. Evaluation of the IEP for a solid body, in particular for an implant surface, is not straightforward. Bearing in mind that all metallic biomaterials used for bone repair are passive, that is become covered by a thin oxide layer, the properties of the oxides forming the passive layer become relevant. IEPs for metal oxides and related materials have recently been compiled.[54] Values for oxides that are present in the passive layers of the metallic biomaterials (or as coatings) are: 8.8–9.5 for Al_2O_3, 6.7 for Cr_2O_3 and 3.5–6.7 for TiO_2. Consequently, most of the alloys used for orthopaedic implants exhibit at their surface a net negative charge at physiological pH.[55]

Surface energy

Surface wettability, a measurement of surface energy, influences the degree of contact with the physiologic environment and is considered to be one of the most important parameters affecting the biological response to an implanted material.[56,57] Wettability affects protein adsorption, platelet adhesion/activation, blood coagulation and cell bacterial adhesion.[58] Generally the cellular attachment is poor on any hydrophobic surface and high on moderately hydrophilic surfaces.

Surface energy is dictated by composition of the surface but not by topography (including roughness).[59] It was suggested that wettability, expressed in terms of contact angle and related time-dependent non-equilibrium phenomena, should be correlated with crystalline structure and the chemical composition of the oxide films that form on the surfaces.[60] Titanium surfaces, covered by Ti-rich oxide films, are hydrophilic owing to the high polarity of the Ti–O bond, although surface contamination, such as by carbon or hydrocarbon adsorption, produces higher values of water contact. Recently it has been reported that thermal oxidation of NiTi alloys enhances the hydrophilic character and statistically increases both albumin and fibronectin adsorption.[61] A significant decrease in the contact angle has been also observed after UV radiation of Ti-6Al-4V and Ti-6Al-4V oxidized alloy.[62]

One further issue is that cleaning and sterilization methods of the implants produce significant changes in contamination and surface energy.[63]

6.5 Trends in the development of metallic biomaterials

Metallic biomaterials have been the most suitable for bone replacement up to now. In the past, they were basically borrowed from other fields of applications, mostly the aerospace industry. After the World War II, a number of high-performance materials originally developed for military purposes became available for clinical use. In the 20th century, efforts to enhance their biological response have been focused on their surface modification by using physical, chemical or biological methods. Additionally, the research and development of titanium alloys without toxic elements lead to the production of Ti-6Al-4Nb, the first alloy specifically developed for medical applications.

Nowadays there have been many approaches to designing the next generation of bone implants. These can be grouped as proposals for new compositions, with non-toxic and non-allergic elements, or for new microstructures obtained through the introduction of novel processing techniques.

6.5.1 Materials with a lower Young's modulus

Common metallic biomaterials have a modulus that is much higher than that of bone (see Table 6.4). Assuming isoelastic behaviour of the implant/bone system during service, the implant takes over a considerable part of the mechanical load, thereby shielding the remaining bone that surrounds the implant. Reduction of physiological loads on the bone induces resorption mechanisms that lead to a drop in bone density. In addition, tissue resorption increases micromotions at the bone–implant interface facilitating the formation and migration of wear debris via biological fluid transport. All these features yield premature failures of the implant that overall are associated with the 'stress yielding' phenomena.

The elastic modulus of common Ti and Ti-base alloys is lower than that of Co-base alloys and stainless steel, but it is still much higher than that of cortical bone (Table 6.4). Thus a reduction in the Young's modulus is regarded as a high priority in the overall strategy of the design of Ti alloys for biomedical applications, which is focused on a new generation of β type titanium alloys.[64–70] These are composed of non-toxic elements such as Nb, Ta, Zr, Mo and Sn that stabilise the bcc β-phase preserving the light weight character of Ti alloys. As can be seen in Table 6.5, the Young's modulus of β type titanium alloys is much smaller than that of α + β type titanium alloys. Two promising biomedical alloys are Ti-35Nb-7Zr-5Ta (TNZT)[71] and Ti-12Mo-6Zr-2Fe (TMZF)[72] which offer an elastic modulus of about 55 and 80 GPa, respectively. These materials do not reveal any toxicity versus osteoblastic cells and have a high corrosion resistance.[68, 69] In addition to solid solution, mechanical strength can be enhanced by cold working or by precipitation of secondary phases (α and ω), although in this case the Young's moduli tend to increase with increasing precipitation. Volume fractions of precipitates can be controlled by proper thermomechanical processing.[73, 74] On the other hand, the strength of β type alloys is comparable or superior to those of aged α+β alloys.[64]

A further decrease in Young's modulus can be achieved by the use of foams as porous implants [75] or implants with a porous surface layer. An open porosity would also permit good attachment of tissues to the surface allowing the tissue ingrowth (see later section on metallic scaffolds). A decrease in the Young's modulus of the metal will favour the load transfer to the ingrown bone, stimulating new bone formation.

6.5.2 Ni-free Fe-based alloys

Austenitic stainless steels, such us 316L, and CoCr alloys are biocompatible materials widely used to produce permanent implants or parts which merely come into contact with the human body. They are widely used because of the excellent compromise between their various characteristics, such as intrinsic mechanical strength, and wear resistance. Austenitic stainless steel must contain a nickel content in the range 9–15 wt% to ensure an austenitic

Table 6.5 Mechanical properties of Ti, Ti-based alloys and some representative β type titanium alloys developed for biomedical applications

Alloy	Microstructure	Young's modulus *E* (GPa)	Yield strength (MPa)	Tensile strength (MPa)
cpTi	α	105	170–485	240–760
Ti-6Al-4V	α + β	110	760–895	900–970
Ti-6Al-7Nb	α + β	105	921	1024
Ti-13Nb-13Zr	β	79	900	1030
Ti-12Mo-6Zr-2Fe (TMZF)	β	74–85	1000–1060	1060–1100
Ti-15Mo-5Zr-3Al	β	82	771	812
	Aged β + α	100	1215	1310
Ti-35Nb-7Zr-5Ta (TNZT)	β	55	530	590

state at room temperature for the high Cr content (>18 wt%) used. Co base alloys, used for heavily loaded joints (wrought products), usually contain nickel contents below 0.5%, although much higher values of up to about 37 wt% are sometimes present in hip or knee prosthesis components (F562).

It has been known for a number of years that nickel ions leach into the human body and can lead to localized irritation and infection, even in the absence of any evident corrosion mechanism. Contact dermatitis and toxicity caused by nickel and its salts have been well documented.[76, 77] As a matter of fact, intracutaneous tests have shown that in Europe 10–15% of adult females and 1–3% of adult males can be susceptible to allergic reactions to nickel.[78] Consequently, the trend in legislation in a number of countries is currently towards limiting or even eliminating nickel from alloys which come into contact with skin or which are used to manufacture temporary or permanent prosthetic material.

Fortunately, nickel is not alone in being an austenite former. Ni-free austenitic stainless steels with a large amount of nitrogen (up to 4.2 at%) and manganese (up to 23 at%) have been recently developed to enhance the strength, corrosion resistance and biocompatibility of conventional stainless steels.[79–82] On the other hand, Ni-free austenitic stainless steels without manganese but with a higher N content (up to 5.1 at%) have been also developed.[83] One of these new types of steel has been subjected to biological studies and shown promising results.[84] ASTM F2229 is a Ni-free (< 0.05% Ni) austenitic stainless steel with a nominal composition of 23Mn-21Cr-1Mo and about 1.0% N. The higher N content contributes to high levels of corrosion resistance and strength when compared to type 316 L.[1]

Ni-free Fe-base ODS (oxide dispersion strengthened) alloys have been developed as potential biomaterials for surgical implants. Evidence of good biocompatibility was found *in vitro* when challenging different types of cells to the alloy either as fine particles [85] or solid samples.[86] The soft ferromagnetic behaviour makes the alloy a useful candidate for the preparation of medical devices where biocompatible and soft magnetic materials are sought.[21]

A further achievement concerns the development of new FeAlCr intermetallic alloys. Their major advantages are their low density (< 6 g cm^{-3}), low raw materials cost and low content of strategic elements. Biocompatibility was evaluated *in vitro* by testing human osteoblast-like Saos2 cells with mechanically alloyed particles[85] or solid samples.[87] Overall, none of the investigated new alloys was found to be cytotoxic. Instead, a good level of biocompatibility was assessed.

6.5.3 Nanostructured alloys

Another recent approach to improving orthopaedic implants has centred on the development of alloys with an extremely fine grain size. Grain boundaries of metals and alloys delimit crystals of different orientation. The high degree of disorder along a grain boundary naturally is more permeable to diffusing materials and the extra strain energy in the immediate neighbourhood of the boundary increases the chemical activity locally. In recent years, development of nanotechnology in material science and engineering has gained increased interest owing to the possibility of obtaining improved properties compared with conventional coarse-grained materials. Compared to respective micro-sized counterparts most nanoscale bone implant ceramics (alumina, titania, hydroxyapatite)[88–90] or polymers (PLGA (polylactic-co-glycolic acid), polyurethane)[88] have been shown to enhance bone cell responses and functions including cellular adhesion, proliferation, synthesis of alkaline phosphatase and calcium deposition. The mechanism(s) of these responses involve proteins since, in the absence of serum, osteoblast adhesion was greatly reduced and independent of ceramic grain size.[88] The applicability of nanostructured materials for biomedical applications has logically triggered off a considerable interest in a number of devices and systems.[91, 92]

As the name suggests, nanostructured materials refer to materials with structures falling in the 1–100 nm range. In the case of metals, the finest microstructures with potential applications as structural materials are obtained by 'top-down' techniques based on severe plastic deformation (SPD) such as equal channel angular pressing (ECAP) and high pressure torsion (HPT). A common feature is to use multiple passes of deformation or to impose the large strains needed for refinement of the microstructure.[93] Conventional SPD techniques are mostly performed at elevated temperatures where the increased ductility and yield strength reduction facilitate large-strain deformation. The relative high temperature during processing facilitates recrystallization and, therefore, 'coarsening' of the microstructure cannot be avoided. Most common microstructures fall in the 250–1000 nm range and thus the term 'ultrafine-grain size' is often used. The advantages of developing ultrafine grained (UFG) metallic materials are known in terms of chemical[94] and mechanical [95–97] properties. It is therefore not surprising that the biological response is affected too.

Recently, Yao *et al.*[98] have shown an enhanced osteoblast adhesion on UFG pure Ti in comparison to its regular grained counterpart after a 4-hour exposure. UFG pure Zr, however, was found to exhibit an osteoblastic response essentially identical to conventional grained Zr.[99] The UFG Zr has an average grain size of about 250 nm, which is well below the size scale of the investigated cells. Therefore, in theory, cells could have noticed the variation in the hierarchical structure of the surface. However, the *in vitro* results did not show any significant effect of the grain size reduction on the biological response. Therefore, the truly fundamental microstructural aspects behind this improvement of UFG Ti remain unclear.

Investigations into the osteoblast response to nanostructured metals are limited to HPT-processed titanium. It has been associated with increased surface wettability and improved pre-osteoblast attachment and growth rate *in vitro*.[100, 101] Cytoskeletal and extracellular matrix activity is also increased. Interestingly, the morphological and histochemical pattern of the fibronectin self-assembly, aggregation and fibrillar network seems similar to that observed on hydroxyapatite-coated titanium, which is known for its high osteoinductivity.

Therefore, the introduction of novel technologies to obtain nanostructured metals provides a promising alternative for enhancing the mechanical properties of the bulk material, associated with the grain size decrease but they may be very useful for understanding the physicochemical mechanisms controlling the cell–substrate interaction in materials modified by severe surface plastic deformation (SSPD) techniques such as grit blasting and shot peening. For instance, it has been recently reported that ageing of sandblasted Ti develops a nanocrystalline structure at the surface layer that significantly improves the corrosion resistance.[102]

6.5.4 Biodegradable alloys

Stainless steels and titanium alloys are widely used in internal fixations because of their strength and toughness. For young patients, it is generally recommended that these devices be removed to avoid adverse physiological responses associated with stress yielding. In the case of children, removal is definitively required in order to allow developmental bone growth. Degradable metallic implants are a new category of implants aimed to degrade *in vivo*, eliminating the need for a second operation to remove the implant. From a historical point of view, this concept breaks the paradigm requiring biomaterials to be corrosion resistant.

Magnesium alloys were introduced into orthopaedic and trauma surgery in the first half of the 20th century.[103]

The main advantages in comparison to other metallic biomaterials are related to their low density (1.7–2.0 g cm^{-3}). In addition, fracture toughness is greater than in ceramic materials, while Young's modulus (41–45 GPa) is closer to that of natural bone (Table 6.4). Although biocompatibility is good, degradation of magnesium is too fast, losing mechanical integrity before the tissue has sufficiently healed and producing hydrogen gas in the corrosion process at a rate that produces an accumulation of hydrogen as subcutaneous gas bubbles (about one litre of hydrogen per gram of magnesium). Moreover, such implants could not maintain mechanical integrity over a period that was long enough for sufficient bony union to develop. Owing to these problems, their use was abandoned when stainless steels became available.

In order to control the corrosion rate in body fluids, complex alloys containing aluminium (2–10 wt%) and minor amounts of zinc and manganese (AZ31, AZ91) or with addition of rare earth elements (WE43, LAE442) have been investigated.[104] Achievements with new alloys developed for orthopaedic applications have been recently reviewed.[105] Biodegradable magnesium alloys provide a twofold higher tensile strength and fourfold higher Young's modulus than degradable polymeric implant materials that are used, like polyglycolic acid (PGA) and polylactic acid (PLA). Surface modifications by alkali-heat treatment or non-toxic coatings can also be applied to improve the corrosion resistance.[106]

6.5.5 Bioactive materials

The conventional metallic alloys used for bone replacement are appreciated for their good mechanical properties and reasonable biocompatibility. After implantation into the living body, they become spontaneously encapsulated, without direct contact with bone, by a fibrous tissue with a thickness that is proportional to the amount and toxicity of the dissolution products. This granulomatous hypertrophic tissue allows diffusion of ions and microparticles and impairs the mechanical and biological stability of the interface. It is interesting to note that bioinert materials, as titanium or its alloys, may elicit a minimal fibrous encapsulation, whereas biotolerant materials, like stainless steel and CoCr alloys, give rise to a thicker fibrous capsule (up to about 2 μm thick).

Encapsulation of the implant is not observed in the case of some bioactive ceramics, used to repair bones, which promote an increase in the formation of new mineralized bone although their low mechanical properties limit their use in loading applications. Therefore, the search for biomaterials that facilitate the osseointegration is one of the key objectives in the development of a new generation of dental and orthopaedic implants. Continuous efforts have been addressed by developing surface modifications or coating by using chemical or biological methods that are out of the scope of this chapter.

6.5.6 Metallic scaffolds

The first generation of modern biomaterials (mid-20th century) selected for medical applications were high-performance industrial materials originally developed for airplane components. The goal was to achieve a minimal response from the host tissue; therefore, they were intended to be bioinert. In the 1980s, the trend was to induce a controlled reaction with the tissues, which yielded the second generation of biomaterials which were considered to be bioactives. The third generation of biomaterials is intended to regenerate the tissue rather than its replacement. A key concept is the use of scaffolds, in which cells could be seeded, proliferated and differentiated *in vitro* for subsequent implantation *in vivo*. They should have an open cellular structure.

With regard to the bone regeneration, it is important to note that bone tissue is an extremely strong and dense material suited to its role in providing load-bearing support for the body. It can be considered to have two different types of structures corresponding to the cortical bone, which is quite dense (5–25% of porosity), and cancellous or trabecular bone, which is highly porous (40–95% of porosity). Trabecular bone is found at the ends of long bones (surrounded by a thin layer of cortical bone) and in bones like skull and vertebra. The optimal pore size for attachment, differentiation and growth of osteoblasts and vascularization is in the range 200–500 μm. To mimic the complex architecture of bone, gradients of pore size must be generated within scaffolds by special arrangement of the pore size.

To ensure the biomechanical properties of natural bone, considerable efforts have been made in the production of porous implants. The effect of porosity on the elastic modulus has resulted in the derivation of a large number of empirical and semi-empirical equations that allow the stiffness of the implant to be tailored. Variation of Young's modulus with increasing porosity can be estimated in the case of spherical pores by using the equation:[107]

$$E_p = E_0 (1 - 1.21p)^{2/3} \qquad [6.1]$$

where p is the porosity and E_0 and E_p, denote Young's modulus for the bulk and porous material, respectively. Figure 6.12 shows this variation for most of the biomaterials in use. One popular approach to engineering bone tissue has involved seeding bioresorbable polymers in a porous configuration. A major limitation is that Young's modulus becomes lower than that for bone making them unsuitable for load-bearing applications. As can be seen, only metals offer a good combination of porosity and stiffness. Consequently, a large number of metallic materials have been recognized as very promising materials for bone implants, presumably strong enough to resist handling during implantation and *in vivo* loading.[108, 109] Titanium structures that have a porosity of 30–35% exhibit a modulus identical to human bone. In order to increase the contact surface area, functionally macroporous graded Ti coatings have been developed.[110] The pore size and the porosity are gradually increased from the substrate to the outermost layer where pores in the range of 100–400 μm allow bone tissue ingrowth. Since titanium alloys are known to be notch sensitive, the fatigue strength of implants with porous surface layers will be diminished.

NiTi shape memory alloy foam is also an excellent candidate for reconstructive orthopaedic applications, ranging from spinal fixation to acetabular hip prosthesis, dental implants, permanent osteosynthesis plates, and so on.[111] It can match bone density and allow the ingrowth of living tissues withstanding short- and long-term physiological loads.[112] Thermal oxidation

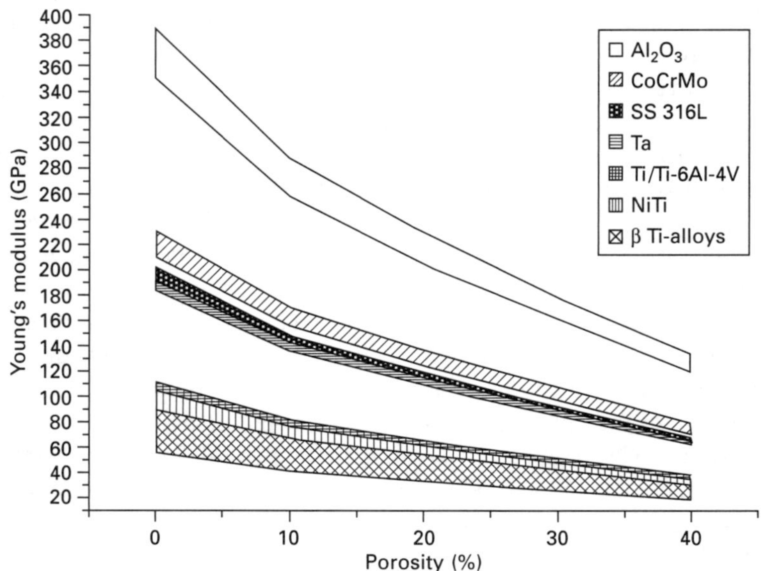

6.12 Variation of Young's modulus as a function of porosity of alumina and common metallic biomaterials of interest for the fabrication of scaffolds.

of NiTi foams significantly improves corrosion resistance and decreases nickel ion release, while barely affecting transformation temperatures.[113]

Hirschhorn and Reynolds[114] explored the use of totally porous CoCrMo implants that had an elastic modulus closer to that of bone, but the porosity made the strength insufficient for the load. Another approach was to fabricate porosity-graded composite structures that favour the mechanical anchorage of cementless joint prostheses.[115, 116] The level of porosity can be graded from a highly porous to a dense core, giving the component suitable strength to withstand the physiological loadings while having a porous surface layer that allows tissue ingrowth.

Recently, Lotus-type porous high nitrogen nickel-free stainless steels have been successfully fabricated using high temperature nitriding.[117] The porosity of the samples oscillated between 44 and 48% and the mean pore size was in the biomedical field desired range (145–374 μm). When the pores are aligned perpendicular to the load direction, the mechanical properties are near to the human cortical bone.

Strongly bonded assemblies of short ferritic fibres constitute an interesting class of highly porous, permeable materials (Fig. 6.13). It has been recently proposed that if ferromagnetic fibres are employed, the material can be actuated by the imposition of a magnetic field.[118] The resultant deformation of the fibre array generates a shape change, which can be predicted for a given

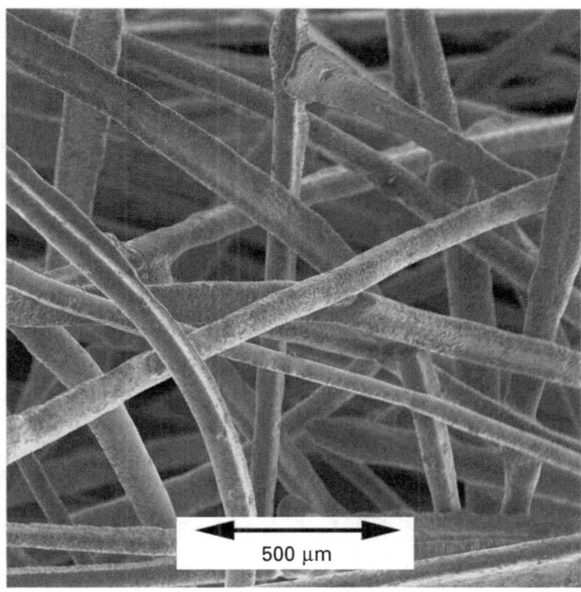

6.13 Scanning electron micrograph of a bonded array of ferromagnetic fibres used for magneto-mechanical stimulation of bone growth (courtesy of A.E. Markaki and T.W.T. William Clyne).

fibre orientation distribution and fibre segment aspect ratio. Moreover, the new bone located in the inter-fibre space will be mechanically strained by these fibre deflections. Since the stiffness of this material – less than about 1 GPa – will be lower than that of bone, it was proposed to attach an outer layer of a porous bonded-fibre material to a fully dense metallic core of a prosthetic implant, tailoring the overall stiffness of the device to minimize stress shielding effects while ensuring magneto-mechanical bone growth stimulation.

Porous tantalum has been developed as biological scaffold for new bone formation in several orthopaedic applications, including hip and knee arthroplasty, spine surgery and bone graft substitute, as illustrated in Fig. 6.14. With approximately 70–80% porosity, it exhibits a characteristic appearance similar to cancellous bone.[119–121] This trabecular metal has been shown to be highly biocompatible in several animal models. Studies have demonstrated substantial cortical bone ingrowth between the trabecular network, as well as high levels of bone growth onto the scaffold itself. The initial stability of the trabecular metal itself is also higher than that of standard materials, such as cobalt chrome. Furthermore, this new material offers better osteoconduction than other technologies used for biological fixation. Data on the clinical applications of this biomaterial in the form of a monoblock acetabular component are also promising. The pore size and high volume

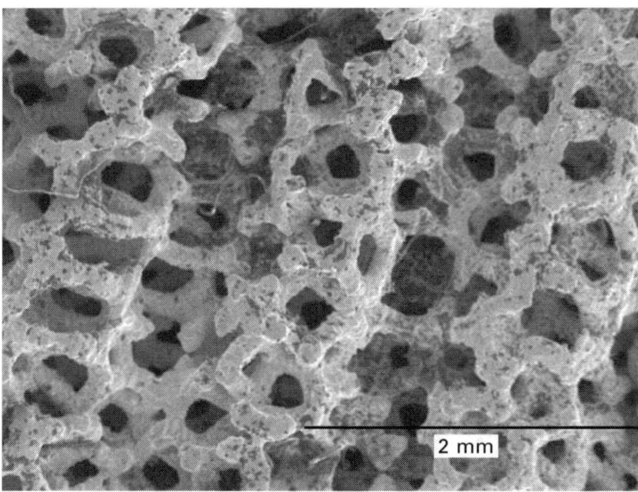

6.14 Scanning electron micrograph of porous tantalum developed as scaffold (courtesy of F.J. Gil Mur).

porosity of trabecular metal supports vascularization and rapid, secure soft tissue ingrowth. Approximately 7000 of these acetabular components have been implanted in Europe since 1997 and no revisions for aseptic loosening have been reported.

6.6 Conclusions

This chapter has attempted to give an overview of metallic materials used for bone repair. It is evident that the continuous development of orthopaedic materials during the 20th century has led to a remarkable improvement in the quality of life for millions of aged patients. The challenge for this millennium is the shift from the replacement to the *in situ* regeneration of bone, which will bring great benefit especially for young patients. Till now it has been shown that metals are the materials of choice for many structural implantable device applications and there is no reason to expect a change in the short or medium term. Although initial results with the novel metallic biomaterials are good, it is worth remembering that in the past some developments led to clinical failures despite promising short-term results. Thus further clinical testing and follow-up for most of these materials are needed.

A final consideration of concern is the fact that fabrication of new metallic materials for surgical implants that have shown promising properties at a laboratory scale has been traditionally hindered by a conflict of interest between the manufacturers of the alloys, thinking in terms of production of tons of material, and the biomaterial companies, whose facilities and benefits are mostly related to fabrication of components for medical devices using existing alloys. Alloys manufacturers and biomaterials companies are therefore strongly recommended to combine their efforts in future developments within this research field.

6.7 Acknowledgements

The author would like to thank his research colleagues at CENIM-CSIC and CIBER-BBN, especially Marta Multigner, Jesus Chao, Emilio Frutos, Marcela Lieblich, Maria Luisa González and Nuria Vilaboa for fruitful collaboration and many stimulating discussions.

6.8 References

1 Davis J R, *Handbook of Materials for Medical Devices*. JR Davis (ed.), ASM International, Materials Park, USA, 2003.
2 Breme J and Biehl V, *Handbook of Biomaterials Properties*, Part II, Black J and Hastings G (eds), Chapman & Hall, London, UK, 1998, 135–213.
3 Ratner B D, Hoffman A L, Schoen F J and Lemons J E (eds), *Biomaterials Science. An Introduction to Materials in Medicine*, Elsevier Academic Press, San Diego, CA, 2004.
4 Venable C S and Stuck W G, *The Internal Fixation of Fractures*, Thomas C G, Springfield, Illinois, 1947.
5 Rondelli G, 'Corrosion resistance tests on NiTi shape memory alloys', *Biomaterials*, 1996, **17**, 2003–8.
6 Humbeeck J V, 'Shape memory alloys: a material and a technology', *Adv Eng Mater*, 2001, **3**(11), 837–50.
7 Porter D A and Esterling K E, *Phase Transformations in Metals and Alloys*, Chapman and Hall, London, 1992, 431–7.
8 Michiardi A, Aparicio C, Planell J A and Gil F J, 'New oxidation treatment on NiTi shape memory alloys to obtain Ni-Free surfaces and improve biocompatibility', *J Biomed Mater Res B*, 2006, **77**, 249–56.
9 Michiardi A, Aparicio C, Planell J A and Gil F J, 'Electrochemical behaviour of oxidised NiTi shape memory alloys for biomedical applications', *Surf Coat Technol*, 2007, **201**(14), 6484–8.
10 Shabalovskaya S, Anderegg J and Van Humbeeck J, 'Critical overview of Nitinol surfaces and their modifications for medical applications', *Acta Biomater*, 2008, **4**, 447–67.
11 Narayan R J, Hobbs L W, Jin C and Rabiei A, 'The use of functionally gradient materials in medicine', *JOM*, 2006, **58**, 52–6.
12 OXINIUM™, Smith & Nephew, Memphis, TN, USA.
13 Good V, Widding K, Hunter G and Heuer D, 'Oxidised zirconium: a potentially longer lasting hip implant', *Mater Design*, 2005, **26**, 618–22.
14 Zitter H and Plenk H, 'The electrochemical behaviour of metallic implant materials as an indicator of their biocompatibility', *J Biomed Mater Res*, 1987, **21**(7), 881–96.
15 Matsuno H, Yokoyama A, Watari F, Uo M and Kawasaki T, 'Biocompatibility and osteogenesis of refractory metal implants, titanium, hafnium, niobium, tantalum and rhenium', *Biomaterials*, 2001, **22**(11), 1252–62.

16 Riley M A, Walmsley A D, Speight J D and Harris I R, 'Magnets in medicine', *Mater Sci Technol*, 2002, **18**, 1–12.

17 Watanabe I, Hai K, Tanaba Y, Hisatsune K and Atsuta M, '*In vitro* corrosion behaviour of cast iron-platinum magnetic alloys', *Dent Mater*, 2001, **17**, 217–20.

18 Riley M A, Walmsley A D and Harris I R, 'Magnets in prosthetic dentistry', *J Prosthet Dent*, 2001, **86**, 137–42.

19 Gillings B R D, 'Magnetic retention for complete and partial over-dentures: Part 2', *J Prosthet Dent*, 1983, **49**, 607–18.

20 Takada Y and Okuno O, 'Corrosion behavior of stainless steels and dental precious alloys used for dental magnetic attachments', *J Mag Dent*, 1994, **3**(1), 14–22.

21 Flores M S, Ciapetti G, González-Carrasco J L, Montealegre M A, Multigner M, Pagani S and Rivero G, 'Evaluation of magnetic behavior and *in vitro* biocompatibility of ferritic PM 2000 alloy', *J Mater Sci: Mater Med*, 2004, **15**, 1–7.

22 González-Carrasco J L, García-Alonso M C, Montealegre M A, Escudero M L and Chao J, 'Comparative study of the alumina scale integrity on MA 956 and PM 2000, alloys', *Oxid Met*, 2001, **55**(3/4), 209–21.

23 Laakman R W, Kaufman B, Han J S, Nelson A D, Clampitt M, O'Block A M, Haaga J R and Alfidi R J, 'MR imaging in patients with metallic implants', *Radiology*, 1985, **157**(3), 711–4.

24 Da Rocha S S, Adabo G L, Vaz L G and Henriques G E, 'Effect of thermal treatments on tensile strength of commercially cast pure titanium and Ti-6Al-4V alloys', *J Mater Sci: Mater Med*, 2005, **16**, 759–66.

25 Hall E O, 'The deformation and ageing of mild steel: III Discussion of results', *Proc. Phys. Soc.* (London), 1951, **64B**, 747–53.

26 Petch N J, 'The cleavage strength of polycristals', *J Iron Steel Inst (London)*, 1953, **3**, 25–8.

27 Fleming D G and Feinberg B N (eds), *Handbook of Engineering in Medicine and Biology*, CRC Press, Boca Raton, FL, 1976.

28 Callister W D (ed.), *Materials Science and Engineering. An Introduction*, John Wiley & Sons, New York, 2003.

29 *ASM Metals Handbook, Vol 3: Properties and Selection: Stainless Steels, Tool Materials and Special-purpose Materials*, ASM International, Metals Park, USA, 1985.

30 Turner N G and Roberts W T, 'Fatigue behavior of titanium', *Trans. TMS-AIME*, 1968, **242**, 1223– 30.

31 Kuhlman G W, in: *Microstructure/Property Relationships in Titanium Aluminides and Alloys*, Kim Y-W and Boyer RR (eds), TMS, Warrendale, PA, 1991, p 465.

32 Jaffe R I and Lutjering G, in *Microstructure, Fracture Toughness and Fatigue Crack Growth Rate in Titanium Alloys*, Chakrabarti AK, Chestnut JC (eds), TMS, Warrendale, PA, 1987, p 193.

33 Sivakumar M, Suresh Kumar Dhanadurai K, Rajeswari S and Thulasiraman V, 'Failures in stainless steel orthopaedic implant devices: A survey', *J Mater Sci Lett*, 1995, **14**, 351–4.

34 Chao J and López V, 'Failure analysis of a Ti-6Al-4V cementless HIP prosthesis', *Engineering Failure Analysis*, 2007, **14**(5), 822–30.

35 Viceconti M, Toni A and Giunti A, 'Effects of some technological aspects on the fatigue strength of a cementless hip stem', *J Biomed Mater Res*, 1995, **29**, 875–81.

36 Jiang X P, Wang X Y, Li J X, Li D Y, Man C-S, Shepard M J and Zhai T, 'Enhancement of fatigue and corrosion properties of pure Ti by sandblasting', *Mater Sci Eng A*, 2006, **429**, 30–5.
37 Leinenbach C and Eifler D, 'Fatigue and cyclic deformation behaviour of surface-modified titanium alloys in simulated physiological media', *Biomaterials*, 2006, **27**, 1200–8.
38 Baleani M, Viceconti M and Toni A, 'The effect of sandblasting treatment on endurance properties of titanium alloy hip prostheses', *Artificial Organs*, 2001, **24**(4), 296–9.
39 Gil F J, Planell J A, Padrós A and Aparicio C, 'The effect of shot blasting and heat treatment on the fatigue behavior of titanium for dental implant applications', *Dent Mater*, 2007, **23**(4), 486–91.
40 Clark G C F and Williams D F, 'The effects of proteins on metallic corrosion', *J Biomed Mater Res*, 2004, **16**(2), 125–34.
41 Marcus P, 'On some fundamental factors in the effect of alloying elements on passivation of alloys', *Corros Sci,* 1994, **36**, 2155–8.
42 Sittig C, Hähner G, Marti A, Textor M, Spencer N D and Hauert R, 'The implant materials, Ti6Al7Nb: surface microstructure, composition and properties', *J Mater Sci: Mater Med*, 1999, **10**, 191–8.
43 Zitter H and Plenk Jr, 'The electrochemical behavior of metallic implant materials as an indicator of their biocompatibility', *J Biomed Mater Res*, 1987, **21**, 881–96.
44 Fraker A C, 'Corrosion of metallic implants and prosthetic devices', *Corrosion*, ASM Handbook Vol. 13, ASM International, Metals Park, USA, 1987, 1324–35.
45 Rubio J C, Garcia-Alonso M C, Alonso C, Alobera M A, Clemente C, Munuera L and Escudero M L, 'Determination of metallic traces in kidneys, livers, lungs and spleens of rats with metallic implants after a long implantation time', *J Mater Sci: Mater Med*, 2008, **19**(1), 369–75.
46 Kubashewski O, Evans E Cl and Alcok C B, *Metallurgical Termochemistry*, Pergamon Press, London, 1967.
47 *Biophase Implant Material, Technical Information Publ. N° 3846*, Richards Manufacturing, Memphis, Tennessee, 1980, p 7.
48 Reclaru L, Lüthy H, Ziegenhagen R, Eschler P-Y and Blatter A, 'Anisotropy of nickel release and corrosion in austenitic stainless steels', *Acta Biomater*, 2008, **4**(3), 680–5.
49 Wilson C J, Clegg R E, Leavesley D I and Pearcy M J, 'Mediation of biomaterial-cell interactions by adsorbed proteins: a review', *Tissue Eng*, 2005, **11**, 1–18.
50 Thull R, 'Physicochemical principles of tissue material interactions', *Biomol Eng*, 2002, **19**(2–6), 43–50.
51 Shelton R M, Rasmussen A C and Davies J E, 'Protein adsorption at the interface between charged polymer substrata and migrating osteoblasts', *Biomaterials*, 1988, **9**, 24–9.
52 Davies J E, *Surface Characterization of Biomaterials*, B D Ratner (ed), Elsevier Science Publishers B.V., Amsterdam 1988, p 219.
53 Davies J E, Causton B, Bovell Y, Davy K and Sturt C S, 'The migration of osteoblasts over substrata of discrete surface charge', *Biomaterials*, 1986, **7**(3), 231–3.
54 Kosmulski M, 'pH-dependent surface charging and points of zero charge II. Update', *J Coll Interf Sci*, 2004, **275**, 214–24.
55 Hallab N J, Bundy K J, O'Connor K, Clark R and Moses R L, 'Cell adhesion to

biomaterials: Correlations between surface charge, surface roughness, adsorbed protein, and cell morphology', *J Long Term Eff. Med. Implants*, 1995, **5**, 209–31.

56 Anselme K, 'Osteoblast adhesion on biomaterials', *Biomaterials*, 2000, **21**, 667–81.

57 Zhu X, Chen J, Scheideler L, Reichl R and Geis-Gerstorfer J, 'Effects of topography and composition of titanium surface oxides on osteoblast responses', *Biomaterials*, 2004, **25**, 4087–103.

58 Xu L-C and Siedlecki C A, 'Effects of surface wettability and contact time on protein adhesion to biomaterial surfaces', *Biomaterials*, 2007, **28**, 3273–83.

59 Morra M, Volpe C D and Siboni S, 'Comment on the paper: Enhancing surface free energy and hydrophilicity through chemical modification of microstructured titanium implant surfaces, by Rupp F, Scheideler, Olshanska, de Wild M, Wieland M, Geis-Gerstorfer J', *J Biomed Mater Res A*, 2006, **76**(2), 323–34.

60 Oshida Y, Sachdeva R and Miyazaki S, 'Changes in contact angles as a function of time on some pre-oxidised biomaterials', *J Mater Sci: Mater Med*, 1992, **3**, 306–12.

61 Michiardi A, Aparicio C, Ratner B, Planell J A and Gil J, 'The influence of surface energy on competitive adsorption on oxidised NiTi surfaces', *Biomaterials*, 2007, **28**, 586–94.

62 Pacha-Olivenza M A, Gallardo-Moreno A M, Méndez-Vilas A, Bruque J M, González-Carrasco J L and González-Martín M L, 'Effect of UV radiation on the surface Gibbs energy of Ti-6Al-4V and Ti-6Al-4V oxidised alloys', *J Coll Interf Sci*, 2008, **320**, 117–24.

63 Kasemo B and Lausmaa J, 'Biomaterial and implant surface: on the role of cleanliness, contamination, and preparation procedures', *J Biomed Mater Res*, 1998, **22**, 145–58.

64 Long M and Rack H J, 'Titanium alloys in total joint replacement-A materials Science Perspective', *Biomaterials*, 1998, **19**, 1621–39.

65 Niinomi M, Kuroda D, Fukunaga K, Morinaga M, Kato Y, Yashiro T and Suzuki A, *Mater Sci Eng A*, 1999, **263**, 193–9.

66 Okazaki Y, 'A new Ti-15Zr-4Nb-4Ta alloy for medical applications', *Curr Opin Solid State M*, 2001, **5**, 45–53.

67 Niinomi M, 'Fatigue performance and cyto-toxicity of low rigidity titanium alloy, Ti-29Nb-13Ta-4.6 Zr', *Biomaterials*, 2003, **24**, 2673–83.

68 Guillemot F, Prima F, Bareille R, Gordín D, Gloriant T, Porté-Durrieu M C, Ansel D and Baquey Ch, 'Design of new titanium alloys for orthopaedic applications', *Med Biol Eng Comput*, 2004, **42**, 137–41.

69 Oliveira N T C, Aleixo G, Caram R and Guastaldi A C, 'Development of Ti-Mo alloys for biomedical applications: Microstructure and electrochemical characterization', *Mat Sci Eng A-Struct*, 2006, **452–453**, 727–31.

70 Raabe D, Sander B, Friák M, Ma D and Neugebauer J, 'Theory-guided bottom-up design of β-titanium alloys as biomaterials based on first principles calculations: Theory and experiments', *Acta Mater*, 2007, **55**(13), 4475–87.

71 Ahmed T A, Long M, Silverstri J, Ruiz C and Rack H J, 'A new low modulus biocompatible titanium alloy', *Titanium 95': Sci Technol*, 1996, 1760.

72 Wang K, Gustavson L and Dumbleton J, 'The characterization of Ti-12Mo-6Zr-2Fe. A new biocompatible titanium alloy developed for surgical implants'. *Beta Titanium in the 1990s*. Eylon D, Boyes RR and Koss D A (eds), Mineral, Metals and Materials Society, Warrendale, PA, 1993, 2697.

73 Weiss I and Semiatin S L, 'Thermomechanical processing of beta titanium alloys-an overview', *Mat Sci Eng A-Struct*, 1998, **243**, 46–65.

74 Ankem S and Greene C A, 'Recent developments in microstructure/property relationships of beta titanium alloys', *Mat. Sci. Eng. A-Struct*, 1999, **263**, 127–31.

75 Wen C E, Yamada Y and Hodgson P D, 'Fabrication of novel TiZr alloy foams for biomedical applications', *Mater Sci Eng C*, 2006, **26**(8), 1439–44.

76 Basketter D A, Briatico-Vangosa G, Kaestner W, Lally C and Bontinck W J, 'Nickel, cobalt and chromium in consumer products: a role in allergenic contact dermatitis?', *Contact Dermatitis*, 1993, **28**, 15–25.

77 Yamamoto A, Kohyama Y and Hanawa T, 'Mutagenicity evaluation of forty-one metal salts by the umu test', *J Biomed Mater Res*, 2002, **59**, 176–83.

78 Meding B, Liden C and Berglind N, 'Self-diagnosed dermatitis in adults. Results from a population survey in Stockholm', *Contact Dermatitis*, 2001, **45**, 341– 5.

79 Menzel J, Kirschner W and Stein G, 'High nitrogen containing Ni-free austenitic steels for medical applications', *ISIJ Int*, 1996, **36**, 893–900.

80 Uggowitzer P J, Magdowski R and Speidel M O, 'Nickel free high nitrogen austenitic steels', *ISIJ Int,* 1996, **36**, 901–8.

81 Gebeau R C and Brown R S, 'Biomedical implant alloy', *Adv Mater Proc*, 2001, **159**, 46–8.

82 Montagnon J and Moraux J Y, *Nickel-free Stainless Steel for Biomedical Applications*, US Patent, July 2001, n° 6, 267, 921.

83 Yamamoto A, Kohyama Y, Kuroda D and Hanawa T, 'Cytocompatibility evaluation of Ni-free stainless steel manufactured by nitrogen adsorption treatment', *Mater Sci Eng C*, 2004, **24**, 737–43.

84 Fini M, Aldini N, Torricelli P, Giavaresi G, Borsari V, Lenger H, Bernauer J, Giardino R, Chiesa R and Cigada A, 'A new austenitic stainless steel with negligible nickel content: an *in vitro* and *in vivo* comparative investigation', *Biomaterials*, 2003, **24**, 4929–39.

85 Ciapetti G, González-Carrasco J L, Savarino L, Montealegre M A, Pagani S and Baldini N, 'Quantitative assessment of the response of osteoblast- and macrophage-like cells to Ni-free Fe-base alloy particles', *Biomaterials*, 2005, **26**, 849–59.

86 González-Carrasco J L, Ciapetti G, Montealegre M A, Pagani S, Chao J and Baldini N, 'Evaluation of mechanical properties and biological response of an alumina forming Ni-free ferritic alloy', *Biomaterials*, 2005, **26**, 3861–71.

87 González-Carrasco J L, Ciapetti G, Montealegre M A, Savarino L, Munoz-Morris M A and Baldini N, 'Potential of FeAlCr intermetallics reinforced with nanoparticles as new biomaterials for medical devices', *J Biomed Mater Res Part B Appl Biomater*, 2007, **80B**, 201–10.

88 Webster T J, Siegel R W, and Bizios R, 'Osteoblast adhesion on nanophase ceramics', *Biomaterials*, 1999, **20**, 1221– 7.

89 Webster T J, Ergun C, Doremus R H, Siegel R W, and Bizios R, 'Enhanced functions of osteoblasts on nanophase ceramics', *Biomaterials*, 2000, **21**, 1803–10.

90 Webster T J, Ergun C, Doremus R H, Siegel R W and Bizios R, 'Enhanced osteoclast-like cell functions on nanophase ceramics', *Biomaterials*, 2001, **22**, 1327–33.

91 Xu T, Zhang N, Nichols H L, Shi D and Wen X, 'Modification of nanostructured materials for biomedical applications', *Mater Sci Eng C*, 2007, **27**(3), 579–94.

92 Liu H and Webster T J, 'Nanomedicine for implants: A review of studies and necessary experimental tools', *Biomaterials*, 2007, **28**, 354–69.

93 Furukawa M, Horita Z, Nemoto M and Langdon T G, *Mater Sci Eng A*, 2002, **324**, 82–9.

94 Balyanov A, Kutnyakova J, Amirkhanova N A, Stolyarov V V, Valiev R Z, Liao X Z, ZhaoY H, Jiang Y B, Xu H F, Lowe T C and Zhu Y T, 'Corrosion resistance of ultra fine-grained Ti', *Scripta Materialia*, 2004, **51**, 225–9.

95 Valiev R Z, Islamgaliev R K and Alexandrov I V, 'Bulk nanostructured materials from severe plastic deformation', *Progr Mat Sci*, 2000, **45**, 103–89.

96 Valiev R Z, Stolyarov V V, Rack H J, and Lowe T C, in *Medical Device Materials*, Shrivastava S (ed), ASM, Cleveland, OH, 2004, p 362.

97 Rack H J and Qazi J I, 'Titanium alloys for biomedical applications', *Mater Sci Eng C*, 2006, **26**, 1269–77.

98 Yao C, Qazi J L, Rack H J, Slamovich E B and Webster T J, 'Improved bone cell adhesion on ultrafine grained titanium and Ti-6Al-4V', *Ceramic Nanomaterials and Nanotecnology* III, 106th Acers Transactions, 159, 2004.

99 Saldaña L, Méndez-Vilas A, Jiang L, Multigner M, González-Carrasco J L, Pérez-Prado M T, González-Martín M L, Munuera L and Vilaboa N, 'Osteoblast response to zirconium surfaces', *Biomaterials*, 2007, **28**, 4343–54.

100 Faghihi S, Zhilyaev A P, Szpunar J A, Azari F, Vali H and Tabrizian M, 'Nanonstructuring of titanium material by high pressure torsion improves pre-oesteoblast attachment', *Adv Mater*, 2007, **19**, 1069–73.

101 Faghihi S, Azari F, Zhilyaev A P, Szpunar J A, Vali H and Tabrizian M, 'Cellular and molecular interactions between MC3T3-E1 pre-osteoblasts and nanostructured titanium produced by high-pressure torsion', *Biomaterials*, 2007, **28**, 3887–95.

102 Jiang X P, Wang X Y, Li J X, Li DY, Man C-S, Shepard M J and Zhai T-, 'Enhancement of fatigue and corrosion properties of pure Ti by sandblasting', *Mater Sci Eng A*, 2006, **429**, 30–5.

103 McBride E D, 'Absorbable metal in bone surgery', *J Am Med Assoc*, 1938, **111**(27), 2464–7.

104 Witte F, Kaese V, Haferkamp H, Switzer E, Meyer-Lindenberg A, Wirth C J and Windhagen H, '*In vivo* corrosion of four magnesium alloys and the associated bone response', *Biomaterials*, 2005, **26**, 3557–63.

105 Staiger M P, Pietak A M, Huadmai J and Dias G, 'Magnesium and its alloys as orthopaedic biomaterials: a review', *Biomaterials*, 2006, **27**, 1728–34.

106 Grey J E and Luan B, 'Protective coatings on magnesium and its alloys- a critical review', *J Alloys Comp*, 2002, **336**, 88–113.

107 Ondracek G and Kravchenko I A, 'Composites: general considerations, relationship of the microstructure and effective properties, applications of composites in development of the materials with specific properties. III Relationship of the microstructure and effective properties of materials using Young's modulus as an example', *Powder Metall Metal Ceramics*, 1993, **32**(6), 555–60.

108 Wen C E, Mabuchi M, Yamada Y, Shimojima K, Chino Y and Asahina T. 'Processing of biocompatible porous Ti and Mg', *Scripta Materialia*, 2001, **45**, 1147–53.

109 Oh I, Nomura N and Hanada S, 'Microstructures and mechanical properties of porous titanium compacts prepared by powder sintering', *Mater T JIM,* 2002, **43**(3), 443–6.

110 YangY Z, Tian J M, Tian J T, Chen Z Q, Deng X J and Zhang D H, 'Preparation of graded porous titanium coatings on titanium implant materials by plasma spraying', *J Biomed Mater Res Part A*, 2000, **52**, 333–7.

111 Gil F J, Manero J M and Planell J A, 'Relevant aspects in the clinical applications of NiTi shape memory alloys', *J Mater Sci: Mater Med*, 1996, **7**, 403–6.

112 Barrabés M, Sevilla P, Planell J A and Gil F J, 'Mechanical properties of nickel-titanium foams for reconstructive orthopaedics', *Mater Sci Eng C*, 2008, **28**, 23–7.

113 Barrabés M, Michiardi A, Aparicio C, Sevilla P, Planell J A and Gil F J, 'Oxidized nickel-titanium foams for bone reconstructions: chemical and mechanical characterization', *J Mater Sci: Mater Med*, 2007, **18**, 2123–9.

114 Hirschhorn J S and Reynolds J T, 'Powder metallurgy fabrication of cobalt alloy surgical implant materials', *Research in Dental and Medical Materials*, Korostoff E (ed), Metallurgical Society of AIME Proceedings, Plenum Press, New York, 1969, 137–50.

115 Ozols A, Barreiro M, Forlerer E and Sirkin H R, 'Coating of Co–Cr–Mo alloy for surgical implants by centrifugal spray: Preliminary evaluation', *Surf Coat Tecnol*, 2006, **200**, 5884–8.

116 Dourandish M, Godlinski D, Simchi A and Firouzdor V, 'Sintering of biocompatible P/M Co-Cr-Mo alloy (F-75) for fabrication of porosity-graded composite structures', *Mater Sci Eng A*, 2008, **472**, 338–46.

117 Alvarez K, Sato K, Hyun S K and Nakajima H, 'Fabrication and properties of Lotus-type porous nickel-free stainless steel for biomedical applications', *Mater Sci Eng C*, 2008, **28**, 44–50.

118 Markaki A E and Clyne T W, 'Magneto-mechanical stimulation of bone growth in a bonded array of ferromagnetic fibres', *Biomaterials*, 2004, **25**(19), 4805–15.

119 Bobyn J D, Stackpool G, Toh K K, Hacking S A and Tanzer M, 'Bone ingrowth characteristics of a new porous tantalum biomaterial', *J Bone Joint Surg*, 1999, **81B**, 907–14.

120 Bobyn J D, Toh K K, Hacking S A, Tanzer M and Krygier J J, 'The tissue response to porous tantalum acetabular cups: a canine model', *J Arthroplasty*, 1999, **14**, 347–54.

121 Levine B R, Sporer S, Poggie R A, Della Valle C J and Jacobs J, 'Experimental and clinical performance of porous tantalum in orthopaedic surgery', *Biomaterials*, 2006, **27**, 4671–81.

7
Ceramics as bone repair materials

M. VALLET-REGÍ and A. J. SALINAS,
Universidad Complutense, Spain and CIBER-BBN, Spain

Abstract: In this chapter, ceramics used to repair and regenerate bone are reviewed comprehensively. First, an overview of ceramics used in biomedical applications as well as those formed in living beings by biomineralization is presented. Then, ceramics used for bone repair and other ceramics now under investigation are described. For the sake of clarity, bioceramics are classified by their reactivity in the organism: almost bioinert (i.e. first generation), bioactive and resorbable (i.e. second generation) and third generation bioceramics which are those intending to drive the self-regeneration ability of the human body. Finally, the present state and future perspectives of bioceramics are presented.

Key words: almost bioinert ceramics, bioceramics, degradable and bioactive ceramics, third generation bioceramics.

7.1 Overview of ceramics in biomedical engineering

Ceramic materials are important sources of biomaterials for applications in biomedical engineering. Those ceramics intended to be in contact with living tissues are called bioceramics, and have experienced great development in the last 50 years.[1–5] The medical needs of an increasingly ageing population have driven a great deal of research looking for new materials for the manufacture of implants. These are used to regenerate and repair living tissues damaged by disease or trauma. For specific clinical applications, mainly in orthopaedics and dentistry, bioceramics are playing a key role.

In general, ceramics are inorganic materials that have a combination of ionic and covalent bonding. The use of new ceramic materials represents an evolution in many aspects of the history of mankind. Many millennia ago, the possibility of storing grain in ceramic receptacles allowed man to become a settler instead of a nomadic hunter. Some centuries ago, the use of structural ceramics also brought about great advances in the quality of life of mankind with the possibility of making clay bricks and tiles. Decades ago, ceramics produced a new revolution, with the development of functional ceramics in dielectrics, semiconductors, magnets, piezoelectrics, high temperature superconductors, and so on. In addition, ceramics have also played an important role in improving the quality and length of human life through their use in biomaterials and medical devices.

Figure 7.1 represents the historical evolution of ceramics up until the present bioceramics. As observed, the investigation of bioceramics has also evolved when, as it will be explained later, more restrictive properties for the new ceramics were required. Thus, alumina, zirconia, calcium phosphates and certain glasses and glass–ceramics are genuine examples of bioceramics. Nowadays, new advanced bioceramics are under study including ordered mesoporous silica materials or specific compositions of organic–inorganic hybrids.

Ceramic materials exhibit high melting temperatures, low conduction of electricity and heat and relatively high hardness. Carbon is an element, not a compound, and conducts the electricity in its graphite form, but it is considered a ceramic because of its many ceramic-like properties. Figure 7.2 shows general properties of ceramics conformed as dense pieces that play an important role in their behaviour as biomaterials. With regard to their mechanical behaviour, ceramic materials exhibit great compressive strength

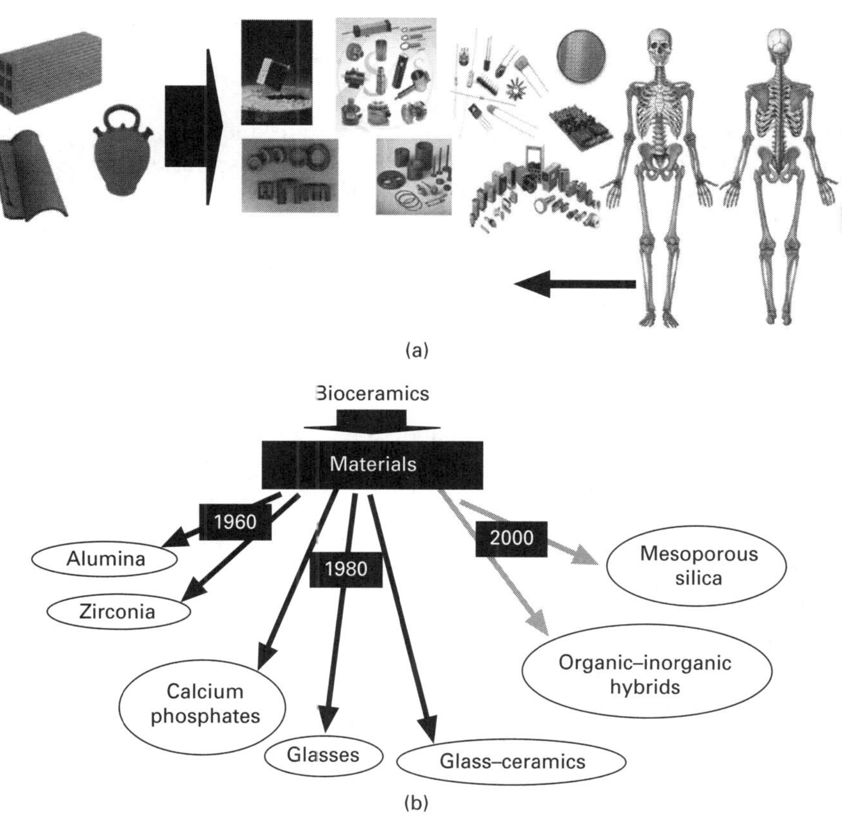

7.1 Historical evolution of ceramics up until bioceramics. (a) Pictorial examples, (b) timeline of bioceramics.

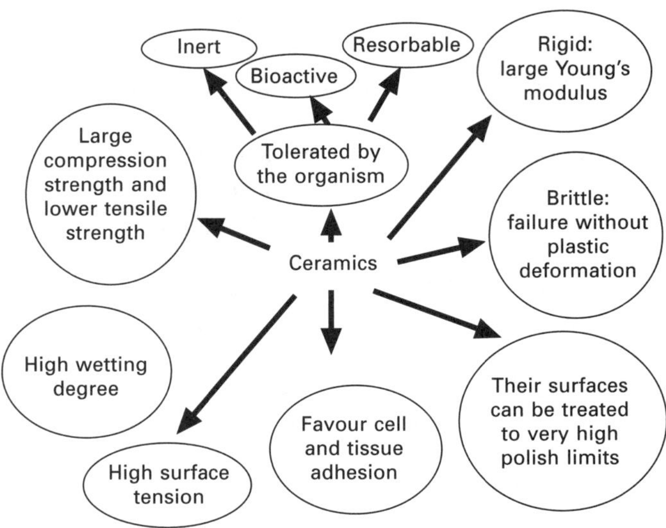

7.2 General properties of ceramics as dense monoliths that make them suitable as implants.

and very much lower tensile strength. In addition, they are stiff materials, with a high Young's modulus, and are brittle because failure takes place without plastic deformation. In relation to their surface properties, ceramics show high degrees of wetting and surface tension which favour the adhesion of proteins, cells and other biological moieties. Furthermore, the ceramic surface can be treated to reach very high polish limits. However, as will be explained latter, nowadays many research efforts are devoted towards ceramics with interconnected porosity and in these cases the mechanical properties will drastically change.

Concerning their reactivity inside the living body, bioceramics are classified as almost bioinert, bioactive and resorbable. Figure 7.3 includes the most important ceramics of each type as well as the clinical applications of bioceramics. Bioactive ceramics are those where a sequence of reactions, restricted only to the material surface, take place yielding a mechanically strong bond between the bioceramic and the living tissues. Almost bioinert ceramics are considered to be first generation bioceramics whereas bioactive and resorbable ceramics are known as second generation bioceramics.[6]

The reactivity is a better criterion for classifying bioceramics than their chemical composition or crystallinity. For instance, in the field of amorphous ceramics, it is possible to obtain glasses that behave as bioinert, bioactive or resorbable in the same chemical system depending on their different compositions.[7] In addition, it is possible to find glasses with identical composition behaving as bioinert when obtained by melting, or bioactive

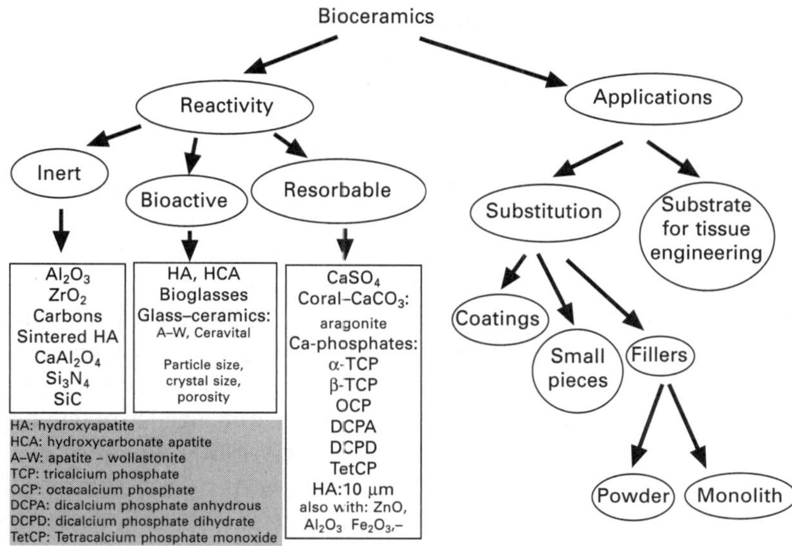

7.3 Main first and second generation bioceramics and their clinical applications.

when they are synthesised by a sol–gel method.[8] Moreover, some glass compositions that are considered to be bioactive can be completely resorbed when used as particulates under a certain size limit, for instance, 90 μm for Bioglass® 45S5.[6] Analogous examples can be found among crystalline ceramics. For instance, the *in vivo* reactivity of hydroxyapatite (HA) can range from almost bioinert, when highly sintered like dense monoliths,[9] to resorbable, when used in powdered form, passing by the bioactive character generally attributed to HA.[10]

When some glass compositions presenting the highest levels of bioactivity were investigated, it was found that they were able to bond to hard and soft tissues, whereas other bioactive materials only bond to hard tissues. To explain these differences in reactivity in 1994 Hench defined two classes of bioactivity: class A, osteoproductive and class B, osteoconductive.[11] The first one, takes place when material obtains extracellular and intracellular responses, whereas in the second one only an extracellular response is obtained. It was explained that the ions released from these bioactive glasses, in particulate form, stimulated regeneration of living tissues mediated by genes. These osteoproductive glasses were considered to be third generation bioceramics[6] and are the basis of actual research efforts looking for new biomaterials that intend to stimulate a cellular response. Nowadays, research efforts are concentrated on porous second generation bioceramics and new advanced bioceramics. In these materials, ceramic plays the role of scaffold of cells and substances with biological activity (growth factors, hormones…)

which are released to the medium in a controlled way. In this way, they are beginning to be used in applications related to tissue engineering.[12]

On the other hand, bioceramics must be biocompatible and functional for the required implantation time. In addition, they must not be toxic, carcinogenic, allergic or inflammatory. In general, because of their ionic bonds and chemical stability, ceramic materials are generally biocompatible.

In this chapter, bioceramics will be studied, divided into first, second and third generations. The study of first generation bioceramics started in the 1960s, when the goal was to have as low a reactivity as possible. The more representative examples of this kind of bioceramics are alumina, Al_2O_3, and zirconia, ZrO_2. They are widely used as biomaterials because of their high strength, excellent corrosion and wear resistance, stability, non-toxicity and *in vivo* biocompatibility. Around the 1980s the objective changed to obtaining favourable interactions with the living body, namely a bioactive response or degradation. Specific compositions of calcium phosphates or sulphates, bioactive glasses and glass–ceramics are examples of second generation bioceramics used for bone tissue augmentation, as bone cements or for metallic implants coating. In the last decade, bioceramics with more demanding properties were required. The studies of third generation bioceramics are more based in biology and follow the purpose of substituting 'replace' tissues by 'regenerate' tissues. This category includes bioceramics based on porous second generation bioceramics, loaded with biologically active substances, and new advanced bioceramics like silica mesoporous materials, mesoporous ordered glasses or organic–inorganic hybrids. Table 7.1 shows important first, second and third generation bioceramics that will be presented in this chapter.

7.1.1 Biological ceramics: biominerals

If we look at how Nature solves the task of fabricating hard tissue, we will find first that biomineralization processes mainly use calcium and silicon combined with carbonates, phosphates and oxides. Figure 7.4 depicts the four most abundant inorganic phases present in different living species.[13] Thus, bone is formed by biomineralization processes, natural sequences of physical–chemical reactions that form hard tissues in vertebrates or protective tissues in invertebrates and inferior zoological species. As a result, natural composites are formed. In this way, materials with exceptional mechanical properties that are impossible to obtain with pure materials are reached.

In this section, we will focus on materials that induce bone formation. However, before dealing with the production of some ceramics in the laboratory, we should recall that the inorganic phase of our bones is an apatite-like phase. Its structure has the special ability to accommodate several different ions in its three sublattices. Bone apatites can be considered to be

Table 7.1 First, second and third generation bioceramics

Type of bioceramic	*In vivo* reactivity	Examples
1st generation:		
Bioinert non-absorbable	Isolated by a non-adherent fibrous capsule	Alumina: Al_2O_3 Zirconia: ZrO_2 Carbons, mainly pyrolytic and as fibres in composites
2nd generation:		
Biodegradable resorbable	Dissolved after a specific time	Calcium phosphates Calcium sulphate Calcium phosphates and sulphates + ZnO, Al_2O_3, Fe_2O_3 Coralline $CaCO_3$
Bioactive surface reactive	Tightly bonded to living tissues	Hydroxyapatite (HA), pure and substituted Hydroxycarbonate apatite (HCA) Glasses: by melting and sol-gel Glass ceramics: A/W glass-ceramic® and Ceravital®
3rd generation: scaffolds of biologically active molecules	Stimulating living tissues regeneration	Bioglass®: in particulate form Porous bioactive and biodegradable ceramics Advanced bioceramics: mesoporous materials, organic–inorganic hybrids

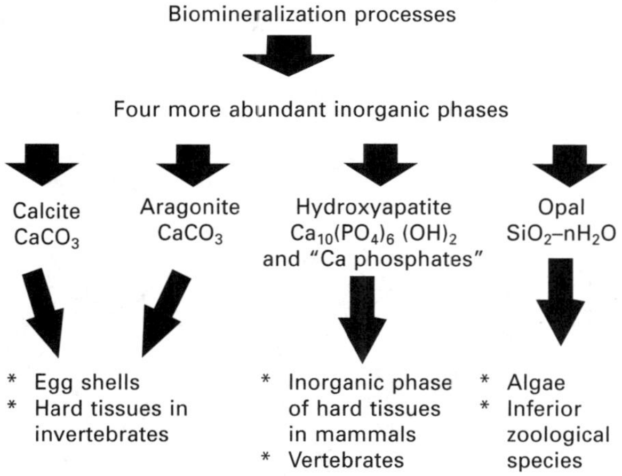

7.4 Four more abundant inorganic phases formed by biomineralization processes.

basic calcium phosphate. As indicated earlier, bones of vertebrate animals are organic–inorganic composite materials whose structure can be briefly described as follows: the inorganic component is a carbonated and calcium-deficient non-stoichiometric hydroxyapatite. These biological apatite crystals exhibit nanometre size, ranging from 25–50 nm.[13, 14] These crystals grow at the mineralization sites of the collagen molecules, which are grouped together forming collagen fibres. Furthermore, a certain hierarchical bone porosity is necessary for several physiological functions performed by the bone.[15] The order of magnitude of biological apatites and bone pores is shown in Fig. 7.5.

7.2 Almost bioinert ceramics: first generation bioceramics

The most widely used almost bioinert ceramics are alumina, Al_2O_3, zirconia, ZrO_2, and diverse forms of carbon, such as low temperature isotropic form (LTI) of pyrolytic carbon (PyC), glassy (vitreous) carbon, ultra-low temperature isotropic (ULTI) form of PyC and carbon fibres. In Table 7.2 important clinical applications of first generation bioceramics are presented. The applications of alumina and zirconia in medicine are similar and are presented together. The main application of these oxides as bioceramics is for fabrication of femoral heads. On the other hand, carbons are mainly used to obtain coatings in applications requiring contact with blood or as fibres in reinforced composites.

According to its almost bioinert character, first generation ceramics, similar to metallic and polymeric biomaterials, elicit a foreign body reaction. Therefore, in spite of being biocompatible, the organism will react against

Biological apatites
$Ca_{8.3\square 0.7}(PO_4)_{4.3}(HPO_4, CO_3)_{1.7}(2OH, CO_3)_{0.15\square 1.7}$

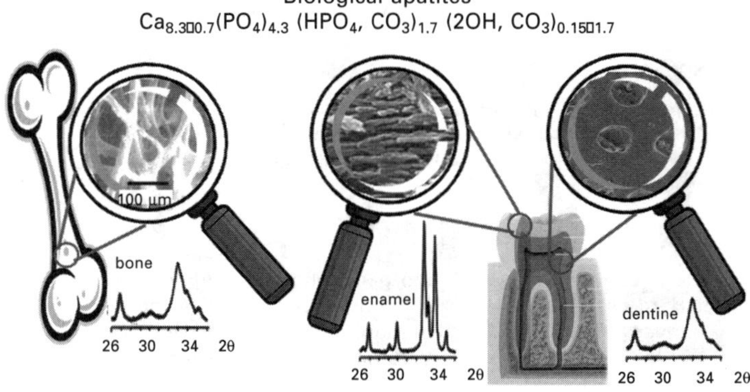

Crystal size biological apatites:	25–50 nm
Pore size needed for:	
Bone physiology:	1–100 µm
Ideal internal growth:	100–350 µm

7.5 Biological apatites are formed by nanometric crystals whereas bone pores are at the micrometre scale. The general formula of biological apatite is included; the rectangles (□) at the top of the figure represent vacancies in the apatite structure.

Table 7.2 Clinical applications of almost bioinert ceramics

Bioinert ceramics	Clinical applications
Alumina Al_2O_3 & Zirconia ZrO_2	Bearing-surface total joint arthoplastia components: hip implants (ball and cup), knee prosthesis Bone screws Maxillofacial and alveolar ridge reconstruction Dental implants, crowns and brackets and inlay Ossicular bone substitutes, cochlear replacement Ophthalmology
Carbons	Heart valve coatings Orthopaedic implants

them in a series of biochemical processes in which macrophages, giant cells, cytokines and collagen fibres are involved. As a final result, the implant is surrounded by an acellular collagen capsule which isolates it from the body.[16] This non-adherent capsule of fibrous tissue provokes interfacial micromovements that grow with time and will eventually produce failure of certain kinds of prosthesis. However, for applications of almost bioinert ceramics, such as bearing surfaces and contact with blood, the foreign body reaction is not an issue.

7.2.1 Alumina, Al_2O_3

The first applications of alumina as a biomaterial were reported in 1963, as a bone substitute,[17] and in 1967, as a dental implant.[18] In addition, the first bioceramic couple (alumina–alumina) was implanted in 1970.[19] The advantage of ceramic-on-ceramic articulating surfaces is their low wear. Alumina has been extensively used in total hip arthoplastia from the 1980s (approved by FDA in 1982). The initial concerns about fracture toughness and wear were avoided by decreasing the grain size of alumina from 10 to 2 μm, increasing purity, lowering porosity and improving the processing methods with the use of hot isostatic pressure. Thus, the performance of alumina ceramic hip balls was significantly improved. However, the hip balls of polycrystalline alumina must have a minimum size of 28 mm owing to strength limitations. Research studies are underway to reduce the ball size to decrease wear and make the prosthesis more appropriate for patients who are shorter in height. Single crystalline alumina might overcome the strength limitation but with excessive cost of manufacture.

Alumina has been also used in dentistry for root analogue, endosteal screws, blades and pine-type dental implants.[20] The root and blade from dental implants used in the 1970s tended to fracture after a few years. Long-term mechanical tests showed functional limitations. However, single crystalline alumina showed mechanical strength superior to polycrystalline alumina, allowing very much higher loads. Alumina can also be used for other dental applications such as ceramic crowns. It must be noted that the term dental implant is used only for materials in contact with bone and soft tissue.

Alumina ceramics have also been used in total knee prosthesis,[21] middle ear implants,[22] ophthalmology[23] and single crystal alumina bone screws.[24] The mechanical properties of alumina and other significant almost inert bioceramics are shown in Table 7.3.

7.2.2 Zirconia, ZrO_2

Partially stabilized (with MgO or Y_2O_3) zirconia was proposed in 1986 as an alternative to alumina in ceramic femoral heads.[25] From then, it has been gaining market because of its enhanced mechanical properties when compared to alumina (See Table 7.3). In 1993, the first dental implant of zirconia was reported.[26] This application is greatly appreciated in comparison with conventional titanium implants for aesthetical considerations, owing to its white colour which is more like the colour of natural teeth. In addition, dental implants of zirconia have a similar mechanical strength, much higher fracture toughness and a lower production cost than single crystalline alumina.

ZrO_2 presents three polymorphs of symmetry, monoclinic (under 1170ºC), tetragonal (1170ºC–2370ºC) and cubic (> 2370ºC), as well as a high pressure orthorhombic phase. Large volume variations of around 5% take place when zirconia transforms from tetragonal to monoclinic. These variations exceed the elastic and fracture limits and cause cracking of zirconia ceramics. To avoid this, additives such as calcia (CaO), magnesia (MgO) or yttria (Y_2O_3) must be added to zirconia to stabilize the material in tetragonal or cubic phases. Partially Stabilized Zirconia (PSZ) is a mixture of cubic, tetragonal and/or monoclinic phases. In contrast, tetragonal zirconia polycrystals (TZP) are 100% in the tetragonal phase. Both PSZ and TZP are suggested for medical applications. Yttria-TZP ceramics have strength and fracture toughness almost twice that alumina. Thus, zirconia heads are less sensitive to stress concentrations at the point of contact with metal cones. Nowadays most medical-grade zirconia is PSZ tetragonal zirconia.

Zirconia ceramics present low micro-hardness and elastic modulus, together with high strength and fracture toughness compared with alumina. The superior mechanical strength provides the possibility for producing ceramic ball heads below 32 mm is size. Moreover, zirconia also presents advantages over alumina in terms of lower friction and wear.

Potential limitations to the use of zirconia as a bioceramic are degradation and radiation. Degradation is due to the phase transformation accelerated in the aqueous body environment. Consequently, studies are taking place to try to understand the zirconia degradation mechanism in a biological environment, particularly under dynamic loadings. On the other hand, radioactive ^{235}U

Table 7.3 Mechanical properties of some almost inert bioceramics and cortical bone

	Bending strength (MPa)	Ultimate strength (MPa)	Young's modulus (GPa)	Fracture toughness (MPa $m^{1/2}$)	Hardness Vickers (HV)	Strain to failure (%)	Density (g cm^{-3})
Oxide ceramics							
Al_2O_3	551	3790c/310t	366	4.0	20–30	0.1	3.9
ZrO_2	1074	7500c/420t	201	6–15	12	–	6.1
ZrO_2 (MgO stabilized)	–	634	200	–	–	–	–
ZrO_2 (Y_2O_3 stabilized)	–	900	200	–	–	–	–
Carbons							
LTI PyC+ 5–12% Si	–	600	30	–	–	2.0	–
Pure PyC	494	–	29.4	–	–	1.6	1.5–2.0
Si-alloyed PyC	408	–	30.5	–	–	–	–
Glassy carbon	171	–	21	–	–	–	1.5
Cortical bone (average)							–
Low strain	114t	150c/90t	15.2	–	–	–	–
High strain	–	400c/270t	40.8	–	–	–	

c: compressive; t: tensile; PyC: pyrolytic carbon.

impurities were detected in some zirconia ceramics. Measured radioactivity levels are low but more work needs to be done on this aspect.

The surface degradation of zirconia balls caused by the phase transformation do not seem significant. However, zirconia femoral heads have a relatively short history and more investigation is required. The mechanical integrity of all ceramic components is dependent on manufacturing quality controls. In general, ceramic particulate debris is chemically stable and biocompatible and causes undesirable biological responses at high concentrations.

Other possible improvements in these almost bioinert ceramics could come from the preparation of alumina/zirconia composites. Alternatively, new advances could come from research into non-oxide bioinert ceramics, such as nitrides and carbides like Si_3N_4 or SiC.

7.2.3 Carbons

They are a group of compounds included in the category of almost bioinert ceramics that can be made in many allotropic forms: graphite, diamond, nanocrystalline glassy carbon and PyC. In addition, carbon fibres have been also used in reinforced biomedical composites. Recently, new variations of carbon, such as nanotubes and bucky-balls, were produced and their potential clinical applications have also been explored. However, the most common form of carbon used in implants is PyC which can be presented in two forms: LTI and ULTI.[27]

From the mid-1960s LTI-PyC received great attention in the biomaterials industry, specifically for mechanical heart valves, because it is highly thromboresistant and exhibits good biocompatibility with blood and soft tissues. Moreover, LTI carbon shows excellent durability, strength and resistance to wear and fatigue. Nowadays over 90% of mechanical heart-valve prostheses utilize components manufactured from silicon alloyed LTI-PyC as a coating on a polycrystalline substrate or as a monolithic material. Up to 20 wt% silicon is added to LTI carbon to improve its mechanical properties without significant changes in biocompatibility. To obtain more complicated shapes and mechanical properties, an impermeable layer of ULTI carbon can be obtained on different substrates by vapour deposition. On the other hand, because of the low density and weakness of the glassy carbons they are used as thick coatings mechanically reinforced by the substrate.

PyC is also used for small orthopaedic joints such as fingers and spinal inserts. Attempts to use carbon in other clinical applications, such as dental implants, vascular, ligaments, tendons and so on, obtained low success rates. Research to improve PyC is devoted towards eliminating the small amounts of silicon carbide in the coatings, which are partially thrombogenic, and to improve its mechanical properties. In addition, a better characterization of the obtained materials is required.

7.3 Biodegradable and bioactive ceramics: second generation bioceramics

As it was indicated in Section 7.1, between almost bioinert and resorbable ceramics, there is another important group of bioceramics whose surface reacts with living tissues. These ceramics are usually referred to as bioactive and, after a series of chemical processes, form a mechanically strong bond with the living tissues. Thus, these bioceramics are suitable for many clinical uses when bonding of the biomaterial and the living tissues is required. In this section, the most important resorbable and bioactive ceramics will be described comparatively. In addition, it must be considered that decreasing the particle size or increasing the hydrophilic character can make a bioactive material resorbable.[2, 28]

The most widely used biodegradable ceramics are based on calcium phosphates and calcium sulphates.[29–32] Indeed, both have in common a certain degree of reactivity that promotes positive interactions with living tissues. Biodegradable ceramics are designed to fulfil specific body functionality for a given period of time, aiding the self-repair processes of the living organism. After that they must be resorbed. This could be an ideal behaviour because it avoids the problems associated with a long residence of a synthetic biomaterial in the body. The critical aspect in the design of biodegradable ceramics is to adjust (slow down) the kinetics of the ceramic degradation, which is usually quicker than that of living tissue formation. Moreover, it must be considered whether the decrease in the mechanical properties of ceramics during the resorption process could impede the required functionality. Table 7.4 includes important second generation bioceramics and their main clinical applications.

The search for bioactive ceramics yielded promising results in the 1980s. Larry Hench pioneered the field when he put an imaginative idea into practice, that is, that certain glasses in contact with living tissue will be able to bond to bone.[33] These bioactive ceramics react with physiological fluids, but only at the level of the surface of material, forming an apatite-like biologically active layer. In the presence of living cells, this apatite can form new bone that tightly bonds bioactive material and osseous tissues. The more characteristic examples of bioactive ceramics are hydroxyapatite and some compositions of glasses and glass–ceramics.[3, 8, 34–38]

For medical applications, bioactive materials are provided in different formats: powder, porous monoliths, dense monoliths, injectable mixtures and coatings. They have excellent features in terms of biocompatibility and bioactivity, but they are brittle, rendering it impossible to use them for repairing large osseous defects. However, these ceramics are excellent for filling small defects, where the rate of bone regeneration is the main concern and where mechanical properties are just a secondary aspect.

Table 7.4 Bioactive and resorbable bioceramics and their current clinical uses as implants

Material	Form	Application	Function
Calcium phosphates	Bulk	Bone graft substitutes, cell scaffolfds	Replace the bone loss
	Coatings	Surface coatings on total joint prosthesis	Provide bioactive bonding to bone
Glasses	Bulk	Endosseous alveolar ridge maintenance	Space filling and tissue bonding
		Middle ear prosthesis	Replacement of part of the ossicular chain
		Orbital floor prosthesis	Repair damaged bone supporting eye
	Powder	Fixation or revision arthoplasty	Restore bone after prostheses loss
		Filler in periodontal defects	Periodontal disease treatment
		Bone graft substitutes & cranial repair	Augmentation after diverse illness or traumas
Glass–ceramics	Bulk	Vertebral prostheses	Replace vertebrae removed by surgery
		Iliac crest prostheses	Substitute bone removed for autogenous graft
	Coatings	Fixation of hip prosthesis	Provide bioactive bonding
Calcium sulphate	Bulk & powder	Bone graft substitutes	Repairing osseous tissues

On the other hand, if a bioactive glass is shaped like a porous monolith, it would exhibit a quicker bioactive response.[39, 40] Also, since the fluid would reach the inner positions more easily, the reactivity of the whole glass would also improve. But the mechanical properties would be even worse. Hence it is important to choose materials depending on the required application. In addition, glasses can also be used as precursors in the production of glass–ceramics.[41] In fact, a particular thermal treatment of a bioactive glass yields a bioactive glass–ceramic, which exhibits mechanical properties closer to natural bone, although a certain decrease in the bioactive response takes place.[42] Using bioactive glasses and glass–ceramics, it is possible to design magnetic materials that fulfil two roles simultaneously: regenerating the bone due to their bioactivity and treating cancer in bone tissues, through hyperthermia treatments.[43]

The use of bioactive ceramics is ideal for situations when a permanent binding of the prosthesis and osseous tissues is desired. The only concern about these materials is the permanence in the living body of the bulk material that does not react with the surrounding tissues. This situation could be a disadvantage for certain applications or an advantage in other cases. It must be taken into account that because the reactivity is only at the surface, the loss of the mechanical properties at the material surface will be very small, facilitating the total functionality of the bioceramic.

Both types of second generation ceramics, that is biodegradable and bioactive, can present different crystallization degrees: ceramics, which are crystalline solids, glasses, which are amorphous solids and glass–ceramics formed by an amorphous glassy matrix with crystallization nuclei. In this section, these bioceramics will be divided by their crystallization states. First, crystalline ceramics will be presented: calcium phosphates, in bulk and as coatings, biphasic mixture compounds and bone cements, then bioactive glasses and finally bioactive glass–ceramics.

7.3.1 Calcium phosphates

Most of the crystalline bioactive and biodegradable ceramics used for bone regeneration are based on calcium phosphates. Here synthetic apatites, pure and substituted, biphasic mixtures of calcium phosphates and calcium bone cements containing calcium phosphates and calcium sulphate will be described.

Synthetic apatites

Hydroxyapatite with the chemical formula $Ca_{10}(PO_4)_6(OH)_2$, (HA) is the synthetic calcium phosphate more studied as biomaterial because of its structural and chemical similarities with the inorganic component of bone.[29] HA with hexagonal symmetry spacial group (SG) $P6_3/m$ and lattice parameters $a = 0.95$ nm and $c = 0.68$ nm, is a biocompatible, bioactive and osteoconductive material. To mimic biological materials, synthetic apatites must present nanometric particle size and contain 4–8 wt% of CO_3^{2-} ions (in the PO_4^{3-} sublattice, type B apatites). Regarding particle size, HA sub-micrometric particles have been obtained by aerosol pyrolysis,[44] precipitation[45, 46] and a liquid mix technique based on the Pechini patent.[47, 48] Regarding carbonate inclusion in HA, high temperatures of synthesis produced type A (non-biological) hydroxycarbonate apatite (HCA), where carbonate ions are in the OH^- sub-lattice.[14, 49] At lower temperatures, HCA of the type B is synthesized, but with a very small content of carbonate ions.[50, 51]

The HA structure can accept many compositional variations in the Ca^{2+}, PO_4^{3-} or OH^- sublattices. Thus, apatite crystals usually present the inclusion of many ions, such as Na^+, K^+, Mg^{2+}, Sr^{2+}, Cl^-, F^-, $HPO_4{}^{2-}$, and so on.[52, 53] All these ions migrate towards the living tissues which are linked to producing an increase in the crystal size. This migration has notable physiological consequences, since the younger, and consequently less crystalline, tissues can develop and grow faster, while storing other elements that the body requires during its growth. Increases in the crystal size of HA make ionic interchanges difficult. Hence, it is worth stressing that the ease of ionic substitutions in the HA structure makes bone an important system for keeping toxic heavy metals out of physiological fluids.

The ability to host ions in this structure allow synthetic calcium phosphates to be designed with improved properties for specific biomedical applications. The ionic substitutions can modify the surface structure and electric charge of HA, with a potential influence on the material in biological environments. In addition, the presence of certain chemical elements that are released during the ceramic resorption facilitates the bone regeneration carried out by osteoblasts. In this sense, amounts of strontium, zinc or silicate stimulate new bone formation. Carbonate and strontium ions facilitate apatite dissolution and, consequently, the resorption of the implant. Silicates in the network increase the mechanical strength of apatite, a very important factor in porous ceramics, and accelerate its bioactive response.[54–56] Thus, the current trend is to obtain synthetic calcium phosphates partially substituted for use in implants.

Biphasic mixtures of calcium phosphates

Most popular materials of this type are based on HA and β-tricalcium phosphate, $\beta\text{-}Ca_3(PO_4)_2$, (β-TCP) mixtures.[57–62] Such mixtures evolve to HCA under physiological conditions. The chemical reactions take place under equilibrium conditions between the more stable HA and the more resorbable β-TCP. The mixture is gradually dissolved, acting as a stem for newly formed bone by the releasing of Ca^{2+} and PO_4^{3-} to the local environment. This material can be injected, used as coating or as bulk in bone replacement: forming of bulk pieces, filling of bone defects, and so on.[63] Moreover, many other biphasic mixtures were investigated including calcium phosphates and other second generation ceramics such as bioactive glasses, calcium sulphates, and so on.[64–66]

Bone cements based on calcium salts

Cements based on calcium phosphates, calcium carbonates or calcium sulphates, have attracted much attention as biomaterials owing to their excellent biocompatibility and bone-repair properties.[67–70] These cements must not be delivered in a prefabricated form and this is a remarkable advantage of the cements over the conventional bioceramics. Most of the injectable calcium phosphates used evolve to an apatitic calcium phosphate during the setting reaction. The physical–chemical properties of these materials, such as the setting time, porosity and mechanical behaviour, depend on cement formulation and the presence of additives.[71–74] These cements cure in field, are biocompatible and can be resorbed slowly. During this gradual process, the newly formed bone grows and replaces the cement. Some aspects that must be improved are related to their mechanical toughness, the curing time, the application technique on the osseous defect and the final biological properties. Research is under way to shorten the curing time, even in contact with blood, and to improve the mechanical toughness. In this book, a complete chapter is devoted to cements where this subject is treated in depth.

Calcium phosphate coatings

The poor mechanical properties of calcium phosphate ceramics impede their use in load-bearing applications. Coatings of HA and other calcium phosphates over metallic substrates were synthesized to overcome this drawback. More common substrates are titanium alloys, Ti6Al4V and commercially pure Ti, because of their low density, good mechanical strength and resistance to cyclic loads.

Commercial implants coated with HA or other calcium phosphates are produced by plasma spray.[75–79] The advantages of the method include a rapid deposition rate and a relatively low cost. However, some problems need to be solved, including the presence of resorbable amorphous calcium phosphate in coatings producing resorption problems. Other aspects to be solved are the adherence to substrate and the instability of HA at high temperatures or at the phase transition of titanium at 1156 K. Thus, the effect of many synthesis parameters in the coatings or of post heat treatment to crystallize the amorphous phases has been investigated.

Other techniques have been used to obtain coatings, including physical vapour deposition (PVD),[80] chemical vapour deposition (CVD),[81] magnetron sputtering,[82] electrophoretic deposition,[83] pulsed laser deposition (PLD),[84, 85] and sol-gel based dip coating.[86, 87] Some of these processes allow greater control of the thickness of coatings and crystallinity of phases. Other processes take place at temperatures lower than those of plasma spray, providing interesting advantages. A recent book reviews the state of art of calcium phosphate coatings.[88]

7.3.2 Glasses

Specific compositions of glasses react with body fluids forming a layer of HCA nanocrystals, which favour the generation of bone matrix and bone growth. These glasses are clinically used for filling osseous cavities, substitution of ear ossicles, maxilofacial reconstruction and dental applications[8] (see Table 7.4). In addition, these glasses which exhibit a high bioactivity are eligible as bioactivity accelerators for mineral apatites or as bioactivity inductors of magnetic materials for hyperthermia treatment of osseous tumors.

Melt glasses

Early bioactive glasses, prepared by quenching a melt, contained SiO_2 and P_2O_5 as network formers and CaO and Na_2O as network modifiers.[33] Many advances in the development of bioactive glasses and other bioactive materials were reached by the *in vitro* assays of bioactivity performed in fluids mimicking human blood plasma. The most common *in vitro* solution to evaluate the bioactive response is so-called simulated body fluid (SBF), proposed by Kokubo *et al.*[89] SBF is an aqueous acellular solution with a composition of inorganic ions almost equal to human blood plasma. In these tests the formation on the glass surface of a layer of HCA nanocrystals is indicative of a positive bioactive response because the glass will bond with the living tissues when implanted.[2] *In vitro* tests allowed comparison of the reactivity of glasses with different kinetics of bioactive response as well as to in depth study of the mechanism of bioactive bond formation. Thus, the essential role of the initial silica-rich layer formed in the glass surface was shown to be due to the ionic interchange of calcium and sodium ions in the glass and protons in the solution. This layer attracted the calcium, phosphate and carbonate ions in solution to form an amorphous calcium phosphate layer, which crystallizes into biologically active HCA nanocrystals. This HCA layer attracts the inorganic moieties that promote new bone formation.[2]

Sol–gel glasses

The sol–gel synthesis of bioactive glasses allows their bioactive response to be tailored and accelerated.[90] In a sol–gel glass (SSG), textural properties can be modified to control their bioactive response. The sol–gel method is more versatile because it allows bioactive coatings, fibres and highly porous monoliths to be used as scaffolds for tissue engineering including growth factors, polypeptides, and so on.

The sol–gel route is more time consuming than the traditional quenching of a melt but requires noticeably lower temperatures. CaO–P_2O_5–SiO_2 has been the most widely system of SSGs studied,[36, 40, 91–97] with some additions, MgO, ZnO, or removals, P_2O_5, to modify mechanical properties, sorption rates or the interaction with osteoblasts.[98–104] CaO plays an essential role in the texture and the bioactive response of a SSG.[105, 106] Ca^{2+} ions leaching from the glass to the medium increase both the silanol (Si–OH) group concentration at the surface, which favours the formation of the HCA layer, and the supersaturation of the solution with respect to apatite. In addition, differences were found in the *in vitro* formation of HCA depending on the presence or not of P_2O_5 in the glass.[107] CaO–SiO_2 glasses exhibit higher initial reactivity. However, HCA nanocrystal formation required 7 days. In contrast, in CaO–P_2O_5–SiO_2 glasses, amorphous calcium phosphate formation is slower, but the HCA nanocrystals are detected quicker than in CaO–SiO_2 glasses. These differences were explained in the nanostructural characterization.[108] P_2O_5-free glasses contain numerous calcium ions in the network that can interchange with protons in the SBF to form additional silanol groups, facilitating amorphous calcium phosphate formation. However, the HCA crystallization required more time. In P_2O_5-containing glasses, calcium is strongly bonded in the Si-doped β-TCP nanocrystals and is difficult to be released to SBF. Thus, the formation of the amorphous calcium phosphate is slower. However, once this phase is formed, Si-doped β-TCP nanocrystals accelerate HCA crystallization. Furthermore, sol–gel glasses exhibited excellent biocompatibility in both cell culture studies[109] and in animal models.[110–112] The high bioactivity of sol–gel glasses makes them excellent candidates to be used in coatings, mixed materials or as porous scaffolds in third generation biomaterials.

Bioactive glass coatings

As it was indicated in the section discussing calcium phosphate coatings above, many techniques can be used to obtain ceramic coatings on metallic substrates including PLD, PVD, CVD, plasma spray and so on. Taking advantage of sol–gel technology, bioactive glass coatings have been obtained by dip coating. This method allows the porosity, roughness and composition of the bioactive film formed to be controlled. Simultaneously, the metallic surface is protected from the biological environment. Coatings of a bioactive glass with a composition of 20%CaO–80%SiO_2 (mol-%) on Ti6Al4V were obtained.[113, 114] After 14 days, the acellular SBF coatings were completely dissolved. First, the calcium ions and then the silica in the coatings leached into the solution. It seems that the extreme reactivity of sol–gel glasses can be a drawback in coatings when compared with HA. However, when analogous studies were performed in the presence of osteoblasts, the coatings remained stable and, simultaneously, an increase of the cellular parameters (adhesion, proliferation, differentiation, spreading) was observed.[115] In addition, the influence of the substrate in the synthesis of sol–gel glasses coatings was also evaluated. When coatings on 316L stainless steel were obtained, the silicon in the glass bonded to chromium in the substrate during the dip coating synthesis, with a subsequent increase in corrosion of the metallic alloy.[116]

Mixed materials containing bioactive sol–gel glasses

Mixed materials systems containing a bioactive SSG to induce or increase bioactivity were investigated including SSG–polymer–drug, SSG–magnetic component and SSG–HA.

SSG–polymer–drug materials were designed to obtain controlled release bioactive systems.[117–122] In this way, osseous integration is improved and drug release is favoured, owing to the ionic interchange between the glass and the medium.

SSG–magnetic glass–ceramic materials were designed to treat osseous tissues affected by tumours. Thus, it should be possible to obtain bioactive materials that are able to regenerate bone, with magnetic behaviour that can be used in hyperthermia treatments. Interstitial hyperthermia, based on the higher sensibility to high temperatures of cancer cells, concentrates the heat treatment to the desired volume without affecting healthy surrounding tissues. Magnetic glass–ceramics act as thermoseeds, whereas SSG induce the bioactivity.[123–130] However, SSG seems to partially inhibit the iron incorporation into crystalline phases of glass–ceramic, consequently decreasing the magnetic behaviour.[129, 130] At the present, the *in vitro* biocompatibility of these mixtures has been established[131] and the *in vivo* behaviour is being studied.

SSG–HA materials were designed to accelerate the bioactive response of HA.[132] Biphasic SSG–HA mixtures exhibit higher bioactivity than pure HA.[133–136] The addition of a 5% bioactive glass noticeably increases the bioactive response of HA. Thus, a mixture 30%CaO–70%SiO_2 glass/HA was covered with a HCA layer after 12 hours in SBF, whereas the surface of pure HA was not modified even after 45 days of immersion. To reach high reactivity in aqueous solutions, HA powders with particle sizes in the range 0.1–50 μm were used. After the sintering process of HA and dry gels, biphasic mixtures with an average particle size around 30 μm were obtained. Another interesting feature of these bioceramics is that the HCA layers formed after the *in vitro* studies are more homogeneous than those formed on pure sol–gel glasses.

7.3.3 Glass–ceramics

Glass–ceramics are crystalline materials nucleated within and from a glass. The formation of these materials is initiated for the addition of nucleating agents that help to nucleate and grow small crystals uniformly distributed within the glass matrix. These nucleating agents can be metals such as Cu, Ag, Au or Pt and oxides like TiO_2, ZrO_2 or P_2O_5. The nucleation process takes place at temperatures lower than the melting temperature and further annealing is conducted at appropriate temperatures to cause uniform crystal growth. The nucleating agents and the heat treatment temperatures help to control grain size to 0.1–1 μm. The resultant glass–ceramic acts as a composite with crystalline phases actuating as a reinforced component, thus, it exhibits superior mechanical properties to the parent glass and to sintered crystalline ceramics. Actually monophase bioactive ceramics, such as glasses or sintered HA, do not show as high a mechanical strength as human cortical bone as is observed in Table 7.5.

Table 7.5 Mechanical properties of some bioactive ceramics and cortical bone

	Bending strength (MPa)	Compressive strength (MPa)	Young's modulus (MPa)	Fracture toughness (MPa $m^{1/2}$)	Hardness Vickers (HV)	Slow crack growth *n*	Density (g cm^{-3})
Glasses							
Bioglass® 45S5	42t	–	35	–	458	–	2.66
S53P4	–	–	–	–	–	–	–
Glass–ceramics							
Ceravital®	–	500	100–150	–	–	–	–
Cerabone® A/W	215	1080	118	2.0	680	33	3.07
Ilmaplant® L1	160	–	–	2.5	–	–	–
Bioverit®	100–160	500	70–88	0.5–1.0	500	–	2.8
Calcium phosphates							
Sintered HA $Ca_{10}(PO_4)_6(OH)_2$	115–200	500–1000	80–110	1.0	600	12–27	3.16
Sintered β-TCP $Ca_3(PO_4)_2$	140–154	460–687	33–90	–	–	–	3.07
Cortical bone (aver.)							–
Low strain	114t	150c/90t	15.2	–	–	–	–
High strain	–	400c/270t	40.8	–	–	–	

c: compressive; t: tensile.

However, glass–ceramics always present a lower surface reactivity than glasses and consequently a lower bioactive response. The reason is the decrease in the number of Si–OH groups at the surface and the more difficult release of calcium ions that are usually entrapped at the crystalline phases. This decrease can be quantified by using the bioactivity index I_B:[137]

$$I_B = 100/t_{0,5bb}\ (d^{-1})$$

Where $t_{0,5bb}$ is the time in days necessary for bonding to bone of 50% of the bioceramic surface after *in vivo* implantation. Using this definition, the higher I_B, the higher the bioactivity. This index can be determined only for bioceramics that have been implanted. Experimental values of I_B of bioceramics used clinically are: 0 for alumina and other almost bioinert ceramics, 2.3 for HA, 3.2 for A/W glass ceramic and 12.5, the maximum value obtained for a synthetic material, for Bioglass® 45S5.

When a large series of new bioceramics are evaluated, their bioactivity can be initially approximated considering the time required for the HCA formation after soaking in SBF. Thus, glass–ceramics with a very quick bioactive response, that are able to be coated by HCA after 1 day in SBF were synthesized by thermal treatment of sol–gel glasses.[42] The mechanical properties of glass–ceramics are clearly better than those of the parent glasses but still lower than cortical bone.[138]

Before describing the third generation ceramics, the clinical applications of first and second generation bioceramics are compared in Table 7.6. As observed, for certain applications bioactive ceramics, such as HA, compete with almost bioinert ceramics, such as Al_2O_3.

7.4 Ceramics in bone regeneration: third generation ceramics

The main purpose of third generation bioceramics is to obtain porous ceramics that act as scaffolds for cells and inducting molecules and that are able to drive self regeneration of tissues. With these requirements, second generation bioceramics with added porosity are being studied, although the design of new advanced ceramics is also explored, with added porosity. This porosity should be in agreement with biological requirements. Apatites, shaped as pieces with interconnected and hierarchical porosity, within the micrometre range, would be a good starting point for fabricating these scaffolds.

The fabrication of ceramic scaffolds for tissue engineering requires a conformation method that yields a material with interconnected porosity and pores in the 2–400 μm range.[139] Therefore, the first step would be to find methods of conformation that yield monoliths with interconnected porosity in the micrometre range.[140–142] This should be possible with the second generation bioceramics discussed previously. Nowadays, there are several conformation

Table 7.6 Clinical applications of first and second generation bioceramics

Ceramic	Clinical application	Examples
Bioinert	Coatings for tissue ingrowth: orthopaedic, dental, maxillofacial	Al_2O_3
	Orthopaedic load bearing applications	Al_2O_3, ZrO_2 , PE-HA- composite
	Artificial heart valves	Pyrolytic carbon coatings
	Artificial tendon and ligament	PLA-carbon fibre composites
Bioactive	Coatings for prosthesis fixation: orthopaedic, dental, maxillofacial	HA, bioactive glasses and glass-ceramics
	Percutaneous devices	Bioactive glasses, bioactive composites
	Periodontal pockets elimination	HA, HA-PLA composite, sodium phosphate, calcium phosphates, bioactive glasses
	Spinal surgery	Bioactive glass–ceramics, HA
Bioinert & bioactive	Dental implants	Al_2O_3 , HA, bioactive glasses
	Alveolar ridge augmentations	Al_2O_3, HA, HA-autogenous bone, bioactive glasses
	Maxillofacial reconstruction	Al_2O_3, HA, HA-PLA composite, bioactive glasses
	Otolaryngological applications	Al_2O_3, HA, glasses, glass–ceramics
	Orthopaedic fixation devices	PLA-carbon fibres, PLA-Ca/P glass fibres
Resorbable	Temporary bone spacers fillers	Calcium phosphates (α and β TCP,...), calcium sulphate

methods that allow monoliths to be obtained at room temperature.[143–146] In addition, working at room temperature it is possible to include molecules with biological activity to treat different diseases, or to improve the treatment of various bone pathologies.

At present, the aim is to find bioceramics which induce the regeneration of osseous tissues stimulating the response of the cells involved. These bioceramics acting as scaffolds must be porous so that the cells can do their job. This porosity implies a certain sacrifice of the mechanical properties. A certain smart behaviour is also required, so that their properties can be modified in response to external stimuli and also to allow biologically active molecules to be loaded onto such ceramics. This is the beginning of what could be termed as third generation bioceramics (see Fig. 7.6). All those ceramics that fulfil the biocompatibility requirements are possible candidates as scaffolds for tissue engineering, where bioceramics particles must be nanometric in size to enhance their reactivity.

Figure 7.7 shows a hierarchy of sizes from the human skeletal (far left, a) which has a size of the order of metres to the hydroxyapatite unit cell (far right, f) with dimensions close to 0.7 nm. Image (b) represents a human femur which is

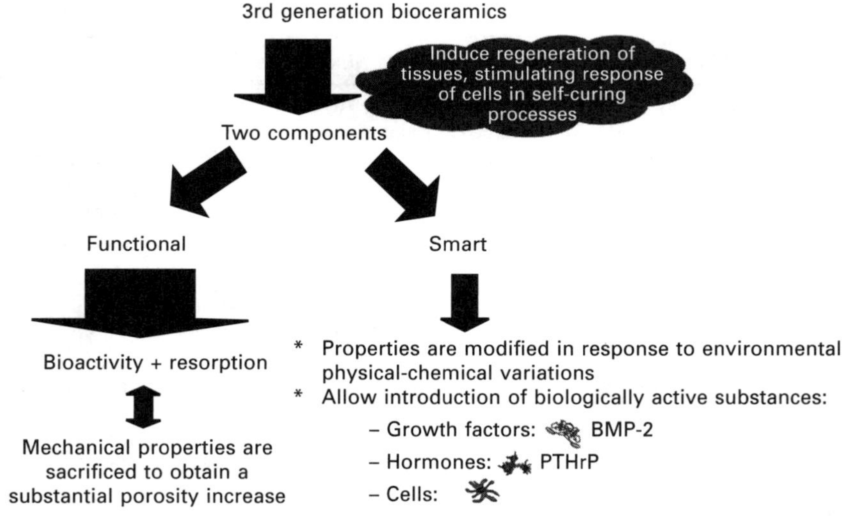

7.6 Functional and smart components of third generation bioceramics. BMP: bone morphogenetic protein, PTHrP: parathyroid hormone related peptide.

mainly made up of collagen fibres reinforced by nanometric size apatite crystals. (c), (d) and (e) (from left to right) are microscopy images of some apatite particles grown in vitro on the surface of bioactive ceramics. These apatites are similar in composition and size to biological ones. Image (c), obtained by scanning electron microscopy (SEM), shows pseudo-spherical particles of around 10 mm. When higher magnification is reached with transmission electron microscopy (TEM) (d), it is possible to verify that the spheres are formed by bundles of needle-like apatite crystals. Image (e) is a higher resolution TEM micrograph of these crystals.

Bearing in mind the natural bone model, an approach for the fabrication of synthetic materials able to regenerate and repair bone would be to combine the organic and inorganic phases so that we could achieve a ceramic with a certain viscoelasticity degree, allowing cell activity and, obviously, being biocompatible.

7.4.1 Silica-based mesoporous materials as bioceramics

Research on the potential use of silica-based ordered mesoporous materials as drug delivery systems for biomedical applications started in 2001,[147] and in 2006 extended to their use as potentially bioactive ceramics.[148] These are, therefore, materials still at an experimental stage but with great expectations in the field of biomaterials.[149, 150]

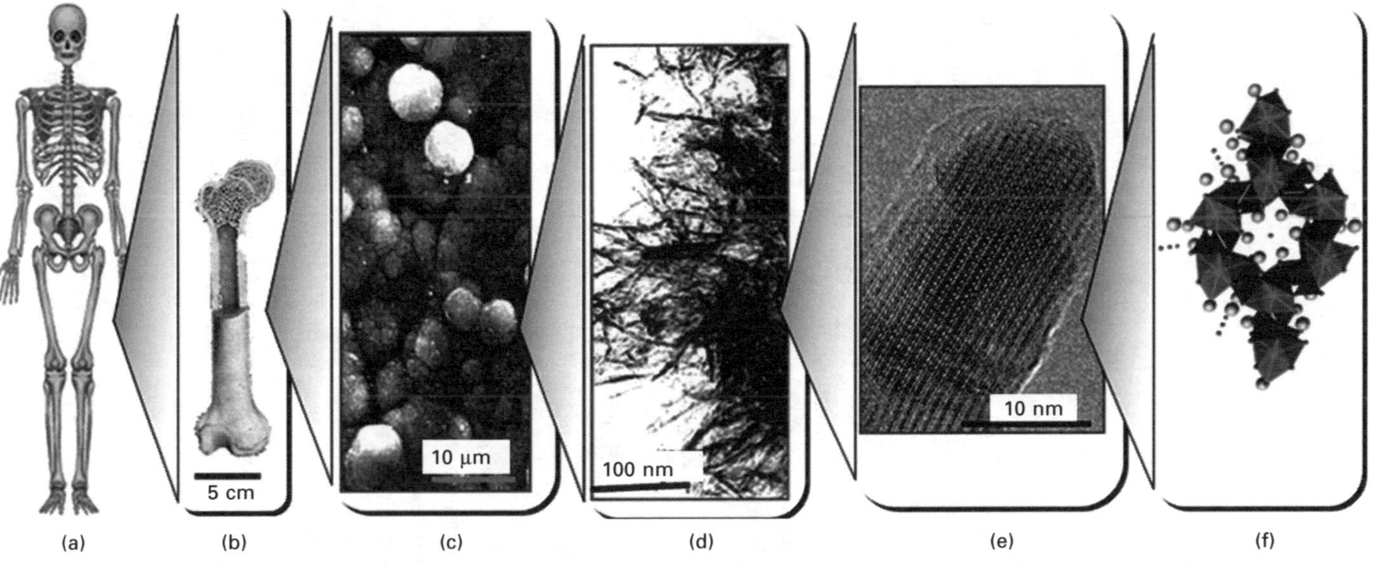

7.7 A hierarchy of sizes from the human skeletal (far left, a) to the hydroxyapatite unit cell (far right, f). From left to right, image (b) is a human femur, image (c) is a SEM micrograph and (d) and (e) are TEM micrographs, all of apatite nanocrystals grown *in vitro* on the surface of bioactive ceramics.

These materials are synthesized using surfactants which play the role of a template, allowing the production of materials with ordered porosity, in the nanometre size range, and amorphous silica pore walls.

The application of this synthesis methodology to the production of bioactive glasses leads to amorphous silica materials, which are highly reactive and have ordered mesoporosity. This stage leads in turn to the synthesis of templated glasses.[151] These templated glasses exhibit spectacular textural properties when compared with traditional bioactive sol–gel glasses; specific surface values, for instance, are twice as large. They are bioactive and, owing to their more open texture, the bioactive response is evidenced after much shorter periods of time; the best bioactive response data in traditional sol–gel glasses is obtained after 3 days, while 1 hour suffices in the mesoporous templated glasses.[151] These templated glasses exhibit high *in vitro* reactivity when in contact with SBF. The transformation path starts with the formation of an amorphous calcium phosphate, which then evolves to octacalcium phosphate and subsequently to calcium deficient carbonate hydroxyapatite. The whole sequence is performed in just 8 hours[152] and its most interesting feature is its similarity to the biomineralization processes which take place in natural bone.

On the other hand, mesoporous microspheres have been recently investigated for biomedical applications. Thus, bioactive glass microspheres with accelerated deposition rates of HCA and hemostatic efficacy[153] and magnetic silica microspheres for drug targeting have been reported.[154, 155]

7.4.2 Organic–inorganic hybrid materials

The synthesis of bioactive organic–inorganic hybrid materials able to bond osseous tissues and to host molecules with biological activity is an important task in the biomedical engineering field.[156] Hybrids are synthesized by sol–gel processes at temperatures close to ambient that do not destroy the organic component. This method makes possible the production of hybrid materials in different forms: as bulk, coatings, fibres, and so on. Inorganic components of hybrids are often based in SiO_2–CaO glasses because they supply many surface silanol groups and release Ca^{2+} ions into solution, both effects promoting the bioactive response. With respect to the organic component, several biocompatible polymers were investigated in order to tailor the hybrid materials properties. For instance, bioactive hybrids with mechanical features comparable to natural bone were obtained.[157] In addition, polymers with specific functionality (i.e. amino groups) able to interact with biological entities, have been used as the organic component of hybrids.[28]

Several organic–inorganic systems were investigated for clinical uses as bioactive or degradable materials. In some hybrid systems, only weak physical interactions between inorganic and organic domains are present. Examples include hybrids containing poly(vinyl alcohol) (PVA),[158, 159] or poly(hydroxyethyl methacrylate) (pHEMA).[160] In other cases, chemical links between both components are formed. This is the case for hybrids containing poly(methyl methacrylate) (PMMA),[161, 162] poly(ε-caprolactone) (PCL)[163, 164] or gelatine.[165–167] To improve the bioactive response, inorganic components, such as TiO_2 or P, were also added to hybrids with poly(dimethylsiloxane) (PDMS)[168–170] or poly(tetramethylene oxide) (PTMO).[171, 172]

Examples of hybrid systems investigated for bone repairing include: (i) CaO–SiO_2–PDMS, obtained as bioactive coatings[173] or as bioactive monoliths pure,[174] or with P additions to accelerate the bioactive response,[170] (ii) CaO–SiO_2–P_2O_5–PVA synthesized as transparent films[158] and as bioactive and degradable monoliths[159] and (iii) CaO–SiO_2-based hybrids with organic polymers with methacriloxy and amino groups,[28] with tailored bioactivity and degradability that has recently been proposed to enable the time release of bioencapsulates.[175]

A family of bioactive organic–inorganic hybrids with amazing mechanical properties is based in the denominated 'star gels' developed by Dupont in 1995.[176] These materials exhibit a singular structure of an organic core surrounded by flexible arms, which are terminated in alkoxysilane groups that can form a silica network through a sol–gel process. The flexibility of the structure at the molecular level yields materials with a macroscopic mechanical behaviour between glasses and rubbers.[177, 178] When Ca^{2+} ions where added to the 'star gels', materials with a bioactive response were obtained.[157] Moreover, these hybrids present fracture toughness comparable to the human tibia, opening up interesting possibilities in the use of these types of materials in implants.

Hybrid materials have been also synthesized as porous scaffolds for tissue engineering.[179] A three-dimensional interconnected pore structure is obtained by using different strategies. Thus, SiO_2–PDMS with 90% porosity and pore sizes about 200–500 μm in diameter were obtained using sieved sucrose particles as the template.[180] These hybrids have been evaluated for scaffold and bioreactor applications and implanted into brain defects. Gelatin–siloxane (3-glicidopropyltrimethoxisilane, GPTMS) hybrid scaffolds with different orders of porosity (5–10, 30–50 and 300–500 μm) were obtained by freeze drying the wet hybrid gels.[166] These hybrid materials have been also evaluated in brain defects without inflammation being observed.[181] Finally, chitosan–GPTMS hybrids with or without calcium with 90% porosity and a pore size of around 100 μm were also prepared by freeze-drying methods and their biocompatibility evaluated in cell cultures.[182]

These results allow organic–inorganic hybrids to be considered, like those presented in this section or others based on dendrimers that are just starting to be investigated, as promising candidates for use as scaffolds in bone tissue regeneration applications.

7.5 Bioceramics today

First and second generation bioceramics, that is, almost bioinert, bioactive and resorbable, are being used today in implants and medical devices. Third generation bioceramics, that is, those driving living tissue regeneration are now under experimentation and represent hope for the future. A interesting example of the actual research interests in biomaterials in general and in bioceramics in particular can be obtained from the programme of the Eighth World Biomaterials Congress that took place in Amsterdam in May–June of 2008. The almost 3000 communications presented were classified into 102 scientific sessions. Twenty were devoted to tissue engineering or regenerative medicine. The words scaffolds, cells, stem cells or cellular appeared in the title of 26 sessions. Six sessions were devoted to surfaces and the prefix 'nano-' appeared in another six as a logical consequence of the interest in nanoscience and nanotechnology. With regards to the type of material, seven were specifically dedicated to bioceramics, and of them four to calcium phosphates, one to glasses, one to glass–ceramics and one to ceramic coatings, and one to dendrimers. In addition, ceramics also appeared as studied materials in sessions devoted to tissue engineering and regenerative medicine, bone, porous matrixes, biomaterials for cancer research, injectable biomaterials, biomechanics, tribology of artificial hip replacements, surface characterization, composite biomaterials and osteoblast–material interactions.

7.6 Acknowledgements

We would like to express our deepest gratitude to all our co-workers and colleagues who have contributed their effort and consideration of these studies over the years and whose names are collected in the reference section.

7.7 References

1 Hench L L, 'Bioceramics: from concept to clinic', *J Am Ceram Soc*, 1991, **74**, 1487–510.

2 Vallet-Regí M, 'Ceramics for medical applications', *J Chem Soc, Dalton Trans*, 2001, 97–108.

3 Vallet-Regí M, 'Revisiting ceramics for medical applications', *Dalton Trans*, 2006, 5211–20.

4 Salinas A J and Vallet-Regí M, 'Evolution of ceramics with medical applications' *Z Anorg Allg Chem*, 2007, 1762–73.

5 Vallet-Regí M, 'Bioceramics: where do we come from and which are the future expectations', *Key Eng. Mater*, 2008, **377**, 1–18.

6 Hench L L and Polak J M, 'Third-generation biomedical materials', *Science*, 2002, **295**, 1014–17.

7 Hench L L and Anderson O, 'Bioactive glasses', in *An Introduction to Bioceramics*, Hench L L and Wilson J (eds.), World Scientific, Singapore, 1993, 41–62.

8 Vallet-Regí M, Ragel C V and Salinas A J, 'Glasses with medical applications' *Eur J Inorg Chem*, 2003, 1029–42.

9 Kumta P N, 'Ceramic Biomaterials', in *An Introduction to Biomaterials*, Guelcher S A and Hollinger J (eds.), CRC Taylor & Francis, Boca Raton, 2006, 311–40.
10 Vallet-Regí M and González-Calbet J, 'Calcium phosphates in the substitution of bone tissue', *Prog Solid State Chem*, 2004, **32**, 1–31.
11 Hench L L, 'Bioactive ceramics: theory and clinical applications', in *Bioceramics 7*, Anderson Ö H, Happonen R-P and Yli-Urpo A (eds.), Butterworth-Heinemann Oxford, 1994, 3–14
12 Langer R and Vacanti J P, 'Tissue engineering', *Science*, 1993, **260**, 920–6.
13 Vallet-Regí M and Arcos-Navarrete D, *Biomimetic Nanoceramics in Clinical Use: From Materials to Applications*, Royal Society of Chemistry, Cambridge, 2008.
14 LeGeros R Z, 'Calcium phosphates in oral biology and medicine', in *Monographs in Oral Science, Vol. 15*, Myers H M (ed.), S. Karger, Basel, 1991.
15 Frieb W and Warner J, 'Biomedical applications', in *Handbook of Porous Solids*, Schuth F, Sing K S W and Weitkamp J (eds.), Wiley-VCH, Weinheim, 2002, 2923–70
16 Ratner B D and Castner D G, 'Biomedical surface science: foundations to frontiers', *Surface Science*, 2002, **500**, 28–60.
17 Smith L, 'Ceramic plastic material as a bone substitute', *Arch Surg*, 1963, **87**, 653–61.
18 Sandhaus S, Bone Implants and Drills and Taps for Bone Surgery, 1967, British Patent 1083769.
19 Boutin P, 'Alumina and its use in surgery of the hip', *Presse Med*, 1971, **79**, 639.
20 Li J and Hastings G W, 'Oxide bioceramics: inert ceramic materials in medicine and dentistry', in: *Handbook of Biomaterial Properties*, Black J and Hastings G (eds.), Chapman Hall, Oxford, 1998, 340–54.
21 Oonishi H, Okabe N, Hamaguchi, T and Nabeshima T, 'Cementless alumina ceramic total knee prosthesis', *Orthopaedic Ceramic Implants 1*, 1981, 11–18.
22 Schulte W, 'The Frialit Tuebingen implant system', in *Osseointegrated Implants Volume II. Implants in Oral and ENT Surgery*, Heimke G. (ed.), CRC Press, Boca Raton, 1990, 1–34.
23 Polack F M and Heimke G, 'Ceramic kerato-prostheses', *Ophtalmology*, 1980, **87**, 693–8.
24 Kawahara H, 'Implant biomaterial and ceramics', *Orthopaedic Ceramic Implants 1*, 1981, 1–10
25 Christel P, Meunier A, Dorlot, J M, Crolet J M, Witvoet, J, Sedel L and Boutin P, 'Biomechanical compatibility and design of ceramic implants for orthopaedic surgery. Bioceramics: material characteristics versus *in vivo* behaviour', *Ann NY Acad Sci*, 1988, **523**, 234–56.
26 Akagawa Y, Ichikawa Y, Nikai H and Tsuru H, 'Interface histology of unloaded and early loaded partially-stabilized zirconia endosseous implant in initial bone healing', *J Prosthet Dent*, 1993, **69**, 599–604
27 Dauskardt R H and Ritchie R O, 'Pyrolytic carbon coatings', in *An Introduction to Bioceramics*, Hench, L L, Wilson J (eds), World Scientific, Singapore, 1993, 261–80.
28 Colilla M, Salinas A J and Vallet-Regí M, 'Amino-polysiloxane hybrid materials for bone reconstruction', *Chem Mater*, 2006, **18**, 5676–83.
29 Elliott J C, *Structure and Chemistry of the Apatites and Other Calcium Orthophosphates*, Elsevier, London, 1994.

30 De Groot K, 'Bioceramics consisting of calcium phosphate salts', *Biomaterials*, 1991, **1**, 47–50.

31 Dorozhkin S V and Epple M, 'Biological and medical significance of calcium phosphates', *Angew Chem-Int. ed*, 2002, **41**, 3130–46.

32 Pietrzak W S and Ronk R, 'Calcium sulphate bone void filler: A review and a look ahead', *J Craniofac Surg*, 2000, **11**, 327–34.

33 Hench L L, Splinter R J, Allen W C and Greenlee T K, 'Bonding. mechanisms at the interface of ceramic prosthetic materials', *J Biomed Mater Res*, 1971, **2**, 117–41.

34 Hench L L and Wilson J, 'Surface-active biomaterials', *Science*, 1984, **226**, 630–6.

35 Yuan H P, Kurashina K, de Bruijn J D, Li Y B, de Groot K and Zhang X D, 'A preliminary study on osteoinduction of two kinds of calcium phosphate ceramics', *Biomaterials*, 1999, **20**, 1799–806.

36 Vallet-Regí M, Romero A M, Ragel C V and LeGeros R Z, 'XRD, SEM-EDS and FTIR studies of *in vitro* growth of an apatite-like layer on sol–gel glasses', *J Biomed Mater Res*, 1999, **44**, 416–21.

37 Livingston T, Ducheyne P and Garino J, '*In vivo* evaluation of a bioactive scaffold for bone tissue engineering', *J Biomed Mater Res*, 2002, **62**, 1–13.

38 Kokubo T, Kim H M and Kawashita M, 'Novel bioactive materials with different mechanical properties', *Biomaterials*, 2003, **24**, 2161–75.

39 Vallet-Regí M and Rámila A, 'New bioactive glass and changes in porosity during the growth of a carbonate hydroxyapatite layer on glass surface', *Chem Mater*, 2000, **12**, 961–5.

40 Vallet-Regí M, Arcos D and Pérez-Pariente J, 'Evolution of porosity during *in vitro* hydroxycarbonate apatite growth in sol–gel glasses', *J Biomed Mater Res*, 2000, **51**, 23–8.

41 Roman J, Padilla S and Vallet-Regí M, 'Sol–gel glasses as precursors of bioactive glass-ceramics', *Chem Mat*, 2003, **15**, 798–806.

42 Padilla S, Roman J, Carenas A and Vallet-Regí M, 'Influence of the phosphorus content on the bioactivity in sol–gel glass ceramics', *Biomaterials*, 2005, **26**, 475–83

43 del Real R P, Arcos D and Vallet-Regí M, 'Implantable magnetic glass-ceramic based on (Fe, Ca) SiO_3 solid solutions', *Chem Mater*, 2002, **14**, 64–70.

44 Vallet-Regí M, Gutiérrez-Ríos M T, Alonso M P, de Frutos M I and Nicolopoulos S, 'Hydroxyapatite particles synthesized. by pyrolysis of an aerosol', *J Solid State Chem*, 1994, **112**, 58–64.

45 Narasaraju T S B and Phebe D E, 'Some physico-chemical aspects of hydroxyapatite', *J Mater Sci*, 1996, **31**, 1–21.

46 Vallet-Regí M, Rodríguez Lorenzo L M and Salinas A J, 'Synthesis and characterisation of calcium deficient apatite', *Solid State Ionics*, 1997, **101–03**, 1279–85.

47 Pechini M P, *Method of preparing lead and alkaline earth titanates and niobates and coating method using the same to form capacitor*, (July 11, 1967) U. S. Patent 3,330,697.

48 Peña J and Vallet-Regí M, 'Hydroxyapatite, tricalcium phosphate and biphasic materials prepared by a liquid mix technique', *J Eur Ceram Soc*, 2003, **23**, 1687–96.

49 Elliott J C, Bonel G and Tombe J C, 'Space group and lattice-constants of $Ca_{10}(PO_4)_6CO_3$', *J Appl Crystallog*, 1980, **13**, 618–21.

50 Okazaki M, Matsumoto T, Taira M, Takakashi J and LeGeros R Z, 'CO3-Apatite preparation with solubility gradient: potential degradable biomaterials', in *Bioceramics 11*, LeGeros R Z and LeGeros J P (eds.), World Scientific, New York, 1998, 85–8.
51 Doi Y, Shibutani T, Moriwaki Y, Kajimoto T and Iwayama Y J, 'Sintered carbonate apatites as bioresorbable bone substitutes', *J Biomed Mater Res*, 1998, **39**, 603–10.
52 LeGeros R Z , 'Effect of carbonate on the lattice parameters of apatite', *Nature*, 1965, **206**, 403–4.
53 Jha L J, Best S M, Knowles J C, Rehman I, Santos J D and Bonfield W, 'Preparation and characterization of fluoride-substituted apatites', *J Mater. Sci: Mater Med*, 1997, **8**, 185–91.
54 Vallet-Regí M and Arcos D, 'Silicon substituted hydroxyapatites. A method to upgrade calcium phosphate based implants', *J Mater Chem*, 2005, **15**, 1509–16.
55 Boyer L, Carpena J and Lacout J L, 'Synthesis of phosphate silicate apatites at atmospheric pressure', *Solid State Ionics*, 1997, **95**, 121–9.
56 Gibson I R, Best S M and Bonfield W, 'Chemical characterization of silicon substituted hydroxyapatite', *J Biomed Mater Res*, 1999, **44**, 422–8.
57 Daculsi G, 'Biphasic calcium phosphate concept applied to artificial bone, implant coating and injectable bone substitute', *Biomaterials*, 1998, **19**, 1473–8.
58 Tancred D C, McCormack B A O and Carr A J, 'A synthetic bone implant macroscopically identical to cancellous bone', *Biomaterials*, 1998, **19**, 2303–11.
59 Kivrak N and Tas A C, 'Synthesis of calcium hydroxyapatite-tricalcium phosphate (HA-TCP) composite bioceramic powders and their sintering behavior', *J Am Ceram Soc*, 1998, **82**, 2245–52.
60 Gauthier O, Goyenvalle E, Bouler J M, J. Guicheux, Pilet P, Weiss P and Daculsi G, 'Macroporous biphasic calcium phosphate ceramics versus injectable bone substitute: a comparative study 3 and 8 weeks after implantation in rabbit bone', *J Mater Sci Mater Med*, 2001, **12**, 385–90.
61 Sánchez-Salcedo S, Werner J and Vallet-Regí M, 'Hierarchical pore structure of calcium phosphate scaffolds by combination of the gel casting and multiple tape casting methods', *Acta Biomaterialia*, 2008, **4**, 913–22
62 Sánchez-Salcedo S, Arcos D and Vallet-Regí M, 'Upgrading calcium phosphate scaffolds for tissue engineering applications', *Key Eng Mater*, 2008, **377**, 19–42.
63 Grimandi G, Wiss P, Millot F and Daculsi G, '*In vitro* evaluation of a new injectable calcium phosphate material', *J Biomed Mater Res*, 1998, **39**, 660–6.
64 Cabañas M V, Rodríguez-Lorenzo L M and Vallet-Regí M, 'Setting behavior and *in vitro* bioactivity of hydroxyapatite/calcium sulphate cements', *Chem Mater*, 2002, **14**, 3550–5.
65 Ragel C V, Vallet-Regí M and Rodríguez-Lorenzo L M, 'Preparation and *in vitro* bioactivity of hydroxyapatite/sol–gel glass biphasic material', *Biomaterials*, 2002, **23**, 1865–72.
66 Rámila A, Padilla S, Muñoz B and Vallet-Regí M, 'A new hydroxyapatite/glass biphasic material: *in vitro* bioactivity', *Chem Mater*, 2002, **14**, 2439–43.
67 Coetzee A S, 'Regeneration of bone in the presence of calcium sulphate', *Arch Otolaryngol*, 1980, **106**, 405–9.
68 Lemâitre J, Mirtchi A A and Mortier A, 'Calcium phosphate cements for medical use: state of the art and perspectives of development', *Silic Ind*, 1987, **9–10**, 141–6.

69 Chow L C, 'Development of Self-Setting Calcium Phosphate Cements', *J Ceram Soc Jpn*, 1991, **99**, 954–64.

70 Constantz B R, Ison I C, Fulmer M, Poser R D and Smith S T, 'Skeletal repair by *in situ* formation of the mineral phase of bone', *Science*, 1995, **267**, 1796–9.

71 Ginebra M P, Driessens F C M and Planell J A, 'Effect of the particle size on the micro and nanostructural features of a calcium phosphate cement: a kinetic analysis', *Biomaterials*, 2004, **25**, 3453–62.

72 Otsuka M, Matsuda Y, Suwa Y, Fox J L and Higuchi W, 'Effect of particle size of metastable calcium phosphates on mechanical strength of a novel self-setting bioactive calcium phosphate cement', *J Biomed Mater Res*, 1995, **29**, 25–32.

73 Miyamoto Y, Ishikawa K, Takechi M, Toh T, Yuasa T, Nagayama M and Suzuki K, 'Basic properties of calcium phosphate cement containing atelocollagen in its liquid or powder phases', *Biomaterials*, 1998, **19**, 707–15.

74 Nilsson M, Fernández E, Sarda S, Lidgren L and Planell J A, 'Characterization of a novel calcium phosphate/sulphate bone cement' *J Biomed Mater Res*, 2002, **61**, 600–7.

75 Koch B, Wolke J G and de Groot K, 'X-ray diffraction studies on plasma-sprayed calcium phosphate-coated implants', *J Biomed Mater Res*, 1990, **24**, 655–67.

76 Garcia-Sanz F J, Mayor M B, Arias J L, Pou J, Leon B and Perez-Amor M, 'Hydroxyapatite coatings: a comparative study between plasma-spray and pulsed laser deposition techniques', *J Mater Sci Mater Med*, 1997, **8**, 861–5.

77 Tsui Y C, Doyle C and Clyne T W, 'Plasma sprayed hydroxyapatite coatings on titanium substrates Part 1: Mechanical properties and residual stress levels', *Biomaterials*, 1998, **19**, 2015–29.

78 Sun L M, Berndt C C, Gross, K A and Kucuk A, 'Material fundamentals and clinical performance of plasma-sprayed hydroxyapatite coatings: A review' *J Biomed Mater Res*, 2001, **58**, 570–92.

79 Yan L L, Leng Y and Weng L T, 'Characterization of chemical inhomogeneity in plasma-sprayed hydroxyapatite coatings', *Biomaterials*, 2003, **24**, 2585–92.

80 Park Y S, Yi K Y, Lee I S, Han C H and Jung Y C, 'The effects of ion beam-assisted deposition of hydroxyapatite on the grit-blasted surface of endosseous implants in rabbit tibiae', *Int J Oral Maxillofac Implants*, 2005, **20**, 31–8.

81 Cabañas M V and Vallet-Regí, M, 'Calcium phosphate coatings deposited by aerosol chemical vapour deposition', *J Mater Chem*, 2003, **13**, 1104–7.

82 Wolke J G C, de Groot K and Jansen J A, 'Subperiosteal implantation of various RF magnetron sputtered Ca-P coatings in goats', *J Biomed Mater Res*, 1998, **43**, 270–6.

83 Kannan S, Balamurugan A and Rajeswari S, 'Development of calcium phosphate coatings on type 316L SS and their *in-vitro* response', *Trends Biomater Artif Organs*, 2002, **16**, 8–11.

84. Arias J L, Mayor M B, Pou J, Leng Y, León B and Pérez-Amor M, 'Micro- and nano-testing of calcium phosphate coatings produced by pulsed laser deposition', *Biomaterials*, 2003, **24**, 3403–8.

85 Hashimoto Y, Kawashima M, Hatanaka R, Kusunoki M, Nishikawa H, Hontsu S and Nakamura M, 'Cytocompatibility of calcium phosphate coatings deposited by an ArF pulsed laser', *J Mater Sci: Mater Med*, 2008, **19**, 327–33.

86 Hijón N, Cabañas M V, Izquierdo-Barba I and Vallet–Regí M, 'Bioactive carbonate-hydroxyapatite coatings deposited onto Ti6Al4V substrate', *Chem Mater*, 2004, **16**, 1451–5.

87 Hijon N, Cabañas M V, Izquierdo-Barba I, Garcia M A and Vallet-Regi M, Nanocrystalline bioactive apatite coatings', *Solid State Sci*, 2006, **8**, 685–9.

88 León, B and Jansen J A (Eds.), *Thin Calcium Phosphate Coatings for Medical Implants*, 2008, Springer.

89 Kokubo T, Kushitani H, Sakka S, Kitsugi T and Yamamuro T, 'Solutions able to reproduce *in vivo* surface-structure changes in bioactive glass-ceramic A-W', *J Biomed Mat. Res*, 1990, **24**, 721–34.

90 Li R, Clark A E and Hench L L, 'An investigation of bioactive glass powders by sol-gel processing', *J Appl Biomat*, 1991, **2**, 231–9.

91 Pereira M M, Clark A E and Hench L L, 'Calcium-phosphate formation on sol–gel-derived bioactive glasses *in-vitro*', *J Biomed Mater Res*, 1994, **28**, 693–8.

92 Peltola T, Jokinen M, Rahiala H, Levänen E, Rosenhold J B, Kangasniemi I and Yli-Urpo A, 'Calcium phosphate formation on porous sol–gel-derived SiO_2 and CaO-P_2O_5-SiO_2 substrates *in vitro*', *J Biomed Mater Res*, 1999, **44**, 12–21.

93 Vallet-Regí M, Izquierdo-Barba I and Salinas A J, 'Influence of P_2O_5 on crystallinity of apatite formed in vitro on surface of bioactive glasses', *J Biomed Mater Res*, 1999, **46**, 560–5.

94 Vallet-Regí M, Pérez-Pariente J, Izquierdo-Barba I and Salinas A J, 'Compositional variations in time calcium phosphate layer growth on gel glasses soaked in a simulated body fluid', *Chem Mater*, 2000, **12**, 3770–5.

95 Salinas A J, Vallet-Regí M and Izquierdo-Barba I, 'Biomimetic apatite deposition on calcium silicate gel glasses', *J Sol-Gel Sci Techn*, 2001, **21**, 13–25.

96 Balas F, Arcos D, Pérez-Pariente J and Vallet-Regí M, 'Textural properties of SiO_2–CaO–P_2O_5 glasses prepared by the sol–gel method', *J Mater Res*, 2001, **16**, 1345–8.

97 Arcos D, Greenspan D and Vallet-Regí M, 'Influence of the stabilization temperature on textural and structural features and ion release in SiO_2–CaO–P_2O_5 sol–gel glasses', *Chem Mater*, 2002, **14**, 1515–22.

98 Pérez-Pariente J, Balas F, Román J, Salinas A J and Vallet-Regí M, 'Influence of composition and surface characteristics on the *in vitro* bioactivity of SiO_2–CaO–P_2O_5–MgO sol–gel glasses', *J Biomed Mater Res*, 1999, **47**, 170–5.

99 Vallet-Regí M, Salinas A J, Román J and Gil M, 'Effect of magnesium content on the in vitro bioactivity of CaO–MgO–SiO_2–P_2O_5 sol–gel glasses', *J Mater Chem*, 1999, **9**, 515–18.

100 Pérez-Pariente J, Balas F and Vallet-Regí M, 'Surface and chemical study of $SiO_2P_2O_5CaO(MgO)$ bioactive glasses', *Chem Mater*, 2000, **12**, 750–5.

101 Du R L and Chang J, 'Preparation and characterization of Zn and Mg doped bioactive glasses', *J Inorg Mater*, 2004, **19**, 1353–8.

102 Oki A, Parveen B, Hossain S, Adeniji A and Donahue H, 'Preparation and *in vitro* bioactivity of zinc containing sol–gel-derived bioglass materials', *J Biomed Mater Res*, 2004, **69A**, 216–21.

103 Day R M and Boccaccini A R, 'Effect of particulate bioactive glasses on human macrophages and monocytes *in vitro*', *J Biomed Mater Res*, 2005, **73A**, 73–9.

104 Du R N, Chang J, Ni S Y and Zhai N Y, 'Characterization and *in vitro* bioactivity of zinc-containing bioactive glass and glass-ceramics', *J Biomater Appl*, 2006, **20**, 341–60.

105 Martínez A, Izquierdo-Barba I and Vallet-Regí M, 'Bioactivity of a CaO-SiO_2 binary glasses system', *Chem Mater*, 2000, **12**, 3080–8.

106 Vallet-Regí M, Salinas A J, Martínez A, Izquierdo-Barba I and Pérez-Pariente J,

'Textural properties of CaO-SiO_2 glasses for use in implants', *Solid State Ionics*, 2004, **172**, 441–4.

107 Salinas A J, Martín A I and Vallet-Regí M, 'Bioactivity of three CaO–P_2O_5–SiO_2 sol–gel glasses', *J Biomed Mater Res*, 2002, **61**, 524–32.

108 Vallet-Regí M, Salinas A J, Ramírez-Castellanos J and González-Calbet J M, 'Nanostructure of bioactive sol–gel glasses and organic inorganic hybrids', *Chem Mater*, 2005, **17**, 1874–9.

109 Olmo N, Martín A I, Salinas A J, Turnay J, Vallet-Regí M and Lizarbe M A, 'Bioactive sol–gel glasses with and without a hydroxycarbonate apatite layer as substrates for osteoblast cell adhesion and proliferation', *Biomaterials*, 2003, **24**, 3383–93.

110 Meseguer-Olmo L, Ros-Nicolás M J, Clavel-Sainz M, Vicente-Ortega V, Alcaraz Baños M, Lax-Pérez A, Arcos D, Ragel C V and Vallet-Regí M, 'Biocompatibility and *in vivo* gentamicin release from bioactive sol–gel glass implants', *J Biomed Mater Res*, 2002, **61**, 458–65.

111 Gil-Albarova J, Garrido-Lahiguera R, Salinas A J, Román J, Bueno-Lozano A L, Gil-Albarova R and Vallet-Regí M, 'The in vivo performance of a sol–gel glass and a glass–ceramic in the treatment of limited bone defects', *Biomaterials*, 2004, **25**, 4639–45.

112 Gil-Albarova J, Salinas A J, Bueno-Lozano A L, Román J, Aldini-Nicolo N, García-Barea A, Giavaresi G, Fini M, Giardini R and Vallet-Regí M, 'The *in vivo* behaviour of a sol–gel glass and a glass-ceramic during critical diaphyseal bone defects healing', *Biomaterials*, 2005, **26**, 4374–82.

113 Izquierdo-Barba I, Asenjo A, Esquivias L and Vallet-Regí M, 'SiO_2–CaO vitreous films deposited onto Ti6Al4V Substrates', *Eur J Inorg Chem*, 2003, 1608–13.

114 Izquierdo-Barba I, Rojo J M, Blanco E, Vallet-Regí M and Esquivias L, 'The role of precursor concentration on the characteristics of SiO_2-CaO films', *J Sol–Gel Sci Techn*, 2003, **26**, 1179–82.

115 Izquierdo-Barba I, Conde F, Olmo N, Lizarbe M A, García M A and Vallet-Regí M, 'Vitreous SiO_2-CaO coatings onto Ti6Al4V alloys: reactivity in acellular solution vs osteoblast cell culture', *Acta Biomater*, 2006, **2**, 445–55.

116 Vallet-Regí M, Izquierdo-Barba I and Gil F J, 'Localized corrosion of 316L Stainless Steel with SiO_2-CaO films obtained by means of sol–gel treatment', *J Biomed Mater Res*, 2003, **67A**, 674–8.

117 Arcos D, Cabañas M V, Ragel C V, Vallet-Regí M and San Román J, 'Ibuprofen release from hydrophilic ceramic–polymer composites', *Biomaterials*, 1997, **18**, 1235–42.

118 Granado S, Ragel C V, Cabañas V, San Román J and Vallet-Regí M, 'Morphology and particle size on drug release from ceramic/polymer composites', *J Mater Chem*, 1997, **7**, 1581–5.

119 Vallet-Regí M, Granado S, Arcos D, Gordo M, Cabañas M V, Ragel C V, Salinas A J, Doadrio A L and San Román J, 'Preparation, characterization, and *in vitro* release of ibuprofen from Al_2O_3/PLA/PMMA composites', *J Biomed Mater Res*, 1998, **39**, 423–8.

120 Vallet-Regí M, Gordo M, Ragel C V, Cabañas M V and San Román J, 'Synthesis of ceramic/polymer/drug biocomposites at room temperature', *Solid State Ionics*, 1997, **101–103**, 887–92.

121 del Real R P, Padilla S and Vallet-Regí M, 'Gentamicin release from OHAp/PEMA/PMMA composites', *J Biomed Mater Res*, 2000, **52**, 1–7.

122 Padilla S, del Real R P and Vallet-Regí M, '*In vitro* release of gentamicin from OHAP/PEMA/PMMA samples', *J Control Release*, 2002, **83**, 343–52.

123 Ohura K, Ikenaga M, Nakamura T, Yamamuro T, Ebisawa Y, Kokubo T, Kotoura Y and Oka M, 'A heat-generating bioactive glass ceramic for hyperthermia', *J Appl Biomater*, 1991, **2**, 153–9.

124 Ebisawa Y, Sugimoto Y, Hayashi T, Kokubo T, Ohura K and Yamamuro T, 'Crystallization of (FeO, Fe_2O_3)-CaO-SiO_2 glasses and magnetic-properties of their crystallized products'. *J Ceram Soc Jpn*, 1991, **99**, 7–13.

125 Ikenaga M, Ohura K, Yamamuro T, Kotoura Y, Oka M and Kokubo T, 'Localized hyperthermic treatment of experimental bone-tumors with ferromagnetic ceramics', *J Orthop Res*, 1993, **11**, 849–55.

126 Ebisawa Y, Miyaji F, Kokubo T, Ohura K and Nakamura T, 'Surface reaction of bioactive and ferrimagnetic glass–ceramics in the system FeO–Fe_2O_3–CaO–SiO_2, *J Ceram Soc Jpn*, 1997, **105**, 947–51

127 Ebisawa Y, Miyaji F, Kokubo T, Ohura K and Nakamura T, 'Bioactivity of ferrimagnetic glass-ceramics in the system FeO–Fe_2O_3–CaO–SiO_2', *Biomaterials*, 1997, **18**, 1277–84.

128 Arcos D, del Real R P and Vallet-Regí M, 'A novel bioactive and magnetic biphasic material', *Biomaterials*, 2002, **23**, 2151–8.

129 Arcos D, del Real R P and Vallet-Regí M, 'Biphasic materials for bone grafting and hyperthermia treatment of cancer', *J Biomed Mater Res*, 2003, **65A**, 71–8.

130 Ruiz E, Serrano M C, Arcos D and Vallet-Regí M, 'Glass–glass ceramic thermoseeds for hyperthermic treatment of bone tumours, *J Biomed Mater Res: Part A*, 2006, **79A**, 533–43.

131 Serrano M C, Portolés M T, Pagani R, Sáez de Guinoa J, Ruíz-Hernández E, Arcos D and Vallet-Regí M, '*In vitro* positive biocompatibility evaluation of glass–glass ceramic thermoseeds for hyperthermic treatment of bone tumors', *Tissue Eng: Part A*, 2008, **14**, 617–27.

132 Oonishi H, Hench L L, Wilson J, Sugihara F, Tsuji E, Matsuura M, Kim S, Yamamoto T and Mizokawa S, *J Biomed Mater Res*, 2000, **51**, 233.

133 Rámila A, Padilla S, Muñoz B and Vallet-Regí M, 'A new hydroxyapatite/glass biphasic material: *In vitro* bioactivity', *Chem Mater*, 2002, **14**, 2439–43.

134 Vallet-Regí M, Rámila A, Padilla S and Muñoz B, 'Bioactive glasses as accelerators of the apatites bioactivity'. *J Biomed Mater Res*, 2003, **66**, 580–5.

135 Padilla S, Sánchez-Salcedo S and Vallet-Regí M, 'Bioactive and biocompatible pieces of HA/sol–gel glass mixtures obtained by the gel casting method', *J Biomed Mater Res*, 2005, **75A**, 63–72.

136 Padilla S, Román J, Sánchez-Salcedo S and Vallet-Regí M, 'Hydroxyapatite/ SiO_2–CaO–P_2O_5 materials: *in vitro* bioactivity and biocompatibility', *Acta Biomater*, 2006, **2**, 331–42.

137 Hench L L, 'Bioceramics'. *J Am Ceram Soc'*, 1998, **81**, 1705–28.

138 Vallet-Regí M, Román J, Padilla S, Doadrio J C and Gil F J, Bioactivity and mechanical properties of SiO_2–CaO–P_2O_5 glass–ceramics, *J Mater Chem*, 2005, **15**, 1353–9.

139 Sánchez-Salcedo S, Nieto A and Vallet-Regí M, 'Hydroxyapatite/ß-tricalcium phosphate/agarose macroporous scaffolds for bone tissue engineering', *Chem Eng J*, 2008, **137**, 62–71.

140 Karp J M, Dalton P D and Schoichet M S, 'Scaffolds for tissue engineering', *MRS Bulletin*, 2003, **28**, 301–6.

141 Gibson L J, 'Cellular solids', *MRS Bulletin*, 2003, **28**, 270–1.
142 Gibson L J and Ashby M J, *Cellular Solids: Structure and Properties*, second edition, Cambridge University Press, Cambridge, 1997.
143 Peña J, Izquierdo-Barba I, García M A and Vallet-Regí M, 'Room temperature synthesis of chitosan/apatite powders and coatings', *J Eur Ceram Soc*, 2006, **26**, 3631–8.
144 Cabañas M V, Peña J, Román J and Vallet-Regí M, 'Room temperature synthesis of pieces with tailored interconnected porosity', *J Biomed Mat Res*, 2006, **78A**, 508–14.
145 Peña J, Izquierdo-Barba I, Martínez A and Vallet-Regí M, 'New method to obtain chitosan/apatite materials at room temperature', *Solid State Sci*, 2006, **8**, 513–19.
146 Román J, Cabañas M V, Peña J, Doadrio J C and Vallet-Regí M, 'An optimised ß-tricalcium phosphate and agarose scaffold fabrication technique', *J Biomed Mater Res A*, 2008, **84A**, 99–107 .
147 Vallet-Regí M, Rámila A, del Real R P and Pérez-Pariente J, a new property of MCM-41: drug delivery system, *Chem Mater*, 2001, **13**, 308–11.
148 Vallet-Regí M, Ruiz-González M L, Izquierdo-Barba I and González-Calbet J M, 'Revisiting silica based ordered mesoporous materials: medical applications', *J Mater Chem*, 2006, **16**, 26–31.
149 Vallet-Regí M, 'Ordered mesoporous materials in the context of drug delivery systems and tissue engineering', *Chem Eur J*, 2006, **12**, 5934–43.
150 Vallet-Regí M, Balas F and Arcos D, 'Mesoporous materials for drug delivery', *Angew Chem Int Ed*, 2007, **46**, 7548–58.
151 López-Noriega A, Arcos D, Izquierdo-Barba I, Sakamoto Y, Terasaki O and Vallet-Regí M, 'Ordered mesoporous bioactive glasses for bone tissue regeneration', *Chem Mat*, 2006, **18**, 3137–44
152 Izquierdo-Barba I, Arcos D, Sakamoto Y, Terasaki O, López-Noriega A and Vallet-Regí M, 'High performance mesoporous bioceramics mimicking bone mineralization', *Chem Mater*, 2008, **20**, 3191–8.
153 Ostomel T A, Shi Q H, Tsung C K, Liang H J and Stucky G D, 'Spherical bioactive glass with enhanced rates of hydroxyapatite deposition and hemostatic activity', *Small*, 2006, **2**, 1261–5.
154 Ruíz-Hernández E, López-Noriega A, Arcos D, Izquierdo-Barba I, Terasaki O and Vallet-Regí M, 'Aerosol-assisted synthesis of magnetic mesoporous silica spheres for drug targeting', *Chem Mater*, 2007, **19**, 3455–63.
155 Ruiz-Hernández E, López-Noriega A, Arcos D and Vallet-Regí M, 'Mesoporous magnetic microspheres for drug targeting', *Solid State Sci*, 2008, **10**, 421–6.
156 Vallet-Regí M and Arcos D, 'Nanostructured hybrid materials for bone tissue regeneration', *Curr Nanosci*, 2006, **2**, 179–89.
157 Manzano M, Arcos D, Delgado M R, Ruiz E, Gil F J and Vallet-Regí M, 'Bioactive star gels', *Chem Mater*, 2006, **18**, 5696–703.
158 Pereira A P V, Vasconcelos W L and Oréfice R K, 'Novel multicomponent silicate-poly(vinyl alcohol) hybrids with controlled reactivity', *J Non-Cryst Solids*, 2000, **273**, 180–5.
159 Martín A I, Salinas A J and Vallet-Regí M, 'Bioactive and degradable organic-inorganic hybrids', *J Eur Ceram Soc*, 2005, 2**5**, 3533–8.
160 Schiraldi C, D'Agostino A, Oliva A, Flamma F, De la Rosa A, Apicella A, Aversa R and De la Rosa M, 'Development of hybrid materials based on hydroxyethylmethacrylate

as supports for improving cell adhesion and proliferation', *Biomaterials*, 2004, **25**, 3645–53.

161 Wei Y and Jin D, 'A new class of organic-inorganic hybrid dental materials', *Polym Prep*, 1997, **38**, 122–3.

162 Rhee S and Choi J, 'Preparation of a bioactive poly(methyl methacrylate)/silica nanocomposite', *J Am Ceram Soc*, 2002, **85**, 1318–20.

163 Tian D, Blacher S, Dubois P, Pirard J P and Jerome R, 'Porous silica obtained from biodegradable and biocompatible inorganic- organic hybrid materials', *J Sol–Gel Sci Techn*, 1998, **13**, 415–9.

164 Rhee S H, 'Bone-like apatite-forming ability and mechanical properties of poly(ε-caprolactone)/silica hybrid as a function of poly(ε-caprolactone) content', *Biomaterials*, 2004, **25**, 1167–75.

165 Ren L, Tsuru K, Hayakawa S and Osaka A, 'Synthesis and characterization of gelatin-siloxane hybrids derived through sol–gel procedure', *J Sol-Gel Sci Techn*, 2001, **21**, 115–21.

166 Ren L, Tsuru K, Hayakawa S and Osaka A, 'Novel approach to fabricate porous gelatin-siloxane hybrids for bone tissue engineering', *Biomaterials*, 2002, **23**, 4765–73.

167 Coradin T, Bah S and Livage J, 'Gelatine/silicate interactions: from nanoparticles to composite gels', *Colloid Surface B*, 2004, **35**, 53–8.

168 Chen Q, Miyaji F, Kokubo T and Nakamura T, 'Apatite formation on PDMS-modified $CaO–SiO_2–TiO_2$ hybrids prepared by sol–gel process', *Biomaterials*, 1999, **20**, 1127–32.

169 Chen Q, Miyaji F, Kokubo T and Nakamura T, 'Bioactivity and mechanical properties of PDMS-modified $CaO–SiO_2–TiO_2$ hybrids prepared by sol–gel process', *J Biomed Mater Res*, 2000, **51**, 605–11.

170 Manzano M, Salinas A J and Vallet-Regí M, 'P-containing ormosils for bone reconstruction', *Prog Solid State Chem*, 2006, **34**, 267–77.

171 Miyata N, Fuke K, Chen Q, Kawashita M, Kokubo T and Nakamura T, 'Apatite-forming ability and mechanical properties of PTMO-modified $CaO–SiO_2$ hybrids prepared by sol–gel processing: effect of CaO and PTMO contents', *Biomaterials*, 2002, **23**, 3033–40.

172 Miyata N, Fuke K, Chen Q, Kawashita M, Kokubo T and Nakamura T, 'Apatite-forming ability and mechanical properties of PTMO-modified $CaO–SiO_2–TiO_2$ hybrids derived from sol–gel processing', *Biomaterials*, 2004, **25**, 1–7.

173 Hijón N, Manzano M, Salinas A J and Vallet-Regí M, 'Bioactive $CaO–SiO_2$–PDMS coatings onto Ti6Al4V substrates', *Chem Mater*, 2005, **17**, 1591–6.

174 Salinas A J, Merino J M, Gil F J, Babonneau F and Vallet-Regí M, 'Microstructure and macroscopic properties of $CaO–SiO_2$ PDMS hybrids for use in implants', *J Biomed Mater Res B*, 2007, **81B**, 274–82.

175 González B, Colilla M and Vallet-Regí M, 'Time-delayed release of bioencapsulates: a novel controlled delivery concept for bone implant technology', *Chem Mater*, 2008, **20**, 4826-34.

176 Michalczyk M J and Sharp K G, *Single component inorganic/organic network and precursors thereof*, US Patent 5378790, 1995.

177 Sharp K G and Michalczyk M J, 'Star gels: New hybrid network materials from polyfunctional single component precursors', *J Sol–Gel Sci Techn*, 1997, **8**, 541–6.

178 Sharp K G, 'Inorganic/organic hybrid materials', *Adv Mater*, 1998, **10**, 1243–8.

179 Tsuru K, Hayakawa S and Osaka A, 'Cell proliferation and tissue compatibility of organic-inorganic hybrid materials', *Key Eng Mater*, 2008, **377**, 167–80.
180 Yabuta T, Bescher E P, Mackenzie J D, Tsuru K, Hayakawa S and Osaka A, 'Synthesis of PDMS-based porous materials for biomedical applications', *J Sol–Gel Sci Techn*, 2003, **26**, 1219–22.
181 Deguchi K, Tsuru K, Hayashi T, Takaishi M, Nagahara M, Nagotani S, Sehara Y, Jin G, Zhang H, Hayakawa S, Shoji M, Miyazaki M, Osaka A, Huh N-H and Abe K, 'Implantation of a new porous gelatin-siloxane hybrid into a brain lesion as a potential scaffold for tissue regeneration', *J Cereb Blood Flow Metab*, 2006, **26**, 1263–73.
182 Shirosaki Y, Tsuru K, Hayakawa S and Osaka A, 'Biodegradable chitosan-silicate porous hybrids for drug delivery', *Key Eng Mater*, 2008, **361–363**, 1219–22.

8
Polymers for bone repair

M. A. MATEOS-TIMONEDA, Institute for Bioengineering of Catalonia (IBEC), CIBER-BBN, Spain

Abstract: The use of polymeric materials for bone repair applications has attracted a great deal of attention for many years, particularly for total hip replacement prostheses and bone defect fillers. In this chapter, the most used polymers in the field of bone replacement, both biodegradable and non-degradable, are reviewed. Special attention is paid to properties/application relationship for each of the materials described.

Key words: acrylic polymers, biodegradable polymers, bone cement, bone repair, polymers, prostheses, UHMWPE.

8.1 Introduction

The substitution of tissues owing to tumours, pathologies or traumatic accidents is well known and different branches of surgery perform this kind of surgery on a daily basis with relative ease. The substitution of bone tissue is especially relevant as it contributes to the structural stability of the body.

Bone tissue is composed of an organic matrix, a mineral component and water in approximately similar volumes. The combination of these elements forms a composite material with different hierarchical levels in its microstructure. It is still not possible to reproduce this highly hierarchical structure.

Historically, articular prostheses have been made of metallic materials owing to the high mechanical tensions that they will suffer once implanted, as well as their good fatigue resistance and tenacity. Lately, the use of polymeric materials has attracted a great deal of attention, although they have not yet arrived to the market. On the other hand, the choice of a material for filling bone defects or bone cavities is greater, ranging from biodegradable polymers to calcium phosphate cements and ceramics.

The role of polymers in bone substitution is relevant but limited to a few applications, such as articulating bearing surfaces of joint replacements, both hip and knee, and as interpositional cementing material between the implant surface and bone. In the first application, the ultimate choice is ultra-high molecular weight polyethylene (UHMWPE) and in the second one the most used polymer is poly(methyl methacrylate) (PMMA). Recently, the use of biodegradable polymers has grown significantly in applications dealing with the support structures needed for the normal movement of articulating joints.

In this chapter, the most used polymers in orthopaedic applications will be described. Especial emphasis will be given to their physical and chemical properties.

8.2 Ultra high molecular weight polyethylene (UHMWPE)

Ultra-high molecular weight polyethylene (UHMWPE) is a unique polymer with outstanding physical and mechanical properties, such as its chemical inertness, lubricity, impact resistance and abrasion resistance. It is the gold standard in articulating bearing surfaces of joint replacements.

Polyethylene is a polymer formed from ethylene (C_2H_4), which is a gas which has a molecular weight of 28. The generic chemical formula for polyethylene is $-(C_2H_4)_n-$, where n is the degree of polymerization.[1] A schematic of the chemical structures of ethylene and polyethylene is shown in Fig. 8.1.

There are several kinds of commercial polyethylene (low-density polyethylene: LDPE; linear low-density polyethylene: LLDPE; high-density polyethylene: HDPE; ultra high molecular weight polyethylene: UHMWPE) which are synthesized with different molecular weights and chain architectures. LDPE and LLDPE refer to low-density polyethylene and linear low-density polyethylene, respectively. The molecular weight of these polyethylenes is typically lower than 50 000 g mol^{-1}. The only difference between them is the architecture, LDPE has a branch architecture whereas LLDPE has a linear architecture. HDPE is a linear polymer with a molecular weight of up to 200 000 g mol^{-1}. UHMWPE, in comparison, has a molecular weight of up to 6 million g mol^{-1} with as many as 200 000 ethylene units. The physical and mechanical properties of UHMWPE and HDPE are summarized in Table 8.1.

The better packing of linear chains with the resulting increased crystallinity in the UHMWPE form provides the improved mechanical properties required for orthopaedic use even though there is a decrease in both ductility and fracture toughness.

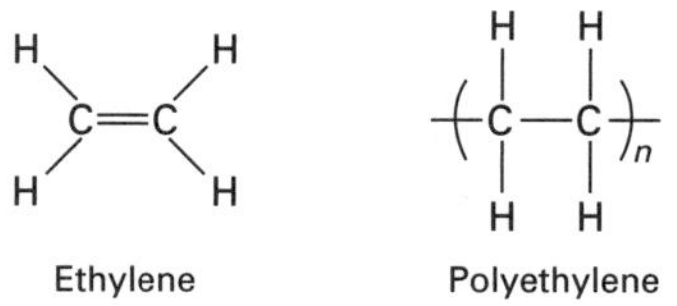

Ethylene Polyethylene

8.1 Chemical structure of ethylene and polyethylene.

Table 8.1 Typical average physical properties of HDPE and UHMWPE[a]

Property	HDPE	UHMWPE
Molecular weight (10^6 g mol^{-1})	0.05–0.25	2–6
Degree of crystallinity (%)	60–80	39–75
Poisson's ratio	0.40	0.46
Tensile modulus of elasticity* (GPa)	0.4–4.0	0.8–1.6
Tensile yield strength* (MPa)	26–33	21–28
Tensile ultimate strength* (MPa)	22–31	39–48
Tensile ultimate elongation* (%)	10–1200	350–525

*Testing conducted at 23°C
[a]Edidin and Kurtz.[2]

8.2.1 Synthesis of UHMWPE and manufacture of the implant

The synthesis of UHMWPE from ethylene gas in the presence of a Ziegler–Natta catalyst produces a white powder with particle size of 45–500 μm and a molecular weight of 2.9 to 6 million g mol^{-1}.[3]

In a second step, the polymerized UHMWPE, in the form of resin powder, needs to be consolidated into a sheet, rod or near-net shaped implant. Finally, in most instances, the UHMWPE implant needs to be machined into its final shape. A small subset of implants are consolidated into their final form directly, in a process known as direct compression molding (DCM), without need of additional machining.

Each of these three principal steps produces a subtle alteration of the properties of UHMWPE.[4] In some cases, such as machining, the change in the material may occur only in the topography and appearance of the surface. On the other hand, changes in the polymerization and conversion of the UHMWPE can have an impact on the physical and mechanical properties of the entire implant.[5]

Another important factor in the later performance of the device is the sterilization method employed.[6] The most common method is the gamma irradiation of the devices, however, two main opposing effects over the material have been detected. The gamma irradiation provokes the cross-linking of the UHMWPE chains, which leads to an improvement in the material properties, such as its fatigue resistance. Unfortunately, the oxidation of the polymer, which compromises its function in the long term owing to the formation of wear debris, is also observed.[7]

8.2.2 Properties and structure of polyethylene

UHMWPE presents very interesting physical and chemical properties which render it unique for its use in articular prostheses. UHMWPE shows the highest resistance to abrasion of all the thermoplastic materials. Furthermore, it has high impact and fatigue resistance, low friction coefficient, autolubricant properties and high capacity to dissipate mechanical energy.[8]

From the structural point of view, UHMWPE is presented in three different phases: orthorhombic crystalline, approximately 60% in proportion, monoclinic crystalline, around 10% of the material, and an amorphous phase, which accounts for approximately 30%. In contrast to the relatively short chains of HDPE, the long chains of UHMWPE hamper the formation of crystalline layers, thus limiting the amount of crystalline material. The crystalline phase is formed by lamellae with thicknesses ranging from 10 to 50 nm and 1 to 50 μm in length with tie molecules connecting these lamellae,[5] where the amorphous phase is embedded (Fig. 8.2). The average spacing between lamellae is 50 nm.[9]

8.2.3 Thermal properties and transitions

One of the distinguishing characteristics of polymeric materials is the temperature dependence of their properties. In general terms, polymers undergo three major thermal transitions: the glass transition temperature (T_g), the melting temperature (T_m), and the flow temperature (T_f).[10]

The glass transition (T_g) is defined as the temperature below which the polymer chains behave like a brittle glass. Below T_g, the polymer chains

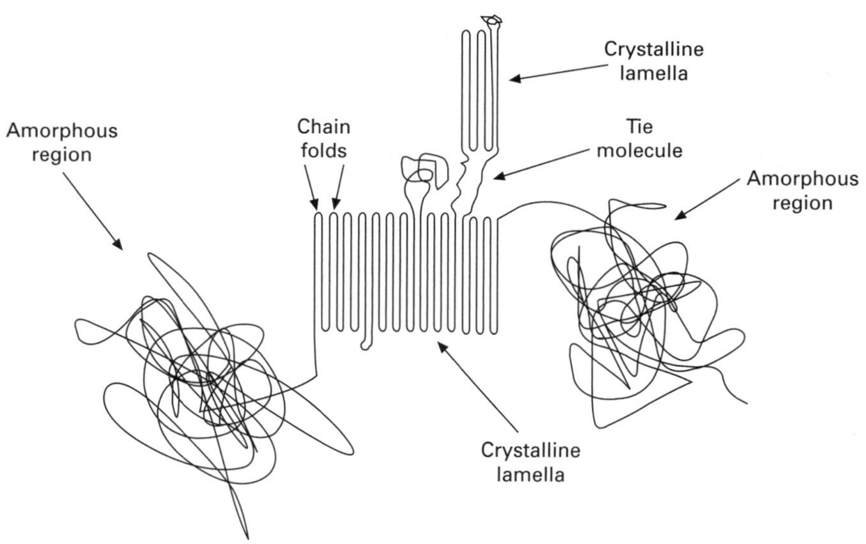

8.2 Morphological features of UHMWPE showing the presence of crystalline lamellae and the amorphous phase embedded in the crystalline phase.

have insufficient thermal energy to slide past one another and the only way for the material to respond to mechanical stress is by stretching (or rupture) of the bonds constituting the molecular chain. In UHMWPE, the glass transition occurs at around –160°C. As the temperature is raised above T_g, the amorphous regions within the polymer gain increased mobility. When the temperature of UHMWPE rises above 60–90°C, the smaller crystalline lamellae begin to melt. The melting behaviour of semicrystalline polymers, including UHMWPE, is typically measured using differential scanning calorimetry (DSC).[11] DSC measures the amount of heat needed to increase the temperature of a polymer sample. The DSC trace for UHMWPE shows the peak of the melting temperature (T_m), which occurs at around 137°C and corresponds to the point at which the majority of the crystalline regions have melted. The melting temperature reflects the thickness of the crystals as well as their perfection. Thicker and more perfect polyethylene crystals will tend to melt at a higher temperature than smaller crystals.

In addition, the area underneath the melting peak is proportional to the crystallinity of the UHMWPE. DSC provides a measure of the total heat energy per unit mass (also referred to as the change in enthalpy, ΔH) required to melt the crystalline regions within the sample. By comparing the change in enthalpy of an UHMWPE sample to that of a perfect 100% crystal, one can calculate the degree of crystallinity of the UHMWPE.

If the temperature is raised above the melt temperature, the polymer may undergo a flow transition and become liquid. This phenomenon is only observed for polyethylenes with a molecular weight lower than 500 000 g mol^{-1}. For UHMWPE, the entanglement of the immense polymer chains prevents it from showing a flow transition (T_f).

8.2.4 Mechanical properties of UHMWPE

The mechanical behaviour of UHMWPE is closely related to its average molecular weight, which is routinely calculated from its intrinsic viscosity (IV).[12] Other methods for molecular weight measurement of UHMWPE are sequential extraction[13] and gel permeation chromatography (GPC), a type of size exclusion chromatography.[14]

The bulk impact strength and abrasive wear resistance of UHMWPE after conversion to bulk form are related to the molecular weight and thus to the IV, although the relationships are non-linear. The maximum impact strength is found between 16 and 20 IV, which is equivalent to a molecular weight range of 2.4 million to 3.3 million g mol^{-1}. As the IV increases, abrasive wear resistance increases, as measured by sand slurry testing, reaching a plateau for IV greater than 20.

The static fracture response, as well as the mechanical behaviour at large strains, is also influenced by the molecular weight of UHMWPE.[15] For example, beyond the polymer yield point, the hardening or cold drawing portion behaviour in uniaxial tension is sensitive to the molecular weight. Under biaxial drawing conditions of the small punch test,[16] the large deformation mechanical behaviour of polyethylene also displays strong molecular weight dependence.

8.2.5 Wear of UHMWPE in total joint replacements

The generation of wear debris is a key issue in the longevity of total joint replacements, owing to the subsequent tissue reaction to such debris. Particulate debris of UHMWPE generated by wear, fragmentation or fretting induces the formation of an inflammatory process in order to resorb the polymer particles. This process promotes a foreign-body granulation tissue response that has the ability to invade the bone–implant interface. It results in a progressive local bone loss that compromises the fixation of the device.[17–19]

Wear involves the erosion and loss of material in particulate form as a consequence of relative motion between two surfaces.[20] The particles (wear debris) may be lost from the system. There are three principal wear processes: (1) adhesive wear is also known as scoring, galling or seizing and it occurs when two solid surfaces slide over one another under pressure; (2) abrasive wear occurs when material is removed by contact with hard particles; (3) surface fatigue by which the surface of a material is weakened, and ultimately subsurface cracks will appear and propagate to form particles that are shed form the surface, by cyclic loading and unloading.

In general, in the most popular joint replacement (cobalt-based alloy head and UHMWPE cup), the UHMWPE component wears almost exclusively. The wear rate of this couple is generally in the order of 0.1 mm/year, with particulate generation in the order of 1×10^6 particles per step or per cycle. In clinical studies, the wear rate of UHMWPE implants has been found to increase with the following processes: (1) physical activity and weight of the patient; (2) size of the femoral head and (3) oxidation of the UHMWPE.[17]

8.2.6 New UHMWPEs: highly cross-linked UHMWPEs

As it has been mentioned earlier in the text, the cross-linking of UHMWPE by gamma irradiation or other methods leads to a decrease in polymer wear with potential for less wear debris and therefore less bioreactivity/osteolisis.[5, 21] Three important processing steps are necessary to produce highly cross-linked polyethylene for hip bearings. These steps are an irradiation step to promote cross-linking, an intra or post-irradiation thermal processing step to increase the level of cross-linking and remove residual stress and a sterilization step. In the irradiation step, gamma radiation produces free radicals (unpaired electrons) in the polyethylene, which in secondary chemical reactions leads to a combination of cross-linking and chain scission. Cross-linking is beneficial for reducing wear. Chain scission produces a decrease in molecular weight, with a concomitant reduction in wear resistance and mechanical properties. Thus, it is very important to control the conditions under which gamma irradiation is used. For instance, when irradiation is conducted in the presence of oxygen, scission predominates over cross-linking. However, when conducted in an inert environment, such as nitrogen, cross-linking predominates over scission.[22]

The cross-linking of UHMWPE increases the wear performance of the material. However it adversely affects uniaxial ductility and the uniaxial failure strain of UHMWPE decreases linearly with increasing radiation dosage.[23] Even though there are a few disadvantages of cross-linked UHMWPE, it is now by far the most widely used alternative to conventional UHMWPE, especially in the USA.

8.3 Acrylic polymers as bone cement

The acrylic polymers, or polyacrylates, are compounds with a high molecular weight. Their chemical and physical properties depend on the lateral substituents of the polymeric chains. These materials have an excellent light transmittance, making them good materials for intraocular lenses and contact lenses, both hard and soft.

The most common acrylic compound used for bone repair is poly(methyl methacrylate) (PMMA), also known as 'Plexiglas' (Fig. 8.3). PMMA is a hydrophobic, linear chain polymer that is transparent, amorphous and glassy at room temperature. It is obtained by an addition polymerization (chain reaction) of methyl methacrylate (MMA) in the presence of an initiator of the radical polymerization and an activator for the formation of free radicals.[24]

The PMMA is used as bone cement in joint arthroplasty. Bone cements are used for the fixation of artificial joints. The cements fill the free space between the prosthesis and the bone and constitute a very important zone. Owing to their optimal rigidity, the cements can evenly buffer the forces acting against the bone. The close connection between the cement and the

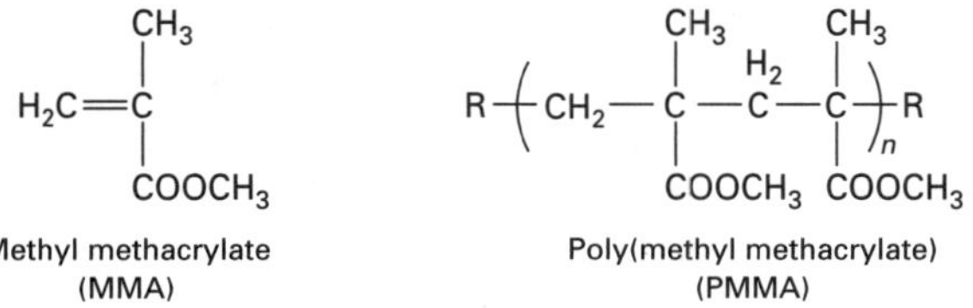

Methyl methacrylate (MMA)

Poly(methyl methacrylate) (PMMA)

8.3 Chemical structure of monomer MMA and PMMA.

bone as well as cement and the prosthesis leads to an optimal distribution of the stresses and interface strain energy.[25]

Bone cement based on PMMA consists of two components: a powder component (mainly PMMA) and a liquid component (mainly the monomer MMA), and it was first introduced by Charnley in 1958.[26]

8.3.1 Synthesis of bone cement based on poly (methyl methacrylate)

As it has been previously mentioned, the bone cements based on PMMA consists of two components, a liquid and a powder component.[27]

The polymer powder component mainly consists of PMMA. Additionally, it contains benzoyl peroxide (BPO), as initiator of the radical polymerization, included in the polymer beads or simply admixed to the powder. The powder also may contain a radiopacifier and optionally an antibiotic. Thus bone cements can provide the function of the carrier matrix. The radiopacifier is needed to monitor and identify failures in the bone cement.

In the liquid component, the monomer MMA is the main ingredient. As an activator for forming radicals, the liquid contains an aromatic amine, such as *N,N*-dimethyl-*p*-toluidine (DmpT). Additionally, it contains an inhibitor, to avoid premature polymerization during storage, and optionally a coloring agent.

Upon mixing the liquid and powder component, reaction between the initiator and the activator occurs. The DmpT (liquid component) causes the decomposition of BPO (powder component) in a reduction/oxidation process by electron transfer resulting in benzoyl radicals. These are reactive, short-lived chemical entities that are able to start the polymerization by adding themselves to the reactive C=C double bond of the MMA (see Initiation, Fig. 8.4). Because of the large amount of radicals, a large number of rapidly growing polymer chains is generated, reaching molecular weights of 100 000 to 1 000 000 g mol^{-1} (see Chain growth, Fig. 8.4). With the increasing viscosity of the dough, the mobility of the monomer is reduced and via recombination of two radical chains, the system is depleted of radicals and the polymerization ends (see Chain recombination, Fig. 8.4).[28] This polymerization is an exothermic chemical reaction with a polymerization heat of 57 kJ mol^{-1} (13.8 kcal mol^{-1}) MMA.

The molecular weight of the cured cement depends mainly on the molecular weight of the polymer in the powder component and its sterilization method. The molecular weight is very important because it has a significant influence on the swelling property, the fatigue properties, the cement viscosity and the working time. The sterilization method of choice is gamma irradiation because its high penetration depth allows the material to be sterilized in the final package. However, it leads to a reduction of the molecular weight

Initiation

BPO + H_3C–DmpT → Benzoyl radical

BPO

DmpT

Benzoyl radical

Chain growth

$$R\bullet + H_2C{-}C(CH_3)(COOCH_3) \longrightarrow H_3C{-}C\bullet(CH_3)(COOCH_3) \xrightarrow{+nH_2C{=}C(CH_3)(COOCH_3)} R{-}\!(CH_2{-}C(CH_3)(COOCH_3))_n{-}\overset{H_2}{C}{-}C\bullet(CH_3)(COOCH_3)$$

Chain recombination

$$2R{-}\!(CH_2{-}C(CH_3)(COOCH_3))_n\bullet \longrightarrow R{-}\!(CH_2{-}C(CH_3)(H_3CCOOC){-}C(CH_3)(COOCH_3){-}\overset{H_2}{C})_n{-}R$$

8.4 Synthesis of PMMA-based bone cements.

of the cement, thus it is necessary for irradiated polymers to have a much higher molecular weight before the sterilization.[29]

Another important factor is the shrinkage of the bone cement.[30] This is the reason why it is not possible to use only MMA for bone cements, as the polymerization shrinkage would be extremely high. For example, pure MMA shrinks by 21%, which means that 1 litre of MMA results in 790 ml PMMA. On the other hand, the use of a pre-polymerized powder component leads to a theoretical shrinkage of 6–7% which in reality is lower owing to the cement porosity.

8.3.2 Thermal properties and transitions

As has been previously discussed, plastics change their physical state with rising temperature from glass-like/brittle to rubber-elastic. The temperature range in which this change occurs is characterized by the glass transition temperature (T_g).

In the dry state, PMMA bone cements have a relatively high glass transition temperature (about 90–100°C) compared to the body temperature. However, water uptake by the polymer softens the polymer and therefore T_g decreases. The softening effect is due to micro-Brownian movement and leads to a change in the elasticity modulus, heat conduction and thermal expansion. This effect is known as plasticizing and will cause the T_g of bone cements to drop by 20°C. With this temperature clearly above body temperature, safe use of the cements is assured.[29]

8.3.3 Mechanical properties of PMMA-based bone cements

The function of bone cements in cemented hip arthroplasty is to locate the implant components in the bony skeleton and to transmit loads through the joint into the bone and muscle surrounding the joint over very long periods of time. Bone cement is subjected to high stresses since the forces transmitted through the hip joint are high and, in addition, it has to function in the relatively aggressive environment of the body.[31, 32]

As has been mentioned before, PMMA bone cement is a thermoplastic polymer and its properties change as temperature changes. Similarly, the water in the surroundings will act as a plasticizer and change the characteristic properties of the cement.[33] Therefore, bone cement must be tested in conditions that replicate the body environment as far as possible.[34]

There are five mechanical properties of bone cement that should be measured by testing samples in the laboratory.[35] These are tensile strength, shear strength, compressive strength, bending strength and modulus of elasticity.[25, 36, 37] The average results for these different properties are:

- tensile strength: 35.3 MPa
- shear strength: 42.2 MPa
- compressive strength: 93.0 MPa
- bending strength: 64.2 MPa
- bending modulus: 2.55 GPa.

In addition to the five elastic mechanical properties described above, there are three long-term viscoelastic properties that are of importance. These properties are creep, stress relaxation and fatigue.

Creep is defined as the change in strain with time in a sample held at constant stress.[34] All PMMA cements creep and the creep rate is affected by the environment, ageing of the cement (creep rate reduces with age of the cement), temperature and stress level (an increase of the temperature and/or stress level will increase the creep rate).

Stress relaxation is defined as the change in stress with time under constant strain (deformation).[38] Stress relaxation in bone cement takes place by a similar molecular relaxation process within the polymer to that which causes creep. Similarly, the same effects as for creep are observed for stress relaxation, that is environment, ageing of the cement, temperature and stress level. Creep and stress relaxation increase the compressive stress in the cement and at the cement–bone interface which leads to long-term stability of the total replacement hip joint.

Finally, fatigue is the effect of repeated load cycles below the level needed to fail the material in a single load application.[38] Polymers do not have an endurance limit (level of stress below which the material will not fail) and consequently they will always fail after sufficient load cycles have been applied. Fatigue failure normally originates at a point of high tensile stress concentration.[39] Nevertheless, tensile stresses in bone cements can be relaxed very rapidly. It is this stress relaxation that provides a form of self-protection for the entire bone cement.

8.3.4 PMMA-based antibiotic loaded acrylic cements (ALAC)

The addition of antimicrobial agents to acrylic bone cement was begun as early as 1969.[40] It is very useful because it reduces the risk of infection. PMMA bone cement is a meshwork of PMMA chains and consequently antibiotics enclosed in these meshes are released by elution from the bone cement. The elution properties of acrylic bone cements correlate directly with the ability to absorb water during bone cement preparation.[41] For this application, the antibiotics need to present a certain physicochemical profile that allows them to be eluted from the bone cement. Among these properties are high solubility in water, heat stability during the polymerization reaction, no chemical interaction with PMMA or mediators of the polymerization, low effect on the mechanical strength of the bone cement and finally good release from the bone cement.[42]

There are two main uses of antibiotic loaded acrylic cements (ALAC), both prophylaxis and therapy. Prophylactic use is determined by the pathogens expected at the site of the prosthesis. Gentamicin, a well-known antibiotic, turned out to be a suitable agent for prophylactic use in ALAC.[42] On the other hand, for the therapy of periprosthetic infection, the pathogen must be identified prior to revision surgery so that appropriate antibiotics can be selected in advance according to the susceptibility pattern of the individual bacterial strain for application in ALAC.

8.4 Biodegradable polymers

The biodegradable polymers are a class of polymers that will degrade and therefore resorb once they are in contact with tissues and fluids of the body. The main advantages of these polymers are: (1) once their function has been accomplished they will disappear and (2) the tissue will grow after their disappearance. For these same reasons, they must fullfil stringent requirements in terms of their biocompatibility. In addition to the potential problem of toxic substances leaching from the implant (residual monomer, initiators), the potential toxicity of the degradation products is another problem.

A biodegradable polymer may be derived from either natural or synthetic sources. Natural polymeric materials, such as collagen and heparin, have been used as medical devices.[43] However, the use of synthetic polymers in general offers greater advantages over natural materials in that they can be tailored to give a wider range of properties and have more predictable lot-to-lot uniformity than materials from natural sources. Also, a more reliable source of raw materials is obtained with synthetic polymers that are free of concerns about immunogenicity.[44]

Most synthetic biodegradable polymers have functional groups which are sensible to hydrolytic processes such as ester, carbonate, anhydride, urethane, orthoester or amide. The most used are the polymers that contain esters of carboxylic acids, such as poly(lactic acid) (PLA) or poly(glycolic acid) (PGA). Their applications range from suture materials to osteosynthesis materials (needles, screws or plaques).

8.4.1 Types of synthetic biodegradable polymers

The chemical structure of several synthetic polymers is shown in Fig. 8.5.

Polyanhydrides

These are among the most reactive and unstable polymers currently used as biomaterials. Aliphatic polyanhydrides degrade within days, whereas aromatic polyanhydrides degrade over several years. Thus, it is possible to control their degradation via copolymerization of different ratios of monomer (aliphatic/aromatic).[45]

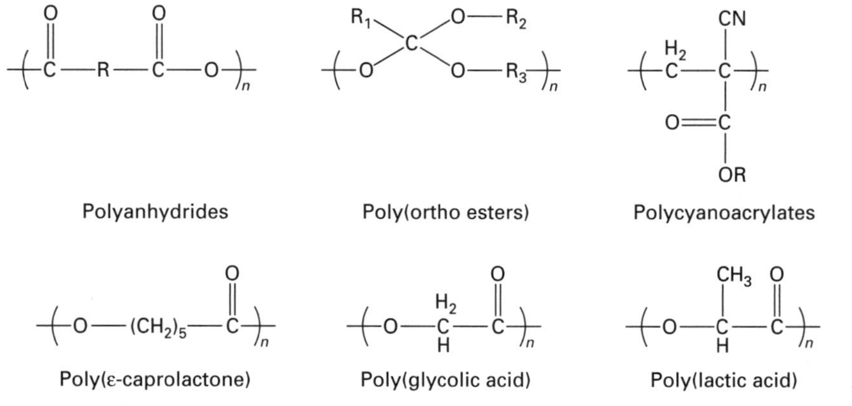

Polyanhydrides

Poly(ortho esters)

Polycyanoacrylates

Poly(ε-caprolactone)

Poly(glycolic acid)

Poly(lactic acid)

8.5 Chemical structure of several synthetic biodegradable polymers.

Poly(ortho esters)

These are a family of synthetic, degradable polymers that have been under evaluation for a number of years.[46] The addition of appropriate excipients into the polymeric matrix made them to erode by 'surface erosion', which makes them very useful for controlled-release drug delivery applications.[47]

Polycyanoacrylates

These are used as bioadhesives. However, they have limiting properties, such as the monomers are very reactive and have significant toxicity and their degradation compounds (formaldehyde) provoke an intense inflammatory response in the surrounding tissue. In spite of these limitations, they have been used as ocular drug delivery systems.[48]

Poly(amino acids)

The rational behind the use of poly(amino acids) in biomedical applications is because proteins are composed of amino acids. They show a low systemic toxicity, owing to their degradation to amino acids. However, they have found limited application since most of them are highly insoluble and non-processible materials.

Polycaprolactone

This is a semicrystalline polymer with a very low glass transition temperature (T_g = –60°C) and low melting point (59–64°C). These characteristics, as well as its high solubility and ability to form blends, make it a good candidate for applications as a biomaterial. Polycaprolactone is a hydrophobic polymer, therefore it degrades very slowly (up to 1 year). The release characteristics of polycaprolactone have been investigated for their use as an implantable contraceptive (Capronor®).[49]

Poly(α-hydroxy acids): poly(glycolic acid) (PGA), poly(lactic acid) (PLA) and their copolymers (PLG)

PGA and PLA are the most widely used synthetic, biodegradable polymers. PGA is the simplest linear polyester. It is highly crystalline and consequently it presents a high melting point and low solubility in organic solvents. It has been processed as a material for sutures (Dexon®). The limitation of these sutures is that they tend to lose their mechanical properties over a period of 2–4 weeks after implantation. To overcome this problem, the use of copolymers of PGA and PLA has been studied. The introduction of the more hydrophobic PLA into the polymeric structure limits the water uptake and reduces the rate of backbone hydrolysis.

Lactic acid is a chiral molecule (i.e. a molecule that is not superimposable on its mirror image), it exists in two stereoisomeric forms that give rise to four morphologically different polymers: D-PLA, L-PLA, DL-PLA and meso-PLA. The crystalline properties differ from polymer to polymer. Both D and L polymers are semicrystalline materials, whereas the optically inactive DL-PLA is always amorphous. For this reason, L-PLA is preferred for application where high mechanical strength and toughness are needed.

Other biodegradable polymers

Polyphosphazenes are at the interface between inorganic and organic polymers as their backbone consists of nitrogen–phosphorus bonds. The main applications of polyphosphazenes are in the field of drug delivery and in skeletal tissue regeneration.[50, 51] Polydioxanone (PDS) is a poly(ether ester) with interest for the medical field owing to its degradation to low toxicity products. It was the first polymer to be used as monofilament suture.

In view of the importance of PGA, PLA and their copolymers poly(lactic-co-glycolic acid) (PLG) in the field of biomaterials, a more detailed description of their properties will be given.

8.4.2 Synthesis of poly(glycolic acid), poly(lactic acid) and copolymers poly(lactic-co-glycolic acid)(PLG)

These polymers are synthesized by ring opening polymerization (ROP) of the corresponding monomers or mixtures of the monomers in different ratios (Fig. 8.6).

The use of ROP of glycolide and/or lactide instead of direct polymerization of the corresponding acid (glycolic acid and lactic acid, respectively) is because the latter leads to low molecular weight polymers and therefore poor mechanical properties. For example, the molecular weight of PLA, obtained via direct polymerization, is approximately 10 000–20 000 g mol^{-1}, while via ring opening polymerization it rises to 500 000 g mol^{-1} or even higher.

8.4.3 Physical properties of poly(glycolic acid), poly(lactic acid) and copolymers PLG

PGA is highly crystalline (45–55%) with a high melting point (220–225°C) and a glass transition temperature of 35–40°C.[52] PGA polymers exhibit high tensile strength and low elongation and consequently have a high modulus (Table 8.2). The homopolymer of L-lactide (L-PLA) is a semicrystalline polymer

Glycolide → PGA

Lactide → PLA

Glycolide + Lactide → PLG

8.6 Ring opening polymerization of PGA, PLA and PLG.

Table 8.2 Physical, mechanical and degradation properties of PGA, PLA and PLG polymers

Polymer	Melting point (°C)	T_g(°C)	Modulus (GPa)[b]	Elongation (%)	Degradation time (months)[c]
PGA	225–230	35–40	7.0	15–20	6–12
50/50 DL-PLG	Amorphous	45–50	2.0	3–10	1–2
65/35 DL-PLG	Amorphous	45–50	2.0	3–10	3–4
75/25 DL-PLG	Amorphous	50–55	2.0	3–10	4–5
85/15 DL-PLG	Amorphous	50–55	2.0	3–10	5–6
L-PLA	173–178	60–65	2.7	5–10	> 24
DL-PLA	Amorphous	55–60	1.9	3–10	12–16

[a]Middleton and Tipton[58]
[b]Tensile or flexural modulus
[c]Time to complete resorption

(37%) with a melting point of 175–178°C and a T_g of 60–65°C.[53, 54] On the other hand, poly(D,L-lactide) (DL-PLA) is an amorphous polymer. It presents a random distribution of both isomeric forms of lactic acid and accordingly is unable to be arranged in a crystalline organized structure. Consequently, this material has lower tensile strength and higher elongation and much more rapid degradation time than L-PLA (Table 8.2). The semicrystalline poly(L-lactide) has a modulus about 25% higher than poly(DL-lactide) and a degradation time of the order of 3 to 5 years. The amorphous poly(DL-lactide) has a degradation time of 12 to 16 months.[55]

The copolymers of L-lactide and glycolide are amorphous owing to the disruption of the regularity of the polymer chain by the other monomer.[56] It is important to note that there is no linear relationship between the copolymer composition and the mechanical and degradation properties of the materials. For example, a copolymer of 50% glycolide and 50% DL-lactide degrades faster than either homopolymer.[57]

8.4.4 Degradation of the polymers

Simple chemical hydrolysis of the hydrolytically unstable backbone is the prevailing mechanism for the polymer degradation (Fig. 8.7).

There are two different mechanisms for this polymer degradation to occur: surface erosion and bulk erosion. In surface erosion, the process is limited to the surface of the device. The polymeric device will become thinner with time while maintaining its bulk integrity.[59] Polyanhydrides and poly(ortho esters) suffer this type of erosion. Alternatively, in bulk erosion, the rate at which water penetrates the device exceeds that at which the polymer is converted into water-soluble materials (resulting in erosion throughout the device). This process occurs in two steps. In the first one, water penetrates the bulk

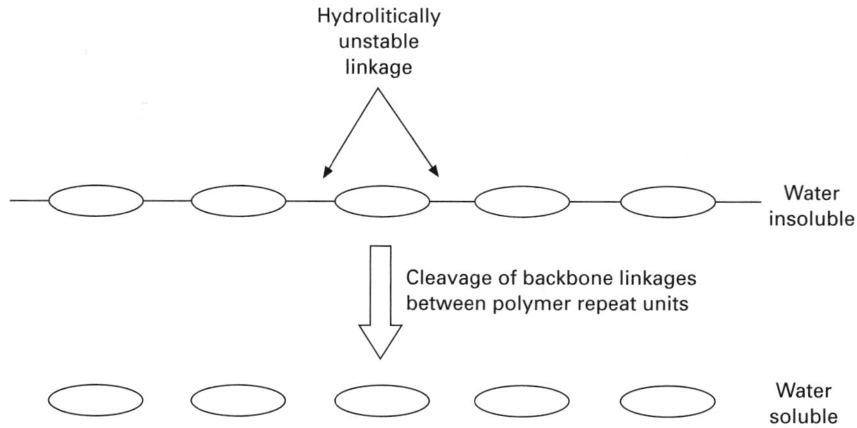

8.7 Degradation of the polymers by cleavage of hydrolytically unstable linkages in the polymer backbone, followed by solubilization of the low molecular weight fragments.

of the device mainly cleaving the hydrolytically unstable chemical bonds in the amorphous phase and converting long polymer chains into shorter, ultimately water-soluble fragments. In the second phase, enzymatic attack of the fragments occurs.[55] This type of erosion is found for semicrystalline polymers such as PGA and L-PLA.

The main factors that determine the rate of erosion are the chemical stability of the polymer backbone, the hydrophilic/hydrophobic balance of the repeating units, the morphology of the polymer (semicrystalline/amorphous) and the molecular weight and molecular weight distribution of the polymer. PGA, PLA and copolymers PLG have ester bonds as linkages between the repeating units, thus they should all degrade at the same rate if the chemical stability of the polymer backbone is the only factor affecting the rate of erosion. However, the hydrophilic versus hydrophobic character of the repeating units have influence in the ability of the water molecules to penetrate into the polymeric matrix. Therefore, PGA erodes much faster than the more hydrophobic PLA. Moreover, the morphology of the polymer is of crucial importance. In the crystalline state, water cannot penetrate into the crystalline domains because the polymer chains are densely packed and organized. Consequently, backbone hydrolysis tends to take place in the amorphous regions and in the surface of the crystalline domains. This phenomenon is illustrated by the rate of erosion of L-PLA and DL-PLA. Although these two polymers have the same backbone linkages and identical degree of hydrophobicity, DL-PLA degrades much faster than L-PLA because the stereoregular polymer is semicrystalline, while the racemic DL-PLA is an amorphous polymer.[60]

8.5 Conclusions

In this chapter, the most used polymers in the field of orthopaedic and bone repair have been shown. In spite of the fact that many of these materials are the gold standard for the different applications, such as bone cement and total joint replacement prostheses, they still present problems associated with their use. However, major changes in the area are being made with advances in the processing techniques of polymers that are in use nowadays and the possible future development of absorbable polymers and composites.

8.6 References

1 S. M. Kurtz. 'A primer in UHMWPE'. *The UHMWPE Handbook: ultra-high molecular weight polyethylene in total joint replacement*. S. M. Kurtz (ed.), Elsevier Academic Press, San Diego, 2004.

2 A. A. Edidin and S. M. Kurtz. 'The influence of mechanical behaviour on the wear of four clinically relevant polymeric biomaterials in a hip simulator'. *J Arthroplasty*, 2000, **15**, 321–31.

3 H. W. Birnkraut. 'Synthesis of UHMWPE'. *Ultra-high Molecular Weight Polyethylene as a Biomaterial in Orthopedic Surgery.* H.G. Willert, G.H. Buchhorn and P. Eyerer (eds), Hogrefe & Huber, New York, 1991.
4 S. M. Kurtz. 'From ethylene gas to UHMWPE component: the process of producing orthopedic implants'. *The UHMWPE Handbook: ultra-high molecular weight polyethylene in total joint replacement.* S. M. Kurtz (ed.), Elsevier Academic Press, San Diego, 2004.
5 S. M. Kurtz, O. K. Muratoglu, M. Evans and A. A. Edidin. 'Advances in the processing, sterilization, and crosslinking of ultra-high molecular weight polyethylene for total joint arthroplasty'. *Biomaterials*, 1999, **20**, 1659–88.
6 M. D. Ries. 'Enhanced polyethylene implants: have we been there before?' *Instr. Course Lect*, 2005, **54**, 189–92.
7 C. Atienza and W. J. Maloney. 'Highly cross-linked polyethylene bearing surfaces in total hip arthroplasty'. *J Surg Orthop Adv*, 2008, **17**, 127–33.
8 L. A. Pruitt. 'Deformation, yielding, fracture and fatigue behavior of conventional and highly cross-linked ultra high molecular weight polyethylene'. *Biomaterials*, 2005, **26**, 905–15.
9 A. Bellare, H. Schnablegger and R. E. Cohen. 'A small-angle X-ray scattering study of high-density polyethylene and ultra-high molecular weight polyethylene'. *Macromolecules*, 1995, **17**, 2325–33.
10 S. L. Cooper, S. A. Visser, R. W. Hergenrother and N. M. K. Lamba. 'Polymers'. *Biomaterials Science: an introduction to materials in medicine*. B. D. Ratner, A. S. Hoffman, F. J. Schoen, J. E. Lemons (eds), Elsevier, London, 2004.
11 K. S. K. Karuppiah, A. L. Bruck, S. Sundararajan, J. Wang, Z. Q. Lin, Z. H. Xu and X. D. Li. 'Friction and wear behavior of ultra-high molecular weight polyethylene as a function of polymer crystallinity'. *Acta Biomaterialia*, 2008, **4**, 1401–10.
12 P. Eyerer, A. Frank and R. Jin. 'Characterization of ultrahigh molecular weight polyethylene (UHMWPE): Extraction and viscometry of UHMWPE'. *Plastverarbeiter*, 1985, **36**, 46–54.
13 R. P. Kusy and J. Q. Whitley. 'Use of a sequential extraction technique to determine the MWD of bulk UHMWPE'. *J Appl Poly Sci*, 1986, **32**, 4263–9.
14 H. L. Wagner and J. G. Dillon. 'Viscosity and molecular weight distribution of ultra-high molecular weight polyethylene'. *J Appl Poly Sci*, 1988, **36**, 567–82.
15 S. M. Kurtz, L. Pruitt, C. W. Jewett, R. P. Crawford, D. J. Crane and A. A. Edidin. 'The yielding, plastic flow, and fracture behavior of ultra-high molecular weight polyethylene used in total joint replacements'. *Biomaterials*, 1998, **19**, 1989–2003.
16 A. A. Edidin and S. M. Kurtz. 'Development and validation of the small punch test for UHMWPE used in total joint replacements'. *Functional Biomaterials*, N. Katsube, W. Soboyejo, and M. Sacks (eds), Trans Tech Publications, Winterthur, 2001.
17 J. J. Jacobs, A. Shanbhag, T. T. Glant, J. Black and J. O. Galante. 'Wear debris in total joints'. *J Am Acad Orthop Surg*, 1994, 2, 212–20.
18 J. Jacobs, R. M. Urban, J. L. Gilbert, A. Skipor, J. Black, M. J. Jasty and J. O. Galante. 'Local and distant products from modularity'. *Clin Orthop*, 1995, **319**, 94–105.
19 J. J. Jacobs, K. A. Roebuck, M. Archibeck, N. J. Hallab and T. T. Glant. 'Osteolysis: basic science'. *Clin Orthop*, 2001, **393**, 71–7.
20 G. Lewis. 'Polyethylene wear in total hip and knee arthroplasties'. *J Biomed Mater Res*, 1997, **38**, 55–75.

21 O. K. Muratoglu and S. M. Kurtz. 'Alternative bearing surfaces in hip replacement'. *Hip Replacement: Current trends and controversies*. R. Sinha (ed), Marcel Dekker, New York, 2002.

22 L. Costa and P. Bracco. 'Mechanisms of crosslinking and oxidative degradation of UHMWPE'. *The UHMWPE Handbook: ultra-high molecular weight polyethylene in total joint replacement.* S. M. Kurtz (ed.), Elsevier Academic Press, San Diego, 2004.

23 S. M. Kurtz, M. L. Villarraga, M. P. Herr, J. S. Bergstrom, C. M. Rimnac and A. A. Edidin. 'Thermomechanical behavior of virgin and highly crosslinked ultra-high molecular weight polyethylene used in total joint replacements'. *Biomaterials*, 2002, **23**, 3681–97.

24 C. P. R. Nair and G. Clouet. 'Thermal iniferters – Their concept and application in free-radical polymerization'. *J Macromol Sci Rev Macromol Chem Phys*, 1991, **C31**, 311–40.

25 K. D. Kühn. *Bone Cements*. Springer, Berlin, 2000.

26 J. Charnley. 'Anchorage of the femoral head prostheses of the shaft of the femur'. *J Bone Joint Surg*, 1960, **42**, 28–30.

27 K. D. Kühn. 'Properties of bone cement: what is bone cement?' *The Well-Cemented Hip Arthroplasty: Theory and Practice*. S. J. Breusch, H. Malchau (eds), Springer, Heidelberg, 2005.

28 D. A. Nussbaum, P. Gailloud and K. Murphy. 'The chemistry of acrylic bone cements and implications for clinical use in image-guided therapy'. *J Vasc Intervent Rad*, 2004, **15**, 121–6.

29 W. Ege, K. D. Kühn, C. Tuchscherer and H. Maurer. 'Physical and chemical properties of bone cements'. *Biomaterials in Surgery*, G. H. I. M. Walenkamp (ed.), Georg Thieme, Stuttgart, 1998.

30 K. Draenert and Y. Draenert. 'Properties of bone cement: the three interfaces'. *The Well-Cemented Hip Arthroplasty: Theory and Practice*. S. J. Breusch and H. Malchau (eds), Springer, Heidelberg, 2005.

31 G. Bergmann, F. Graichen and A. Rohlmann. 'Hip joint loading during walking and running, measured in two patients'. *J Biomechanics*, 1993, **26**, 969–90.

32 N. Berme and J. P. Paul. 'Load actions transmitted by implants'. *J Biomed Eng*, 1979, **1**, 268–72.

33 A. J. C. Lee, R. S. M. Ling and S. S. Vangala. 'Some clinically relevant variables affecting the mechanical behaviour of bone cement'. *Arch Orthop Traumat Surg*, 1978, **92**, 1–18.

34 A. J. C. Lee, R. S. M. Ling, S. Gheduzzi, J.-P. Simon and R. J. Renfro. 'Factors affecting the mechanical and viscoelastic properties of acrylic bone cement'. *J Mater Sci Mater in Med*, 2002, **13**, 723–33.

35 C. Lee. 'Properties of bone cement: The mechanical properties of PMMA bone cement'. *The well-cemented hip arthroplasty: Theory and Practice*. S. J. Breusch, H. Malchau (eds), Springer, Heidelberg, 2005.

36 G. Lewis. 'Properties of acrylic bone cement: state of the art review'. *J Biomed Mater Res*, 1997, **38**, 155–82.

37 S. Saha and S. Pal. 'The mechanical properties of bone cement: a review'. *J Biomed Mater Res*, 1984, **18**, 435–62.

38 W. D. Callister. *Materials Science and Engineering: an introduction*. John Wiley & Sons, New York, 2007.

39 O. R. Eden, A. J. C. Lee and R. M. Hooper. 'Stress relaxation modelling of polymethylmethacrylate bone cement'. *Proc Inst Mech Eng*, 2002, **216**, 195–9.

40 H. W. Buchholz, R. A. Elson and H. Lodenkämper. 'The infected joint implant'. *Recent Advances in Orthopaedics*, B. McKibbin (ed), Curchhill Livingston, New York, 1979.

41 H. A. T. Low, R. H. Fleming, M. F. X. Gilmore, I. D. McCarthy and S. P. F. Hughes. '*In vitro* measurement and computer modelling of the diffusion of antibiotic in bone cement'. *J Biomed Eng*, 1986, **8**, 149–55.

42 K. Adams, I. Couch, G. Cierny, J. Calhoun and J. T. Mader. 'In vitro and in vivo evaluation of antibiotic diffusion from antibiotic-impregnated polymethymethacrylate beads'. *Clin Orthop*, 1992, **278**, 244–52.

43 I. V. Yannas. 'Natural materials'. *Biomaterials Science: an introduction to materials in medicine*. B. D. Ratner, A. S. Hoffman, F. J. Schoen, J. E. Lemons (eds), Elsevier, London, 2004.

44 T. H. Barrows. 'Degradable implant materials: a review of synthetic absorbable polymers and their applications'. *Clin Mater*, 1986, **1**, 233–57.

45 J. A. Tamada and R. Langer. 'Erosion kinetics of hydrolytically degradable polymers'. *Proc Natl Acad Sci USA*, 1993, **90**, 552–6.

46 J. Heller, R. V. Sparer and G. M. Zentner. 'Poly(ortho esters)'. *Biodegradable Polymers as Drug Delivery Systems*. M. Chasin, R. Langer (eds), Marcel Dekker, New York, 1990.

47 J. Heller, J. Barr, S. Y. Ng, K. S. Abdellauoi and R. Gurny. 'Poly(ortho esters): synthesis, characterization, properties and uses'. *Adv Drug Delivery Rev*, 2002, **54**, 1015–39.

48 A. A. Desphande, J. Heller and R. Gurny. 'Bioerodible polymers for ocular drug delivery'. *Crit Rev Thera Drug Carrier Syst*, 1998, **15**, 381–420.

49 C. G. Pitt. 'Poly-ε-caprolactone and its copolymers'. *Biodegradable Polymers as Drug Delivery Systems*. M. Chasin and R. Langer (eds), Marcel Dekker, New York, 1990.

50 H. R. Allcock. 'Polyphosphazenes as new biomedical and bioactive materials'. *Biodegradable Polymers as Drug Delivery Systems*. M. Chasin, R. Langer (eds), Marcel Dekker, New York, 1990.

51 C. T. Laurencin, M. E. Norman, H. M. Elgendy, S. F. El-Amin, H. R. Allcock, S. R. Pucher and A. A. Ambrosio. 'Use of polyphosphazenes for skeletal tissue regeneration'. *J Biomed Mater Res*, 1993, **27**, 963–73.

52 S. W. Shalaby and R. A. Johnson. 'Synthetic absorbable polyesters'. *Biomedical Polymers. Designed to degrade systems*. S. W. Shalaby (ed), Hanser, New York, 1994.

53 A. U. Daniels, M. K. O. Chang, K. P. Andriano and J. Heller J. 'Mechanical properties of biodegradable polymers and composites proposed for internal fixation of bone'. *J Appl Biomater*, 1990, **1**, 57–78.

54 C. M. Agrawal, G. G. Niederauer, D. M. Micallef and K. A. Athanasiou. 'The use of PLA–PGA polymers in orthopedics'. *Encyclopedic Handbook of Biomaterials and Bioengineering Part A. Materials, Vol. 2*. D. L. Wise, D. J. Trantolo, D. E. Altobelli, M. J. Yaszemski, J. D. Greser, E. R. Schwartz (eds), Marcel Dekker, New York, 1995.

55 W. S. Pietrzak, D. R. Sarver and B. S. Verstynen. 'Bioabsorbable polymer science for the practicing surgeon'. *J Craniofaxial Surg*, 1997, **2**, 87–91.

56 D. K. Gilding and A. M. Reed. 'Biodegradable polymers for use in surgery -polyglycolic/poly(lactic acid homo- and copolymers: 1'. *Polymer*, 1979, **20**, 1459–64.

57 R. A. Miller, J. M. Brady and D. E. Cutright. 'Degradation rates of oral implants

(polylactates and polyglycolates): rate modification with changes in PLA/PGA copolymer ratios'. *J Biomed Mater Res*, 1977, **11**, 711–19.

58 J. C. Middleton and A. J. Tipton. 'Synthetic biodegradable polymers as orthopedic devices'. *Biomaterials*, 2000, **21**, 2335–46.

59 J. Kohn, S. Abramson and R. Langer. 'Bioresorbable and bioerodible materials'. *Biomaterials Science: an introduction to materials in medicine*. B. D. Ratner, A. S. Hoffman, F. J. Schoen and J. E. Lemons (eds), Elsevier, London, 2004.

60 Y.-K. Han, P. G. Edelman and S. J. Huang. 'Synthesis and characterization of crosslinked polymers for biomedical composites'. *J Macromol Sci Pure Appl Chem*, 1988, **25**, 5-7, 847–69.

9
Composite biomaterials for bone repair

R. DE SANTIS, V. GUARINO and L. AMBROSIO,
IMCB-CNR Institute of Composite and Biomedical Materials, Italy

Abstract: Surgical strategies used for bone repair are based on two different approaches: restoring bone through synthetic permanent biomaterials or through degradable biomaterials. In this chapter, the mechanical behaviour of permanent and biodegradable composites for bone repair are investigated. Preliminarily, a definition of composite material and the state of the art of surgical approaches are illustrated. The second section deals with composite materials used for bone repair up until the present time by distinguishing between non-degradable and biodegradable materials. Finally, the last section is divided into two sub-sections dealing in fibre-reinforced and inorganic particle filled degradable composites.

Key words: bioactive particles, biodegradable composite, bone repair, fibre reinforcement, filament winding.

9.1 Introduction

Advanced structural design for connective tissues restoration demands materials with complex and unusual combinations of mechanical properties. Tailored stiffness, high strength and toughness, resistance to impact, abrasion and corrosion, represent a combination of properties required by biomechanical design of synthetic prostheses. Adequate transparency to electromagnetic waves for diagnostic purposes, lightness of large prostheses and artificial limbs and long life resistance, are other relevant properties of non-degradable biomedical devices. The complexity of combining properties increases as the design deals with materials for tissue regeneration, such as scaffolds for tissue engineering. These materials require multifunctional properties in order to provide a suitable substrate for cell attachment, migration, proliferation and differentiation. Moreover, programmed biomechanical properties need to be satisfied, since the load-bearing function has to be transferred from the engineered material to the growing extracellular matrix. With this aim in mind, degradable and partially degradable materials are considered. As materials science and technology stands today, the only possible way of satisfying the compelling multifunctional needs and extend material property combinations relies on the development of composite materials.

9.2 Basic concept of composite material

Traditionally, a composite is a material composed of two or more phases. For the sake of simplicity, focusing on a two component composite, a continuous phase, a dispersed phase and an interface can be distinguished. The continuous phase is generally referred as the matrix and polymers represent the material mostly used as its components. The dispersed phase can be discontinuous (i.e. platelet or filler) or continuous (i.e. fibres) and it is generally stiffer than the matrix, thus it is considered to be the reinforcement component of the composite since it enhances the mechanical properties of the matrix (i.e. stiffness, strength). However, examples of a dispersed phase softer than the matrix which enhance the toughness of the composite also exist (i.e. rubber-like reinforcement in a ductile brittle polymer matrix or metal reinforcement in a ceramic matrix).

The interface between the matrix and the reinforcement plays a major role in determining the mechanical performance and environmental stability of composite materials. The mechanical features of the composite rely on the load transfer at the interface. The quality of adhesion between reinforcement and matrix depends on the interactions between the composite constituents, which can be chemical and/or mechanical. Mechanical bonding strongly depends on the surface topography or morphology of the reinforcement, whereas chemical bonding is preferentially promoted by surface treatments or coatings such as the silanization process (Arends, 1993). To a certain extent, the definition given to composite materials depends upon the level of analysis, as all materials may be considered heterogeneous if the scale of interest is sufficiently small. However, connective tissues show a composite structure at all hierarchical levels and the effects of the structure organization on the mechanical properties are evident at a larger micro-mechanical scale. Moreover, living tissues manifest a marked viscoelastic behaviour. To date, polymers represent the only technological solution to bio-inspired composite (Barbucci, 2002)

9.2.1 Mechanical tailoring

Reinforced polymers have gained an increasingly important role in the development of new generation biomedical materials since they can be engineered more accurately than monolithic structures (single phase materials), thus allowing the development of more effective tissue substitutes. The main font of inspiration for designing new high performance and multifunctional materials arises from the observation and study of biological materials. For example, the basic constituents of connective hard tissues are the extracellular matrix (i.e. collagen, apatite and water) and cells (namely osteocytes in bone and odontoblast in dentine) which control and adapt the structure performance based on mechano-sensitivity processes (Fung, 1993). The soft and ductile collagen and the stiff and brittle apatite crystals represent the constituent materials of a composite; more specifically, collagen fibrils of about 100 nm in diameter are reinforced by platelet apatite crystals at a nanostructural level (Rho *et al.*, 1998). Since the elastic properties of collagen and hydroxyapatite are about 1.5 GPa and 110 GPa, respectively, then it is not surprising that in mineralized tissues these constituents are conveniently organized allowing them to cover a wide range of properties (De Santis *et al.*, 2007a). Enamel, basically constituted of apatite prismatic crystals, is the stiffer hard tissue showing a Young's modulus of about 100 GPa. On the other hand, spongy bone presents lower Young's modulus values (Rho *et al.*, 1993). However, trabecular bone is a porous material and experimental values of elastic modulus have to be interpreted as apparent values. In fact, true trabecular tissue properties suggest an elastic modulus between 10 GPa and 20 GPa (Bonfield and Grynpas, 1997; Weiner and Wagner,1998; Ziouposet *et al.*, 1999; Silver *et al.*, 2002) which is similar to compact bone and dentine elastic modulus. Table 9.1 reports the Young's modulus of human compact bone measured through tensile tests according to the loading direction.

Fibre and particulate reinforced polymeric composites represent the engineering response to mineralised tissue analogues. Continuous fibre reinforcement is particularly indicated as mechanical tailoring involves anisotropy.

Figure 9.1 illustrates the micromechanical design capability of particle and fibre reinforced composite. An upper limit for the elastic modulus can be distinguished for each type of reinforcement, E_1 and E_2, respectively. E_2 also represents the Young's modulus in the transverse direction of unidirectional continuous fibre reinforced material. Taking into account the anisotropy and gradients of biological structures, composite materials represent the only approach for manufacturing biomimetic replacements. The adequate definition of the relative volume fraction of the matrix and reinforcement (V_m and V_f, respectively) and fibre orientation allows mechanical tailoring over a wide range. Table 9.2 shows the anisotropy of human trabecular bone measured through compression testing.

Table 9.1 Young's modulus (*E*) of cortical bone from human femur measured in tension

E longitudinal direction (GPa)	*E* transverse direction (GPa)	Reference
17.7	12.8	Reilly and Burstein, 1975
22.5	13.4	Dabestani and Bonfield, 1988

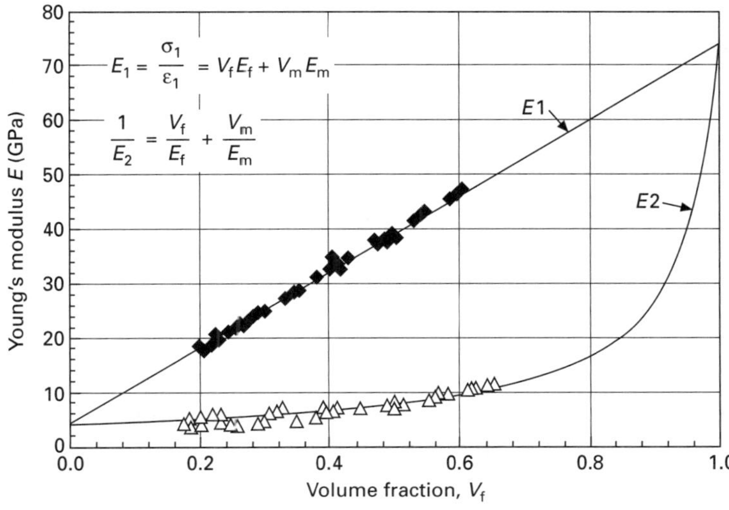

9.1 Rule of mixtures and micromechanical design capability of particle and fibre reinforced composites.

Table 9.2 Mechanical anisotropy of human trabecular bone according to the site and organ

Organ	Site	E_3/E_2	E_3/E_1	Reference
Vertebra	Central body L4	3.8	3.2	Nicholson *et al.*, 1998
	Central body L1	2.5	2.2	Augat *et al.*, 1998
	Vertebral body	1.8	1.8	Hengsberger *et al.*, 2002
Femur	Proximal femur	2.3	2.5	Augat *et al.*, 1998
	Proximal femur	2.5	2.2	Majumdar *et al.*, 1998
	Femoral head	2.2	4.0	Deligiann *et al.*, 1991
Mandible	Incisal	2.0	18	O'Mahony *et al.*, 2000
	Canine	2.0	2.8	
	First premolar	1.5	5.1	
	Second premolar	11.0	19.8	
	Condyle	3.4		Giesen *et al.*, 2001

9.3 Composite biomaterials in bone repair

Bone defect treatments represent a significant medical and socioeconomic challenge involving about one million cases per year which require bone graft procedures for the care of skeletal defects. The socioeconomic consequences of treating bone fracture patients are a major concern for both the USA and EU and will increase in the foreseeable future owing to the ageing of their populations (Petite *et al.*, 2000). Traditionally, bone treatments have been based upon the use of bone grafts, in particular autologous and autogenous grafts, or on replacement by prosthesis using metal and ceramic materials systems (Spitzer *et al.*, 2002). Autologous bone graft, involving the implantation of natural bone taken from another part of the patient's own body, represented for a long time the gold standard for osteogenic bone replacement in osseous defects, because of the reduced negative host response (Kneser *et al.*, 2006; Williams, 1999; Gazdag *et al.*, 1995). Even with a good success rate, this procedure allows the treatment of only a restricted group of clinical cases, mainly owing to the limited amount of autograft tissue available compared to the total requirement (Sassard *et al.*, 2000).

Allografts, involving the implantation of natural bone removed from another human body, may represent a valid alternative solution in bone surgery. However, the rate of graft incorporation here is lower than with the autograft, increasing the risks of rejection, owing to the transmission of pathogen infections from donor to host in the implant site after the transplantation. Finally, processed xenogenic bone grafts, which are implants from different animal species, are also commonly used for the repair of osseous defects when autologous transplantation is not applicable (Arrington *et al.*, 1996; Banwart *et al.*, 1995). Although the initial properties of allogenic or xenogenic grafts resemble those of autologous bone in terms of biomechanical stability and elasticity, the lack of osteogenicity represents a limitation, even when osteoinductive factors are preserved during processing (Lobo Gajiwala *et al.*, 2003; Aho *et al.*, 1994).

In the last few years, alloplastic bone grafts made completely from synthetic materials are receiving increased interest owing to their off-the-shelf availability, ease of use and lack of immunogenicity (Roy *et al.*, 2003). The development of materials for any replacement application should be based on the understanding of the structure to be substituted. Specifically, the demands upon the material properties largely depend on the site of application and the function it has to restore. How Nature designs the complex structures of tissues may be evaluated through comprehension of the intricate phenomena (processing routes) that lead to the final shape and structure (from the macro to the ultrastructural level) by establishing the basic relationships between the physicochemical mechanisms and ideal structure properties (Black, 1992). This approach is particularly true in substitution medicine for bone and mineralized tissues. The bone could be considered as a natural anisotropic composite structure with higher mechanical properties (stiffness, tensile strength) than the soft tissues (blood vessels, cartilage, skin). For instance, during daily activities, bones are subjected to a stress of approximatively 4 MPa and, more importantly, these stresses are repetitive and fluctuate depending on activities like standing, sitting, jogging, stretching and climbing (Black and Hastings, 1998). The stress state, as well as the patient's condition and activities and the pH of the body fluids, which may vary in the range from 1 to 9 in various tissues, are all factors contributing to the definition of the biological environment in which the biomaterials need to survive.

In the near future, the challenge of the material scientist will consist in engineering replacement materials which are able ideally to mimic the living tissue from a mechanical, but also, from the chemical, biological and functional point of view. Starting from the example of the best materials scientist there is, namely Nature, the material scientist has to provide the design of smart structural components that respond, *in situ*, to exterior stimuli adapting the microstructure and corresponding properties and taking into account phenomena that occur owing to the specific mechanisms involved in bone tissue formation such as the biomineralization.

The demand that there is mechanical compatibility with hard tissue historically led to metals and ceramics being considered more suitable than polymers for these types of application. However, this approach is not completely acceptable in many cases, because of mismatches with properties of natural mineralized tissues. Specifically, metals are preferred for high strength, ductility and their wear resistance but may offer some problems in terms of low biocompatibility, corrosion, too high stiffness compared to the natural tissue, high densities and release of metal ions with possible allergic tissue reactions.

On the other hand, unreinforced polymers are typically more ductile but not stiff enough to be used to replace hard tissues in load-bearing applications. In this context, polymer-based composites are a very convenient solution for bone repair providing a wider set of options and possibilities in implant design. Specifically, they may be designed to meet stiffness and strength requirements for hard tissue substitution.

9.4 Non-degradable composites

Composite biomaterials such as the hip prostheses, fixation plates and screws, dental post, bone and dental cements represent efforts to find advanced engineering structures for hard tissue analogues. Carbon and glass fibre reinforced thermoset polymers (Fig. 9.2) such as epoxy resins were the first choice for composite orthopaedic prostheses (Ambrosio *et al.*, 1987). Polymer matrices include poly(sulphone) (PS), poly(ether-etherketone) (PEEK) and poly-etherimide (PEI) (Evans and Gregson, 1998; Alexander, 1996; Yildiz *et al.*, 1998; Akay and Aslan, 1995; Shirandami and Esat, 1990; Kettunen *et al.*, 1998). These engineering polymers are characterized by high mechanical properties, thermal stability, very marginal water absorption and relatively easy processing. In addition, their high level of solvents and thermal resistance allows the production of sterilizable medical devices. Moreover, the selected materials have demonstrated, at the same time, both positive and negative properties for specific applications. For instance, PEEK has

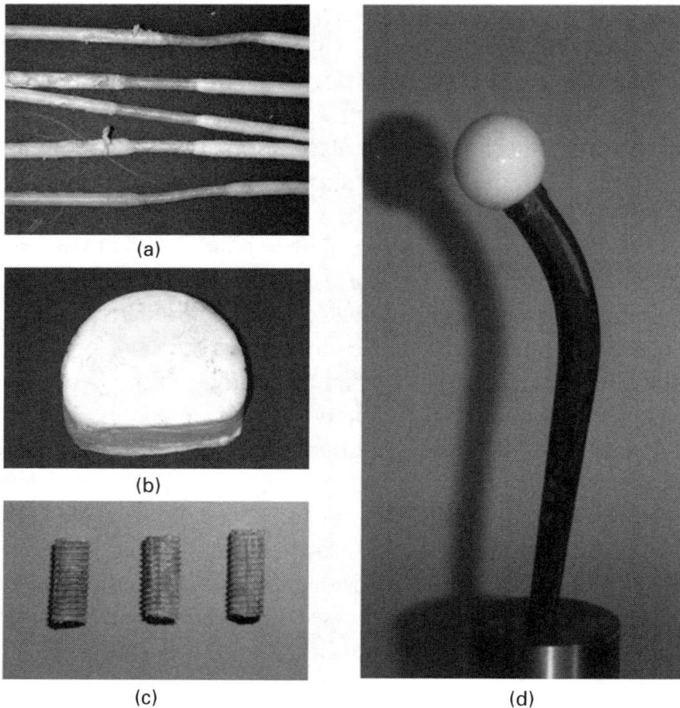

9.2 Examples of continuous fibre reinforced polymers for biomedical applications: ligament (a), intervertebral disc (b), spinal cage (c) and hip prostheses (d).

excellent mechanical stability but critical processing conditions owing to its temperature-sensitive semi-crystalline structure. Polysulphone has shown a reduction of mechanical properties following saturation in Ringer's solution. *In vitro* and *in vivo* studies (Merolli *et al.*, 1999) have shown that PEI is an excellent substrate for cell spreading and growth, eliciting no cytotoxic response or haemolysis, coupled with both easy processability and resistance to sterilization capability (γ rays and autoclave). Using PEI reinforced with drop-off plies of carbon and glass fibres a composite hip prosthesis has been developed in order to provide an adequate stress transfer between the prosthesis and bone (De Santis *et al.*, 2000).

Material–structural designs for advanced prostheses requiring a stem fitting into a canal (i.e. long bone or dental root canals) may differ, although a common challenge is to make a stem more flexible than those made of metal in order to improve proximal stress transfer and to avoid stress-shielding effects (Svensson *et al.*, 1977; Wilke *et al.*, 1994; Chang and Perez, 1990). By tailoring the stiffness of the prosthesis, both along its length and through its thickness, it is possible to change the pattern of load transfer between the prosthesis and the bone. Finite element models (FEM) combined with a mathematical description of adaptive bone remodelling suggest high performances of composite prostheses in terms of mechanical stability and tissue conservation (Van Rietbergen *et al.*, 1993; Mihalko *et al.*, 1992; Kuiper and Huiskes, 1997; Apicella *et al.*, 1994; Peluso *et al.*, 1994).

Based on the rapid prototyping, silicon mould and filament winding technology, a replica of a human mandible has been obtained. The spongy bone is simulated by using poly(methylmethacrylate) (PMMA) bone cement. The cortex of the mandible has been replicated by using a glass fibre reinforcement. The orientation of the windings are chosen according to the osteons' orientation of a human mandible, mainly oriented at 45° in the ramous and at 0° in the mandible arch (De Santis *et al.*, 2004, 2005, 2007b).

Early examples of composite biomimetic design are also well documented for dense connective tissues, ligaments and intervertebral disc. Hydrogel consisting of poly(hydroxyethylmethacrylate) PHEMA and poly(caprolactone) PCL reinforced with PET fibres was used to mimic the intervertebral disc. Using a filament winding machine, samples with a softer and more hydrophilic inner part (i.e. nucleus) and a harder and less hydrophilic outer part (i.e. annulus) were made. By varying the composition of the hydrogel matrix, the winding angle and the quantity of PET (polyethylenetelephthalate) fibres, it has been possible to modulate the hydrophilicity and the mechanical properties of intervertebral disc prosthesis (Ambrosio *et al.*, 1996, 1998a, 1998b). Composite structures based on a polyurethane matrix (HydroThaneTM) reinforced with PET fibres were designed and realised by filament winding in order to model the morphology and mechanical properties of natural ligaments and to reproduce the typical J-shaped stress–strain curve, displayed by natural tendons and ligaments (De Santis *et al.*, 2004). By using a PEI matrix reinforced with carbon fibres through filament winding technology, a composite cage has also been developed (Manto *et al.*, 2005).

9.5 Biodegradable composites

Currently, much research work has been addressed to the production of bioresorbable surgical devices for hard tissue repair. In fact they avoid the employment of surgical operations for their removal, reducing the pain of the patients and the total cost of the treatment with a significant advantage in terms of life quality of the patients (Daniels *et al.*, 1990).

Traditionally, metals such as stainless steel, titanium and Co/Cr alloys were commonly used for fracture fixation. Although they provide the right strength and rigidity to align and control bone motion during healing, they are much stiffer than bone (E_M = 100–200 GPa and E_B = 6–20 GPa) carrying the majority of the load. As result of the large difference in stiffness between bone and metals, a stress protection effect usually may occur causing the bone to atrophy over the long-term period. As consequence, the stress-shielded bone does not heal completely and is susceptible to re-fracture after removal of the metallic implant (Codran, 1969; Tormala *et al.*, 2002). Moreover, the metal chemical composition may evoke an allergic reaction by electrical potential difference which may promote an escalation of uncontrolled corrosion phenomena (Tonino *et al.*, 1976). More specifically, ion release may cause local adverse tissue reactions as well as allogenic responses with negative effects on the bone mineralization and adverse systemic responses like local tumour formation (Lamovec *et al.*, 1988; Martin *et al.*, 1988). To provide a less rigid system with minor problems of corrosion and a reduced need for removal, biodegradable polymeric composites and polymer/ceramic composites have been investigated for potential use in intramedullary rods, bone plates, fixation pins and screws, and bone regenerative scaffolds.

In the case of biodegradable composite, the stress-shielding phenomena associated with the use of rigid metallic implants may also be drastically reduced. Indeed, the continuous degradation of the implant causes a gradual load transfer to the healing tissue, preventing stress-shielding atrophy by stimulation of healing and bone remodelling.

9.5.1 Partially and totally degradable fibre reinforced composites

Some requirements must be fulfilled by ideal prosthetic biodegradable materials, such as biocompatibility, adequate initial strength and stiffness, retention of mechanical properties throughout a sufficient time to assure its biofunctionality and non-toxicity of degradation by-products. From the mechanical point of view, degradable polymers and composites have to possess a modulus of elasticity much closer to bone, one which decreases over time as the healing bone becomes stronger and stiffer (Flahiff *et al.*, 1996). It has been demonstrated that synthetic resorbable polymers like polylactide and polyglycolide fulfil several demands of ideal ostheosynthesis materials in term of biocompatibility and suitable stiffness, ensuring a progressive transfer of stresses to healing bone, obviating the need for a removal operation. However, they are too weak and flexible for safe clinical use in bone surgical applications. To overcome the limited mechanical response of non-reinforced materials based on aliphatic polyesters like PLA (i.e. low bending stiffness up to 4–6 GPa in the dry state at room temperature), the addition of thermoplastic fibres may promote the adjustment of the bending modulus up to 50 GPa as a function of the fibre content and their orientation (Kulkarni *et al.*, 1971).

In the last 30 years, partially resorbable composites have been obtained by combining a degradable polymeric matrix with high modulus fibres that are not resorbable (glass, carbon, aramides) in a continuous or chopped fibre form. The easy processability caused by thermal stability at high temperature combined with the use of economical and versatile processes (i.e. injection moulding) rapidly enabled the market to be captured in the last decade for devices (i.e. pins, screws, wires, plates) for fracture fixation applications. In general, partially resorbable composites comprising copolymers of methylmethacrylate and N-vinyl-pyrrolidone reinforced with polyamide fibres showed quite good mechanical properties (i.e. bending modulus 3–20 GPa) (Belykh *et al.*, 1981). However, the long-term effect of bio-inert, biostable or slowly degradable fibres is not well documented in living tissue and recent studies have demonstrated the presence of an acute or chronic inflammatory reaction in some cases under specific conditions with the detection of a thin encapsulating membrane of mature connective tissues around the implant region.

In this context, totally degradable reinforced composites may represent the main goal in the design of new fixation materials because of the drastic decay of long-term problems induced after their digestion by living tissues (Ambrosio *et al.*, 2001). More specifically, an interesting strategy may be the development of composite scaffolds composed of polymers with different degradation rates. The capability to control composite morphology by the selection of materials with well-known degradation kinetics, certainly offer a significant opportunity to guide tissue formation within the composite after their implant. To date, several approaches are investigating the ability to overcome these limitations even if the most promising strategy provides the development of composites with either dicarboxylic acid or an organic polymer (Pal *et al.*, 1995). Manifold processes such as pultrusion and compression moulding are more complicated and less economical than other techniques, limiting their application in highly advanced technologies. Instead, improved mechanical properties with constrained costs may be obtained by filament winding technologies (Dauner *et al.*, 1998).

In this direction, Ambrosio and co-workers proposed a composite structure obtained by merging a Hydrotane matrix with continuous fibres of PLA and PGA helically wound by filament winding technique in order to design porous and non-porous tubular constructs (Fig. 9.3a). The approach consists of applying the composite theory to design composite biodegradable systems able to mimic the structural organization and performance of living tissue (Ambrosio *et al.*, 2001). Continuous fibres are preliminarily preimpregnated into a Hydrotane/DMAC (dimethylacetammide) solution and then helically wound on the polyethylene (PE) hoses with the desired outer diameter. After winding, once removed from the machine, the composite is inserted in an ethyl alcohol bath to remove the solvent. Finally, the PE hose was removed to obtain three-dimensional (3D) composite constructs with a tubular shape.

Similarly, fibre reinforced composite scaffolds may be fabricated by the

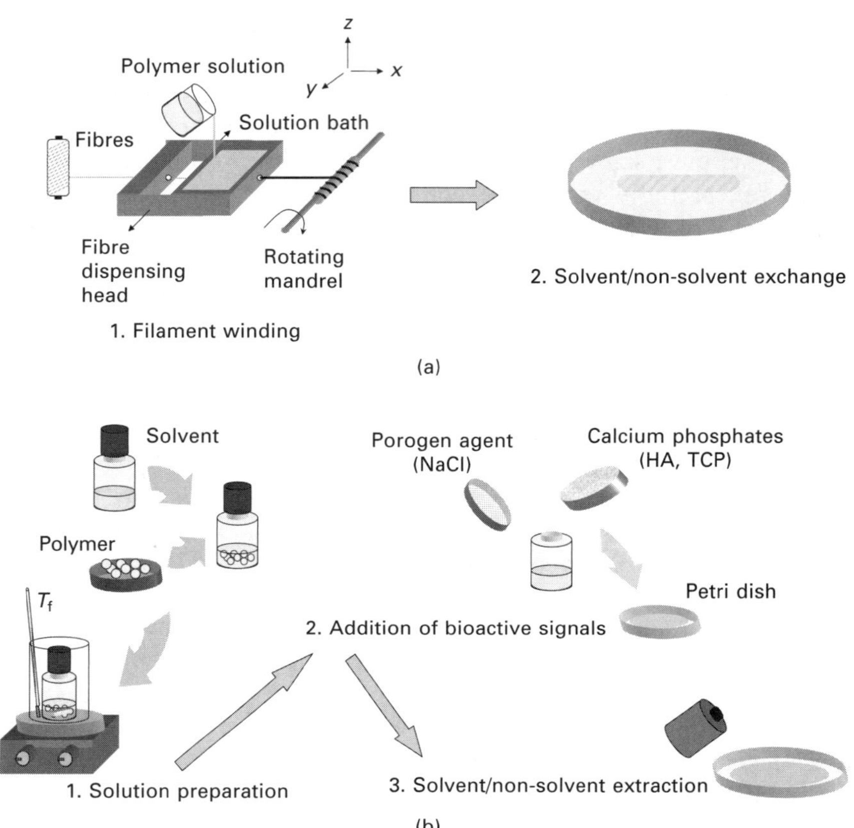

9.3 Scheme of preparation of different typologies of composites. (a) fibre reinforced composites; (b) inorganic filler reinforced composites.

integration of hydrophilic PLA continuous fibres into a hydrophobic PCL matrix in order to obtain highly porous scaffolds for bone regeneration (Guarino *et al.*, 2006). In these fibrous composites (Fig. 9.4a), degradation preferentially occurs at the fibre-polymer interface, resulting in a higher rate of degradation than for either material alone. Usually, the characteristic degradation rate of composites is too high and not totally adequate for clinical applications such as bone fracture fixation which require strength retention in the long term (i.e few weeks up to several months). However, a continuous fibre reinforced composite made of two interconnecting phases which mimic the bone structural organization better, assures a strong mechanical interlocking between two phases which, in turn, assures the retention of some of its properties if breakdown occurs at the interface. The main difficulty in the design of composite materials is referred to the optimization of the adhesion between matrix and reinforcement. An interfacial bond able to promote

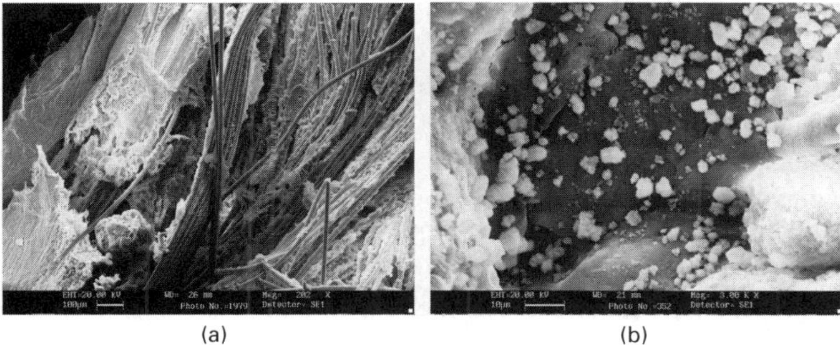

(a) (b)

9.4 Biodegradable composites with degradable polymeric matrix: (a) Fibre reinforced composites composed of a PCL matrix integrated to PLLA fibres; (b) PCL matrix loaded with HA micrometric particles.

more rapid diffusion of fluids at the matrix/fibre interface and also capable of not limiting mechanical strength and fatigue properties offers an optimal compromise condition for improving the final composite properties.

This aspect could be further compromised by the 3D architecture of the substitute (i.e. porosity) and its interaction with the surrounding tissue (Agrawal and Ray, 2001). It is worth noting that properly designed composite materials with high controlled degradation are able to provide new bone growth thanks to the right balance between vascularization promotion and mechanical support. The, final biological behaviour is first determined by the presence of a multi-scale porosity with tailored characteristics, in terms of pore interconnections and pore size, as the degradation mechanisms proceed. A well-organized pore network within the scaffold may potentially control cell colonization and fluid transport through its peculiar geometry (Van Eden and Ripamonti, 1994). The increased amount of open space combined with the progressive formation of channels within the biodegradable matrix caused by polymeric fibre degradation allows all cited mechanisms to be supported thanks to more rapid degradation mechanisms. However, some studies demonstrated that an excessive presence of open spaces may have led to premature fibrous tissue formation before new bone had a chance to infiltrate the scaffold. Furthermore, a large pore volume fraction negatively affects the mechanical performance of the composite, drastically reducing its ability to support static and cyclic loads.

9.5.2 Inorganic filler reinforced composites with a degradable matrix

In recent years, many favourable reports have been published on the use of bioactive materials such as hydroxyapatite (HA) as a substitute for defective bones or teeth in dental, maxillofacial and orthopaedic surgery. From a chemical point of view, they are known to be biocompatible, bioactive (i.e. have the ability to form a direct chemical bond with surrounding tissues), osteoconductive, non-toxic, non-inflammatory and non-immunogenic agent (Hench, 1991). Furthermore, it has been demonstrated that HA prepared at the nano-level may play a significant role in various biomedical applications owing to its unique functional properties, referable to a high particle surface area to volume ratio and an ultra fine structure similar to biological apatite, which has a great impact on cell–biomaterial interaction (Webster *et al.*, 2000). In detail, it has been verified that mineralized bone may be produced in close contact with the nanometric Hap coated surface independently of the morphology of the substrate on the submicrosmetric scale (De Bruijn *et al.*, 1992; Rosa *et al.*, 2002). For these reasons, HA is largely used in particulate form for the treatment of periodontal osseous defects and alveolar ridge augmentation because of its easy fabrication, handling and close surface contact with the surrounding tissue (Doi and Horiguchi, 1996).

However, the employment of HA-based systems was not entirely satisfactory because of the possible mobilization of loose HA particles from the implant site with their possible migration beyond the intended area. In particular, particle instability is often encountered when mixing particles in saline or patient's blood where a significant migration from the implanted site may occur into surrounding tissues, causing damage to healthy tissue (Miyamato and Shikawa, 1998).

To overcome these problems, common alloplastic materials including polyglycolic–lactic acid (PLGA), poly-L-lactic acid (PLLA) and polycaprolactone (PCL) have been combined with hydroxyapatite (HA) and tricalcium phosphates (α-TCP, β-TCP) particles to form composite materials (Guarino *et al.*, 2007). They are especially attractive because they combine the controlled degradation kinetics of the polymer phase, involving the formation of low molecular weight products, easily eliminated in a physiological environment, with the high bioactive potential induced by the employment of ceramic materials which promote the formation of mineralization sites. Moreover, the addition of more materials based on degradable natural (Zhao *et al.*, 2002) and synthetic polymers (Wang *et al.*, 2002) in conjugation of the HA particles allows the mechanical response of the medical device to be improved. More specifically, the brittle behaviour directly ascribable to the ceramic phase can be softened by coupling with the polymeric phase with an overall increase of the composite toughness, offering a more valid solution to mimic the complex behaviour of natural tissues to external mechanical stimuli.

Highly stiff metallic materials, traditionally implanted into bone defects are often encapsulated by a fibrous tissue and do not adhere to bone owing to a lack of bioactivity and, thus are isolated from the surrounding bone and remain as a foreign body (Kokubo *et al.*, 2003). To date, a proposed approach involving the combination of a polymer matrix and ceramic rigid particles allows an excellent balance to be reached between strength and toughness, usually improving specific characteristics compared to their separate components (Ramakrishna *et al.*, 2001) with strong enhancement of the biological response of the implanted device.

Causa *et al.* proposed a particle-reinforced composite consisting of a PCL matrix loaded with micrometric HA rigid particles in order to improve the osteoconductivity of the polymer (Fig. 9.3b). HA addition to the plain polymer strongly enhances the mechanical performance of the PCL scaffold by exhibiting a hardening function offered by the fine dispersion of particles inside the polymer matrix of PCL, which shows a significant increase in the mechanical resistance and up to a three-fold increase in the elastic modulus (Causa *et al.*, 2006). From a structural point of view, the strengthening mechanism of HA within PCL samples is first ascribed to the stiffer mechanical properties of HA in the composite material (Guarino *et al.*, 2008), even if the HA particle clustering ascribable to a not-homogeneous distribution of rigid particles within a polymer matrix may play a negative role by hampering the composite stiffness, as confirmed by a theory of the composite materials (Fig. 9.4b)

Afterwards, the potential of rigid particles to provide a reinforcement system is strongly conditioned by their reactivity in biological environment. In detail, HA is a stable phase, far less resorbable compared to other bioceramics like tricalcium phosphate, even if their resorbability can be slightly improved with some ceramic oxides and ionic doping agents (Murugan and Ramakrishna, 2003).

On the basis of these considerations, recent studies have extended the large number of composites obtained by coupling degradable polymers with reactive calcium phosphates (Roy *et al.*, 2003; Giordano *et al.*, 2006; Schmitt *et al.*, 2002) for the repair or the regeneration of a wide set of hard mineralized tissues as a function of the specific properties of the final material. Sanginario *et al.* (2006) proposed the development of a new injectable bone substitute material as a bone filler in orthopaedic and dental applications by combining a ceramic material like α-TCP or HA with the organic phase of HYAFF11®. It is well known that the attractive characteristic of the calcium phosphates is their ability to form a strong direct bond with the host bone, resulting in a strong dynamic interface compared to bio-inert or biotolerant materials which form a fibrous interface. The addition of the hydrophilic phase allows the cement workability to be modulated during its injection and the mechanical properties to be modulated during the hardening reaction of the ceramic phase giving, in a clinically acceptable time, suitable mechanical strength within the range for cancellous bone for short-term tissue functional recovery. In perspective, biodegradable composite hydrogels could be efficaciously used to deliver appropriate drugs into the application sites with controlled kinetic release.

Roy *et al.* (2003) have studied the performance of biodegradable composites for bone repair by the integration of β-tricalcium phosphate (β-TCP) particles in the PLGA porous matrix, providing evidence for a role of the ceramic phase in the degradation mechanisms of the polymer matrix. The relatively low molecular weight of the 50:50 PLGA (only 50 kDa) promotes a fast hydrolytic degradation *in vivo*, with rapid mechanical failure owing to loss of structure. During the PLGA degradation via bulk erosion, the release of acidic degradation products leads to a local decrease in pH, which rapidly causes local tissue damage, that is bone resorption and fibrous tissue formation. The presence of reactive calcium phosphates such as α- and β-TCP may enable the decay in pH to be buffered, influencing the final polymer degradation. In this direction, several studies related to *in vitro* degradation of PLA composites with various additive charges of TCP particles have highlighted a pH drop at the most of up to 5, corresponding to the approximate pH for activated macrophages, indicating the occurrence of probable bone resorption (Holy *et al.*, 1999; Lin *et al.*, 1999).

9.6 References

Agrawal CM and Ray RB (2001), 'Biodegradable polymeric scaffolds for musculoskeletal tissue engineering', *J Biomed Mater Res*, **55**, 141–50.

Aho AJ, Ekfors T, Dean PB, Aro HT, Ahonen A and Nikkanen V (1994), 'Incorporation and clinical results of large allografts of the extremities and pelvis'. *Clin Orthop Relat Res*, (**307**), 200–13.

Alexander H (1996), *Biomaterial Science*, Ratuer BD (ed.), Academic Press, San Diego, 94–105.

Akay M and Aslan N (1995), 'An estimation. of fatigue life for a carbon fibre/polyether ether ketone hip joint prosthesis', *Proc Inst Mech Engrs, Part H*, **229**, 93–103.

Ambrosio L, Caprino G, Nicolais L, Nicodemo L, Huang SJ, Guida G and Ronca D (1987), *Composite Structures*, Marshall IH (ed.), Elsevier Applied Science, London and New York, Vol. **2**, 2.337–2.344.

Ambrosio L, Netti PA, Iannace S, Huang SJ and Nicolais L (1996), 'Composite hydrogels for intervertebral disc prostheses', *J Mater Sci: Mater Med*, **7**, 251–4.

Ambrosio L, De Santis R and Nicolais L (1998a), 'Composite hydrogels for implants', *J Proc Instn Mech Engrs*, **212**(H), 93–9.

Ambrosio L, De Santis R, Iannace S, Netti PA and Nicolais L (1998b), 'Viscoelastic behavior of composite ligament prostheses', *J Biomed Mater Res*, **42**, 1, 6–12.

Ambrosio L, Netti PA, Santaniello B and Nicolais L (2001), 'Composite materials as scaffolds for tissue engineering', *Biomedical Polymers and Polymer Therapeutics*, Chiellini *et al.* (eds), Kluwer Academic/Plenum USA Part 1, 227–33.

Apicella A, Liguori A, Masi E and Nicolais L (1994), *Experimental Techniques and Design in Composite Materials*, Found MS (ed.), Academic Press, Sheffield, 323–38.

Arends CB (1993), *Polymer Toughening, Foundations of Materials Science and Engineering*. Smith WF (ed.), 2nd edition, McGraw Hill, New York.

Arrington ED, Smith WJ, Chambers HG, Bucknell AL and Davino NA (1996), 'Complications of iliac crest bone graft harvesting', *Clin Orthop Relat Res*, **329**, 300–9.

Augat P, Link T, Lang TF, Lin JC, Majumdar S and Genant HK (1998), 'Anisotropy of the elastic modulus of trabecular bone specimens from different anatomical locations', *Med Eng Phys*, **2**, 124–31.

Banwart JC, Asher MA and Hassanein RS (1995), 'Iliac crest bone graft harvest donor site morbidity. A statistical evaluation', *Spine*, **1**(20), 1055–60.

Barbucci R (2002), *Integrated Biomaterials Science*, Kluwer Academic/Plenum Publishers, New York, USA.

Belykh SI, Davydov AB, Khromov GL, Monschensky AD, Movshovich LA, Roitberg GI, Voskresensky GL, Pershin GG and Moskvitin VA (1981), *Biodestructive Material for Bone Fixation Elements*, US Patent no. 4263185.

Black J (1992), *Biological Performance of Materials: Fundamentals of Biocompatibility*. Marcel Dekker, New York.

Black J and Hastings GW (1998), *Handbook of Biomaterials Properties*, Chapman and Hall, London.

Bonfield W and Grynpas MG (1997), 'Anisotropy of the Young's modulus of bone', *Nature*, **270**, 453–4.

Causa F, Netti PA, Ambrosio L, Ciapetti G, Baldini N, Pagani S, Martini D and Giunti A (2006), 'Polycaprolactone/hydroxyapatite composites for bone regeneration: *in vitro* characterization and human osteoblast response', *J Biomed Mater Res*, **76A**, 151–62.

Chang FK and Perez JL (1990), 'Stiffness and strength tailoring of a hip prosthesis made of advanced composite materials', *J Biomed Mater Res*, **24**, 873–99.

Codran GVB (1969), 'Effects of the internal fixation plates on mechanical deformation of bone', *Surg Forum*, **20**, 469–71.

Dabestani M and Bonfield W (1988), 'Elastic and anelastic microstrain measurement in human cortical bone', *Implant Materials in Biofunction*, de Putter C, de Lange GL, de Groot K and Lee AJC (eds), Elsevier Science Publisher, Amsterdam, 435–40.

Daniels AU, Chang MK and Andriano KP (1990), 'Mechanical properties of biodegradable polymers and composites proposed for internal fixation of bone', *J Appl Biomater*, **1**, 57–78.

Dauner M, Planck H, Caramano L, Missirlis Y and Panagiotopoulos E (1998), 'Resorbable continuous-fibre reinforce polymers for osteosynthesis', *J Mater Sci: Mater Med*, **9**, 173–9.

De Bruijn JD, Klein CPAT, de Groot K and van Blitterswijk CA (1992), 'The ultrastructure of bone-hydroxyapatite interface *in vitro*', *J Biomed Mater Res*, **26**, 1365–82.

Deligiann DD, Missirlis YF, Tanner KE and Bonfield W (1991), 'Mechanical behaviour of trabecular bone of the human femoral head in females', *J Mater Sci: Mater Med*, **2**,168–75.

De Santis R, Ambrosio L and Nicolais L (2000), 'Polymer based composite hip prostheses', *J Inorga Biochemi*, **79**, 97–102.

De Santis R, Sarracino F, Mollica F, Netti PA, Ambrosio L and Nicolais L (2004), 'Continuous fibre reinforced polymers as connective tissue replacement', *Comp Sci Tech*, **64**, 861–78.

De Santis R, Mollica F, Ambrosio L and Nicolais L (2005), 'An experimental and theoretical composite model of the human mandible', *J Mater Sci: Mater Med*, **16**, 1191–7.

De Santis R, Ambrosio L, Mollica F, Netti PA and Nicolais L (2007a), 'Mechanical properties of human mineralised connective tissues', *Modeling of biological materials*, Mollica F, Preziosi L and Rajagopal KR (eds), Birkhauser, Boston, 211–61.

De Santis R, Mollica F, Zarone F, Ambrosio L and Nicolais L (2007b), 'Biomechanical effects of titanium implants with full arch bridge rehabilitation on a synthetic model of the human jaw', *Acta Biomaterialia*, **3**, 121–6.

Doi Y and Horiguchi T (1996), 'Formation of apatite–collagen complexes', *J Biomed Mater Res*, **31**, 43–9.

Evans SL and Gregson PJ (1998), 'Composite technology in load-bearing orthopaedic implants', *Biomaterials*, **19**, 1329–42.

Flahiff CM, Blackwell AS, Hollis JM and Feldman (1996), 'Analysis of a biodegradable composite for bone healing', *J Biomed Mater Res*, **32**, 419–24.

Fung YC (1993), *Biomechanics*, Springer-Verlag, New York.

Gazdag AR, Lane JM, Glaser D and Forster RA (1995), 'Alternatives to autogenous bone graft: efficacy and indications', *J Am Acad Orthop Surg*, **3**, 1–8.

Giesen EB, Ding M, Dalstra M and van Eijden TM (2001), 'Mechanical properties of cancellous bone in the human mandibular condyle are anisotropic', *J Biomech*, **34**(6), 799–803.

Giordano C, Sanginario V, Ambrosio L, Di Silvio L and Santin M (2006), 'Chemical–physical characterization and in vitro preliminary biological assessment of hyaluronic acid benzyl ester–hydroxyapatite composite', *J Biomater Appl*, **20**, 237–53.

Guarino V, Gloria A, Causa F, De Santis R and Ambrosio L (2006), 'Scaffolds for connective tissue regeneration', *Biomed Pharmacother*, **60**, 471.

Guarino V, Causa F and Ambrosio L (2007), 'Bioactive scaffolds for bone and ligament tissue', *Expert Rev Med. Devices*, **4**(3), 406–18.

Guarino V, Causa F, Netti P.A, Ciapetti G, Pagani S, Martini D, Baldini N and Ambrosio L (2008), 'The role of hydroxyapatite as solid signal on performance of PCL porous scaffolds for bone tissue regeneration', *J Biomed Mater Res Part B: Appl Biomater*, **86B**(2), 548–57.

Hench LL (1991), 'Bioceramics from concept to clinic', *J Am Ceram Soc*, **74**, 1487–510.

Hengsberger S, Kulik A and Zysset P (2002), 'Nanoindentation discriminates the elastic properties of individual human bone lamellae under dry and physiological conditions', *Bone*, **30**, 178–84.

Holy CE, Dang SM, Davies JE and Shoichet MS (1999), '*In vitro* degradation of a novel poly(lactide-co-glycolide) 75/25 foam', *Biomaterials*, **20**, 1177–85.

Kettunen J, Makela EA, Miettinen H, Nevalainen T, Heikkila M, Pohjonen T, Tormala P and Rokkanen P, (1998), *Biomaterials*, **19**, 1219–28.

Kneser U, Schaefer DJ, Polykandriotis E and Horch RE (2006), 'Tissue engineering of bone: the reconstructive surgeon's point of view', *J Cell Mol Med*, **10**(1), 7–19.

Kokubo T, Kim HM and Kawashita M (2003), 'Novel bioactive materials with different mechanical properties', *Biomaterials*, **24**, 2161–75.

Kuiper JH and Huiskes R (1997), 'Mathematical optimization elastic properties: application to cementless hip stem design', *J Biomech Eng*, **119**, 166–74.

Kulkarni RK, Moore EG, Hegyeli AF and Leonard F (1971), 'Biodegradable poly(lactid acid) polymers', *J Biomed Mater Res*, **5**, 169–81.

Lamovec J, Zidar A and Cucek M (1988), 'Synovial sarcoma associated with total hip replacement', *J Bone Joint Surg*, **70A**, 1558–60.

Lin FH, Chen TM, Lin CP and Lee CJ (1999), 'The merit of sintered PDLLA/TCP composites in management of bone fracture internal fixation', *Artif Organs*, **23**, 186–94.

Lobo Gajiwala A, Agarwal M, Puri A, Lima C and Duggal A (2003), 'Reconstructing tumour defects: lyophilised, irradiated bone allografts', *Cell Tissue Bank*, **4**, 109–18.

Majumdar S, Kothari M, Augat P, Newitt DC, Link TM, Lin JC, Lang T, Lu Y and Genant

HK (1998), 'High-resolution magnetic resonance imaging: three-dimensional trabecular bone architecture and biomechanical properties', *Bone*, **22**, 445–54.

Manto L, De Santis R, Carrillo G, Ambrosio G, Ambrosio L and Nicolais L (2005), 'Novel composite intervertebral disc cage for spine fusion', *J Bone Joint Surg, British Volume, Orthopaedic Proceedings*, **87–B**(Issue SUPP I), 68.

Martin A, Bauer MT, Manley MT and Marks KE (1988), 'Osteosarcoma at the site of total hip replacement', *J Bone Joint Surg*, **70A**, 1561–8.

Merolli A, Perrone V, Tranquilli Leali P, Ambrosio L, De Santis R, Nicolais L and Gabbi C (1999), 'Response to polyetherimide based composite materials implanted in muscle and in bone', *J Maert Sci: Mater Med*, **10**, 256–68.

Mihalko WM, Beaudoin AJ, Cardea JA and Krause WR (1992), 'Finite-element modelling of femoral shaft fracture fixation techniques post total hip arthroplasty', *J Biomech*, **25**, 469–76.

Miyamato Y and Shikawa KI (1998), 'Basic properties of calcium phosphate cement containing atelocollagen in its liquid or powder phases', *Biomaterials*, **19**, 707–15.

Murugan R and Ramakrishna S (2003), 'Effect of zirconia on the formation of calcium phosphate bioceramics under microwave irradiation', *Mater Lett*, **58**, 230–4.

Nicholson PH, Muller R, Lowet G, Cheng XG, Hildebrand T, Ruegsegger P, van der Perre G, Dequeker J and Boonen S (1998), 'Do quantitative ultrasound measurements reflect structure independently of density in human vertebral cancellous bone', *Bone*, **23**, 425–31.

O'Mahony AM, Williams JL, Katz JO and Spencer P (2000), 'Anisotropic elastic properties of cancellous bone from human edentulous mandible', *Clin Oral Impl Res*, **11**, 415–21.

Pal A, Rawat N and Pal S (1995), 'Characterisation of hydroxyapatite based composites for bone repair', *Engineering in Medicine and Biology Society, 1995 and 14th Conference of the Biomedical Engineering Society of India. An International Meeting, Proceedings of the First Regional Conference*, IEEE Publication.

Peluso G, Petillo O, Ambrosio L and Nicolais L (1994), *J Mater Sci: Mater Med*, **5**, 738–42.

Petite H, Viateau V, Bensaid W, Meunier A, de Pollak C, Bourguignon M, Oudina K, Sedel L and Guillemin G (2000), 'Tissue engineered bone regeneration', *Nature Biotech*, **18**, 959.

Ramakrishna S, Majer J, Wintermantel E and Leong KW (2001), 'Biomedical applications of polymer-composite materials: a review', *Composites Sci Technol*, **61**, 1189–224.

Reilly DT and Burstein AH (1975), 'The elastic and ultimate properties of compact bone tissue', *J Biomech*, 8, 393–405.

Rho JY, Ashman RB and Turner CH (1993), 'Young's modulus of trabecular and cortical bone materials: ultrasonic and microtensile measurements', *J Biomech*, **2**, 111–19.

Rho JY, Kuhn-Spearing L and Zioupos P (1998), 'Mechanical properties and the hierarchical structure of bone', *Med Eng Phys*, **2**, 92–102.

Rosa AL, Beloti MM and Olivera PT (2002), 'Osteointegration and osteoconductivity of Hydroxyapatite of different microporosities', *J Mater Sci Mat Med*, **13**, 1071–5.

Roy TD, Simon JL, Ricci JL, Rekow ED, Thompson VP and Russell Parsons J (2003), 'Performance of degradable composite bone repair products made via three-dimensional fabrication techniques', *J Biomed Mater Res*, **66A**, 283–91.

Sanginario V, Ginebra MP, Tanner KE, Planell JA and Ambrosio L (2006), 'Biodegradable and semi-biodegradable composite hydrogels as bone substitutes: morphology and mechanical characterization', *J Mater Sci: Mater Med*, **17**, 447–54.

Sassard WR, Eidman DK, Gray PM, Block JE, Russo R, Russell JL and Taboada EM (2000), 'Augmenting local bone with Grafton demineralized bone matrix for posterolateral lumbar spine fusion: avoiding second site autologous bone harvest', *Orthopedics*, **23**, 1059–64.

Schmitt M, Weiss P, Bourges X, Amador Del Valle G and Daculsi G (2002), 'Crystallization at the polymer/calcium-phosphate interface in a sterilized injectable bone substitute IBS', *Biomaterials*, **23**, 2789–94.

Shirandami R and Esat II (1990), 'New design of hip prosthesis using carbon fibre reinforced composite', *J Biomed Eng*, **12**, 19–22.

Silver FH, Seehra GP, Freeman JW and DeVore D (2002), 'Viscoelastic properties of young and old human dermis: a proposed molecular mechanism for elastic energy storage in collagen and elastin', *J Appl Polym Sci*, **86**, 1978–85.

Spitzer R, Perka C, Lindenhayn K and Zippel H, (2002), 'Matrix engineering for osteogenic differentiation of rabbit periosteal cells using alpha-tricalcium phosphate particles in a three-dimensional fibrin culture', *J Biomed Mater Res Part A*, **59**(4), 690–6.

Svensson NL, Valliapan S and Wood RD (1977), 'Stress analysis of human femur with implanted Charnley prosthesis', *J Biomech*, **10**, 581–8.

Tonino AJ, Davidson CL, Klopper PJ and Linclau LA (1976), *J Bone Joint Surg*, **58**, 107–13.

Tormala P, Juutilainen T, Partio EK and Rokkanen P (2002), 'Bioabsorbable composite implants for treatment of bone fractures and osteotomies', *Tech Health Care*, **10**(3–4), 245–53.

Van Eden SP and Ripamonti U (1994), 'Bone differentiation in porous hydroxyapatite in baboons is regulated by the geometry of the substratum: Implications for reconstructive craniofacial surgery', *Plast Reconstr Surg*, **93**, 959–66.

Van Rietbergen B, Huiskes R, Weinans H, Sumner DR, Turner TM and Galante JO (1993), 'The mechanism of bone remodeling and resorption around press-fitted THA stems', *J Biomech*, **26**, 369–82.

Wang X, Li Y, Wei J and De Groot K (2002), 'Development of biomimetic nano-hydroxyapatite and poly(hexamethylene adipamide) composites', *Biomaterials*, **23**, 4787–91.

Webster TJ, Siegel RW and Bizios R (2000), 'Enhanced functions of osteoblasts on nanophase ceramics', *Biomaterials*, **21**, 1803–10.

Weiner S and Wagner HD (1998), 'The material bone: Structure-mechanical function relations', *Ann Rev Mater Sci*, **28**, 271–98.

Williams DF (1999), *Bone Engineering*, 1st edition, Em squared, Toronto, p 577.

Wilke HJ, Seiz RS, Bombelli M, Claes L and Durselen L (1994), 'Biomechanical and histomorphological investigations on a isoelastic prosthesis', *J. Mater Sc Mater Med*, **5**, 384–6.

Yildiz H, Chang FK and Goodman S (1998), 'Composite hip prosthesis design. II. Simulation', *J Biomed Mater Res*, **39**, 102–19.

Zhao F, Yin Y, Lu WW, Leong JC, Zhang W, Zhang J, Zhang M and Yao K (2002), 'Preparation and histological evaluation of biomimetic three-dimensional hydroxyapatite/chitosan-gelatin network composite scaffolds', *Biomaterials*, **23**, 3227–34.

Ziouposet P, Currey JD and Hamer AJ (1999), 'The role of collagen in the declining mechanical properties of aging human cortical bone', *J Biomed Mater Res*, **45**, 108–16.

10
Cements as bone repair materials

M. P. GINEBRA, Technical University of Catalonia (UPC), Spain

Abstract: Bone cements can be defined as biomaterials obtained by mixing a powder phase and a liquid phase, which can be moulded and implanted as a paste and have the ability to set once implanted within the body. They are widely used in different applications of orthopaedic surgery. The possibility of injecting them extends their use to minimally invasive surgical techniques. The chapter describes the two main families of bone cements, namely, acrylic bone cements and calcium phosphate bone cements. The basic physicochemical, mechanical and biological properties of these two types of bone cement are reviewed and the most relevant clinical applications are described.

Key words: bone cements, calcium phosphates, hydroxyapatite, polymethyl methacrylate.

10.1 Definition and advantages of bone cements in orthopaedic surgery

Bone cements can be defined as a family of materials that consist of a powder phase and a liquid phase which, after mixing, form a plastic paste which has the ability to self-set once implanted in the body. This means that the material is mouldable, which ensures perfect fit at the implant site and good bone–material contact, even in geometrically complex defects. On the other hand, the fact that the cements undergo a setting reaction once implanted, forming a solid body, guarantees a certain level of mechanical support, although as will be described in the following sections, the mechanical properties achieved are different in different types of bone cement.

Recent advances in orthopaedic surgery are related to the application of minimally invasive surgical techniques. In this field it is crucial to have injectable materials available and, in this sense, bone cements can play a determinant role, provided injectable cements are developed. An example is the implementation of some minimally invasive surgical procedures, namely vertebroplasty and kyphoplasty, to repair vertebral compression fractures, where bone cements are injected into the vertebral body.

The desirable properties that a bone cement should have are summarized in Table 10.1. An 'ideal' cement should fulfil all of them. However, there is no 'ideal' bone cement and all bone cements used nowadays have some limitations. At present the most frequently used bone cements can be classified

Table 10.1 Desirable properties for a bone cement

Ease of handling
Injectability
In vivo setting and hardening with appropriate times
Low setting temperature
Near neutral pH during setting
No disintegration in early contact with body fluids
No shrinkage during setting
Appropriate mechanical strength
High radiopacity
No toxicity
Biocompatibility
Bioactivity
Porosity

in two groups, namely acrylic bone cements (ABCs) and calcium phosphate bone cements (CPCs). The description of their composition, properties and applications will be the object of the following sections.

10.2 Calcium phosphate versus acrylic bone cements: historical perspective and present applications

The term 'bone cement' was initially applied to acrylic bone cements (ABCs), widely used in orthopaedic surgery since the 1960s, especially for arthroplasty fixation, when Sir John Charnley presented the preliminary results of a new method for the fixation of joint prostheses to bone.[1–3] The idea was borrowed from the field of dentistry. Self-curing polymethylmethacrylate (PMMA) was used as a grouting material to fix the femoral stem and the acetabular component in place and to distribute the contact stresses between the implant and the bone over a large area. This strategy represented an important breakthrough in the field of orthopaedics and led to the development of a technique that was successful worldwide, which provides excellent primary fixation and an even load distribution between the implant and the bone, allowing the patient a fast recovery. At present it is still one of the most frequently performed orthopaedic procedures in the world and there are numerous ABC formulations currently commercially available.[4]

Moreover, injectable ABCs are also used in other applications such as vertebroplasty and kyphoplasty after vertebral compression fractures, with the aim of stabilizing bone and restoring it to its functional state.[5, 6] The ABCs used for this application can be either the same commercially available material that is used for cemented arthroplasties, to which an additional amount of radiopacifier is added by the surgeon, or commercially available brands that are specifically formulated for this application.[5]

ABCs are polymeric materials, which cure through a polymerization reaction and produce a stable, non-resorbable material. The main function of ABCs is mechanical. However, ABCs have some drawbacks. In some cases aseptic loosening occurs with time, which is attributed to causes such as the lack of secondary fixation or the mechanical failure of the cement. On the other hand, although once cured the ABC is a non-toxic and biologically inert material, the heat liberated during the setting stage can induce bone necrosis. Moreover, wear particles and debris which could come from the bone cement can cause foreign body reaction inducing osteolysis. The toxicity of the liquid monomer of the cement is another disadvantage. ABCs still have a long way to go but also have a future, mainly when the moderate success of alternative techniques is taken into account.

Calcium phosphate cements (CPCs) were discovered by Legeros[7] and Brown and Chow[8] in the early 1980s. They demonstrated the formation of hydroxyapatite in a monolithic form at room or body temperature by means of a cementitious reaction. This was an important breakthrough in the field of bioceramics research, since it supplied a material which was mouldable and therefore could adapt to the bone cavity, presenting a good fixation and the optimum tissue–biomaterial contact necessary to stimulate the bone ingrowth. Thus, this new family, in common with the ABCs, had the capacity to be moulded into a shape and cured inside the body, allowing their implantation in a paste form. In the last few decades, calcium phosphate cements have attracted much attention and different formulations have been put forward[8–12] and many commercial products exist on the market.[13, 14]

Even if both can be classified as bone cements, the nature, properties and applications of ABC and CPCs are very different, as summarized in Table 10.2, and described in the following sections.

CPCs are not polymeric, but hydraulic cements, which means that water is used as the liquid phase of the cement and their hardening is not due to a polymerization reaction, but to a dissolution and precipitation process. Unlike in the case of ABCs, the heat evolved during setting is very low and it does not provoke problems of necrosis by hyperthermia.[15] Among the main advantages of CPCs are their excellent biocompatibility and bioactivity. This means that they have the capacity to form a direct bond with bone and that they are osteoconductive materials. Moreover, they can be resorbable, with a resorption rate which depends on their composition and microstructural features. The properties mentioned give CPCs high bone regeneration potential. On the other hand, they have some limitations related to their poor mechanical properties.

Like most ceramic materials, CPCs are brittle and, in addition, owing to the fact that they are intrinsically porous materials, their strength is in general lower than that of acrylic cements and therefore they cannot be used for the fixation of articular prostheses. In fact, the first commercial

Table 10.2 Comparison of the composition, properties, applications and functions of acrylic bone cements versus calcium phosphate bone cements

	Acrylic bone cements	Calcium phosphate bone cements
Material type	Polymer	Ceramic
Liquid phase	Mainly methyl methacrylate	Water or aqueous solutions
Powder component	Polymer beads (PMMA/ copolymers). Some inorganic filler can be added as radiopacifier	Calcium phosphate powders
Setting reaction mechanism	Polymerization	Dissolution and precipitation reaction
Reaction products	Mainly polymethyl methacrylate	Calcium phosphates, usually hydroxyapatite or brushite
Exothermic peak temperature during setting (ISO standard 5833)	50–90°C	37°C
Stability	Non-resorbable	Resorbable (low or high resorption rate depending on composition and microstructure)
Biocompatibility	Acceptable although some drawbacks are high exothermy during setting and monomer toxicity	Excellent
Bioactivity	Non-bioactive	Bioactive
Applications	Moderate load-bearing applications: arthroplasty fixation, vertebroplasty	Bone regeneration. Non-load-bearing applications
Function	Primary fixation of the metallic components and even load distribution ('fill and fit')	Cavity filling and enhancement of bone regeneration

apatitic CPCs were introduced in the market in the 1990s and subsequently brushite cements were also commercialized. They are used for different bone regeneration applications, such as (a) maxillofacial and craniofacial reconstruction (cranioplasty, cranial recontouring, cranial flap augmentation, augmentation genioplasty, on-lay grafting, skull base defect repair),[16] (b) treatment of several fracture defects, such as distal radius, proximal and distal tibia, calcaneus, proximal and distal femur, proximal humerus, acetabulum,[17] (c) treatment of surgically or traumatically created osseous defects, filling of cystic lesions and augmentation of screws, (d) more recently, for the treatment of spinal fractures and vertebroplasty (with or without the aid of a kyphoplasty balloon).[18–20] This last application is common with ABCs and even if the nature and properties of the two types of cements are very different, some results reported in the literature about *ex vivo* biomechanical studies show no significant differences between the two materials.[21–26]

CPCs are also used to fabricate pre-set granules and blocks, which have some advantages in comparison to sintered ceramic granules or blocks. The advantages arise from the low-temperature and wet processing method intrinsic to CPCs. Indeed, the apatite CPC products are micro/nanocrystalline, have high specific surface area and, therefore, are much more reactive than sintered ceramics. In addition, CPCs enable the fabrication of low temperature calcium phosphates, such as brushite, octacalcium phosphate or calcium deficient hydroxyapatite, which cannot be obtained by high temperature sintering and which are much closer to the calcium phosphates found in living tissues.

10.3 Acrylic bone cements

10.3.1 Chemical composition

ABCs are based on PMMA which is accepted as a biocompatible polymer when cured. The bone cement is prepared by mixing two components, a liquid phase and a powder phase.

- Liquid component: transparent, volatile and with a characteristic smell. Its viscosity is low and its boiling temperature is approximately 100°C at 760 mm Hg. Its density is 0.94 g cm^{-3}. It contains three basic ingredients:
  - MMA monomer ($CH_2C(CH_3)COOCH_3$): 97% v/v approximately;
  - N,N-Dimethyl-*p*-toluidine (*p*-$N(CH_3)C_6H_4CH_3$): 2.7% v/v approximately; acts as accelerant of the polymerization reaction which activates the initiator mixed with the powder;
  - Hydroquinone (OHC_6H_4OH): 750 ppm; acts as an inhibitor, which prevents the premature polymerization of the monomer.
- Solid component: it contains three basic ingredients:
  - PMMA ($[CH_3C(CH_2)COOCH_3]_n$): 89% w/w approximately. In some instances, instead of PMMA beads, other polymers or copolymers are used. The diameter of most PMMA particles in the cement ranges between 30 and 150 μm and their shape depends on the manufacturing process used;
  - Benzoyl peroxide ($COC_6H_5OOCC_6H_5O$)(BP): 0.75% w/w approximately; acts as initiator, producing free radicals when it reacts with the amine N,N-dimethyl-*p*-toluidine (DMT) of the liquid phase;
  - Barium sulphate ($BaSO_4$) or zirconium dioxide (ZrO_2): 10% w/w; added in order to obtain radiopacity.

Figure 10.1(a) shows the morphology of the powder of an ABC. Both PMMA beads and smaller $BaSO_4$ powder particles are visible.

10.3.2 Processing parameters and setting properties of acrylic bone cements

At the moment of mixing the solid and liquid components, the polymerization of the liquid monomer starts, as a typical reaction of addition polymerization towards curing the paste. The final product, after the polymerization of the liquid phase, consists of a multiphase material, with the PMMA beads embedded in a PMMA matrix which also contains the inorganic radiopacifying fillers. This microstructure can be observed in Fig. 10.1(b), where a SEM picture of a fracture surface of a cured ABC is shown.

Figure 10.2(a) represents schematically the reactants and the product obtained after the polymerization reaction. Both physical and chemical phenomena take place simultaneously, affecting the setting process as well as the microstructure and the mechanical properties of the set material, which depend on variables such as the chemical composition and concentration of the initial powder and liquid components, the physical mixing method and chemical environment (Table 10.3).

The time elapsed from the moment in which the powder and liquid components are mixed until the cement is set is known as the setting time. If the evolution of the temperature with time is recorded, the setting time is the time when the temperature of the polymerizing mass is: $T_{amb} + (T_{max} - T_{amb})/2$, where T_{amb} is the ambient temperature, taken as 23 ± 1°C and

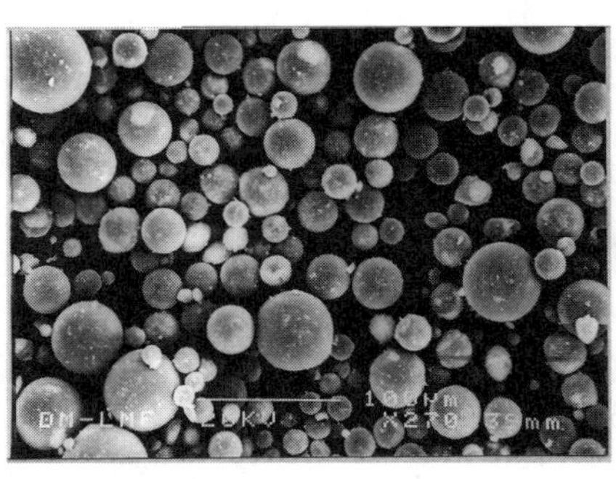

(a)

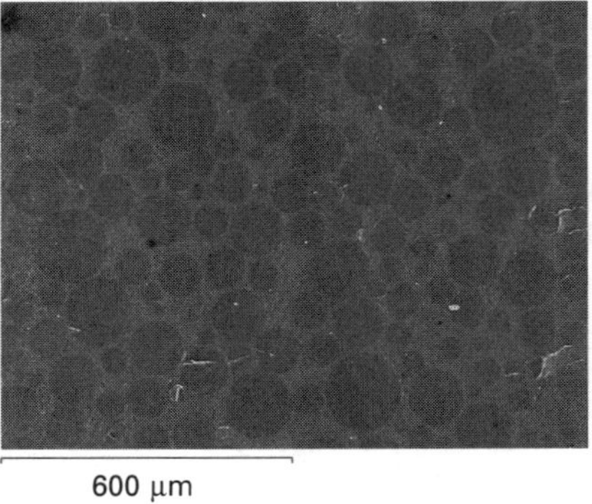

(b)

10.1 (a) Morphology of the powder phase of an acrylic bone cement: PMMA beads and small barium sulphate white particles are visible, (b) SEM image of the fracture surface of a cured acrylic bone cement. PMMA beads are embedded in a PMMA matrix. Scale bar: 600 µm.

Powder
Polymer: PMMA/copolymers
Initiator: BPO
Radiopacifier: ZrO_2
$BaSO_4$
Liquid
Monomer: MMA
Activator: DMT
Stabilizer: hydroquinone

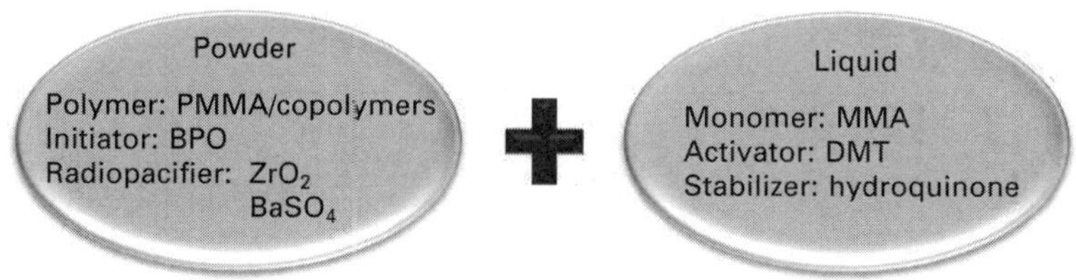

Reaction of addition polymerization

Set cement: multiphase polymeric material

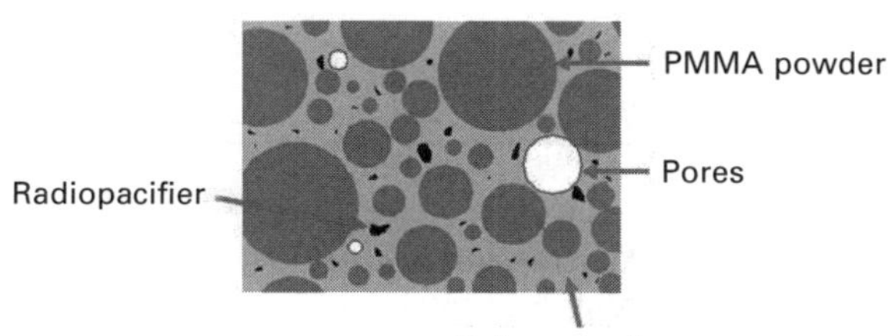

(a)

Powder
One or several
calcium phosphates
Liquid
Water or aqueous solution

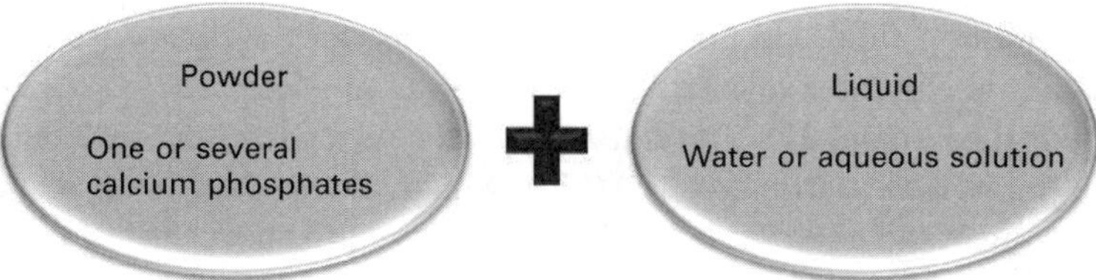

Reaction of dissolution and precipitation

Set cement: entangled calcium phosphate crystals

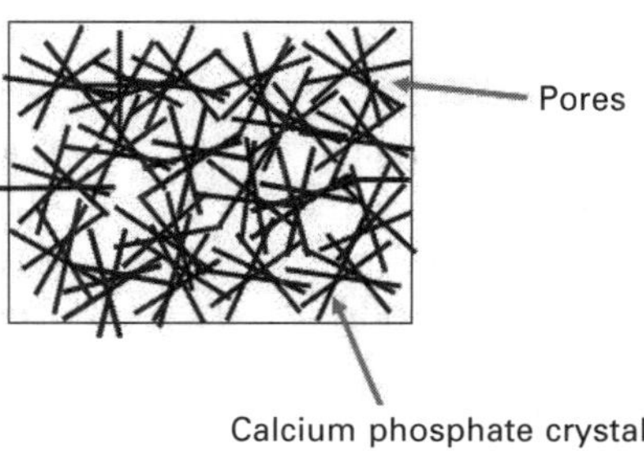

(b)

10.2 Constituents, final product and setting mechanism of (a) acrylic bone cement and (b) calcium phosphate bone cement.

Table 10.3 Processing parameters that affect the properties of a bone cement

Powder phase	Chemical composition Relative proportion of the constituents Additives (seeds, accelerants, retarders, etc) Particle size distribution of the powder
Liquid phase	Additives (accelerants, retarders) pH
Mixing parameters	Liquid/powder ratio Mixing protocol (time, speed, etc) Delay time before implantation
Environmental factors	Temperature Humidity pH

T_{max} is the maximum temperature reached by the polymerizing cement in °C.[27–29] The peak temperature is produced by exothermic propagation reactions which take place during polymerization. The cement sets before the peak temperature is reached. The time at which the mixed cement mass no longer adheres to a surgically gloved finger is known as the dough time. Finally, the difference between the setting time and the dough time is called the handling time and corresponds to the period of time during which the cement is workable and has to be implanted.

For the cement to be produced, it is necessary for the liquid monomer to wet the powder particles of PMMA, which should then swell and allow the diffusion of the liquid into the organic matrix of the particles. Simultaneously, it is necessary for the initiator contained in the powder (BP) to be completely diluted into the liquid. Monomer evaporation during these early stages of mixing occurs and the clinical consequences have been considered.[30, 31] The chain entanglement of the polymer powder and the polymerized monomer at the interface ensures good adhesion between the polymerized monomer and the PMMA particles in the set cement. Several physical processes, such as swelling of the powder, diffusion of the monomer, dilution of the BP into the liquid and polymer–polymer interdiffusion determine the setting dynamics and the final properties of the ABC.

The BP-DMT reaction produces other free radicals or by-products different from the benzoyl peroxide free radical. The kinetics of the free radicals and their slow decay have been well studied.[32] It has been suggested that unreacted radicals and residual components in the set mass may affect the biocompatibility of the cement and its eventual degradation.[33]

Another very important residual component is the monomer which is left unpolymerized after the cement has set and which excludes the unreacted monomer that evaporated before the cement sets and cools down to its environmental temperature. The amount of residual monomer left in the cement mass depends on the type of cement, since different commercial brands give different results, but in all cases it decreases with time. The actual values reported depend on the environment in which the specimens are kept, ranging between 0.05% and 1.3% after 21 days in water at 37°C.[33]

The polymerization process is strongly dependent upon the environmental temperature at which the reaction takes place.[34, 35] Moreover, both dough time and setting time depend not only on chemical composition and concentration of the liquid, but also on the size and size distribution of the powder particles[36] and on environmental factors such as relative humidity or kneading frequency of the mixing. In order to be able to compare, the ASTM and ISO Standards on ABCs state that the dough time and the setting time evaluation should be conducted at a room temperature of 23°C ± 1°C and a relative humidity of 50% ± 10% and allow a maximum dough time of 5 minutes and a setting time ranging from 5–15 minutes. The idea of accelerating the polymerization process has been proposed and the use of preheated implants has been considered.[37]

A parameter which has a very strong effect on the working time of the cement and which is under the control of the manufacturer is the liquid-to-powder ratio of the product. This is taken as the ratio between the weight of the powder in grams and the volume of the liquid in millilitres. As the liquid-to-powder ratio increases, the peak temperature decreases.[29, 34, 38] These results can be understood in terms of the relative amounts of initiator and monomer present in the various liquid-to-powder ratios and the role played by unreactive particles in absorbing heat.

With respect to the molecular weight of the set ABC, it should be noticed that in most cases the molecular weight of the cement is higher than that of the PMMA powder. This means that the polymerized monomer forms longer molecular chains than those present in the initial PMMA powder.[39] This is relevant because it is well known that the molecular weight and the molecular weight distribution of linear polymers play a strong role in their mechanical properties. However, it is usually accepted for PMMA that most mechanical properties are practically independent of molecular weight when this is higher than 1 to 1.5×10^5, although even then the molecular weight distribution may have an effect.[40–43]

10.3.3 Mechanical properties

ABCs mainly perform a mechanical task, by distributing evenly the contact forces and transfer them from the prosthesis to the bone. This is the reason why mechanical properties of bone cements have been measured and reported by many authors. First of all, it has to be kept in mind that ABC is a self-cured multi-phase material when compared to industrial PMMA. These microstructural and process differences explain their poorer mechanical properties. Good reviews of the mechanical properties of ABCs can be found in Kühn[4], Saha and Pal[44] and Lewis.[45]

Since ABCs are based on PMMA, an amorphous thermoplastic polymer with a glass transition temperature T_g of 110°C, their mechanical properties will be very sensitive to the environmental temperature and strain rate will greatly affect their mechanical behaviour owing to their viscoelastic nature. From a practical point of view, creep and stress relaxation will be very important parameters when assessing the life in service of ABCs. The creep behaviour seems to be correlated with the molecular weight distribution and the glass transition temperature. It has been shown that creep resistance increases with density and large PMMA powder particle size. Residual monomer, radiopaque fillers and a plasticizing environment like water, decrease the creep resistance.[46] Creep will also depend upon the polymerizing process of the cement and the temperature at which the test is carried out.[47] Different models to represent creep behaviour of ABCs have been proposed.[48, 49]

Strength and elastic modulus

The strength and modulus of elasticity of ABCs have been measured using different kinds of tests such as tension, compression, bending, torsion and shearing, and controlling different parameters such as temperature, environment, crosshead speed of the testing machine and specimen geometry and size. Consequently, a wide variety of results is available. Moreover, the results reported refer to different commercial cement brands. Other factors related to the manufacture of the specimens contribute to the scatter of results. The values reported in the literature for the elastic modulus range between 1.5–4.1 GPa in tension and 1.9–3.2 GPa in compression, whereas the ultimate strength ranges between 24 and 49 MPa in tension, 73–117 MPa in compression and 12–74 MPa in four-point bending.[45]

Fracture and fatigue behaviour

The fracture features of bone cements have been studied in depth, although some fracture mechanisms have not yet been well explained. The bone cements are taken as linear elastic solids, since PMMA behaves as a brittle material and fracture toughness K_{IC} can be easily evaluated. Fracture toughness has been measured using different kinds of specimen. The results reported range between 1.03 to 2.32 MPa $m^{1/2}$.[45, 50] The brittleness of ABCs is apparent since the K_{IC} are even lower than those of ceramic materials. Note that the highest fracture toughness reported is about double the lowest one. This means that the type of cement, the preparation, moulding conditions and the type of test conducted will play a major role in the values obtained.

Fatigue failure of the cement is currently understood to be one of the most important causes of loosening of cemented joint prostheses.[51] In fact, the fractographic analysis of ABCs explanted from patients during their revision operation compares very well with those obtained from *in vitro* fatigue tests and shows that fatigue crack growth is most likely to be the leading *in vivo* failure mechanism.[52]

The most common approach taken when studying the fatigue failure of ABCs has been to assess the fatigue endurance at a given number of cycles. *S–N* curves have been obtained in rotating bending fatigue,[52, 53] in tension–tension,[54, 55] in tension–compression,[56] in three-point bending,[52] in four-point bending[57] and even in compression,[58] usually under load control. Tests have been also carried out on tension–compression under strain control.[59] Most authors carry out their tests under sinusoidal loading, although this information is not always reported.

In commercial bone cements fatigue endurances at 10^6 cycles, values of 6–20 MPa have been reported in bending[53, 54, 58] and another study found fatigue endurances at 10^7 cycles of 15–26 MPa in bending.[57] Such a wide scatter of results will depend not only on the type of cement used, but also on its preparation process and its final microstructure. Since fatigue has a statistical nature and the probability that two specimens of a same batch exhibit different behaviour is high, a possible approach is to analyse the fatigue results using the Weibull distribution of survival probability, the failure probability or reliability at a given number of cycles, for a constant stress amplitude and a defined frequency.[52, 54] Here again there is also a scatter of results because different authors use different fatigue tests, the type and geometry of the specimens is different and the maximum stresses and frequencies used are also different.

All the tests reported above have been conducted with unnotched specimens, which means that the fatigue failure process requires a crack nucleation stage and a crack propagation stage. The number of cycles required for the nucleating stage will depend on the smoothness and the lack of porosity of the surface. In fact when the cement sets in service, it should be expected that its surface will not be smooth and porosity and voids at the metal–cement and the bone–cement interfaces should be expected. This means that surface flaws exist that will be responsible for fast crack nucleation. Therefore, the fatigue behaviour of bone cement in service may be dominated by the crack propagation behaviour[45, 60–62] as in most of engineering structural components. Fatigue crack propagation in bone cements behaves according to the Paris law:

$$da/dN = A\ (\varnothing \mathrm{K})^m$$

where da/dN is the crack propagation rate in one cycle, $\varnothing K$ is the amplitude of the stress intensity factor which depends on the load applied, the crack length and the geometry of the crack, and A and m are constants which depend on the material and the environment.

10.3.4 Some factors affecting the microstructure and mechanical properties of acrylic bone cements

ABCs can be interpreted as multi-phase materials consisting of PMMA beads, polymerized monomer and radiopacifier particles, as represented in Fig. 10.2(a). In addition, there are some factors related to mixing technique, the presence of blood, grease or body fluids, or possible delaminations produced when introducing the cement in the bone cavity, which will affect the bulk and the interfacial microstructure of the cements and consequently their mechanical behaviour.

Porosity

The presence of porosity in bone cements depends strongly on the mixing technique used. It is convenient to reduce the porosity of bone cements in order to improve the mechanical performance of ABCs and, in fact, the improvement of the mixing techniques has undergone a fast and spectacular evolution. The techniques used to reduce porosity include mechanical or ultrasound mixing, pressurization of the cement, centrifugation of the mixture and vacuum mixing. All these techniques result in a reduction of porosity from about 8% which is achieved by conventional hand mixing to values below 1% for vacuum mixing. Good reviews and discussions about the results on the fight against porosity have been published.[63, 64]

Although most of the reported results show that mechanical properties improve as porosity is decreased, some authors find that certain mechanical properties do not improve at all, mainly fracture toughness and the fatigue crack propagation rate.[63, 65] The main argument used to explain the detrimental effect of porosity is that pores act as stress concentrators. However, it has to be borne in mind that under a tensile state of stress, polymers have a maximum inherent flaw size which will control the fracture load of the material. On the other hand, the main deformation mechanism of PMMA in tension is crazing and therefore, the crack will propagate with a Dugdale plastic region ahead of it, which will account for the crazed region. This model of crack propagation in bone cements would explain that the size of the largest pore in the plane of the advancing crack is more important than porosity. A pore can blunt the tip of the crack, depending on the Dugdale zone size and the size of the pore.

Physiological environment

The influence of body fluids and body temperature (37°C) properties is significant in different properties of the cement. Uptake of liquids has been shown to affect some of the properties of the cement after implantation. Sorption of water generally lowers its mechanical properties.[61, 66–68] However, fracture mechanics studies show that the crack velocity is slower in water than in air and that fracture toughness is about 15–20% higher in water than in air.[69] Other results show that the work to fracture increases with the time of storage of the cement in liquids such as water, Ringer's solution and lipids, although in each case the work to fracture after storage at 21°C is higher than after storage at 37°C.[70] Water in ABCs acts as a plasticizer.

Additives

The main additives usually found in bone cements are radiopacifier particles like $BaSO_4$ and ZrO_2, and antibiotics. It has been shown that these radiopacifying agents have a significant effect on the mechanical properties of acrylic bone cements, which depend on their size and morphology. Indeed, whilst the addition of $BaSO_4$ produces a decrease in the tensile strength of about 10%,[34, 43, 71] the addition of ZrO_2 does not affect this parameter. On the other hand, it has been reported that the fracture toughness, which is unaffected by the inclusion of $BaSO_4$, is increased by around 20% by the addition of ZrO_2.[72] Moreover, both inorganic radiopacifiers enhanced the fatigue crack propagation resistance of the cement.[62, 72] This behaviour can be explained in terms of the morphology of the radiopacifying agent particles and their interaction with the polymeric matrix. Since there is no chemical adhesion between the inorganic particles and the PMMA, it could be interpreted that the filler particles behave like pores when a tensional state of stress is applied to the cement. However, at this point the morphology of the particles plays a determinant role with respect to the mechanical behaviour of the cement. Indeed, the ZrO_2 particles, which have a cauliflower-like shape, can anchor mechanically to the matrix, reinforcing it to a certain extent. This effect does not take place in the case of the smaller and more regular $BaSO_4$ particles.[72]

Other studies have also shown that the addition of radiopaque agents to PMMA enhances the macrophage–osteoclast differentiation and therefore they may contribute to bone resorption and aseptic loosening.[73] Furthermore, these agents evoke a significant pathological response in the surrounding tissue. Barium sulphate has been shown to intensify the release of inflammatory mediators in response to PMMA particles [74]. There is also evidence that the release of the radiopacifier particles in the surrounding tissues can cause damage to the articulating surfaces and a marked increased in the production of polyethylene wear debris if they enter the joint space.[75–77] In order to overcome these limitations, some iodine-containing monomers have been investigated as potential substitutes for the inorganic radiopacifying agents, with improved biological and mechanical characteristics.[71, 72, 78]

Several commercial ABCs also include antibiotics in their powder phase, which after implantation progressively dissolve and leach to the surrounding tissues, with the aim of avoiding post-operative infections. It seems clear that the addition of antibiotics to ABCs reduces their mechanical properties, although the reduction depends very strongly on the amount of antibiotic added.[56, 79–81]

Other additives have also been investigated with the objective of improving the mechanical properties of ABCs, by reinforcing the cement matrix either with particles or with fibres. In relation to particle addition, three main directions can be described. First, reinforcement with hard particles such as glass beads[82, 83] or glass ceramic particles,[84] second, reinforcement with tough or rubber toughened particles[61, 68, 85] and finally the reinforcement with bioactive particles, such as inorganic bone and demineralized bone matrix[86, 87] and hydroxyapatite or other calcium phosphates, which could improve both the mechanical properties of the bulk cement and the interfacial bone–cement strength, by giving rise to a direct bonding between these bioactive particles and the surrounding bone.[88–91] Fibre reinforcement of bone cements has followed two main paths: reinforcement with metallic fibres[92, 93] and reinforcement with polymeric fibres, including carbon fibres.[94–97]

10.3.5 Biocompatibility

The three major concerns relating to the biological performance of ABCs are exothermal polymerization of the cement, the residual liquid monomer and the exposure of medical personnel to the fumes of the liquid monomer.[5]

There is extensive discussion in the literature about the role of exothermic polymerization in the necrosis of the surrounding bone. The amount of heat released depends on the weight of reacting monomer in the mixture and the peak temperature reached depends on the volume of cement and its surface to volume ratio, in other words its thickness in service. More important than the temperature reached by the cement is the temperature at the bone–cement interface, since bone necrosis will occur if the temperature reaches values over 56°C, which corresponds to the onset of coagulation of albumin.[98] However, it seems that this temperature should not be taken as a threshold since cell damage is not only a question of temperature but also of time. A wide variety of temperatures at the bone–bone cement interface have been reported depending on the thickness and the position of the thermocouple.

Certain clinical complications have been associated with the use of bone cement and particularly to monomer release.[99] A large amount of information regarding hypotension, hazards, local tissue damage and even the burn of the sciatic nerve caused by bone cements have been reported by different authors.[100–103]

On the other hand, some studies show that the products of wear and fracture or fragmentation of bone cement, as well as the wear debris of polyethylene from the articulating surface, may cause a foreign body response consisting of a macrophage, giant cell foreign body granulomatous reaction. This tissue can produce a variety of chemical mediators of inflammation and eventually bone resorption. This process of osteolysis induced by bone cement fragmentation may be the biological cause for the loosening of the cemented joint prostheses.[104–105]

A wide variety of possible modifications of the formulation of ABCs, aiming at improving their biological properties, has been investigated. Some examples are the substitution of initiators, accelerators[106–108] or radiopacifying agents[71, 72, 78] by more biocompatible compounds, or the addition of other monomers to the liquid phase,[106, 109–113] that improve the biological performance of ABCs.

10.4 Calcium phosphate bone cements

10.4.1 Chemistry of calcium phosphate bone cements

CPCs are formed by a combination of one or more calcium orthophosphates, which upon mixing with a liquid phase, usually water or an aqueous solution, form a paste which is able to set and harden after being implanted within the body. The cement sets as a result of a dissolution and precipitation process, as represented in Fig. 10.2(b). The entanglement of the precipitated crystals is responsible for cement hardening.

Calcium orthophosphates are the calcium salts derived from orthophosphoric acid. Their names, abbreviations, chemical formulae and Ca/P molar ratio are summarized in Table 4.[114] Some of these calcium orthophosphates can be obtained by precipitation from an aqueous solution at low temperature, whilst others can only be obtained at high temperature. All of them can be used as reactants for CPCs, but only those calcium orthophosphates that can precipitate at low temperature in aqueous systems can be theoretically obtained as a result of the CPC setting reaction. However, despite the large number of possible formulations, the CPCs developed up to now only have two different end products, precipitated hydroxyapatite (PHA) or brushite (DCPD). This is a predictable situation since hydroxyapatite is the most stable calcium phosphate at $pH>4.2$ and brushite the most stable one at $pH< 4.2$.

The driving forces controlling dissolution and precipitation reactions are related to the respective super or under saturation levels defined with regard to

Table 10.4 List of the different calcium orthophosphates

Compound	Abbreviation	Formula	Ca/P
Compounds which can precipitate at room temperature in aqueous systems			
Monocalcium phosphate monohydrate	MCPM	$Ca(H_2PO_4)_2{\cdot}H_2O$	0.50
Dicalcium phosphate dihydrate (brushite)	DCPD	$CaHPO_4{\cdot}2H_2O$	1.00
Octocalcium phosphate	OCP	$Ca_8H_2(PO_4)_6{\cdot}5H_2O$	1.33
Precipitated hydroxyapatite	PHA	$Ca_{10}(PO_4)_6(OH)_2$	1.67
Calcium deficient hydroxyapatite	CDHA	$Ca_{10-x}(HPO_4)_x(PO_4)_{6-x}(OH)_{2-x}$	1.50–1.67
Amorphous calcium phosphate	ACP	–	1.35–1.5
Compounds obtained at high temperature			
Monocalcium phosphate anhydrous	MCPA	$Ca(H_2PO_4)_2$	0.50
Dicalcium phosphate (monetite)	DCP	$CaHPO_4$	1.00
α-Tricalcium phosphate	α-TCP	$\alpha\text{-}Ca_3(PO_4)_2$	1.50
β-Tricalcium phosphate	β-TCP	$\beta\text{-}Ca_3(PO_4)_2$	1.50
Sintered hydroxyapatite	SHA	$Ca_{10}(PO_4)_6(OH)_2$	1.67
Oxyapatite	OHA	$Ca_{10}(PO_4)_6O$	1.67
Tetracalcium phosphate	TTCP	$Ca_4(PO_4)_2O$	2.00

the thermodynamic solubility product and, therefore, the thermodynamics of calcium phosphate salts in an aqueous solution at room or body temperature is the basis for understanding the manufacturing technology involved in CPCs for clinical applications.[14, 115, 116] Moreover, it has to be considered that in addition to thermodynamic factors, kinetic factors can also control both phase dissolution and the precipitation of new phases and can determine the final products obtained in a CPC setting reaction.[117, 118] Therefore, the conclusions that can be derived from the solubility and relative stability diagrams of the different calcium phosphates must be taken as a first approximation, but not as an exhaustive explanation of what is actually happening during the setting reaction.

Apatite calcium phosphate bone cements

The mineral phase of bone has an apatitic structure, which can exist in a range of compositions. Non-stoichiometric or calcium deficient hydroxyapatite (CDHA) can be obtained at low temperatures, with a composition which can be expressed as $Ca_{10-x}(HPO_4)(PO_4)_{6-x}(OH)_{2-x}$, where x ranges from 0 to 1, being 0 for stoichiometric hydroxyapatite (HA) and 1 for fully calcium deficient hydroxyapatite. In fact, biological apatite is a carbonate containing calcium deficient hydroxyapatite, which in addition contains several other ionic substitutions such as Na^+, K^+, Mg^{2+}, F^- and Cl^-.

Apatitic CPCs can form either precipitated HA (PHA) or CDHA through a precipitation reaction. Their fabrication process allows the incorporation of different ions in the lattice depending on the composition of the starting materials. The formation of hydroxyapatite through a cement-type reaction takes place at body temperature and in a physiological environment, as happens when bone is formed or remodelled. This can account for the fact that the hydroxyapatite formed in the setting of CPCs is much more like biological apatites than those obtained when high temperature sintering processes are applied to fabricate ceramic hydroxyapatite.

The CPCs leading to the formation of PHA or CDHA can contain either a single compound or a mixture of reactants in the powder phase. The only cement system that contains a single calcium phosphate was first reported by Monma *et al.*[119, 120] and was further optimized and characterized by Ginebra *el al.*[121–126] This system is based on the hydrolysis of α-TCP to CDHA according to equation [10.1]:

$$3\alpha\text{-}Ca_3(PO_4)_2 + H_2O \rightarrow Ca_9(HPO_4)(PO_4)_5(OH) \qquad [10.1]$$

Since the Ca/P ratio of the initial and final calcium phosphates is the same, no acid or base is released as by-products.

CPCs can also be formed by two reactants, an acidic calcium phosphate and a basic calcium phosphate, which set following an acid–base reaction. The basic component is normally TTCP, since it is the only calcium phosphate that has a Ca/P ratio higher than PHA. From a theoretical point of view, any calcium phosphate more acidic than PHA can react directly with TTCP to form PHA or CDHA. The most widely studied combinations are the TTCP+DCPD and TTCP+DCP mixtures, which were first developed by Brown and Chow[8,127] and have been the object of extensive research.[117, 118, 128–131] These mixtures produce cements that set at body temperature in a pH range around neutral, according to equations [10.2] and [10.3]:

$$Ca_4(PO_4)_2O + CaHPO_4 \rightarrow Ca_5(PO_4)_3OH \qquad [10.2]$$

$$Ca_4(PO_4)_2O + CaHPO_4{\cdot}2H_2O \rightarrow Ca_5(PO_4)_3OH + 2H_2O \qquad [10.3]$$

Other salts can also be added as reactants in CPCs, such as calcium or strontium carbonate or magnesium phosphates. An example is the product developed by Norian Corporation (Norian SRSTM, Skeletal Repair System),[132] where mixtures of calcium phosphates with a Ca/P ratio lower than PHA are used and $CaCO_3$ is added as an additional source of calcium ions. Specifically this system is formed by using a mixture of α-TCP, MCPM and $CaCO_3$. The initial setting process involves the formation of DCPD, while the final setting product is dahllite, a carbonated hydroxyapatite with a Ca/P ratio between 1.67 and 1.69, and with a carbonate ion content similar to bone mineral.[132]

Brushite calcium phosphate bone cements

Some CPCs have been designed that give brushite (DCPD) as the end-product. Brushite is an acidic calcium phosphate, which is metastable under physiological conditions.[114] For this reason, brushite CPCs are much more quickly resorbable than apatite CPCs, although it has been shown that *in vivo* DCPD tends to convert into PHA.[133]

All brushite CPCs are obtained as a result of an acid–base reaction. Several compositions have been proposed for brushite cements, e.g. β-TCP + MCPM,[134] β-TCP + H_3PO_4,[135, 136] and TTCP + MCPM + CaO.[133] In the first of them (β-TCP + MCPM), the reaction responsible for the setting of the cement is reported in equation [10.4].

$$\beta\text{-}Ca_3(PO_4)_2 + Ca(H_2PO_4)_2{\cdot}H_2O + 7H_2O \rightarrow 4CaHPO_4{\cdot}2H_2O \qquad [10.4]$$

The paste of brushite CPCs is acidic during setting because brushite can only precipitate at a pH lower than 6.[114] After setting, the pH of the cement paste slowly changes towards the equilibrium pH, which depends on the singular points of the phases present in the cement.[137]

10.4.2 Processing parameters and setting properties of calcium phosphate bone cements

Processing parameters

As mentioned for the case of ABCs, the properties of a cement system depend on, and therefore can be tailored by, several processing parameters, which are summarized in Table 10.3. The most important are the following:

- The composition of the solid phase: This can vary with the setting reactions desired. Normally they are chosen between the orthophosphates, listed in Table 10.4. On the other hand, those calcium orthophosphates containing biocompatible components like Na^+, K^+, Mg^{2+}, Zn^{2+}, CO_3^{2-}, SO_4^{2-} or Cl^- are also suitable as constituents of CPC powders and calcium carbonate is also added in some formulations.
- The particle size of the starting powder plays an important role in the setting and final properties of the cement. As mentioned before, the setting reaction occurs through a dissolution–precipitation process. Hence, the fineness of the powder will increase the rate of hardening since smaller particles will dissolve faster than bigger particles and the precipitation of a new phase will begin earlier.[126]
- The addition of crystal nucleators in the powder phase: Another strategy that can be used to produce cement with good setting characteristics is the use of seed crystals to act as a 'nucleator' for the precipitation reaction. Several parameters can be modified, such as the amount of seed

added, its crystallinity and crystal size. Although the effects of seeds under different conditions are not entirely clarified, it seems that their main effect is to reduce the setting time of the cement.

- The composition of the liquid phase: The primary role of the liquid phase is to function as a vehicle for dissolution of the reactants and precipitation of products. The liquid phase in CPCs is always water or an aqueous solution. Water solutions ranging from plain water to simulated body fluid have been used. In some cases, some soluble phosphate salts such as NaH_2PO_4 and/or Na_2HPO_4 are added as a source of phosphate ions in solution, because it is known that common ions can have an accelerating effect on the setting reaction.[138] Therefore, neutral salts dissolved in the liquid phase can be used to shorten the setting time exhibited by the cement, for instance in apatitic cements.[124] In some cases, water-soluble polymers can be added providing scope to modify the cohesion of the cement paste or its rheological properties.
- The liquid to powder ratio is a factor that increases the initial plasticity of the paste and consequently its injectability and setting times. The final strength is also affected by this parameter since the porosity of the set specimen is directly correlated to the liquid-to-powder ratio used. Therefore, reducing the liquid-to-powder ratio within the limits of workability would be a means of improving the strength of CPCs.

Several properties must be taken into account in relation to the applicability of the CPCs as bone substitutes. Among them, we can mention setting and cohesion times, the injectability, the hardening rate, the mechanical strength and pH evolution during setting. All of these depend on the composition and the processing parameters that are chosen for each formulation.

Setting properties

Setting properties include the setting time, the cohesion time and injectability.

The setting time of a CPC can be defined as the time required for the initial setting of the cement paste, which is reflected in a loss of plasticity. Usually it is measured following mechanical methods, as a fast way of determining whether a reaction occurs upon making a paste of the mixture of reactants with water. The most common methods are based on the assessment of the ability of the cement paste to resist a mechanical load applied to its surface. Two examples are the Vicat needle and the use of two Gillmore needles. In the first, a single needle is applied to the cement surface. The rationale for the two Gillmore needles, as proposed by Driessens and co-workers[123] is that with the light-and-wide needle one, the initial setting time can be measured, indicating the end of mouldability without serious damage to the cement structure, whereas with the heavy-and-fine needle the final setting time can be measured, beyond which it is possible to touch the cement without causing serious damage. As far as clinical applications are concerned, the proposed ranges were $4 < I < 8$ minutes for the initial setting time and $10 < F < 15$ minutes for the final setting time.[123]

In general, setting times of apatite CPCs are too long and several strategies have to be applied to reach the clinical requirements.[139] Among the parameters that can be adjusted to accelerate the setting of apatitic cements are (i) the liquid-to-powder ratio (a smaller amount of liquid reduces the setting time), (ii) the reduction of the powder size (smaller size, shorter setting time), (iii) the addition of calcium or phosphate ions either pre-dissolved in the liquid phase or as highly soluble salt (common ion effect: the higher the concentration, the shorter the setting time), (iv) the addition of seed materials, which act as crystal nuclei (the more nuclei, the shorter the setting time).

On the other hand, brushite CPCs tend to set too quickly. The setting time of brushite CPCs is controlled by the solubility of the basic phase: the higher the solubility, the faster the setting time.[134] In brushite CPCs, setting retarders are often used and a common approach to increase the setting time is the addition of inhibitors of DCPD crystal growth.[140]

The cohesion time. CPCs are designed to be implanted whilst in a paste state. This means that the paste is in contact with blood or other physiological fluids. Cohesion can be defined as the capacity of a CPC to set in a fluid without disintegrating. It has to be clarified that, in fact, several terms have been used to describe this property, such as non-decay ability, anti-washout, compliance, swelling or stability, and some studies have been devoted to this topic.[141–147] In general, this property was evaluated by an immersion test in water, Ringer's solution or simulated body fluid. The addition of some water-soluble polymers has been proven to be very effective in enhancing the cohesion of CPC pastes.[143, 144] However, the approach followed up to now has been very empirical and there is a need for more understanding of the underlying mechanisms concerning cohesion. It is indeed an important topic since if a CPC has no cohesion at all it will not be able to form a solid body when implanted, or, in the case of poor cohesion, calcium phosphate particles can be released, which can elicit harmful reactions such as inflammation or blood clotting.[146, 147]

Injectability. The capability to inject the cement in the surgical site is an important property, since it can minimize the surgical invasion and permit complex-shaped defects to be filled adequately. All CPCs are mouldable materials and in some cases their processing parameters can be adjusted to obtain injectable CPCs. The injectability of a CPC paste can be defined as its ability to be extruded through a needle without demixing. Of course, this will depend on the diameter and length of the needle (2 mm diameter and 10 mm length are illustrative values).[148] A common problem with CPC injection is demixing or filter pressing, which occurs when the mixing liquid separates from the powder phase, that is, it is expelled through the needle without the CaP particles. Driessens and co-workers[149] defined an injectability coefficient as the percentage by weight of the amount of a CPC paste which could be extruded from a syringe with respect to the total mass of the cement introduced in the syringe, when it was extruded at a compression rate of 15 mm min^{-1} up to a maximum force of 100 N. The experimental setup to measure injectability of a CPC is shown in Fig. 10.3.

Injectability depends on the rheological properties of the paste. The characterization of the rheological properties of CPCs is a complex issue, since they have transient rheological properties caused by the setting reaction that is taking place from the beginning of mixing the liquid and the powder.[150]

There are several ways of modifying the viscosity of a CPC paste, which in turn will affect its injectability. The most relevant are the liquid-to-powder ratio, the particle size of the powder phase and the addition of ionic and non-ionic additives. For example, some studies have been performed on the effect

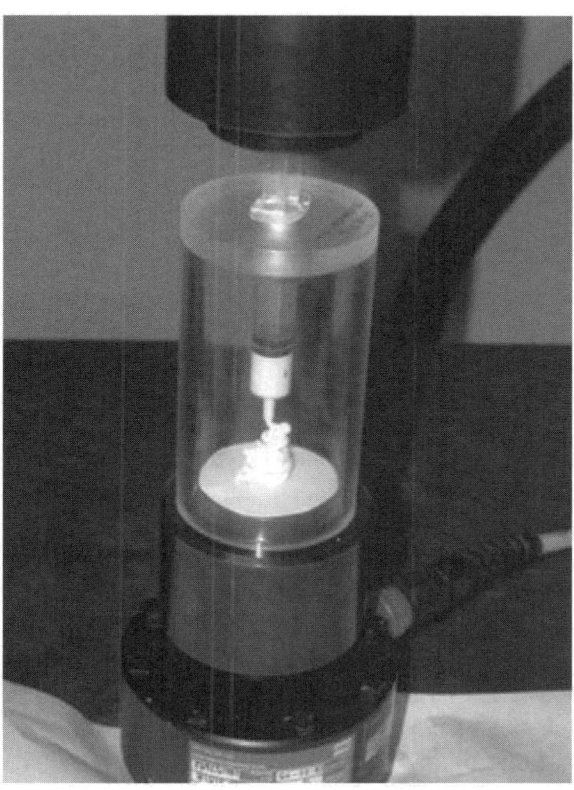

10.3 Experimental setup to measure the injectability of a CPC.

of citric acid and its salts on the rheological properties of CPCs.[151, 152] Citric acid and sodium citrate have been shown to make the surface charge of the particles more negative, acting as a dispersant of the paste and acting as a liquefying agent. This allows the amount of water used in the cement to be reduced, and therefore decreases significantly the porosity and improves the mechanical properties. Another approach is based on the addition of soluble polymers, such as polysaccharides, that is sodium alginate, sodium hyaluronate or chondroitin sulphate[13, 146, 153] or even some polymeric drugs.[154]

10.4.3 Properties of set calcium phosphate bone cements

Microstructure and porosity

The setting reaction of a CPC consists of the dissolution of one or more constituents of the cement powder and the precipitation of a different calcium phosphate. Physically, it takes place by the entanglement of the crystals of the precipitating calcium phosphate. A precipitation reaction will only lead to a considerable strength in these materials under the following two conditions: (i) the precipitate grows in the form of clusters of crystals which have a fair degree of rigidity, (ii) the morphology of the crystals of the precipitate enables the entanglement of the clusters.[121] The evolution of the microstructure of a CPC during the setting reaction is shown in Fig. 10.4. This cement consists of α-TCP as starting product. Once mixed with water, the α-TCP particles dissolve and CDHA crystals start to precipitate. The entanglement of these precipitated crystals is responsible for the progressive hardening of the CPC.

Interestingly, as previously mentioned, many apatite cements involve a reaction in water between acidic dicalcium phosphates (DCP or DCPD) and basic TTCP or α-TCP. No water is consumed during the setting of these CPCs, as it can be seen in equations [10.2] and [10.3], and liquid is required only to make the reactants workable and to allow homogeneous reaction. In other cases, when a hydration reaction takes place (see for instance equation [10.1], some water is consumed, but much less than the total amount added to make a workable paste. Hence, water is a major contributor to the origin of porosity in this system and therefore CPCs are intrinsically porous materials. Figure 10.4(d) shows the microstructure of an apatitic cement after setting and it can be clearly seen that CPCs develop a highly micro/nanoporous structure. The porosity of the set CPC is closely related to the liquid-to-powder ratio used and it normally varies between 30% and 50%, although even higher values can be reached. The pores are normally micro or nanometric in size and the particle size distribution of the starting powder can modify the size of the precipitated crystals and also the pore size distribution.[126]

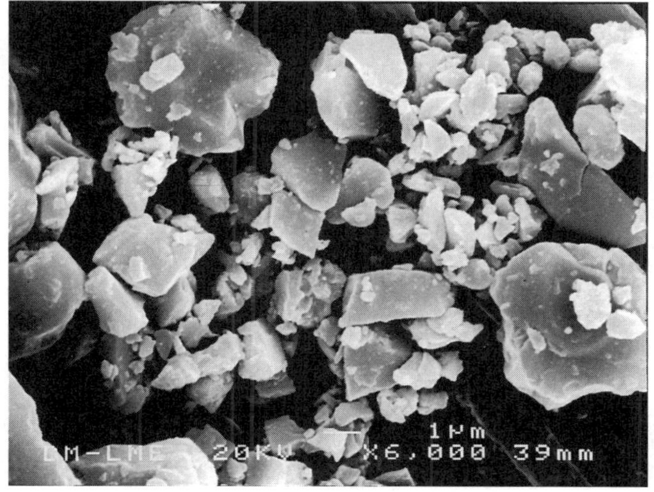

(a)

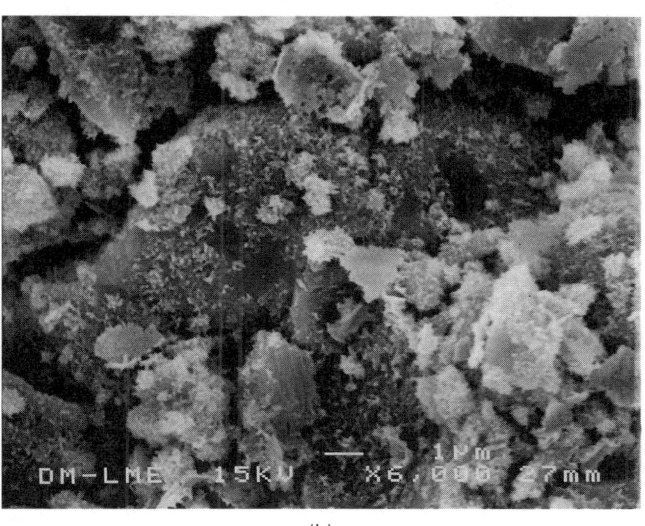

(b)

10.4 Microstructural evolution monitored by SEM of a CPC during the setting reaction. (a) α-TCP powder, which is the reactant of the cement; (b) microstructure after 2 hours setting. Small CDHA precipitated crystals are visible covering the initial α-TCP particles; (c) microstructure after 8 hours setting. The amount of CDHA has increased, although the larger α-TCP particles still remain; (d) after complete setting, α-TCP has completely dissolved and the CPC has transformed to CDHA entangled crystals.

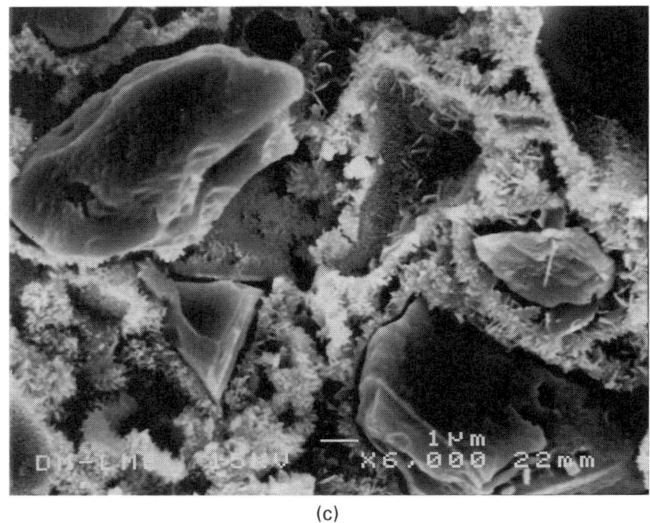

(c)

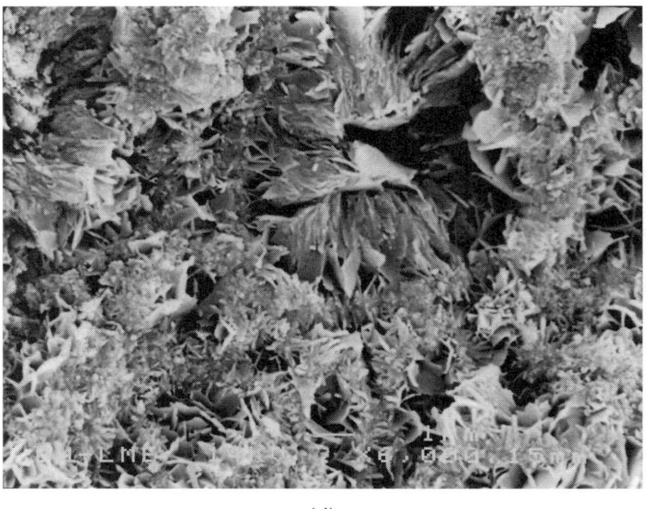

(d)

10.4 Cont'd

Mechanical properties

Compressive strength is the property most often used to characterize the mechanical behaviour of CPCs.[155] Since these materials are conceived as bone substitutes, it is important to keep in mind as reference values that the compressive strength of human cortical bone ranges between 90 and 209 MPa,[156, 157] and that of the cancellous bone between 1.5 and 45 MPa.[158]

Owing to the intrinsic porosity of CPCs, their strength is lower than that of calcium phosphate ceramics.[115] The liquid-to-powder ratio, the particle size of the reactants, the crystallinity and amount of seed and the use of liquid accelerators are factors that affect the strength of the CPC. A wide range of values can be found in the literature, depending on the composition and processing parameters, and it is difficult to make comparisons between them owing to a lack of consistency in specimen dimensions, testing protocols and sample pre-treatments. As indicative values, the compressive strength of apatite cements normally ranges between 20 and 50 MPa[121, 126, 132, 142–145] although lower and higher values for some formulations have also been reported.[159] Brushite CPCs are in general weaker than apatite CPCs and compressive strengths of 25 MPa have been reported.[160]

The reduction of porosity in CPCs has been explored as a way to increase their strength. Reducing the amount of added water and improving particle packaging can reduce the porosity of the cements. Compaction of the cement paste during setting has been demonstrated to increase the compressive strength of apatitic CPCs,[161–163] and values as high as 118 MPa have been reported.[163] The addition of water-reducing or liquefying agents, such as sodium citrate, allows for a further densification of the paste and values of 180 MPa in wet conditions have been reported.[163] However, it has to be considered that this compaction cannot be applied if the cement is implanted or injected within the bone tissue and therefore at present it can be used only to fabricate pre-set substrates or scaffolds for bone regeneration. A two-step protocol, including pre-compaction of a paste followed by a conventional application has been suggested as an alternative for potential clinical use.[163]

The evolution of the CPC strength after implantation has also been studied. The mechanical properties of apatite CPCs are reported to increase,[164] whilst those of brushite CPCs tend to decrease,[165] owing to the higher solubility of DCPD compared with that of PHA. Only after a few weeks of implantation, when bone growth is significant, the mechanical properties of brushite CPCs increase.[165]

10.4.4 Biological performance of calcium phosphate bone cements: present and future strategies

As mentioned previously, CPCs are highly biocompatible osteoconductive materials and can stimulate tissue regeneration.[14, 132, 133, 166–175] The biodegradability of apatite CPCs is larger than that of sintered hydroxyapatite, but it is still slow. It has been shown, for instance, that some CPCs could remain as long as 78 weeks when implanted in dog femurs.[171] Most of the apatitic cements are resorbed via cell-mediated processes. In these processes osteoclastic cells degrade the materials layer by layer, starting at the bone–cement interface throughout its inner core.[14]

Brushite CPCs are resorbed *in vivo* much faster than apatitic cements,[172–174] owing to the fact that brushite is metastable in physiological conditions. However, it has been reported that brushite CPCs tend to transform to PHA *in vivo*, this transformation reducing its overall degradation rate. The addition of magnesium salts can be used to avoid, or at least delay, this transformation.[175]

There are several factors that affect the degradation rate of CPCs, in addition to their chemical composition, such as the crystallinity of the final product, the specific surface area and the porosity of the set cement. One strategy proposed in recent years in a bid to accelerate resorption of apatite CPCs is the incorporation of macroporosity, which is envisaged as a method to facilitate bone ingrowth, not only from the external surface, but throughout the whole bulk of the material. This would accelerate its resorption and its transformation in newly formed bone tissue.

Presently, two different strategies have been adopted to introduce macroporosity in CPCs. The first approach aims to produce the macropores after the cement has set. Different porogenic agents have been suggested, which are added within the CPC paste and after the setting, degrade faster than the cement itself, creating the macroporosity, such as sugars,[176, 177] PLA fibres or particles[178, 179] or frozen sodium phosphate solution particles[180]. However, it is necessary to add a large amount of porogenic agent to guarantee interconnectivity of the porosity, thus compromising the excellent bioactivity and biocompatibility of CPCs. In a second approach, macroporosity is created before the cement sets. The cement paste is foamed while it has a viscous consistency and its setting creates a solid macroporous construct. The macroporosity can be produced by two main routes (i) the addition of some gas-generating compounds, such as hydrogen peroxide[181] or sodium bicarbonate,[182–184] although it has to be taken into account that the liberation of gas after the implantation of the cement paste could have harmful effects for the organism and (ii) the use of biocompatible foaming agents.[185, 186] This last approach has allowed the development of injectable macroporous CPCs, which maintain the macroporosity after injection.[185] *In vivo* studies have shown that this strategy can be effective in accelerating CPC resorption.[186]

In this context, CPCs are also used to fabricate pre-set hydroxyapatite porous blocks acting as scaffolds for guiding *in vitro* or *in vivo* tissue regeneration, which is one of the main goals of tissue engineering.[180, 181, 185] Figure 10.5 shows a CDHA macroporous scaffold obtained by foaming a CPC. These three-dimensional (3D) macroporous constructs satisfy several requirements, such as osteoconductivity, adequate mechanical properties, formability and high interconnected macroporosity, ensuring cell colonization and flow transport of nutrients and metabolic waste. In addition, the apatite foams combine interconnected macroporosity with the intrinsically high micro-nanoporosity of CPCs .[181] Recently, it has also been shown that CPCs can

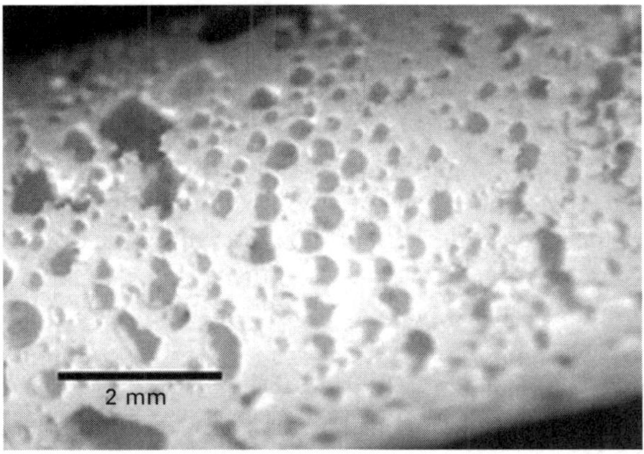

10.5 Macroporus hydroxyapatite scaffold obtained by foaming and setting a CPC.

be used in rapid prototyping techniques and, specifically, low-temperature 3D powder printing can be used to fabricate calcium phosphate structures with simultaneous control of geometry and organic molecule incorporation in three dimensions.[187]

Another application where CPCs have great potential and which can influence strongly the biological performance of CPCs is drug delivery. Most drug delivery materials are polymeric in nature. However, calcium phosphate based materials have an added value owing to their bioactive character in the specific field of the pharmacological treatment of skeletal disorders. An important property of calcium phosphates is their unique ability to adsorb different chemical species on their surfaces. This affinity of hydroxyapatite for these various active molecules can extend the application of CPCs, not only as bone substitutes, but as carriers for local and controlled supply of drugs in treatment of different skeletal diseases, such as bone tumours, osteoporosis or osteomyelitis, which normally require long and painful therapies.[188]

Unlike calcium phosphate ceramics employed as drug delivery systems, where the drugs are usually absorbed on the surface, in CPCs the drugs can be incorporated throughout the whole material volume, by adding them into one of the two cement phases. This can facilitate the release of drugs for more prolonged periods.

Certain factors need to be taken into consideration with reference to the incorporation of drugs in CPCs.[188, 189] In the first instance, it is necessary to verify that the addition of the drug (either to the liquid or the solid phases of the cement), does not interfere in the setting reaction, modifying the physicochemical properties, not only in terms of the setting and hardening mechanisms, but also with respect to the rheological behaviour. Secondly, it is necessary to characterize the kinetics of drug release *in vitro*. Subsequently, the effectiveness of the cement to act as carrier for drug delivery *in vivo*, must be assessed. And finally, the clinical performance of the drug delivery system must be evaluated. Up to the present time, the first three aspects have been extensively studied, but the application of CPCs as drug delivery systems has not yet reached clinical application. Major attention has been paid to antibiotics, owing to their wide areas of application: either as prophylactics to prevent infections produced during surgical interventions, or in general in the treatment of bone infections. Other types of drugs incorporated in cements include anti-inflammatory drugs, anticancer drugs and even hormones have been studied. In recent years the inclusion of growth factors that are able to stimulate bone regeneration, such as bone morphogenetic proteins (BMP) or transforming growth factors β (TGF-β) have been considered for controlled delivery from CPCs.[189]

Although the research carried out to date has shown the great potential of CPCs as carriers for controlled release and vectoring of drugs, the industrial use of CPCs for drug delivery is not yet a reality. Two main causes can be identified. First, implant companies selling CPCs do not generally have the know how to deal with drugs and pharmaceutical companies do not have any know how about CPCs. Second, the infections are not always produced by the same microorganisms and, therefore, it would be necessary to design versatile systems, which could combine a given CPC with many different drugs, in a way that the surgeon could choose the drug just before implantation. Since various drugs have various effects on CPC properties, this represents a serious drawback for technology implementation. Therefore, much work still has to be done to be able to obtain reproducible and predictable systems and to adjust the use of CPCs to different therapeutical needs.

10.5 References

1. Charnley J 'Anchorage of the femoral head prosthesis to the shaft of the femur', *J Bone Joint Surg*, 1964, **42B**, 28.
2. Charnley J 'Bonding of prosthesis to bone by cement', *J Bone Joint Surg*, 1964, **46B**, 518.
3. Charnley J *Acrylic Cement in Orthopaedic Surgery*, E & S Livingstone, London, 1970.
4. Kühn KD *Bone Cements*, Springer Verlag, Berlin Heidelberg, Germany, 2000.
5. Lewis G 'Injectable bone cements for use in vertebroplasty and kyphoplasty: state-of-the-art review', *J Biomed Mater Res Part B: Appl Biomater*, 2006, **76B**, 456–68.
6. Hernández L, Gurruchaga M and Goñi I 'Injectable acrylic bone cements for vertebroplasty based on a radiopaque hydroxyapatite. Formulation and rheological behavior', *J Mater Sci: Mater Med*, 2009, **20**, 89–97.
7. LeGeros R, Chohayeb A and Shulman A 'Apatitic calcium phosphates: possible dental restorative materials', *J Dent Res*, 1982, **61**, 343.

8. Brown WE and Chow LC 'A new calcium phosphate setting cement', *J Dent Res*, 1983, **62**, 672.
9. Tofighi A, Mounic S, Chakravarthy P, Rey C and Lee D 'Setting reactions involved in injectable cements based on amorphous calcium phosphate', *Key Eng Mater*, 2000, 192–5, 769–72.
10. Constantz BR, Ison IC, Fulmer MT, Poser RD, Smith ST, VanWagoner M, Ross J, Goldstein SA, Jupiter JB and Rosenthal DI 'Skeletal repair by *in situ* formation of the mineral phase of bone', *Science*, 1995, **267**, 1796–9.
11. Freche M, Lacout JL and Hatim Z *Method for Preparing a Biomaterial based on Hydroxyapatite, Resulting Biomaterial and Surgical or Dental Use*. FR Patent No. 2776282, 1999.
12. Driessens FCM, Boltong MG, Bermudez O, Ginebra MP, Fernández E and Planell JA 'Effective formulations for the preparation of calcium phosphate bone cements', *J Mater Sci: Mater Med*, 1994, **5**, 164–70.
13. Bohner M, Gbureck U and Barralet JE 'Technological issues for the development of more efficient calcium phosphate bone cements: A critical assessment', *Biomaterials*, 2005, **26**, 6423–9.
14. Ishikawa K 'Calcium phosphate cement', in *Bioceramics and Their Clinical Applications*, Kokubo T (ed), Woodhead Publishing, Cambridge, England, 2008.
15. Fernández E, Ginebra MP, Bermudez O, Boltong MG, Driessens FCM and Planell JA 'Dimensional and thermal behaviour of calcium phosphate cements during setting compared to PMMA bone cements', *J Mater Sci Lett*, 1995, **14**, 4–5.
16. Gómez E, Martín M, Arias J and Carceller F 'Clinical applications of Norian SRS (calcium phosphate cement) in craniofacial reconstruction in children: Our experience at Hospital La Paz since 2001', *J Oral Maxillofac Surg*, 2005, **63**, 8–14.
17. Hidaka N, Yamano Y, Kadoya Y and Nishimura N 'Calcium phosphate bone cement for treatment of distal radius fractures: a preliminary report', *J Orthop Sci*, 2002, **7**, 182–7.
18. Turner TM, Urban RM, Singh K, Hall DJ, Renner SM, Lim TH, Tomlinson MJ and An HS. 'Vertebroplasty comparing injectable calcium phosphate cement compared with polymethylmethacrylate in a unique canine vertebral body large defect model', *Spine J*, 2008, **8**, 482–7.
19. Takemasa R, Kiyasu K, Tani T and Inoue S 'Validity of calcium phosphate cement vertebroplasty for vertebral non-union after osteoporotic fracture with middle column involvement', *The Spine Journal*, 2007, **7**, 148S.
20. Tomita S, Kin A, Yazu M and Abe M 'Biomechanical evaluation of kyphoplasty and vertebroplasty with calcium phosphate cement in a simulated osteoporotic compression fracture', *J Orthopaed Sci*, 2003, **8**, 192–7.
21. Tomita S, Molloy S, Jasper L, Abe M and Belkoff S 'Biomechanical comparison of kyphoplasty with different bone cements', *Eur Spine J*, 2003, **12**(Suppl 1), S37.
22. Wilke HJ, Mehnert U, Boszczyk BM, Bierscneider M, Jaksche H and Claes L 'Biomechanical evaluation of vertebro- and kyphoplasty with PMMA or calcium phosphate cement under cyclic loading', *Eur Spine J*, 2003, **12**(Suppl 1), S75.
23. Lim T-H, Brebach GT, Renner SM, Kim W-J, Kim JG, Lee RE, Andersson GBJ and An HS 'Biomechanical evaluation of an injectable calcium phosphate cement for vertebroplasty', *Spine*, 2002, **27**, 1297–302.
24. Belkoff SM, Mathis JM, Erbe EM and Fenton DC 'Biomechanical evaluation of a new bone cement for use in vertebroplasty', *Spine*, 2000, **25**, 1061–4.

25. Heini PF, Berlemann U, Kaufmann M, Lippuner K, Fankhauser C and van Landuyt P 'Augmentation of mechanical properties in osteoporotic vertebral bones. A biomechanical investigation of vertebroplasty efficacy with different bone cements', *Eur Spine J*, 2001, **10**, 164–71.
26. Belkoff SM, Mathis JM, Deramond H and Jasper LE 'An *ex vivo* biomechanical evaluation of a hydroxyapatite cement for use with kyphoplasty', *Am J Neuroradiol*, 2001, **22**, 1212–16.
27. ISO International standard 5833/2: *Implants for Surgery-Acrylic Resin Cements*, Orthopaedic Application, 1992.
28. ASTM Standard, *Medical Devices*, Section 13, 13.01, Philadelphia, 1986.
29. Meyer PR, Lautenschlager EP and Moore BK 'On the setting properties of acrylic bone cement', *J Bone Joint Surg*, 1973, **55-A**(1), 149.
30. Bayne SC, Lautenschlager EP, Greener EH and Meyer PR 'Clinical influences on bone cement monomer release', *J Biomed Mater Res*, 1977, **11**, 859.
31. Gentil, B, Paugam, C, Wolf, C, Lienhart, A and Augereau B 'Methylmethacrylate plasma levels during total hip arthroplasty', *Clin Orthop Rel Res*, 1993, **287**, 112.
32. Turner RC 'Free radical decay kinetics in PMMA bone cement', *J Biomed Mater Res*, 1984, **18**, 467.
33. Trap B, Wolff P and Jensen JS 'Acrylic bone cements: Residuals and extractability of methacrylate monomers and aromatic amines', *J Appl Biomater*, 1992, **3**, 51.
34. Haas SS, Brauer GM and Dickson G 'A characterization of polymethyl methacrylate bone cement', *J Bone and Joint Surg*, 1975, **57–A**(3), 380.
35. Noble PC 'Selection of acrylic bone cements for use in joint replacement', *Biomaterials*, 1983, **4**, 94.
36. Pascual B, Vázquez B, Gurruchaga M, Goñi I, Ginebra MP, Gil FJ, Planell JA, Levenfeld B and San Román, J 'New aspects of the effect of size and size distribution on the setting parameters and mechanical properties of acrylic bone cement', *Biomaterials*, 1996, **17**, 509–16.
37. Dall DM, Miles AW and Juby G 'Accelerated polymerization of acrylic bone cement using preheated implants', *Clin Orthop Rel Res*, 1986, **211**, 148.
38. Lautenschlager EP, Stupp SI and Keller JC 'Structure and properties of acrylic bone cement', in *Functional Behaviour of Orthopaedic Biomaterials. Volume II. Applications*, Ducheyne P and Hastings GW (eds), CRC Press, Boca Raton, Florida, 1984.
39. Bayne SC, Lautenschlager EP, Compere CL and Wildes R 'Degree of polymerization of acrylic bone cement', *J Biomed Mater Res*, 1975, **9**, 27.
40. Berry J 'Fracture processes in polymeric materials. V. Dependence of the ultimate properties of polymethylmethacrylate on molecular weight', *J Polymer Sci A*, 1964, **2**, 4069.
41. Brauer GM, Termini DJ and Dickson G 'Analysis of the ingredients and determination of the residual components of acrylic bone cements', *J Biomed Mater Res*, 1977, **11**, 577.
42. Kusy RP and Katz MJ 'Effect of molecular weight on the fracture surface energy of poly(methyl methacrylate) in cleavage', *J Mater Sci*, 1976, **11**, 1475.
43. Kusy RP 'Characterization of self-curing acrylic bone cements', *J Biomed Mater Res*, 1978, **12**, 271.
44. Saha S and Pal S 'Mechanical properties of bone cement: A review', *J Biomed Mater Res*, 1984, **18**, 435.

45. Lewis G 'Properties of acrylic bone cement: State of the art review', *J Biomed Mater Res: Appl Biomater*, 1997, **38**, 155–82.
46. Treharne RW and Brown N 'Factors influencing the creep behavior of poly(methyl methacrylate) cements', *J Biomed Mater Res Symp*, 1975, **6**, 81.
47. Oysaed H and Ruyter IE 'Creep studies of multiphase acrylic systems', *J Biomed Mater Res*, 1989, **23**, 719.
48. Norman TL, Kisch V, Blaha JD, Gruen TA and Hustosky K 'Creep characteristics of hand and vacuum mixed acrylic bone cement at elevated stress levels', *J Biomed Mater Res*, 1995, **29**, 495–501.
49. Verdonschot N and Huiskes R 'Dynamic creep behavior of acrylic bone cement', *J Biomed Mater Res*, 1995, **29**, 575–81.
50. Lewis G 'The fracture toughnes of biomaterials: I. Acrylic bone cements', *J Mater Ed*, 1989, **11**, 429–79.
51. Krause W and Mathis R 'Fatigue properties of acrylic bone cements: Review of the literature', *J Biomed Mater Res*, 1988, **22**, 37.
52. Topoleski LDT, Ducheyne P and Cuckler JM 'A fractographic analysis of in vivo poly(methyl methacrylate) bone cement failure mechanisms', *J Biomed Mater Res* 1990, **24**, 135.
53. Freitag TA and Cannon SL 'Fracture characteristics of acrylic bone cements. II. Fatigue', *J Biomed Mater Res*, 1977, **11**, 609.
54. Krause W, Mathis R and Grimes L 'Fatigue properties of acrylic bone cement: S-N, P-N and P-S-N data', *J Biomed Mater Res*, 1988, **22**(A3), 221.
55. Johnson JA, Provan JW, Krygier JJ, Chan KH and Miller J 'Fatigue of acrylic bone cement. Effect of frequency and environment', *J Biomed Mater Res*, 1989, **23**, 819.
56. Davies JP, O'Connor D, Burke D and Harris W 'Influence of antibiotic impregnation on fatigue life of Simplex P and Palacos R acrylic bone cements with and without centrifugation', *J Biomed Mater Res*, 1989, **23**, 379.
57. Soltész U and Ege W 'Fatigue behavior of different acrylic bone cements', *Proceedings of the 4th World Biomaterials Congress*, Berlin, 1992, 90.
58. Jaffe WL, Rose RM and Radin EL 'On the stability of the mechanical properties of self-curing acrylic bone cement', *J Bone Joint Surg*, 1974, **56–A**(8), 1711.
59. Carter DR, Gates EI and Harris WH 'Strain-controlled fatigue of acrylic bone cement', *J Biomed Mater Res*, 1982, **16**, 647.
60. Wright TM and Robinson RP 'Fatigue crack propagation in polymethylmethacrylate bone cements', *J Mater Sci*, 1982, **17**, 2463–8.
61. Vila MM, Ginebra MP, Gil FJ and Planell JA 'effect of porosity and environment on the mechanical properties of acrylic bone cement modified with acrylonitrile–butadiene–styrene particles: Part II. fatigue crack propagation', *J Biomed Mater Res: Appl Biomat*, 1999, **48**, 128–34.
62. Molino LN and Topoleski LDT 'Effect of $BaSO_4$ on the fatigue crack propagation rate of PMMA bone cement', *J Biomed Mater Res*, 1996, **31**, 131–7.
63. Wang CT and Pilliar RM 'Fracture toughness of acrylic bone cements', *J Mater Sci*, 1989, **24**, 3725.
64. Wixson RL 'Do we need to vacuum mix or centrifuge cement?', *Clin. Orthop Rel Res*, 1992, **285**, 84.
65. Rimnac C, Wright T and McGill D 'The effect of centrifugation on the fracture properties of acrylic bone cements', *J Bone Joint Surg*, 1986, **68A**, 281.
66. Bargar WL, Brown SA, Paul HA, Voegli T, Hseih Y and Sharkey N '*In vivo* versus

in vitro polymerization of acrylic bone cement: effect on material properties', *J Orthop Res*, 1986, **4**, 86.

67. Looney MA and Park JB 'Molecular and mechanical property changes during aging of bone cement *in vitro* and *in vivo*', *J Biomat Mater Res*, 1986, **20**, 555.
68. Vila MM, Ginebra MP, Gil FJ and Planell JA 'Effect of porosity and environment on the mechanical properties of acrylic bone cement modified with acrylonitrile–butadiene–styrene particles: Part I. Fracture toughness', *J Biomed Mater Res: Appl Biomat*, 1999, **48**, 121–7.
69. Beaumont PWR and Young RJ 'Slow crack growth in acrylic bone cement', *J Biomed Mater Res*, 1975, **9**, 423.
70. Hailey JL, Turner IG, Miles AW and Price G 'The effect of post-curing chemical bone changes on the mechanical properties of acrylic bone cement', *J Mater Sci Mater Med*, 1994, **5**, 617–21.
71. Ginebra MP, Aparicio C, Albuixech L, Fernández-Barragán E, Gil FJ, Planell JA, Morejón L, Vázquez B and San Román J 'Improvement of the mechanical properties of acrylic bone cements by substitution of the radio-opaque agent', *J Mater Sci Mater Med*, 1999, **10**, 733–7.
72. Ginebra MP, Albuixech L, Fernández-Barragán, Aparicio C, Gil FJ, San Román J, Vázquez B and Planell JA 'Mechanical performance of acrylic bone cements containing different radiopacifying agents', *Biomaterials*, 2000, **23**(8), 1873–2.
73. Sabokbar A, Fujikawa Y, Murray DW and Athanasou NA 'Radio-opaque agents in bone cement increase bone resorption', *J Bone Joint Surg*, (*Br.*), 1997, **79-B**, 129–34.
74. Lazarus MD, Cuckler JM, Schumacher HR, Ducheyne P and Baker DG 'Comparison of the inflammatory response to particulate polymethylmethacrylate debris with and without barium sulphate', *J Orthop Res*, 1994, **12**, 532–41.
75. Isaac GH, Atkinson JR, Dowson D, Kennedy PD and Smith MR 'The causes of femoral head roughening in explanted Charnley hip prostheses', *Eng Med*, 1987, **16**, 167–73.
76. Caravia L, Dowson D, Fisher J and Jobbins B 'The influence of bone and bone cement debris on counterface roughness in sliding wear tests of ultra-high molecular weight polyethylene on stainless steel', *Proc Inst Mech Eng*, 1990, **204**, 65–70.
77. Cooper JR, Dowson D, Fisher J and Jobbins B 'Ceramic bearing surfaces in total artificial joints: resistance to third body wear damage from bone cement particles', *J Med Eng Technol*, 1991, **15**, 63–7.
78. Vázquez, B, Ginebra, MP, Gil, FJ, Planell, JA, López Bravo, A, San Román, J, 1999, Radiopaque acrylic cements prepared with a new acrylic derivative of yodo-quinoline, *Biomaterials*, **20**, 2047–53.
79. Nelson RC, Hoffman RO and Burton JA 'The effect of antibiotic addition on the mechanical properties of acrylic cement', *J Biomed Mater Res*, 1978, **12**, 473.
80. Lautenschlager EP, Jacobs JJ, Marshall GW and Meyer PR 'Mechanical properties of bone cements containing large doses of antibiotic powders,' *J Biomed Mater Res*, 1976, **10**, 929.
81. Davies JP and Harris WH 'Effect of hand-mixing tobramycin on the fatigue strength of Simplex P', *J Biomed Mater Res*, 1991, **25**, 1409.
82. Beaumont PWR 'The strength of acrylic bone cements and acrylic cement-stainless steel interfaces. Part I: The strength of acrylic bone cement containing second phase dispersions', *J Mater Sci*, 1977, **12**, 1845.
83. Guida G, Riccio V, Gatto S, Migliaresi C, Nicodemo L, Nicolais L and Palomba C

'A glass bead composite acrylic bone cement', in *Biomaterials and Biomechanics*, Ducheyne P, Van der Perre G and Aubert AE (eds), Elsevier Science, Amsterdam, 1984, 19.

84. Henning W, Blencke BA, Brömer H, Deutscher KK, Gross A and Ege W 'Investigations with bioactivated polymethylmethacrylates', *J Biomed Mater Res*, 1979, **13**, 89.
85. Murakami A, Behiri JC and Bonfield W 'Rubber-modified bone cement', *J Mater Sci*, 1988, **23**, 2029.
86. Liu YK, Park JB, Njus GO and Steinstra D 'Bone particle impregnated bone cement I. *In vitro* studies', *J Biomed Mat Res*, 1987, **21**, 247.
87. Henrich DE, Cram AE, Park JB, Liu YK and Reddi H 'Inorganic bone and demineralized bone matrix impregnated bone cement: A preliminary *in vivo* study', *J Biomed Mater Res*, 1993, **27**, 277.
88. Low RF, Hulbert SF and Sogal A 'Mechanical properties of hydroxyapatite–polymethylmethacrylate bone cement composite: hydroxyapatite embedded on surface and throughout cement matrix', *Bioceramics 6*, Ducheyne P and Christiansen D (eds), Butterworth-Heinemann, London, 1993, 339.
89. Dandurand J, Delpech V, Lebugle A, Lamure A and Lacabanne C 'Study of the mineral-organic linkage in an apatitic reinforced bone cement', *J Biomed Mater Res*, 1990, **24**, 1377.
90. Morejón L, Mendizábal E, Delgado JA, Ginebra MP, Aparicio C, Gil FJ, Marsal M, Davidenko N, Ballesteros ME and Planell JA 'Static mechanical properties of hydroxyapatite (HA) powder-filled acrylic bone cements: effect of type of HA powder', *J Biomed Mater Res Part B: Appl Biomater*, 2005, **72B**, 345–52.
91. Vázquez B, Ginebra MP, Gil FJ, Planell JA and San Román J 'Acrylic bone cements modified with β-TCP particles encapsulated with poly(ethylene glycol)', *Biomaterials*, 2005, **26**, 4309–16.
92. Fishbane BM and Pond RB 'Stainless steel fibre reinforcement of polymethylmethacrylate', *Clin Orthop Rel Res*, 1977, **128**, 194.
93. Topoleski LDT, Ducheyne P and Cuckler JM 'The fracture toughness of titanium-fibre reinforced bone cement', *J Biomed Mater Res*, 1992, **26**, 1599.
94. Saha S and Pal S 'Mechanical characterization of commercially made carbon-fibre-reinforced polymethylmethacrylate', *J Biomed Mater Res*, 1986, **20**, 817.
95. Pourdeyhimi B and Wagner HD 'Elastic and ultimate properties of acrylic bone cement reinforced with ultra-high-molecular weight polyethylene fibres', *J Biomed Mater Res*, 1989, **23**, 63.
96. Buckley CA, Lautenschlager EP and Gilbert JL 'High strength PMMA fibres for use in a self-reinforced acrylic cement: fibre tensile properties and composite toughness', *Proceedings of the 17th Annual Meeting of the Society for Biomaterials*, Scottsdale, Arizona, 1991, 45.
97. Pilliar RM, Blackwell R, MacNab I and Cameron HV 'Carbon fibre-reinforced bone cement in orthopaedic surgery', *J Biomed Mater Res*, 1976, **10**, 893.
98. Lehnartz E 'Chemical Physiologie', Springer Verlag, Berlin, 1959, S.87.
99. James ML 'Complicaciones anestésicas y metabólicas', in *Complicaciones de las artroplastias totales de cadera*, Ling RSM (ed), Salvat Editores.
100. Newens AF and Volz RG 'Severe hypotension during prosthetic hip surgery with acrylic bone cement', *Anesthesiology*, 1972, **36**, 298.
101. Milne IS 'Hazards of acrylic bone cement', *Anaesthesia*, 1973, **28**, 538.
102. Linder L and Romanus M 'Acute local tissue effects of polymerizing acrylic bone cement', *Clin Orthop Rel Res*, 1976, **115**, 303.

103. Birch R, Wilkinson MCP, Vijayan KP and Gschmeissner 'Cement burn of the sciatic nerve', *J Bone Joint Surg*, 1992, **74-B**, 731–3.
104. Jasty M, Jiranek W and Harris W 'Acrylic fragmentation in total hip replacements and its biological consequences', *Clin Orthop Rel Res*, 1992, **285**, 116.
105. Willert HG, Bertram H and Buchhorn GH 'Osteolysis in alloarthroplasty of the hip. The role of bone cement fragmentation', *Clin Orthop Rel Res*, 1990, **258**, 108.
106. Brauer GM, Steinberger DR and Stansbury JW 'Dependence of curing time, peak temperature, and mechanical properties on the composition of bone cement', *J Biomed Mater Res*, 1986, **20**, 839.
107. Tanzi MC, Sket I, Gatti AM and Monari E 'Physical characterization of acrylic bone cement cured with new accelerator system', *Clin Mater*, 1991, **8**, 131.
108. Vázquez B, Elvira C, Levenfeld B, Pascual B, Goñi I, Gurruchaga M, Ginebra MP, Gil FX, Planell JA, Liso PA, Rebuelta M and San Román J 'Application of new tertiary amines with reduced toxicity to the curing process of acrylic bone cements', *J Biomed Mater Res*, 1997, **34**, 129–36.
109. Migliaresi C and Capuana P '2-Hydroxyethylmethacrylate modified bone cement', in *Clinical Implant Materials, Advances in Biomaterials 9*, Elsevier, Amsterdam, 1990, 141.
110. Davies JP and Harris WH 'The effect of the addition of methylene blue on the fatigue strength of simplex P bone-cement', *J Appl Biomater*, 1992, **3**, 81.
111. Pascual B, Goñi I and Gurruchaga M 'Characterization of a new acrylic bone cement based on a (methyl methacrylate/1-hydroxypropyl methacrylate) monomer', *J Biomed Mater Res: Appl Biomater*, 1999, **48**, 447–57.
112. Pascual B, Gurruchaga M, Ginebra MP, Gil FJ, Planell JA, Vázquez B, San Román J and Goñi I 'Modified acrylic bone cement with high amounts of ethoxytriethyleneglycol methacrylate', *Biomaterials*, 1999, **20**(5), 453–63.
113. Oyasaed H 'Dynamic mechanical properties of multiphase acrylic systems', *J Biomed Mater Res*, 1990, **24**, 1037.
114. Elliott J *Structure and Chemistry of the Apatites and Other Calcium Orthophosphates.* Elsevier, Amsterdam, 1994.
115. Chow LC 'Development of self-setting calcium phosphate cements', *J Ceram Soc Japan Int. Edition*, 1991, **99**, 927–36.
116. Vereecke G and Lemaitre J 'Calculation of the solubility diagrams in the system $Ca(OH)_2$-H_3PO_4-KOH-HNO_3-CO_2-H_2O', *J Crystal Growth*, 1990, **104**, 820–32.
117. Brown PW and Fulmer M 'Kinetics of hydroxyapatite formation at low temperature', *J Am Ceram Soc*, 1991, **74**, 934–40.
118. Xie L and Monroe EA 'The hydrolysis of tetracalcium phosphate and other calcium orthophosphates', in *Handbook of Bioactive Ceramics, Vol. II, Calcium phosphate and hydroxylapatite ceramics*, Yamamuro T, Hench L and Wilson J (eds), CRC Press, Boca Raton, 1990, 29–37.
119. Monma H and Kanazawa T 'The hydration of α-tricalcium phosphate', *J Ceram Soc Japan (Yogo-kyokai-shi)*, 1976, **84**, 209–13.
120. Monma H, Goto M and Komura T 'Effect of additives on hydration and hardening of tricalcium phosphate', *Gypsum and Lime*, 1984, **188**, 11–16.
121. Ginebra MP, Fernández E, De Maeyer EAP, Verbeeck RMH, Boltong MG, Ginebra J, Driessens FCM and Planell JA 'Setting reaction and hardening of an apatitic calcium phosphate cements', *J Dent Res*, 1997, **76**(4), 905–12.
122. Ginebra MP, Boltong MG, Fernández E, Planell JA and Driessens FCM 'Effects

of various additives and temperature on some properties of an apatitic calcium phosphate cement', *J Mater Sci Mater Med*, 1995, **6**, 612–16.

123. Ginebra MP, Fernández E, Boltong MG, Planell JA, Bermudez O and Driessens FCM 'Compliance of an apatitic calcium phosphate cements with some short-term clinical requirements in bone surgery, orthopaedics and dentistry', *Clin Mater*, 1994, **17**, 99–104.
124. Ginebra MP, Fernández E, Driessens FCM and Planell JA 'The effect of Na_2HPO_4 addition on the setting reaction kinetics of an α-TCP cement', *Bioceramics*, 1998, **11**, 243–6.
125. Ginebra MP, Fernández E, Driessens FCM and Planell JA 'Modeling of the hydrolysis of α-TCP', *J Am Ceram Soc*, 1999, **82**(10), 2008–12.
126. Ginebra MP, Driessens FCM and Planell JA 'Effect of the particle size on the micro and nanostructural features of a calcium phosphate cement: a kinetic analysis', *Biomaterials*, 2004, **25**, 3453–62.
127. Brown WE and Chow LC *Dental Restorative Cement Pastes*, US Patent n°4518430, 1985.
128. Chow LC, Takagi S, Costantino PD and Friedman CD 'Self-setting calcium phosphate cements', *Mat Res Soc Symp Proc*, 1991, **179**, 3–24.
129. Ishikawa K, Takagi S, Chow LC, Ishikawa Y, Eanes ED and Asaoka K 'Behaviour of a calcium phosphate cement in simulated blood plasma *in vitro*', *Dent Mater* 1994, **10**, 26–32.
130. Fukase Y, Eanes ED, Takagi S, Chow LC and Brown WE 'Setting reactions and compressive strengths of calcium phosphate cements', *J Dent Res*, 1990, **69**, 1852–6.
131. Tenhuisen KS and Brown PW 'The kinetics of calcium deficient and stoichiometric hydroxyapatite formation from $CaHPO_4.2H_2O$ and $Ca4(PO_4)_2O$', *J Mater Sci Mater Med*, 1996, **7**, 309–16.
132. Constantz BR, Ison IC, Fulmer MT, Poser RD, Smith ST, VanWagoner M, Ross J, Goldstein SA, Jupiter JB and Rosenthal DI 'Skeletal repair by *in situ* formation of the mineral phase of bone', *Science*, 1995, **267**, 1796–9.
133. Constantz BR, Barr BM, Ison IC, Fulmer MT, Baker J, McKinney LA, Goodman SB, Gunasekaren S, Delaney DC, Ross J and Poser RD 'Histological, chemical, and crystallographic analysis of four calcium phosphate cements in different rabbit osseous sites', *J Biomed Mater Res: Appl Biomater*, 1998, **43**, 451–61.
134. Lemaitre J, Mirtchi A and Mortier A 'Calcium phosphate cements for medical use: state of the art and perspectives of development', *Silicates Industries*, 1987, **9–10**, 141–6.
135. Bohner M, Lemaitre J and Ring T 'Hydraulic properties of tricalcium phosphate-phosphoric acid-water mixtures', in *Third Euro-Ceramics*, Duran P and Fernandez JF (eds), Faenza Editrice Iberica S.L, Castellon de la Plana, Spain, 1993.
136. Bajpai P, Fuchs C and McCullum D 'Development of tricalcium phosphate ceramic cement', in *Quantitative Characterization and Performance of Porous Implants for Hard Tissue Applications*, Lemons J (ed.), ASTM STP 953. American Society for Testing and Materials, Philadelphia, 1987, 377–88.
137. Fernandez E, Gil FJ, Ginebra MP, Driessens FCM, Planell JA and Best SM 'Calcium phosphate bone cements for clinical applications. Part I: Solution chemistry', *J Mater Sci Mater Med*, 1999, **10**, 169–76.
138. Fernández E, Boltong MG, Ginebra MP, Bermudez O, Driessens RCM and Planell JA 'Common in effect on some calcium phosphate cements', *Clin Mater*, 1994, **16**, 99–103.

139. Ginebra MP *Desarrollo y caracterización de un cemento óseo basado en fosfato tricálcico-α para aplicaciones quirúrgicas*, PhD Thesis, Universitat Politècnica de Catalunya, Barcelona, 1996.
140. Bohner M, Van Landuyt P, Trophardy G, Merkle H and Lemaitre J 'Effect of several additives and their admixtures on the physico-chemical properties of a calcium phosphate cement', *J Mater Sci Mater Med*, 2000, **11**, 111–16.
141. Fernández E, Boltong MG, Ginebra MP, Driessens FCM, Bermudez O and Planell JA 'Development of a method to measure the period of swelling of calcium phosphate cements', *J Mater Sci Lett*, 1996, **15**, 1004–5.
142. Driessens FCM, Planell JA, Boltong MG, Khairoun I and Ginebra MP 'Osteotransductive bone cements', *J Eng Med*, 1998, **212**, 427–35.
143. Ishikawa K, Miyamoto Y, Kon M, Nagayama M and Asaoka K 'Non-decay type fast-setting calcium phosphate cement: composite with sodium alginate', *Biomaterials*, 1995, **16**, 527–32.
144. Khairoun I, Boltong MG, Driessens FC and Planell JA 'Effect of calcium carbonate on clinical compliance of apatitic calcium phosphate bone cement', *J Biomed Mater Res*, 1997, **38**(4), 356–60.
145. Khairoun I, Driessens FCM, Boltong MG, Planell JA and Wenz R 'Addition of cohesion promotors to calcium phosphate cements', *Biomaterials*, 1999, **20**, 393–8.
146. Andrianjatovo H and Lemaitre J 'Effects of polysaccharides on the cement properties in the monocalcium phosphate monohydrate/b-tricalcium phosphate system', *Innovation Tech Biol Med*, 1995, **16S1**, 140–7.
147. Miyamoto Y, Ishikawa K, Takechi M, Toh T, Yuasa T, Nagayama M and Suzuki K 'Histological and compositional evaluations of three types of calcium phosphate cements when implanted in subcutaneous tissue immediately after mixing', *J Biomed Mater Res: Appl Biomater*, 1999, **48**, 36–42.
148. Bohner M 'Calcium orthophosphates in medicine: from ceramics to calcium phosphate cements', *Injury Int J Care Injured*, 2000, **31**, S-D37–47.
149. Khairoun I, Boltong MG, Driessens FCM and Planell JA 'Some factors controlling the injectability of calcium phosphate bone cements', *J Mater Sci: Mater Med*, 1998, **9**, 425–8.
150. Bohner M and Baroud G 'Injectability of calcium phosphate pastes', *Biomaterials*, 2005, **26**(13), 1553–63.
151. Gbureck U, Barralet JE, Spatz K, Grover LM and Thull R 'Ionic modification of calcium phosphate cement viscosity. Part I: hypodermic injection and strength imporovement of an apatite cement', *Biomaterials*, 2004, **25**, 2187–95.
152. Barralet JE, Hormann M, Grover LM and Gbureck U 'High-Strength Apatitic Cement by Modification with α-Hydroxy Acid Salts', *Adv Mater*, 2003, **15**, 2091–4.
153. Tanaka S, Kishi T, Shimogoryo R, Matsuya S and Ishikawa K 'Biopex aquires anti-washout properties by adding sodium alginate into its liquid phase', *Dent Mater J*, 2003, **22**(3), 301–12.
154. Ginebra MP, Rilliard A, Fernández E, Elvira C, San Román J and Planell JA 'Mechanical and rheological improvement of a calcium phosphate cement by the addition of a polymeric drug', *J Biomed Mater Res*, 2001, **57**, 113–18.
155. Driessens FCM, Boltong MG, Bermúdez O, Planell JA, Ginebra MP and Fernández E 'Effective formulations for the preparation of calcium phosphate bone cements', *J Mater Sci Mater Med*, 1994, **5**,164–70.
156. Ontañón M, Aparicio C, Ginebra MP and Planell JA 'Structure and mechanical

properties of bone', in *Structural Biological Materials*, Elices M (ed), Pergamon Material Series, Elsevier Science, Oxford, 2000, 31–71.

157. Burstein AH, Reilly DT and Martens M 'Aging of bone tissue: mechanical properties', *J Bone Joint Surg*, 1976, **58A**, 82–6.
158. Carter DR and Hayes WC 'The compressive behavior of bone as a two-phase porous structure', *Clin Orthop Relat Res*, 1977, **59A**, 954–62.
159. Driessens FCM 'Chemistry and applied aspects of calcium phosphate bone cements', *Concepts and Clinical Applications of Ionic Cements*. Meeting of the European Society for Biomaterials, Arcachon, France, 1999.
160. Grover LM, Gbureck U, Wright AJ, Tremayne M and Barralet JE 'Biologically mediated resorption of brushite cement *in vitro*', *Biomaterials*, 2006, **27**, 2178–85.
161. Ishikawa K and Asaoka K 'Estimation of ideal mechanical strength and critical porosity of calcium phosphate cement', *J Biomed Mater Res*, 1995, **29**, 1537–43.
162. Chow LC, Hirayama S, Takagi S and Parry E 'Diametral tensile strength and compressive strength of a calcium phosphate cement: effect of applied pressure', *J Biomed Mater Res: Appl Biomater*, 2000, **53**, 511–17.
163. Barralet J, Hofmann M, Grover LM and Gbureck U 'High-strength apatitic cement by modification with α-hydroxy acid salts', *Adv Mater*, 2003, **15**, 2091–4.
164. Miyamoto Y, Ishikawa K, Fukao H *et al.* 'In vivo setting behaviour of fast-setting calcium phosphate cement', *Biomaterials*, 1995, **16**, 855–60.
165. Ikenaga M, Hardouin I, Lemaitre J, Andrianjatovo H and Flautre B 'Biomechanical characterization of a biodegradable calcium phosphate hydraulic cement: a comparison with porous biphasic calcium phosphate ceramics', *J Biomed Mater Res*, 1998, **40**, 139–44.
166. Kurashina K *et al.* 'In vivo study of calcium phosphate cements: implantation of an α-tricalcium phosphate/dicalcium phosphate dibasic/tetracalcium phosphate monoxide cement paste', *Biomaterials*, 1997, **18**, 539–43.
167. Jansen JA, de Ruijter JE, Schaeken HG, van der Waerden JPC, Planell JA and Driessens FCM 'Evaluation of tricalciumphosphate/hydroxyapatite cement for tooth replacement: an experimental animal study', *J Mater Sci: Mater Med*, 1995, **6**, 653–57.
168. Friedman CD, Costantino PD, Takagi S and Chow LC 'Bonesource hydroxyapatite cement: a novel biomaterial for cranofacial skeletal tissue engineering and reconstruction', *J Biomed Mater Res, Appl Biomater*, 1998, **43**, 428–32.
169. Larsson S and Bauer TW 'Use of injectable calcium phosphate cement for fracture fixation: a review', *Clin Orthop Relat Res*, 2002, **395**, 23–32.
170. Ooms EM, Wolke JGC, van de Heuvel MT, Jeschke B and Jansen JA 'Histological evaluation of the bone response to calcium phosphate cement implanted in cortical bone', *Biomaterials*, 2003, **24**(6), 989–1000.
171. Frankenburg EP, Goldstein SA, Bauer TW, Harris SA and Poser RD 'Biomechanical and histological evaluation of a calcium phosphate cement', *J Bone Joint Surg Am*, 1998, **80**, 1112.
172. Apelt D, Theiss F, El-Warrak AO, Zlinszky K, Bettschart-Wolfisberger R, Bohner M, Matter S, Auer JA and Von Rechenberg B '*In vivo* behavior of three different injectable hydraulic calcium phosphate cements', *Biomaterials*, 2004, **25**, 1439–51.
173. Ohura K, Bohner M, Hardouin P, Lemaitre J, Pasquier G and Flautre B 'Resorption

of, and bone formation from, new betatricalcium phosphate-monocalcium phosphate cements: an *in vivo* study', *J Biomed Mater Res*, 1996, **30**(2), 193–200.

174. Munting E, Mirtchi AA and Lemaıtre J 'Bone repair of defects filled with phospocalcic hyraulic cement: an *in vivo* study', *J Mater Sci: Mater Med*, 1993, **4**, 337–44.
175. Bohner M, Theiss F, Apelt D, Hirsiger W, Houriet R, Rizzoli G, Gnos E, Frei C, Auer JA and von Rechenberg B 'Compositional changes of a dicalcium phosphate dihydrate cement after implantation in sheep', *Biomaterials*, 2003, **24**(20), 3463–74.
176. Markovic M, Takagi S and Chow LC 'Formation of macropores in calcium phosphate cements through the use of mannitol crystals', *Key Eng Mater*, 2000, 192–5, 773–6.
177. Takagi S and Chow LC 'Formation of macropores in calcium phosphate cement implants', *J Mater Sci: Mater Med*, 2001, **12**, 135–9.
178. Xu HHK and Quinn JB 'Calcium phosphate cement containing resorbable fibres for short-term reinforcement and macroporosity', *Biomaterials*, 2002, **23**, 193–202.
179. Ruhé PQ, Hedberg EL, Padron NT, Spauwen PHM, Jansen JA and Mikos AG 'Biocompatibility and degradation of poly(DLlactic-co-glycolic acid)/calcium phosphate cement composites', *J Biomed Mater Res A*, 2005, **74**, 533–44.
180. Barralet JE, Grover L, Gaunt T, Wright AJ and Gibson IR 'Preparation of macroporous calcium phosphate cement tissue engeneering scaffold', *Biomaterials*, 2002, **23**, 3063–72.
181. Almirall A, Larrecq G, Delgado JA, Martınez S, Planell JA and Ginebra MP 'Fabrication of low temperature macroporous hydroxyapatite scaffolds by foaming and hydrolysis of an a-TCP paste', *Biomaterials*, 2004, **25**, 3671–80.
182. Del Real RP, Wolke JGC, Vallet-Regı́ M and Jansen JA 'A new method to produce macropores in calcium phosphate cements', *Biomaterials*, 2002, **23**, 3673–80.
183. Edwards B, Higham P and Zitelli J 'Porous calcium phosphate cement', US Patent 6,670,293 B2, 2003.
184. Georgescu G, Lacout JL and Frèche M 'A new porous osteointegrative bone cement material', *Key Eng Mater*, 2004, 254–6, 201–4.
185. Ginebra MP, Delgado JA, Harr I, Almirall A, Del Valle S and Planell JA 'Factors affecting the structure and properties of an injectable self-setting calcium phosphate foam', *J Biomed Mater Res*, 2007, **80A**: 351–61.
186. Del Valle S, Miño N, Muñoz F, González A, Planell JA and Ginebra MP '*In vivo* evaluation of an injectable macroporous calcium phosphate cement', *J Mater Sci: Mater Med*, 2007, **18**, 353–61.
187. Gbureck U, Hölzel T, Doillon CJ, Müller FA and Barralet JE 'Direct printing of bioceramic implants with spatially localized angiogenic factors', *Adv Mater*, 2007, **19**, 795–800.
188. Ginebra MP, Traykova T and Planell JA 'Calcium phosphate cements: Competitive drug carriers for the musculoskeletal system?', *Biomaterials*, 2006, **27**, 2171–7.
189. Ginebra MP, Traykova T and Planell JA 'Calcium phosphate cements as bone drug delivery systems: A review', *J Controlled Release*, 2006, **113**, 102–10.

11
Bioactive polymer coatings to improve bone repair

G. HELARY and V. MIGONNEY, Institut Galilée, France

Abstract: The aim of this chapter is to describe the concept of bioactivity arising from the observed biological performance of new biomaterials when placed in contact with bone cell tissues. The bioactivity of materials could be summarized as the control of the host response preventing foreign body reaction. It represents one way of improving bone cell interactions. The fixation and osteointegration of biomaterials for bone repair requires specific and strong interactions of bone cell and materials – the stronger the interactions the longer the implant will be integrated and be performing. New biomaterials coatings were recently developed to obtain improved bone repair. They are derived from bioactive polymers which were shown to exhibit a controlled cell response and can be grafted onto different implant material surfaces.

Key words: bioactive polymers, biocompatibility, bone integration, host response, osteoblast response, polymer coating, polymer grafting.

11.1 Introduction: concept of biocompatibility of biomaterials for bone repair

Current developments in biomaterials especially designed for bone cell interaction demand implants that exhibit bioactive surfaces capable of preventing atypical fibrosis as a result of the foreign body response (FBR) and favour osteointegration. Why are these new materials needed? What are the specific requirements for these materials, particularly when they are designated for joint replacement as hip or knee prostheses?

The origin of the failures of biomaterial implants may be found in lack of control of the 'host response' leading to a foreign body response characterized by fibrosis and encapsulation. Indeed, when biomaterials are implanted or placed in contact with bone cell tissue, the 'cascade' of the host response events which has been extremely well described by Ratner and by Anderson[1,2] will occur. These series of events are activated at the wound site as soon as wounded tissue is generated and take place whatever the nature of the tissue and its location. Nevertheless, the intensity and duration of each step is greatly dependent on the extent of the wound, the nature of the wound surrounding tissue and the vascularization of the implantation site tissues.

To summarize, the cascade of 'host response' events is characterized by the following steps: protein adsorption, acute and chronic host inflammatory response, granulation of the tissue and fibrosis and encapsulation. In addition or in parallel to the host response, it is worth noting that infection of the surrounding unhealthy tissues may occur.

Once the biomaterial is implanted in the tissue, it is immediately covered and coated by plasma proteins. The nature and composition of the protein layer varies with the chemical and physical nature of the surface as a result of the 'race for the surface' that is taking place. Moreover, the affinity of the different plasma proteins for the surface which is strongly dependent on the chemical composition of the surface will be one of the determinant parameters controlling protein adsorption.[3] Therefore it appears to be possible to orientate the nature and composition of the adsorbed protein layer by varying the chemistry and/or physicochemistry of the surface.

After the protein adsorption step, the following natural event is the arrival of the monocytes and macrophages at the wound site to interrogate the 'material implant' which is considered to be a 'foreign body'. In response, macrophages which are considered to be the key players in the 'foreign body response' will secrete and produce cytokine signals.[4]

The activation of macrophages resulting in the cytokine secretion contributes to the recruitment of fibroblasts around the wound/biomaterial implanted site. Fibroblasts surrounding the site secrete collagen molecules which are involved in the elaboration of the encapsulation bag.

Actually, as no one material is capable of controlling this series of events, it is a real challenge to gain a good understanding of the mechanisms involved in the wound healing/hostile host response processes, since some of the molecular events at the origin and/or which generate the host response required for the natural wound healing are not well understood whereas other molecular events must be prevented. The host response is a natural response which has to occur in order to lead to the wound healing; whatever the wound, healing has to take place. The main problem when the wound originated in the implant of biomaterial remains the control of the healing response, which should not evolve into fibrosis and encapsulation bag formation. One question concerns the cooperation of fibroblasts and macrophages in this series of events which is quite complex and unclear, their possible role in the dedifferentiation of the cell tissue is also unclear.

11.2 Bioactive materials for bone repair

Therefore, whatever the nature of the cells constituting the tissues, the host response has to be controlled to avoid a FBR. How can this be done? The approaches are various but the aim remains the same, to mimic the entities present in the living system and to mask the synthetic or unnatural origin of the new material responsible for the FBR.

The different approaches suggested by the biomaterials community to reach this goal include elaboration of hybrid materials,[5] coating surfaces with specific proteins, peptides[6–11] or bioactive synthetic macromolecules.[12–14] The first approaches appear to be the smartest ones as well as the best candidates for overcoming the FBR since they involve natural molecules that are less likely to initiate an uncontrolled immunogenic and/or inflammatory response. Nevertheless, taking reported results in the literature into account, the balance between advantages and disadvantages is not in favour of them:

- The coating of biomaterial surfaces with proteins presents some enzymatic instability and may lead to emergence of immunogenicity and to the appearance of susceptibility to infection.
- The grafting or coating of surfaces with peptides is more selective and thus a better candidate for improving the cell/surface interaction but cyclic peptides should preferably be used rather than linear ones because of their lack of specificity.[10, 15] Nevertheless, the cost, instability and enzymatic degradation of the coating may tip the balance away from the advantages of peptide coating of surfaces which favour differentiation of osteoblast cells.

Grafting bioactive synthetic polymers favouring bone cell adhesion, proliferation and differentiation onto surfaces has been developed to enhance osteoblast differentiation, to improve the quality of the bone cell/surface interface and to avoid the problems of enzymatic instability and the cost of the final medical device. In addition, the use of bioactive polymers that have been shown to present the capacity to prevent bacteria adhesion in bone cell repair application appears to be really promising.

The appropriate material for bone cell tissue regeneration could be obtained by grafting biomolecules and/or bioactive polymers on to the surface in order to maintain differentiation of osteoblast cells and to control the host response avoiding its transformation into FBR. Bringing bone cell into contact with biomaterials will give most information about events at the interface.

11.3 Need for bone integration and repair biomaterials

Primary total hip and knee arthroplasties, and revision of the same, have been the major subject of numerous studies and then of the development of bone integration and bone repair materials. During the last 20 years, the occurrence of first intention prostheses has steadily increased, around 10% per year, and it has no reason to stop increasing mainly because of the ageing of the population. On the other hand, revision of total hip or knee prosthesis is also increasing because of the failures of the implants.[16, 17] The problems of patients and the diseases that occur at the origin of primary intention total hip prostheses (THP) are numerous, different and well identified, while revision and/or second intention THP are due to two main causes:

- Aseptic loosening which is a perfect illustration of the failure of biomaterial implants integration: Aseptic loosening generally appears within 10 to 15 years after implantation and results from the progressive establishment of a complex hostile host response which can have partially evolved from a FBR. This ineluctable event is characterized by the progressive replacement of the bone/implant interface with a fibrous tissue/implant interface; the encapsulating tissue surrounding the implant cannot supply the required mechanical performance of healthy osseous tissue. Despite a high rate of success owing to the improvement and development of better designed THP (e.g. nature of the alloy, control of the surface chemistry and/or structuration, hydroxyapatite (HAP) coating, oxidation of the surface, cement or cementless, nature of the head/cotyle couple – alumina/alumina to prevent or avoid wear debris generation and FBR[18]) illustrated by a constant decrease in failure frequency, some prostheses survive for less than 10 years and this becomes a dramatic problem especially in the case of young patients.
- The implant-associated infections of joint prostheses which are a major problem for public health: indeed, despite advances in surgical techniques and antibiotics prophylaxis, up to 1.5% of orthopaedic prostheses will become infected[19–23] and the percentage is not decreasing. The parameters which have to be taken into account in this statement are mainly (i) the recrudescence of antibiotic-resistant bacteria strains[19] and the subsequent difficulties of eradicating bacteria and (ii) the weak integration of implant in bone tissue – bacteria will have a predilection for unhealthy and/or damaged tissue. Thus new prevention strategies are needed. Some tentative work has been done consisting in the coating of the prosthesis with antibiotics or bioactive polymers[21] capable of inhibiting adherence of bacteria.[22] Bacterial adherence evaluated *in vitro* and *in vivo* gave positive and encouraging results (see Fig. 11.1) in both cases: a significant decrease in bacterial adhesion associated with no bacteria resistance. These grafted prostheses could be useful in the prevention of prosthesis infection by antibiotic resistant *Staphylococcus aureus* strains like MRSA (methycillin resistant Staphylococcus aureus).

Therefore the need to develop new bioactive surfaces capable of improving the bone/implant interface and the nature of the anchorage of the implant device to the bone tissue in a strong and reliable manner is still and ever important.

11.4 Available and/or new materials

Today, titanium alloy Ti-6Al-4V (TA6V) remains the gold standard biomaterial for orthopaedic implant applications. Part of its success is due to its good resistance to corrosion and mechanical properties in comparison to stainless steel and other alloys, as well as its good 'biocompatibility'. In

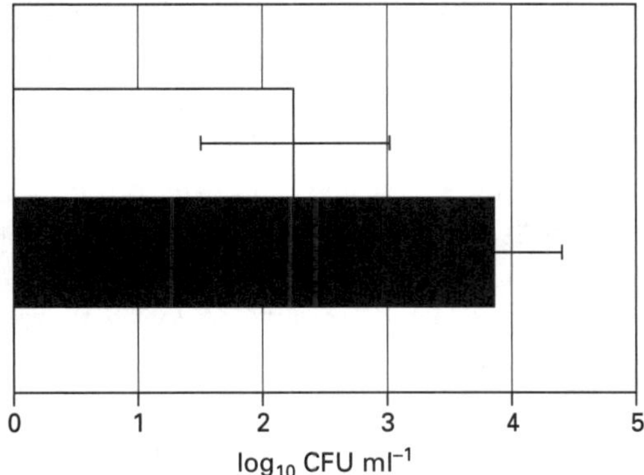

11.1 Comparison of *in vivo* MRSA strain 88244 adhesion on bioactive polymer-coated (□) or control silicone prostheses (■). A double-blind partial knee replacement was performed in 11 rabbits with 6 Q5-coated prostheses and 5 silicone prostheses fitting into the intramedullary canal of the tibia. MRSA 88244 (10^7 CFU) were injected into the knees. The number of bacteria adherent on prostheses was determined 24 h later. Results are means ± SD of 6 Q5-coated and 5 control silicone prostheses (p<0.0035). MRSA : methycillin resistant *Staphylococcus aureus*

fact, despite this displayed property, TA6V cannot be really classified as a 'biocompatible' material for orthopaedic applications since the bone/ TA6V implant interface is not functional, showing weak integration into bone tissue and then limited long-term survival. Moreover, the diffusion of cytotoxic metallic ions in the surrounding tissues may provoke chronic inflammation and then be the cause of severe damage. Various surface modifications have been proposed in order to improve the bone conductivity and the bone/surface cohesion of titanium (Ti) and TA6V alloy surfaces: micro and nanostructuration, coating with HAP or other ceramics[24] and development of bioactive surfaces (proteins coating, RGD peptides coating, chemical and thermal treatment,[25–28] bioactive polymers grafting). In each case, the aim is to enhance osteointegration and thereby the anchorage of the implant in the surrounding osseous tissue, providing a stable and active biointerface strong enough to support functional loading.

Despite the success of Ti alloys in orthopaedic applications, the rate of osteointegration is nevertheless relatively slow, leading to weak anchorage and a poor quality of osseous surrounding tissues (fibrosis). The idea of coating TA6V with bioactive ceramics like HAP and calcium silicate ceramics which are able to enhance osteoblast cell differentiation was smart and showed an interesting improvement of the bone tissue/implant interface as well as bone mineralization and growth. Nevertheless, the good results obtained with HAP-coated surfaces were counterbalanced by several failures mainly caused by the lack of control of the ceramic coating process, leading to ceramic/metal interface bonding of poor quality and to the dissolution of the apatite phase *in vivo*. In addition, the main disadvantage of this technique is the weak cohesion between the coating and the substrate owing to the difference in the thermal expansion properties of HAP coating and TA6V which can lead to micro cracks in the coating layer. Therefore, the bonding strength at the interface of both materials would be not strong enough to allow long-term survival of such coated implants. Recently, a new ceramic coating was developed and proposed by Zreiqat[29] to avoid these interface bonding problems.

The key solution for metallic surfaces for orthopaedic application could be via the bioactivity of surfaces induced by bioactive polymers grafted on to the surfaces.

11.5 Bioactive polymer approach

The idea of controlling the cell response with the aim of avoiding the ineluctable FBR by the control of protein/surface interfaces arose from the observed biological performance of some heparin-like surfaces. Migonney and co-workers[30, 31] demonstrated that the presence of particular chemical carboxylate and sulfonate groups immobilized onto polymer surfaces and randomly distributed along macromolecular chains of poly(styrene) (PS) allowed those surfaces to mimic the catalytic anticoagulant activity of heparin. Moreover, the presence of both carboxylate and sulfonate groups was demonstrated to allow specific adsorption of antithrombin III (AT) molecules with a conformation of the protein onto the surfaces which made available the domains of the protein responsible for quantitative complexation to thrombin (T). Generated thrombin-antithrombin III (TAT) complexes were demonstrated to be quantitatively displaced by antithrombin whereas this catalytic process was not exhibited by surfaces only functionalized by sulfonate groups. The grafting of heparin-like derivatives onto poly(ethylene) (PE) surfaces was shown to allow the development of anticoagulant heparin-like properties originated by the control of the adsorption of AT molecules. This property has been demonstrated *in vitro* and *in vivo*.

The properties of heparin being multiple, surfaces possessing heparin-like properties become of great interest in several biomedical implant applications. In particular, the strong inhibiting properties of heparin towards bacteria strains involved in implant-associated infections like *S. aureus* were demonstrated by Vaudaux.[32] Moreover the role of fibronectin as mediator in the evidenced inhibition was also investigated.[33] Then, adherence of *S. aureus*, responsible for major foreign body infections, was assessed on functionalized poly(methyl methacrylate) (PMMA)-based terpolymers bearing sulfonate and carboxylate groups and onto PMMA as control[22] (see Fig. 11.2) . These terpolymers, have been synthesized by radical copolymerization of methyl methacrylate

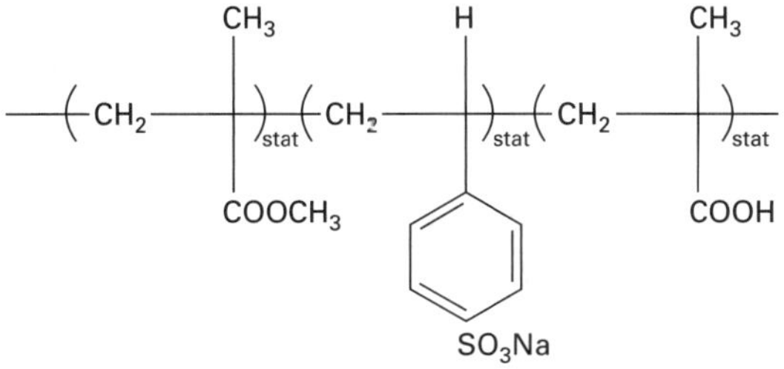

11.2 Schematic representation of functionalized PMMA-based random terpolymer of methyl methacrylate (MMA), comethacrylic acid (MA) and cosodium styrene sulfonate (NaSS).

and two anionic monomers, methacrylic acid (MA) and sodium styrene sulfonate (NaSS), by varying the ratio R = $[COO^-]/[COO^- + SO_3^-]$ from 0 to 1 and keeping the ionic monomer molar content below 15% to avoid polymer solubilization in the physiologic medium.

Adsorption of fibronectin onto PMMA was shown dramatically to promote bacterial adherence, whereas strong inhibition of bacteria adherence (up to 90%) was observed onto functionalized terpolymers containing both carboxylate and sulfonate groups with R at around 0.5–0.6. When terpolymers were predominantly functionalized by a carboxylate group, bacteria adherence was favoured and reached values close to PMMA.[22] These results have been related to the radical copolymerization process of the three monomers, allowing the creation of active sites responsible for specific interactions with fibronectin and inducing modifications of its conformation. The conformation of the adsorbed adhesive protein was then suggested to have an influence on the availability of its interaction sites with bacteria adhesins and therefore on modulation of bacteria adherence. Inhibition of *S. aureus* adherence by functionalized PMMA-based terpolymers was shown to be of great interest in the field of biomedical implants.

The bioactive polymer exhibiting the highest inhibiting properties against *S. aureus* has been covalently grafted onto silicon implants[34] and bacteria adhesion was assessed *in vivo* on rabbits for 24 hours[21] following the 'model of infection' developed by Crémieux and co-workers.[20] Results evidenced the maintainence of the inhibiting properties of the bioactive polymer grafted surfaces in comparison to the non-grafted one under physiological *in vivo* conditions. The observed difference in bacteria adhesion was attributed to differences in the composition of the protein layer adsorbed onto the surfaces during the experiment. Indeed, controlling the host response using bioactive surfaces is generated by controlling the adsorption of proteins; proteins adsorbed onto bioactive surfaces exposed domains favourable, or not, to further interactions with cells and bacteria. By varying the chemistry of the surface – introducing precise functional groups – it is possible to modulate the response of the living system. To illustrate this, grafted and non-grafted silicon implants were implanted in rabbits for 24 hours and then explanted to be incubated with bacteria and to evaluate bacteria adhesion onto surfaces covered with host plasma proteins. In the case of non-grafted surfaces, bacteria strongly adhered, whereas they were 90% inhibited in the case of grafted surfaces (see Fig. 11.3). Control of the composition and conformation of adsorbed proteins is the key solution to developing the biological activity of functionalized surfaces.

The behaviour of different cells types towards these functionalized polymers has been studied extensively.[13, 33, 37] Results showed that it is possible to vary the adhesion, proliferation and activity of cells by varying the composition of carboxylate and sulfonate groups in the copolymers (see Fig. 11.4). It appeared interesting to investigate the osteoblast cell response – adhesion, morphology, proliferation and differentiation – towards these terpolymers in order to investigate their application in orthopaedic applications. Polymers with various compositions of carboxyl and sulfonate groups, R varying from 0 to 1, were synthesized and exposed to osteoblasts from MG 63 and Saos 2 cell lines as well as primary cells (calvaria).[35] Whatever the origin of the osteoblast cells, the results are similar: the cell response strongly varies with the value of the R ratio which illustrates the composition of the polymers with regard to functional groups. The closer the R value to 0.7–0.8 of the bioactive copolymer, the better the differentiation of osteoblasts as illustrated in Fig. 11.5. It is worth noting that the alkaline phosphatase activity (ALP) was shown to reach the highest value for R equaling 0.8 whatever the conditions – supplemented medium or not – and that the mineralization of osteoblast was clearly more homogeneous and more important on the same copolymer in comparison to the other composition. PMMA-based polymers with R equalling 0.7–0.8 are the best candidates to improve the bone cell/

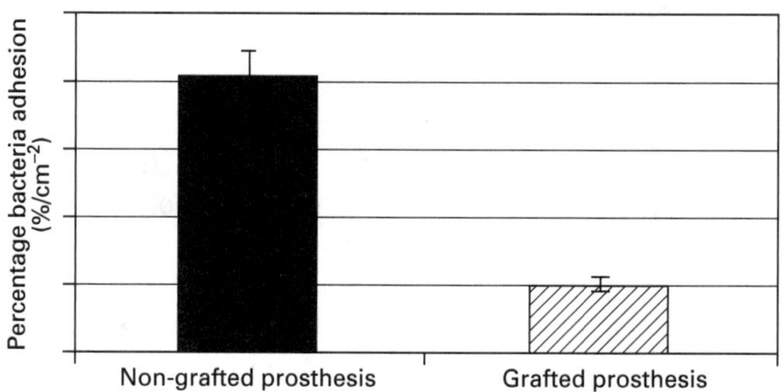

11.3 Ex vivo experiment on rabbits. Adhered bacteria (%) onto silicone prosthesis – virgin and bioactive polymer grafted silicone – previously implanted for 24 hours in the knee of rabbits (n = 6)

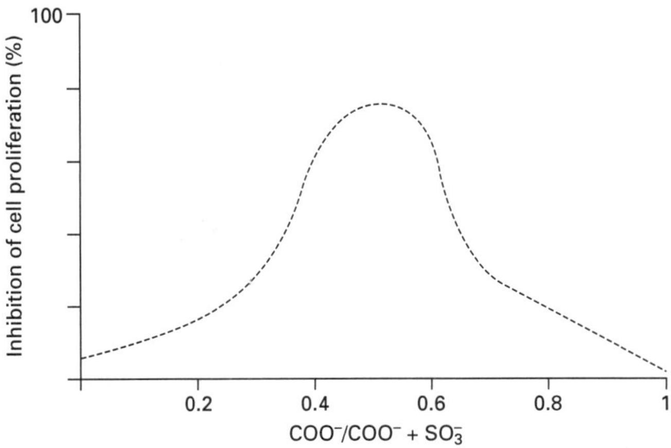

11.4 Inhibition percentage of fibroblast cells onto functionalized PMMA with various compositions.

material interactions and to enhance cell differentiation, mineralization and bone growth. Such bioactive polymers which combine improvement of the osteoblast cell response with properties that inhibit bacteria associated with implant infection are the best candidates to be grafted onto metallic implant surfaces like Ti and TA6V alloys in order to obtain biointegrable and infection preventing orthopaedic implants.

11.6 New approach: grafting bioactive polymers onto titanium implants

The grafting of organic bioactive polymers to metallic surfaces is one of the key solutions for elaborating biocompatible and 'biointegrable' orthopaedic implant surfaces. Indeed, as described above, it is amongst the numerous strategies which have been developed to improve osteointegration of implants: HAP coatings, physical (thermal, laser, shot blasting, etc.) and chemical (etching) treatments. Nevertheless, even if all the strategies were developed with the aim of enhancing protein/cell/surface interactions, none have been demonstrated to exhibit the required long-term biological properties through *in vivo* assays and to be easily reproducible and transferable on the industrial scale.

Recently, new techniques of surface grafting were developed to functionalize biomaterial implants, appearing to be a more promising approach for elaborating bioactive biomaterial surfaces. Grafting techniques have been first developed on polymers like poly(ethylene terephtalate)[7, 11, 14] and then applied to metallic surfaces like titanium Ti and TA6V titanium alloy.[8, 11, 36–40] These surface functionalization techniques consist in covalent bonding

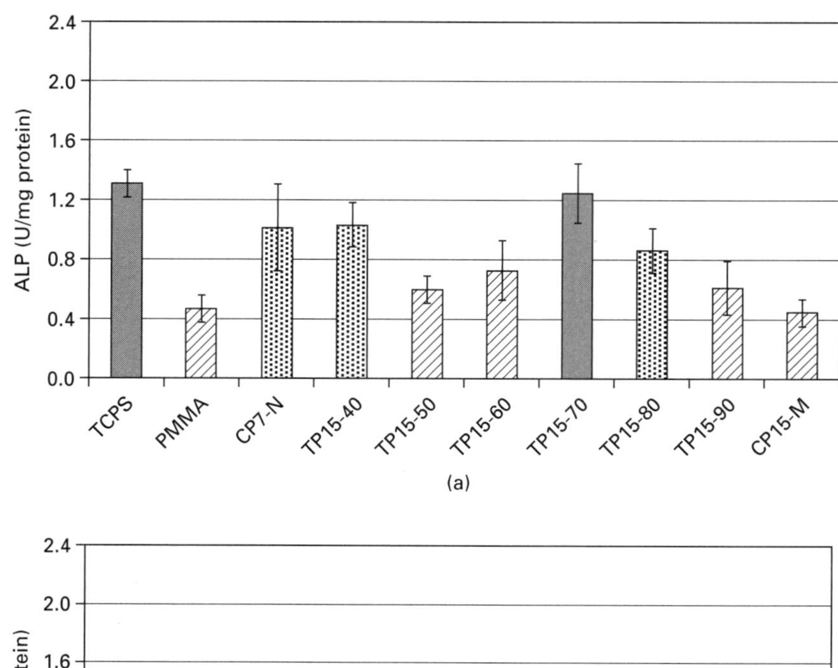

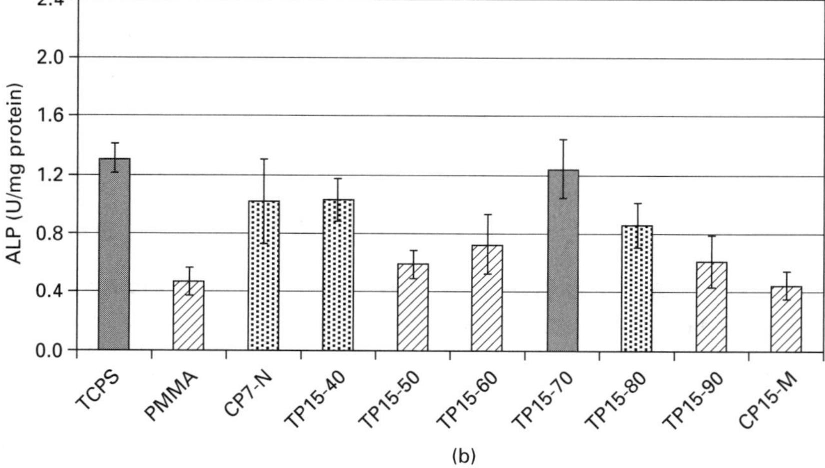

11.5 Alkaline phosphatase activity of MG 63 osteoblast proliferating onto bioactive polymers of various compositions at day 14; (a) non-supplemented and (b) supplemented medium. The best ALP is observed on TP15-70 which has 70% mol of carboxylate groups and 30% mol of sulfonate.

of bioactive – natural or synthetic – molecules which would assure a good resistance to shear stress and a perfect interface cohesion. Nevertheless, as detailed above, the functionalization of surfaces by peptides which at first appeared to be the smartest solution to set up 'bioactive' surfaces but it is less promising since peptides are expensive molecules, they are not specific enough when linear and they are sensitive to enzymatic instability. Moreover the yield and the reproducibility of grafting of peptides are not easy to control (at least at the industrial scale) and the *in vivo* assays are too few to be conclusive.

Therefore, the conclusion that arises from an overview of the literature on the development of bioactive material surfaces enhances the benefits of grafting bioactive polymers onto polymer and metallic implants to endow them with the appropriate biological properties and to control the host response so as to prevent FBR. The 'grafting from' method chosen to functionalize Ti and TA6V alloys requires one activation step to create an active species on the surface that is able to initiate or to allow the copolymerization reaction of the anionic monomers responsible for the observed enhancement of the osteoblast differentiation. Grafting of bioactive polymers has been carried out onto Ti and TA6V alloy using two strategies, 'direct' and 'indirect' grafting.[38–40] Both strategies need an oxidation step which is achieved either chemically or electrochemically.

In the 'direct method', the chemical oxidation of Ti surfaces is performed using a piranha solution, a mixture of hydrogen peroxide and sulfuric acid. The attack induces the formation of a gel at the surface, the structure of which is due to the formation of a Ti(IV)-H_2O_2 complex. The presence of the peroxides –O–O– bonds (detected by IR spectroscopy) allows the generation of radicals by simple heating which will initiate polymerization of the chosen anionic monomers to build the bioactive polymer chains covalently bound to the titanium surfaces.[38–40]

In the indirect method, the first step is electrochemical oxidation which leads to the formation of an oxide layer with hydroxyl groups at the titanium or titanium alloy surface. The generated TiOH hydroxyl groups will react in a silanization reaction with the silanol SiOH groups from the silane derivative-bearing vinyl groups. The next step is radical copolymerization of the vinyl groups of the silane derivatives with the anionic monomer NaSS and MA initiated by a thermal initiator (azobisisobutyronitrile – AIBN). Electrochemical oxidation is a well controlled method that allows perfect control of the depth of the oxide layer. It is routinely used in the fabrication of orthopaedic titanium implants and devices (THP, spine, screw etc.)

In both methods, the oxidation step is followed either by polymerization (direct method) or by silanization and polymerization (indirect method). One of the advantages of both of these methods is that they can be applied to any Ti or TA6V alloy surface whatever its shape. Moreover, it can be easily transferred to an industrial scale. On the other hand, there are some disadvantages that have to be taken into account:[38–40]

- The direct method: this is quite simple and can be carried out but the most important difficulty remains control of the chemical oxidation parameter in order to obtain homogeneous oxidized surfaces. This includes the sequence of addition of the reactants, time to oxidation, temperature and inert atmosphere. Moreover, as the reaction can be very violent, particularly in the case of TA6V, the time to oxidation has to be optimized to prevent undesired roughness of the surface. Smooth surfaces are more easily obtained in case of Ti surfaces by this method.

- The indirect method: the oxidation step is better controlled giving a homogeneous distribution of TiOH groups on the surface and leading to well distributed bioactive sites on the grafted titanium surfaces. The principal inconvenience of this process is the conditions required for the silanization reaction,[39] namely the use of organic solvent and the high temperature of the reaction. Nevertheless this indirect method, even if more complex than the direct one, remains the best controlled chemically and has the advantage of not modifying the rugosity of the surfaces.

Kinetic studies of the oxidation and polymerization steps of bioactive polymer grafting have been recently described[38, 39] and their analysis has allowed the optimal conditions of grafting for both methods to be determined. It is worth noting that the rates of grafting of the bioactive polymers onto Ti surfaces, as determined by toluidin blue (TB) method, fourier transform infrared (FTIR) and X-ray photoelectron spectroscopy (XPS), are very high in comparison to those described in the literature for grafting biomolecules onto titanium and its alloys. It is possible to reach high grafting rate of 5 μg cm^{-2}. In addition to these chemical characterization methods, contact angle measurements correlate with the characterization method. The presence of anionic polymers on the Ti surfaces increases the wettability and then decreases the contact angle of the grafted Ti surfaces compared with non-grafted ones. The grafting of bioactive polymers onto titanium and its alloys has been performed using either one monomer (NaSS or MA) leading to the grafting of homopolymers and two monomers (NaSS and MA) leading to copolymers.

Osteoblast cell interactions were assessed on different grafted and non-grafted surfaces and showed (i) an increase in the adhesion strength of the cell correlated with spread of morphology of the cell when grafted and (ii) a decrease or comparable proliferation and increase in ALP activity as well as mineralization. The presence of anionic bioactive polymers enhances the differentiation of osteoblast cells as well as their anchorage. Whatever the surface, Ti or TA6V alloy, an improvement is observed. This grafting has been performed on TA6V alloy cylinders and implanted in rabbit knee, showing a difference in the host response by varying the chemistry of the Ti alloy surfaces.

The choice of polymer to be grafted on Ti and alloys is greatly dependent on the desired properties of the tailored titanium surface:

- When the best osteoblast differentiation is required, the copolymer to be grafted would be composed of 80% mol MA and 20% mol NaSS. In this case the inhibition properties of bacteria adhesion are not optimized and in the least case, not maximized.

- When the most important property is to prevent infection – in immune depressed patients or in a second intention prosthesis – the homopolymer of NaSS will be grafted. Those bioactive polymers have been grafted on to a TA6V cylinder and *in vivo* assessed in rabbits. Preliminary results showed a difference in the osteoblast response and in osseous regrowth by varying the chemistry confirming the *in vitro* results.

11.7 Conclusion

Despite great progress in elaborating new materials that favour bone cell interaction and repair and the encouraging results described in the literature on osteointegrable materials fields, investigations must continue to improve the host response and to prevent FBR which is the origin of the main failures. Grafting of surfaces by bioactive polymers appears to be an intermediate step, since future solutions will come from developments in tissue engineering and regenerative medicine. These future solutions will allow reproduction of living healthy tissues which will naturally minimize the hostile host response.

11.8 References

1 Ratner BD, 'The engineering of biomaterials exhibiting recognition and specificity', *J Mol Recognit*, 1996, **9**(5–6), 617–25.

2 Brunstedt MR, Anderson JM, Spilizewski KL, Marchant RE and Hiltner A, '*In vivo* leucocyte interactions on pellethane surfaces', *Biomaterials*, 1990, **11**(6), 370–8.

3 Brash JL and Ten Hove P, 'Protein adsorption studies on 'standard' polymeric materials', *J Biomater Sci Polym Ed*, 1993, **4**(6), 591–9.

4 Godek ML, Michel R, Chamberlain LM, Castner DG and Grainger DW, 'Adsorbed serum albumin is permissive to macrophage attachment to perfluorocarbon polymer surfaces in culture', *J Biomed Mater Res A*, 2008, **88**(2), 503–19.

5 Santin M and Ambrosio L, 'Soybean-based biomaterials: preparation, properties and tissue regeneration potential', *Expert Rev Med Devices*, 2008, **5**(3), 349–58.

6 Hubbell J, Fittkau MH, Zilla P, Bezuidenhout D, Lutolf MP, Human P, Hubbell JA and Davies N, 'The selective modulation of endothelial cell mobility on RGD peptide containing surfaces by YIGSR peptides', *Biomaterials*, 2005, **26**(2), 167–74.

7 Chollet C, Chanseau C, Brouillaud B and Durrieu MC, 'RGD peptides grafting onto poly(ethylene terephthalate) with well controlled densities', *Biomol Eng*, 2007, **24**(5), 477–82.

8 Maddikeri RR, Tosatti M, Schuler S, Textor M, Richards RG and Harris LG, 'Reduced medical infection related bacterial strains adhesion on bioactive RGD modified titanium surfaces: A first step toward cell selective surfaces', *J Biomed Mater Res A*, 2008, **84**(2), 425–35.

9 Schürmann K, Roos A, Meyer J, Ries B, Lahann J, Hermanns B, Kulisch A, Vorwerk D, Klee D and Günther RW, 'A novel hirudin coating of vascular endoprostheses: experimental results', *Rofo*, 2003, **175**(2), 262–70.

10 Kessler Hirschfeld-Warneken VC, Arnold M, Cavalcanti-Adam A, López-García M, Kessler H and Spatz JP, 'Cell adhesion and polarisation on molecularly defined spacing gradient surfaces of cyclic RGDfK peptide patches', *Eur J Cell Biol*, 2008, **87**(8–9), 743–50.
11 Rezania A and Healy KE, 'The effect of peptide surface density on mineralization of a matrix deposited by osteogenic cells', *J Biomed Mater Res*, 2000, **52**(4), 595–600.
12 Belleney J, Helary G and Migonney V, 'Terpolymerization of methyl methacrylate, poy(ethylene glycol) methyl ether methacrylate or poly(ethylene glycol) ethyl ether methacrylate with methacrylic acid and sodium styrene sulfonate: determination of the reactivity ratios', *Eur Polym Journal*, 2002, **38**(3), 439–44.
13 El Khadali F, Hélary G, Pavon-Djavid G and Migonney V, 'Modulating fibroblast cell proliferation with functionalized poly(methyl methacrylate) based copolymers: chemical composition and monomer distribution effect', *Biomacromolecules*, 2002, **3**(1), 51–6.
14 Ciobanu M, Siove A, Gueguen V, Gamble LJ, Castner DG and Migonney V, 'Radical graft polymerization of styrene sulfonate on poly(ethylene terephthalate) films for ACL applications: "grafting from" and chemical characterization', *Biomacromolecules*, 2006, **7**(3), 755–60.
15 Kalinina S, Gliemann H, López-García M, Petershans A, Auernheimer J, Schimmel T, Bruns M, Schambony A, Kessler H and Wedlich D, 'Isothiocyanate-functionalized RGD peptides for tailoring cell-adhesive surface patterns', *Biomaterials*, 2008, **29**(20), 3004–13.
16 Kurtz SM, Ong KL, Schmier J, Mowat F, Saleh K, Dybvik E, Kärrholm J, Garellick G, Havelin LI, Furnes O, Malchau H and Lau E, 'Future clinical and economic impact of revision total hip and knee arthroplasty', *J Bone Joint Surg Am*, 2007, **89**(Suppl 3), 144–51.
17 Kurtz SM, Harrigan TP, Herr M and Manley MT, 'An *in vitro* model for fluid pressurization of screw holes in metal-backed total joint components', *J Arthroplasty*, 2005, **20**(7), 932–8.
18 Nizard R, Pourreyron D, Raould A, Hannouche D and Sedel L, 'Alumina-on-alumina hip arthroplasty in patients younger than 30 years old', *Clin Orthop Relat Res*, 2008, **466**(2), 317–23.
19 Lortat-Jacob A, Desplaces N, Gaudias J, Dacquet V, Dupon M, Carsenti H, Dellamonica P and Groupe Tirésias, 'Secondary infection of joint implants: diagnostic criteria, treatment and prevention', *Rev Chir Orthop Reparatrice Appar Mot*, 2002, **88**(1), 51–61 (Review, French).
20 Belmatoug N, Cremieux AC, Bleton R, Volk A, Saleh-Mghir A, Grossin M, Garry L and Carbon C, 'A new model of experimental prosthetic joint infection due to methicillin-resistant Staphylococcus aureus: a microbiologic, histopathologic, and magnetic resonance imaging characterization', *J Infect Dis*, 1996, **174**, 414–17.
21 Cremieux AC, Saleh-Mghir A, Hélary G and Migonney V, 'Bioactive polymers grafted on silicone to prevent *Staphylococcus Aureus* prosthesis adherence: *in vitro* and *in vivo* study', *J Appl Biomater Biomech*, 2003, **1**, 178–85.
22 Berlot S, Aissaoui Z, Pavon-Djavid G, Belleney J, Jozefowicz M, Helary G and Migonney V, 'Biomimetic poly(methyl methacrylate)-based terpolymers: modulation of bacterial adhesion effect', *Biomacromolecules*, 2002, **3**, 63–8.
23 Pavon-Djavid G, Helary G and Migonney V, 'Les biomatériaux inhibiteurs de l'adhérence et de la prolifération bactérienne: un enjeu pour la prévention des infections sur matériel prothétique', *ITBM-RBM*, 2005, **26**(3), 183–91.

24 Wu C, Ramaswamy Y, Soeparto A and Zreiqat H, 'Incorporation of titanium into calcium silicate improved their chemical stability and biological properties', *J Biomed Mater Res A*, 2008, **86**(2), 402–10.
25 Takemoto M, Fujibayashi S, Neo M, So K, Akiyama N, Matsushita T, Kokubo T and Nakamura T, 'A porous bioactive titanium implant for spinal interbody fusion: an experimental study using a canine model', *J Neurosurg Spine*, 2007, **7**(4), 435–43.
26 Yan C and Xue D, 'General, spontaneous ion replacement reaction for the synthesis of micro- and nanostructured metal oxides', *J Phys Chem B*, 2006, **110**(4), 1581–6.
27 Gill FJ, Planell JA, Padrós A and Aparicio C, 'The effect of shot blasting and heat treatment on the fatigue behaviour of titanium for dental implant applications', *Dent Mater*, 2007, **23**(4), 486–91.
28 Barrabés M, Michiardi A, Aparicio C, Sevilla P, Planell JA and Gil FJ, 'Oxidized nickel–titanium foams for bone reconstructions: chemical and mechanical characterization', *J Mater Sci Mater Med*, 2007 **18**(11), 2123–9.
29 Ramaswamy Y, Wu C, Zhou H and Zreiqat H, 'Biological response of human bone cells to zinc-modified Ca-Si-based ceramics', *Acta Biomater*, 2008, **4**(5), 487–97.
30 Migonney V, Fougnot C and Jozefowicz M, 'Heparin-like tubings. III. Kinetics and mechanism of thrombin, antithrombin III and thrombin-antithrombin complex adsorption under controlled-flow conditions', *Biomaterials*, 1988, **9**(5), 413–8.
31 Migonney V, Fougnot C and Jozefowicz M, 'Heparin-like tubings. II. Mechanism of the thrombin-antithrombin III reaction at the surface, *Biomaterials*, 1988, **9**(3), 230–4.
32 Vaudaux P, Avramoglou T, Letourneur D, Lew DP and Jozefonvicz J, 'Inhibition by heparin and derivatized dextrans of Staphylococcus aureus adhesion to fibronectin-coated biomaterials', *J Biomater Sci Polym Ed*, 1992, **4**, 89–97.
33 Que YA, Francois P, Haefliger JA, Entenza JM, Vaudaux P and Moreillon P, 'Reassessing the role of Staphylococcus aureus clumping factor and fibronectin-binding protein by expression in *Lactococcus lactis*', *Infect Immun*, 2001, **69**, 6296–302.
34 Yammine P, Pavon-Djavid G, Helary G and Migonney V, 'Surface modification of silicone intraocular implants to inhibit cell proliferation', *Biomacromolecules*, 2005, **6**(5), 2630–7.
35 Anagnostou F, Debet A, Pavon-Djavid G, Goudaby Z, Hélary G and Migonney V, 'Osteoblast functions on functionalized PMMA-based polymers exhibiting *Staphylococcus aureus* adhesion inhibition', *Biomaterials*, 2006, **27**(21), 3912–9.
36 Zhou J, Pavon-Djavid G, Anagnostou F and Migonney V, 'Inhibition de l'adhérence de Porphyromonas gingivalis sur la surface de titane greffé de poly(styrene sulfonate de sodium)', *ITBM-RBM*, 2007, **28** (1), 42–8.
37 Latz C, Pavon-Djavid G, Hélary G, Evans MD and Migonney V, 'Alternative intracellular signaling mechanism involved in the inhibitory biological response of functionalized PMMA-based polymers', *Biomacromolecules*, 2003, **4**(3), 766–71.
38 Mayingi J, Hélary G, Noirclere F, Bacroix B and Migonney V, 'Grafting of bioactive polymers onto titanium surfaces and human osteoblasts response', *Conf Proc IEEE Eng Med Biol Soc*, 2007, 5119–22.
39 Noirclère F, Mayingi J, Hélary G and Migonney V, 'A new approach to graft bioactive polymers on titanium implants. Improvement of MG 63 cell differentiation onto this coating', *Acta Biomater*, 2009, **5**(1), 124–33.
40 Migonney V, Hélary G and Noiclère F, *Procédé de greffage de polymères bioactifs sur des matériaux prothétiques*, French Patent no FR 06 05 073, June 2006.

12 Long-term performance and failure of orthopaedic devices

D. TAYLOR, Trinity College Dublin, Ireland

Abstract: Most engineering components fail by long-term failure mechanisms such as fatigue and wear, and orthopaedic devices are no exception. This chapter describes the main types of long-term failure, which are fatigue, creep, wear and corrosion cracking. Corrosion and physiological reactions such as adaptation are also considered. Two detailed case studies are presented to illustrate the design procedures typically used. We have come a long way in ensuring the long-term integrity of materials for orthopaedic use, but many exciting challenges remain.

Key words: artificial hip joint, creep, fatigue, UHMWPE, wear.

12.1 Introduction

Most failures in engineering structures and components do not occur immediately, but after some period of time in service. Medical components such as orthopaedic implants and fracture fixation devices are certainly no exception and the problem of designing against failure in these cases is complicated by the fact that they are expected to function for long periods of time without the possibility of preventative maintenance. Thus the responsibility lies with the designer, who is required to estimate the working life of the component, considering all possible failure modes. This is no easy task given the relatively high stresses and strains which implant components experience and the complex responses of the human body.

Implants such as the artificial hip joint (AHJ) have, in recent years, become extremely reliable by the standards normally accepted for engineering components. Following extensive research and development over a 20-year period, AHJs have reached the point where, at least for some designs, failure rates of less than 5% over ten years can be expected (see, for example, the *Swedish Hip Arthroplasty Register* at www.jru.orthop.gu.se). This success has been largely due to an intensive effort on the part of researchers to understand the various long-term failure mechanisms that were found to occur in early designs and to eliminate these using a combination of improved design, better materials and more careful surgical procedures.

Hip joints are a success story, but major challenges still remain for other implantable devices. More complex joint prostheses such as knees and shoulders still experience significant failure rates and there are major difficulties in predicting the performance of custom-made, one-off implants such as those used for spinal surgery and the repair of complex fractures.

This chapter will begin with an overview of the various types of long-term failure in engineering components, giving examples of their occurrence in orthopaedic devices. After a brief note on stress analysis, two case studies illustrate how particular failure modes can be predicted and prevented. The chapter will conclude with some general remarks about the application of failure analysis and prevention methods in the medical field.

12.2 Long-term failure modes

There are essentially four different types of long-term mechanical failure: fatigue, creep, stress-corrosion cracking and wear. In addition we must consider time-dependent chemical effects (corrosion and biochemical reactions) and the functional adaptation reactions of the human body, especially bone resorption. In this section, each type of failure mode will be introduced. For a more detailed treatment the reader is referred to one of the many excellent textbooks on engineering materials, for example Ashby and Jones (1980). The situation is made more complex by the tendency of these failure modes to interact with each other; thus, for example, wear on the surface of a component can lead on to the creation of fatigue cracks, whose growth can be accelerated by corrosion. Much of our understanding of these interactions has been gained in retrospect, by carefully analysing failures that have occurred *in vivo*.

12.2.1 Fatigue

Fatigue is the most common type of mechanical failure in engineering components in general and certainly occurs often in orthopaedic implants. Fatigue is essentially a cracking process: over a period of time in service, small cracks form in the material and gradually grow. In some cases, such as the intramedullary pin shown in Fig. 12.1, a fatigue crack may become long enough to cause total failure of the component. In other cases the effect of cracking is to compromise function in some way; for example, multiple cracking in bone cement causes loss of fixation between implant and bone, leading to loosening (Jasty *et al.*, 1991).

Why do these cracks form and grow? The physics of the process is quite complex but the essential feature is cyclic stress, that is a stress which changes periodically with time. For example an implant in the leg experiences a stress cycle every time the person takes a step during walking. Higher stress cycles occur less frequently, during running and other strenuous activities and, less obviously, during stair climbing, rising from a chair and accidental stumbles and trips (Bergmann *et al.*, 1993). Even though the maximum stress in the

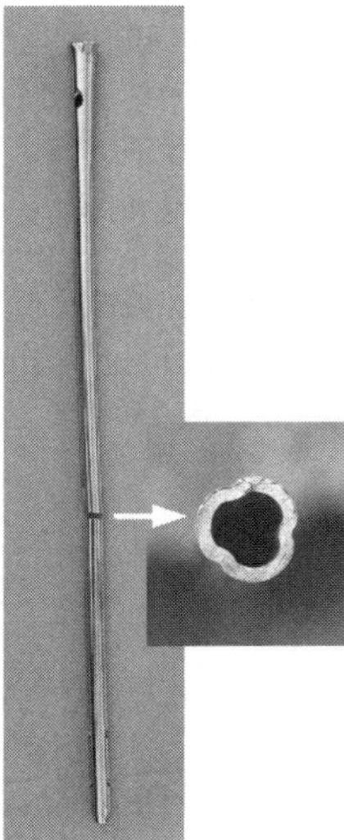

12.1 An intramedullary pin which failed in use owing to fatigue. The insert shows the fracture surface.

cycle is less than the static strength of the material (e.g., less than the ultimate tensile strength), the mere repetition of this cycle, taking the stress off and reapplying it many times, causes microscopic damage processes such as microcracking and non-reversible plasticity, leading to cracks which, once formed, tend to grow because they concentrate stress at their tips (Hertzberg, 1989).

There are two ways to measure and characterise fatigue in a material. The first involves taking a sample of the material and subjecting it to a known cyclic stress. Normally we apply a sinusoidally varying stress of maximum and minimum values σ_{max} and σ_{min}. The test is continued until failure occurs, defined either as complete fracture of the specimen or a significant loss of stiffness owing to the presence of large cracks. Data are plotted as shown in Fig. 12.2(a): the number of cycles to failure N_f as a function of the stress range, Dσ, defined as $\sigma_{max} - \sigma_{min}$. The mean stress (average of σ_{max} and σ_{min}) is also important, though less important than Dσ. Another way to define the cycle (rather than using mean stress) is the stress ratio $R = \sigma_{min}/\sigma_{max}$. In most orthopaedic components, σ_{min} corresponds to the stress in the component at rest and so is close to zero, therefore R will also be close to zero.

This test data is known as an *S*/*N* curve or stress–life curve; in many European countries it is referred to as a Wohler curve after an early pioneer of fatigue research. Its use is fairly obvious: given a certain life requirement (i.e. the total number of cycles to be experienced) one can find a safe operating stress range. This is referred to as the fatigue strength of the material. For

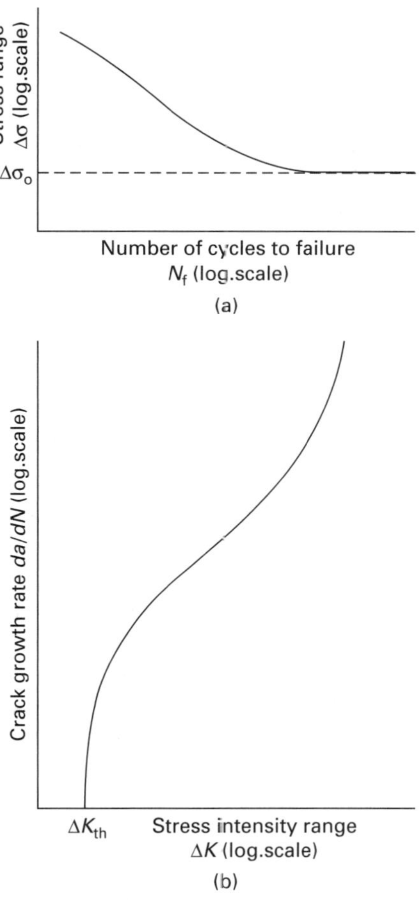

12.2 Fatigue test data is usually expressed in terms of (a) the number of cycles to failure as a function of the applied stress range, or (b) the crack growth rate as a function of applied stress intensity range. Logarithmic scales are normally used: in each case one can define a lower limit (the fatigue strength $\Delta\sigma_0$ or the crack growth threshold ΔK_{th}) below which fatigue failure will not occur.

implantable devices, we are generally interested in very large numbers of cycles, in excess of one million, so it is fortunate that the *S*/*N* curve tends to become more or less horizontal for N_f values in the range 10^6–10^7 cycles, allowing us to define a fatigue limit. Actually, recent research has shown that for some materials the curve can bend downwards again at very high numbers of cycles, resulting in lower fatigue strengths for lives greater than 10^9 cycles which may be relevant for some applications such as cardiovascular stents (cyclically loaded by the beating heart) but probably not for orthopaedic devices.

The fatigue process can be much accelerated if the material already contains cracks or other defects introduced during manufacturing, because the time taken for cracks to initiate is effectively bypassed. Design features which concentrate stress, such as notches and sharp corners, have a similar effect. So it is also useful to carry out tests on specimens which are pre-cracked, measuring the rate of crack growth, defined as the increase in crack length *a* per cycle, usually written d*a*/d*N*. As might be expected, d*a*/d*N* is a function of the applied stress range, but it is also a function of the length of the crack. These two parameters are combined to form the stress intensity range, D*K*; the theoretical derivation of this parameter is beyond the scope of this chapter. The interested reader is referred to textbooks on engineering materials (Ashby and Jones, 1980; Hertzberg, 1989) or fracture mechanics (Janssen *et al.*, 2002). As Fig. 12.2(b) shows, D*K* correlates to the crack growth rate (d*a*/d*N* is also a function of *R* although this is not shown here) so that, knowing the applied stress and crack length, one can estimate how fast the crack will grow at any given point in time and thus, by integration, predict the total life of a pre-cracked component. This approach is commonly used in those structures which can make use of crack-growth monitoring through regular inspection, such as aircraft. Currently this is not possible for orthopaedic devices but the approach can still be a useful way to assess the effect of manufacturing defects and design features. For a more thorough treatment of the effect of stress concentrations in engineering components, the reader is referred to another recent publication (Taylor, 2007).

12.2.2 Wear

Wear, defined as the removal of material caused by contact and relative motion between two surfaces, is a major problem for joint implants such as the hip and knee. The physics of the problem is more complex than for fatigue because there are many different mechanisms of wear. More details can be found in textbooks devoted to the subject of tribology; a recent article by Jin *et al.* gives a very useful introduction to the tribology of implants (Jin *et al.*, 2006). The underlying causes, however, are always the same: if two components are placed in contact, with a relatively low nominal stress between them (defined as the compressive load divided by the contact area), then high local stresses exist owing to the fact that no surface is perfectly flat. At high magnification (Fig. 12.3) the surfaces will be seen to make contact only at their highest points, local stresses can exceed the stress needed to cause yielding or cracking in the material. If relative motion now occurs between the surfaces, shearing forces will cause small particles to break free from one or both surfaces.

If one material is much softer than the other, for example the metal/polymer and ceramic/polymer combinations that are common in joint implants, then

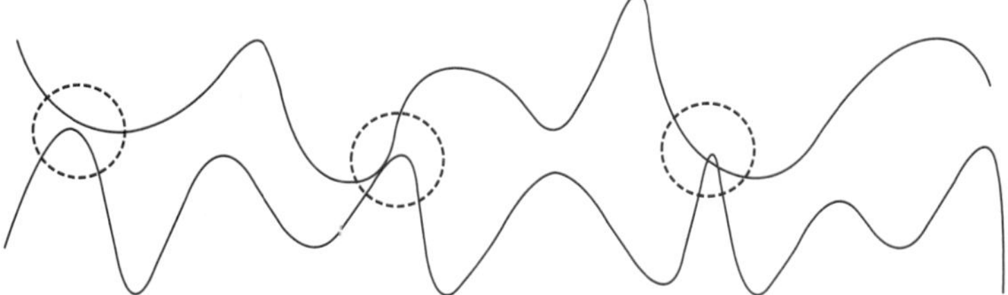

12.3 At high magnification any surface will appear rough, therefore two opposing surfaces will only come into contact at isolated points, where the local stresses will be very high, causing wear.

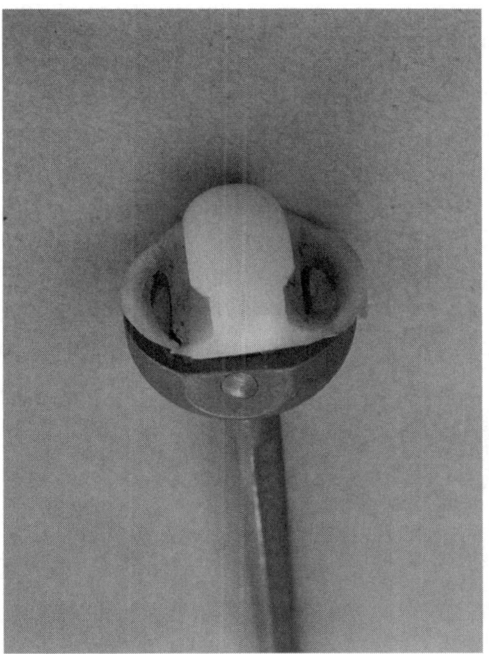

12.4 Excessive wear in an early type of knee joint (the Sheehan knee). In places the polymer material that forms the tibial bearing surface has completely worn away, revealing the metal below. Despite improvements over the years, this kind of massive wear still occurs from time to time in modern knee joints.

abrasive wear occurs in which the harder component ploughs up the softer one, removing material in the form of wear debris. Figure 12.4 shows an example of excessive wear in an early knee joint design: in this case a 4 mm-thick layer of polymer bearing surface has been completely worn away over a period of several years in use, revealing the metal component beneath. Such examples of massive removal of material still occur in knee joints, though thankfully they are less common today. Another mechanism of wear – common in engineering components though not so much in orthopaedic applications – results from local adhesion between the two surfaces, producing wear debris by local fractures when motion occurs. This adhesive wear mechanism usually occurs if the two materials are similar, for example stainless steel screws used to attach a stainless steel fracture plate.

Failures that occur after relatively long periods of time, in good-quality materials chosen for their ability to resist mechanisms such as abrasive and adhesive wear, tend to occur via a fatigue mechanism. Near-surface material is cyclically loaded, for example on each walking step, leading to the creation of small fatigue cracks, usually lying just below the surface. These cracks can grow up to the surface, causing a large piece of material to spall off; alternatively they can grow down through the part, leading to a fatigue failure. Figure 12.5 shows an example of the latter: a knee joint in which the polyethylene component was completely worn through, causing contact between two metal components (the tibial tray and the femoral condyles). A shiny wear patch is visible, from the edge of which a fatigue crack has formed, causing part of the tibial tray to break off. This synergistic combination of wear and fatigue is called fretting fatigue; more details of this kind of failure can be found in specialized engineering publications, for example Lindley (2004).

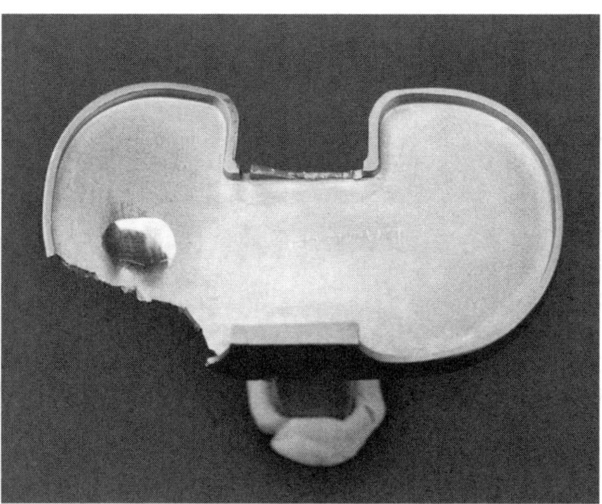

12.5 Fretting fatigue in the tibial tray of a knee joint, seen after removal of the polymer liner. Massive wear of the polymer (as illustrated in Fig.12.4) has resulted in metal-on-metal contact, forming the bright wear patch on the metal surface. Fatigue cracking at the edge of the wear patch has caused part of the tibial tray to detach.

Wear is usually measured in tests such as the pin-on-disc test in which the end of a stationary pin is pressed up against a rotating disc of material. The amount of material removed is calculated by measuring or weighing the parts, allowing one to define a wear rate. Clearly this wear rate will be affected not only by the properties of the base materials but also by surface properties such as roughness. Wear problems are often addressed by modifying the surface via coatings and other treatments, because properties that prevent wear (such as high hardness) are often undesirable in the bulk material.

12.2.3 Creep

In general, the strain experienced by a material is a function not only of the applied stress, but also of the time for which the stress acts. All solid materials possess, to varying degrees, the ability to flow. Therefore, if a constant stress is applied, the strain (be it elastic or plastic) will gradually increase with time. The physical mechanisms at work here are complex and varied but essentially one can say that the material, though solid, possesses some of the properties of a liquid. Not surprisingly then, this effect increases at higher temperatures, as the melting point of the material is approached. A rough rule of thumb is that time-dependent effects are negligible at temperatures less than one-third of the material's melting point (measured in degrees Kelvin). Therefore, at physiological temperatures, metals and ceramics do not display this effect, whilst polymers invariably do.

The phenomenon whereby elastic strain changes with time is termed viscoelasticity; one result is that the measured elastic modulus (also called Youngs modulus, E) becomes a function of the applied strain rate during the test. Removing the applied load will cause the strain to return to zero, but this now will take some finite time. Viscoplasticity refers to a time-dependent change in plastic strain. This is also called creep but the terminology here is somewhat confusing, with polymer scientists frequently using the term creep to apply to both elastic and plastic strain. In fact, it is often difficult to distinguish between the elastic and plastic components, given that the elastic recovery may take a very long time. A typical creep test involves measuring the total strain as a function of time for a constant applied stress.

Figure 12.6 shows typical results: the form of the curve is complex but a creep strain rate can be defined, which will of course be a function of the applied stress and also the temperature. If sufficient plastic strain develops, then complete fracture can occur; more insidiously, creep causes gradual deformation in a structure which can compromise its function. For example, in the AHJ creep in the bone cement (which is a polymer, polymethylmethacrylate PMMA) causes a slow movement of the metal component in the distal direction, termed subsidence. Some prostheses are deliberately designed to subside initially, becoming firmly wedged in place

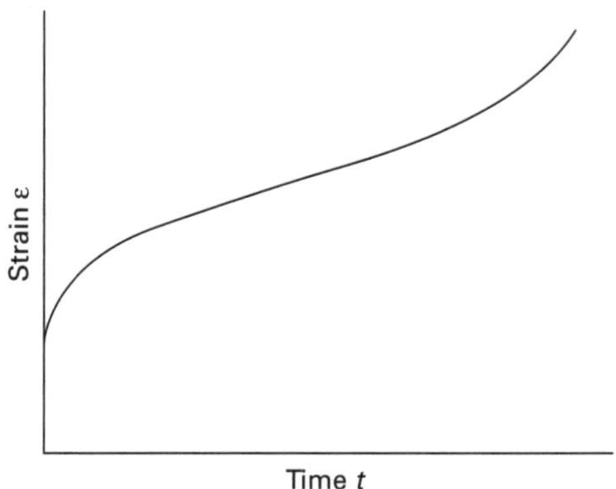

12.6 Creep data is typically recorded in terms of the strain in a sample as a function of time. Some instantaneous elastic strain is followed by a gradual accumulation of plastic strain, until failure occurs.

as time goes on, but in most prostheses subsidence is a bad thing and, in fact, the rate of early subsidence (measured radiographically) has been used as a predictor of eventual failure (Perillo-Marcone *et al.*, 2004). Human body tissues (bone and, to a much greater extent, soft tissues) are subject to creep effects, which must be taken into account when conducting stress analysis of implants (see below).

12.2.4 Stress-corrosion cracking

Stress-corrosion cracking (SCC) has some similarities with fatigue, in that it involves the creation and growth of cracks. The difference is that, whilst in fatigue the essential ingredient is a cyclic stress, SCC can occur under a constant stress, because of interactions between the stress and the chemical environment. Fortunately, SCC only happens under some very specific combinations of material and environment. However, several of those combinations are commonly present in medical devices. For example, stainless steels are susceptible to SCC in saline solutions and some polymers display the phenomenon in the presence of iodine. Ceramic materials, although characterized by chemical inertness, nevertheless can experience SCC. Ceramicists refer to this phenomenon by the rather confusing name of static fatigue.

In principle one can measure SCC in simple tests similar to those used for measuring fatigue: a sample of material can be exposed to a constant stress along with a chemical environment, the time to failure can be recorded, as can the growth rate of cracks. However, it is very difficult to predict SCC in real applications. This is because it proceeds by a variety of different mechanisms and involves a very intimate synergy between the mechanical and chemical factors. So, for example, the rate of growth of a crack may be strongly influenced by the pH of the corroding solution, but this pH will itself change in the rather stagnant region inside the crack. Thus even measuring the local chemical conditions can be a challenge. Normally designers approach this problem by avoiding it, choosing to use material/environment combinations which are not susceptible to SCC. However, there have been some notable exceptions, for example Fig. 12.7 shows a laparoscopic forceps which failed in use: the particular stainless steel alloy was found to be very susceptible to SCC in the presence of chloride ions.

For more detailed discussion of the above issues the reader is referred to some excellent textbooks which compare the various types of mechanical failure and give many examples of their occurrence in engineering components (Wulpi, 1985; ASM, 2002).

12.2.5 Other chemical effects and physiological reactions

It goes without saying that we avoid using materials inside the body if they are known to react strongly with the physiological environment, causing loss of material by corrosion or releasing substances which are toxic. But we should acknowledge the fact that there is probably no material in existence which is completely inert when placed in the human body. Titanium, for example, although it functions very well as an implant material, certainly reacts, as evidenced by the staining of surrounding tissues. Fatigue in most materials is often accelerated by the presence of a chemical environment,

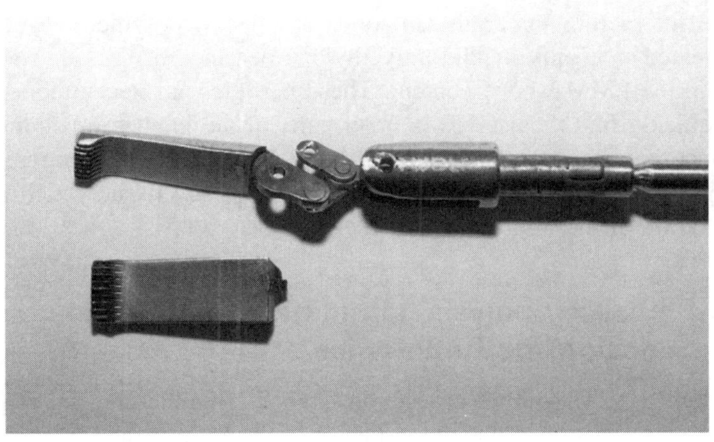

12.7 A laparoscopic forceps which failed during use by stress-corrosion cracking.

leading to so-called corrosion fatigue which is a much more ubiquitous phenomenon than SCC.

Many new materials like bioceramics have indeed been deliberately designed to interact with the body. These are often used as coatings, which work by encouraging bone formation on the surface of an implant; in some cases the original coating is designed to be resorbed by the body and replaced by living tissue. Another example of a reactive material which has a long history is bone graft: a material designed to temporarily fill a defect such as a hole in a fractured bone. Bone graft materials include ground-up pieces of human bone and artificial substitutes based on calcium compounds similar to the body's own, such as hydroxyapatite or tricalcium phosphate. These materials have very inferior mechanical properties but, provided the defect is not too large, they can support the structure for long enough (a few weeks or months) until they are replaced by living bone.

The body's ability to create new bone to fill a defect is just one example of the more general phenomenon of functional adaptation, whereby the structure and properties of bone, and indeed of almost all living tissues, change in response to the mechanical environment. This important phenomenon will be dealt with in another chapter of this book; clearly it must be taken into account when predicting the long-term integrity of implants. One example, which will be discussed below, is the resorption of bone that can occur close to a joint implant as a result of 'stress shielding' by the rather stiff metallic material.

Finally, mention should be made of the important interactions between wear and physiological reactions, because they are the cause of some modes of long-term failure in joint implants which are becoming increasingly important as the lifetime of these implants increases. As mentioned above, wear processes create wear debris: small particles removed from the surfaces of the interacting materials. In joint prostheses, polymer wear particles are created, not only on the polyethylene bearing surfaces, but also from wear in the PMMA bone cement. These particles are very mobile and can very quickly find themselves in other parts of the joint, for example on the interface between bone cement and bone, where they can initiate adverse reactions, leading to the formation of a layer of soft tissue which threatens the fixation of the implant (Ingham and Fisher, 2005).

12.3 Stress analysis, simulations and other design methodologies

Before moving on to some case studies, it is worth reflecting on what will be needed in order to use the above information in a practical way. Assuming that we have access to material data from the various tests mentioned above, this will only be of value if we also know what stresses our materials will be subjected to in service and for what durations: this is known as the stress history of the component. The general situation with regard to stress analysis for engineering components has been greatly aided by the development of computer simulations, especially finite element analysis (FEA) and multi-body analysis. Thanks to these tools and to the increasing power of computers, we can estimate with reasonable accuracy the stresses that arise in many engineering structures, such as a girder in a bridge or a suspension component in a car. The same technology can also be applied to predict the stress histories of orthopaedic devices, but not with the same level of accuracy.

There are a number of reasons for this. First, a typical implant has several mechanical features which, whilst they can be simulated using FEA, create problems which reduce accuracy. These include the presence of interfaces in contact, in conditions in which the properties of the interface (e.g. the friction coefficient) are not well known, and the existence of materials which have anisotropic properties (such as bone) and time dependent properties (such as bone cement and soft biological tissues). Second, the exact geometry of the body components (e.g. the diameter of the medullary cavity of the bone) is poorly known, difficult to measure and varies from one person to another. Third, there is considerable uncertainly about the boundary conditions of the model, for example the forces provided by the various muscle groups surrounding a joint. Finally, unlike the engineering components mentioned above, there is limited scope for conducting experimental measurements that would act as validations of the computer simulations. Significant progress in this area has been made by Bergmann and co-workers who have provided data from instrumented implants *in vivo* (Bergmann *et al.*, 1993).

All this is not to say that computer simulations are useless, far from it. They have provided us with important insights, helped us to understand failures after they have occurred and prevented mistakes being made in new designs. But we should regard these simulations as providing useful general indications of the stresses and strains that arise in components, rather than precise, quantitative results.

The stress history of a component will also tell us about the number of cycles it experiences. Of course this is something which varies considerably from person to person, depending on activity level and lifestyle. For general design purposes, some workers have defined typical activity levels in terms of the number of load cycles per day for walking, running and so on. For example, Table 12.1 gives some data from Whalen *et al.* (1988). We might reasonably assume that a person who has received a joint implant such as an AHJ would be content with a sedentary lifestyle, consisting mainly of low-stress cycles arising from slow walking. However, this author has come across one person who continued working on his farm after receiving an AHJ and another who was very fond of Irish dancing: in fact both of these returned to hospital with fatigue failures in their implants. One major issue in joint implants is the requirement to use them for younger, more active people, who are victims of accidents or early onset arthritis. The magnitude of this problem is realized when one notes, as shown in Table 12.1, that the forces (and therefore stresses) involved in running are much higher than those sustained during slow walking.

12.4 Case study 1: fatigue design in the artificial hip joint

This author makes no apology for returning frequently to the AHJ in this chapter. Because, whilst it was mentioned in the Introduction that the problem of failure in this implant has to a considerable extent been solved, this is thanks to the large body of research which has been conducted and which therefore makes this an excellent example to study. Furthermore, the lessons learned on the hip joint can certainly be applied (though with some additional complications) to other implants and to orthopaedic devices in general.

The development of the AHJ was greatly aided by studies, mostly conducted in the 1980s, which considered the interaction of component shape and material properties in determining the stresses in the implant and ultimately the long-term integrity of the chosen design (Prendergast *et al.*, 1989; Fagan and Lee, 1986; Rohlmann *et al.*, 1987). Figure 12.8(a) shows some results synthesised from these various studies, which illustrate the behaviour of a

Table 12.1 Activity levels as defined by Whalen *et al.* (1988)

Activity	Slow walking (hr/day)	Normal walking (hr/day)	Fast walking (hr/day)	Slow jogging (hr/day)	Distance running (hr/day)
Sedentary	4				
Sedentary plus exercise	4			0.67	
Normal		4	4		
Active		4	8		
Active plus exercise		4	8	0.67	
Athletic		4	4		0.75

Action	Frequency (cycles min^{-1})	Force (normalised by the single-leg stance force)
Slow walking	35	1.01
Normal walking	51	1.17
Fast walking	68	1.33
Slow jogging	84	1.7
Distance running	91	2.62

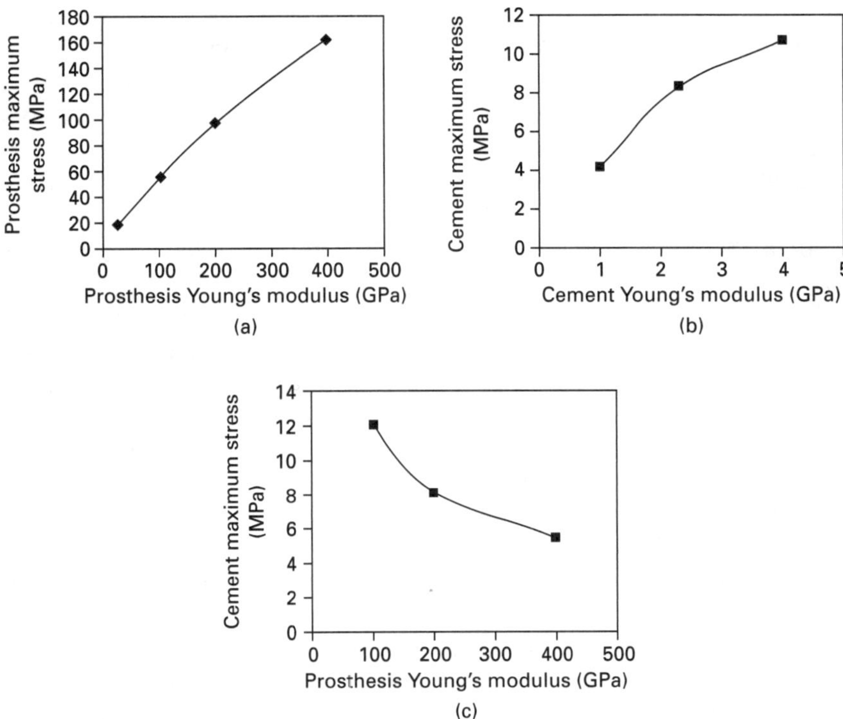

12.8 Results from stress analysis of the artificial hip joint using finite element analysis (Prendergast *et al.*, 1989). (a) The maximum stress in the stem as a function of the Young's modulus (E) of the stem material. (b) The maximum stress in the bone cement as a function of the E value of the cement. (c) The maximum stress in the cement as a function of the E value of the stem. All results obtained for an input load of 3 kN at the femoral head.

typical hip joint. The figure shows the maximum stress experienced in the stem part of the implant, that is, the part which inserts into the femur. The applied force is assumed to be 3 kN, which would be the typical maximum force during walking. By varying the elastic modulus of the implant material we can see how the maximum stress changes when different materials are used. Such analyses have been performed for many different AHJ designs and, despite some variations, they all present the same picture: the stress increases with the elastic modulus (Young's modulus) in a manner which is close to a simple proportionality.

Why should this be? For a component of constant shape, loaded with a constant force, we would not expect the stress to change with the Young's modulus of the material, at least provided the overall deflections are quite small, which they will be in this case. The reason for the effect seen here is that we are dealing with a structure containing more than one material.

The prosthesis stem is inserted into a tube of bone which is relatively stiff, by virtue of its thickness, rather than its Young's modulus. The amount by which this tube bends is determined by the applied load and is almost unchanged by changes in the prosthesis material. Now, since the prosthesis stem is located inside the bone tube, it is forced to bend by the same amount as the tube. Knowing this, we can appreciate that if the prosthesis is made from a relatively stiff material, then high stresses will arise in it. We say that the prosthesis material is under strain control whilst the bone is under stress control.

Figure 12.8(b) shows the maximum stress in the bone cement, as a function of its Young's modulus, assuming a constant Young's modulus for the prosthesis material of 200 GPa. There are various FE analyses in the literature and they show much greater variation in cement stress values than in the prosthesis stress values shown above (see Prendergast *et al.*, 1989 for a summary). Here, this author has deliberately chosen results which give rather high stresses. This variation is largely caused by changes in prosthesis design (some designs cause high local stress concentrations in the bone) and also by variations in the thickness of the cement layer. The data in Fig. 12.8(b) also show an increase of stress with material stiffness, however there is a significant downwards curvature of the line, implying conditions which are intermediate between strain control and stress control. To complete the picture, Fig. 12.8(c) shows that the stress in the cement material (using here a normal PMMA bone cement with $E = 2.3$ GPa) decreases with increasing prosthesis stiffness. This is to be expected since the stress is essentially being shared between the prosthesis and the cement, so if the prosthesis takes more, the cement will have less.

We can use these figures to compare different materials with regard to their long-term performance in the AHJ. For example, Table 12.2 shows a comparison of the fatigue behaviour of some prosthesis materials, calculated by dividing the fatigue limit of each material by the maximum stress to give a safety factor. As well as traditional metallic materials, included here are

Table 12.2 Safety factors for various AHJ stem materials (using standard bone cement)

Material	Young's modulus (GPa)	Fatigue limit (MPa)	Maximum stress in stem (MPa)	Safety factor
Particulate composite	25	30	18	1.7
Fibre composite	50	120	31	3.9
Titanium alloy	100	550	56	9.8
CoCr alloy (cast)	200	300	98	3.1
CoCr alloy (wrought)	200	670	98	6.8
Stainless steel	200	420	98	4.3

two interesting non-metallic candidates: a carbon fibre composite material made using long, continuous fibres and a particulate-reinforced composite material which is interesting because its Young's modulus is similar to that of bone itself.

In theory, all of these materials are suitable for this application because all the factors of safety are greater than unity. However, we should remember that, as discussed above, the accuracy of this analysis is quite low, so materials which give a factor of safety less than 2 should certainly be treated with suspicion, which rules out the particulate composite. The most interesting result from this analysis is that the titanium alloy, though it does not have the highest fatigue limit, does have the highest safety factor, by virtue of its relatively low Young's modulus. The fibre composite material seems to be a plausible candidate, especially because a low Young's modulus is attractive for other reasons (see below), and indeed some AHJs have been made from carbon fibre composites (Christel *et al.*, 1987). The problem is that, in order to get a reasonably high fatigue limit, it is necessary to have long fibres and to arrange them so that they are aligned with the principal stress axes, not an easy task in this rather complex, three-dimensional component.

Almost all cemented hip implants use the same bone cement material, a rather poor-quality version of PMMA. As Table 12.3 shows, this has a low safety factor which accords well with the fact that cement failure is a major cause of loosening. One might consider improving the cement by adding reinforcing fibres and this indeed has been attempted (Pilliar *et al.*, 1976). However Table 12.3 would predict no improvement in the fatigue situation and possibly even a slight disimprovement, because the increase in fatigue limit is less than the increase in stiffness. Rubber would seem to be a much better material and, indeed, with regard to fatigue it would be; however rubber would be unsuitable because it would creep, leading to massive subsidence of the prosthesis. Attempts to improve PMMA by adding particles of rubber have encountered the same type of problem. Given these findings, it is perhaps not surprising that the bone cement of choice for most orthopaedic surgeons has not changed significantly in the last 20 years.

Table 12.3 Safety factors for various AHJ cement materials (using a prosthesis stem with $E = 200$ GPa)

Material	Young's modulus (GPa)	Fatigue limit (MPa)	Maximum stress in stem (MPa)	Safety factor
Standard PMMA	2.3	12	8.4	1.4
PMMA with short carbon fibres added	5.5	16	13	1.7
Rubber	0.1	30	0.4	75

It should be pointed out that the mechanical properties used in this analysis are typical, approximate values only. These properties, especially the fatigue limit, can vary significantly with the chemical composition of the material and manufacturing route used. The objective here was to show that the problem of materials selection for an orthopaedic implant can be approached in a rational, quantitative manner.

12.5 Case study 2: wear in ultra-high molecular weight polyethylene

The choice of materials for the bearing surfaces of joint arthroplasties presents considerable challenges, because these bearings will be subjected to relatively high loads and large motions and are required to function without maintenance for several decades. The most common solution is a metal-on-polymer bearing in which the metal component (for example the femoral condyles of the artificial knee joint) articulates on a nominally stationary plastic liner. Ultra-high molecular weight polyethylene (UHMWPE) is by far the most popular choice for the liner material. This material, originally developed in the 1950s, was quickly adopted for use in early hip joint designs, after an initial flirtation with PTFE proved disastrous: PTFE, although it has a lower coefficient of friction, has a much higher rate of wear. UHMWPE is a modification of the common thermoplastic polyethylene; it owes its mechanical performance to its particularly long polymer chains.

Measurement of the tribological properties of a material, such as friction and wear, is much more complex than the measurement of some other properties such as yield strength or fatigue limit. The reason is that many more factors come into play, some of which are difficult to control or quantify. Simple wear tests usually involve a sample of one material being pressed against the flat, moving face of another. For example, in the pin-on-disc test, wear is created in a flat-ended pin by pressing it against a rotating disc. The amount of wear is most conveniently measured by weighing the pin periodically. Results can be reported in terms of the loss of weight DW or volume DV as a function of the total sliding distance d (i.e. the speed of the moving part multiplied by the time) and the applied load P. These parameters can be combined to produce the so-called wear factor, k, as follows:

$$k = \frac{\Delta V}{Pd} \qquad [12.1]$$

Typical units for k are mm^3/Nm. The use of this normalization implies that the amount of wear is controlled by the applied load between the two components and not the applied stress. At first this seems counterintuitive: one would expect more wear to occur if the contact area was reduced, increasing the pressure between the two surfaces. What equation [12.1] implies is that this effect is exactly cancelled out by the fact that the area available for wearing has also reduced. This convenient relationship is not always correct but seems to be obeyed closely enough in most practical situations. In any case for joint arthroplasty studies it is possible to use loads and areas of contact which are similar in magnitude to those in the actual joints, so we don't need to rely too heavily on this relationship when comparing the test data to the real situation. The other implication of equation [12.1] is that the wear rate is constant, with always the same amount of material being removed per metre of sliding. Although this does sometimes occur, in practice it is quite common for wear rates to be initially high, often settling down to more constant values as the test proceeds. This is a reflection of changes in various influential factors, such as the lubrication conditions, the roughness of the two surfaces and the presence of particles of wear debris which can themselves contribute to further removal of material.

Whilst the results obtained from pin-on-disc machines and other simple test devices are useful for giving a general idea of wear rates and for comparing different materials, it is generally agreed that realistic data can only be obtained using test equipment which reproduces more accurately the geometry and loading conditions of real arthroplasties. Some workers have developed systems which try to reproduce some aspects of the true contact conditions (Schwartz and Bahadur, 2007) but most people accept the fact that there is no substitute for testing actual joint implants loaded under conditions which closely simulate real-life conditions. The design of these simulators involves considerable ingenuity: Fig. 12.9 shows a well-respected example, the Stanmore knee-joint simulator (Walker *et al.*, 1997). One major reason

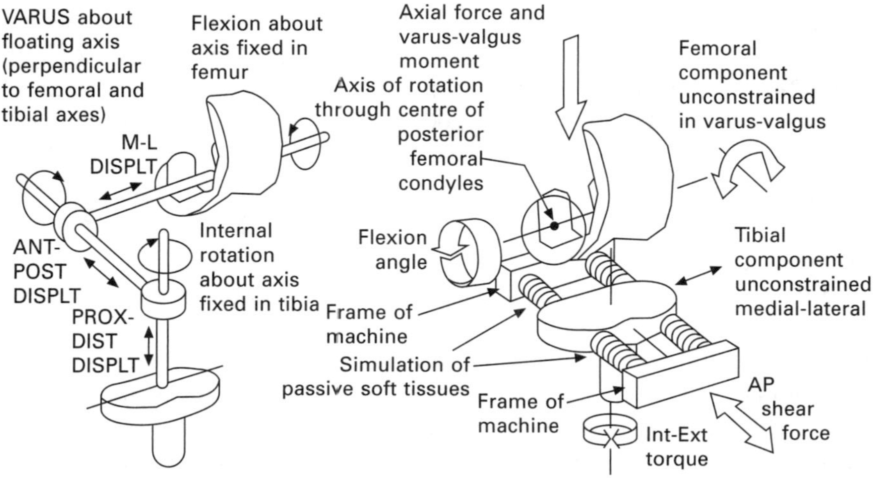

12.9 An example of a joint simulator: the Stanmore knee simulator (Walker *et al.*, 1997), reproduced with permission.

for the difference in results between simple tests and simulators is the local lubrication condition, determined by the exact geometry of the two parts (and especially of the gap between them) and their precise motions (which affect the flow of fluid in the gap).

A typical wear factor for modern UHMWPE in contact with metal is 10^{-7} mm^3/Nm. What does this equate to in terms of loss of material in a joint implant? A typical hip joint will lose about 40 mm^3 of material for every million cycles; given that we typically walk 2 million cycles per year this is quite a lot of material to lose. The wearing away of the joint surface corresponds to about 0.1 mm of depth lost per year, which is just about acceptable for a joint that might be used for several decades, since the total thickness of the polymer liner is typically 5–15 mm. A more worrying aspect of this wear is the large number of particles produced, which contribute to loosening as a result of adverse physiological reactions (see above). The study of wear debris, its size and morphology and how these factors affect physiological responses, is a major area of current research (Jin *et al.*, 2006).

Modifications to the material can have profound effects on wear rate; for example a home-made version of UHMWPE gave wear rates which were a hundred times higher than commercially made material (Roy Chowdhury *et al.*, 2004). A major factor of recent concern is the oxidation of UHMWPE which occurs following sterilization with ionizing radiation. Oxidation occurs over long periods of time, whether the device is in storage or in use, causing the material to become embrittled and to crack easily. A particularly insidious feature of this oxidation reaction is that it occurs preferentially sub-surface, leading to a brittle layer about 1 mm below the surface. Cyclic stresses caused by bearing contact act on this layer, causing cracks by a fatigue mechanism. Eventually these cracks break through to the surface, causing large pieces of material to be lost. Once begun, this process accelerates quickly, leading to massive loss of material in a relatively short time. Rimnac and Kurtz provide a useful overview of this problem (Rimnac and Kurtz, 2005). Reggiani *et al.* (2007) present data for a particular case showing the effect of long periods of storage and Burroughs and co-workers suggest a treatment to reduce oxidation effects which promises a fourfold reduction in wear rates (Burroughs and Blanchet, 2006), at least in pin-on-disc tests.

A new form of UHMWPE, much more highly crosslinked than previous versions, shows considerably less wear in simulator studies and appears to be promising (Herrera *et al.*, 2007), although the improvements are rather less impressive when tested against rougher metal surfaces (Galvin *et al.*, 2006). On the subject of roughness, Des Jardins *et al.* (2006) investigated the role of hyaluronic acid, which is known to be present in joint spaces in the body. Adding this to the lubricating fluid used in the simulator caused corrosion of the Co/Cr alloy head, leading to pitting and roughening of the surface which was similar to that observed clinically. There was a significant increase in wear rate as a result.

Design issues also arise in the context of wear prevention. Different knee joint designs can give rise to greatly varying amounts of wear: even quite subtle design changes can be significant (Mueller-Rath *et al.*, 2007). The history of knee joint design has seen a gradual move away from rather fixed, rigid designs to looser, more mobile implants which more closely reproduce the motions of the natural joint. An inevitable effect of this, however, is an increase in the number and complexity of motions across load-bearing surfaces. Jennings *et al.* (2007) noticed that, in some artificial knee joints, the femoral condyles actually lift off the plastic surface of the tibia: simulator experiments showed that this caused a more than threefold increase in wear rates.

One simple design change, which at first seems counterintuitive, is the reduction of wear in the hip joint by reducing the diameter of the femoral head. This will increase the compressive stress across the joint, but as noted above, it is the load, not the stress, which controls the wear rate. But reducing the head will reduce the sliding distance for a given angular motion of the femur, so we can expect the amount of wear to reduce in proportion to head size. Of course, if we take this too far we will create other problems for ourselves. The high local stresses may cause creep in the polymer, for example; we should always bear in mind that a design change which prevents one type of failure may encourage another. A recent paper by McEwan *et al.* (2005) is recommended for a good comparative study of wear in the knee, showing the interacting effects of design, materials and kinematics.

12.6 Conclusions and future trends

There have been some great successes in the development of implants during the last few decades: examples are hip joints, dental implants and stents. These devices all moved from basic concepts to mass-produced products within a 20-year period. The scientists and engineers who worked on these developments are certainly to be congratulated for quickly overcoming a host of problems which had not previously been faced in other medical devices or in any other kinds of engineering components, for that matter. But many new challenges lie ahead.

Tissue engineering has been suggested as an approach for the fabrication of implants, but progress from laboratory studies to clinical products has been much slower than expected. Certainly the future will see implants which are more active, which integrate more fully with the body's living system. We are already familiar with bioactive coatings on implants, and a great variety of active ceramic and polymeric materials are currently being developed. However, it is worth remembering that implants are often used because the body's own systems have broken down and are no longer able to provide the appropriate materials – cartilage on joint surfaces for example – and that traditional metallic materials such as titanium alloys and stainless steels provide a level of strength and toughness which are unlikely to be matched by any new non-metallic materials. The level of engineering skill which is now being applied to the design and validation of implants is very impressive, including not only 'hard' skills in mechanics, materials and manufacturing technology but also 'soft' skills such as the use of sophisticated optimization methods and pre-clinical testing philosophies. Implant technology has truly developed as a separate and distinct branch of biomedical engineering.

12.7 References

Ashby, M.F. and Jones, D.R.H. (1980) *Engineering Materials*. Pergamon, Oxford, UK.

ASM (2002) *Failure Analysis and Prevention*. ASM International, Ohio USA.

Bergmann, G., Graichen, F. and Rohlmann, A. (1993) 'Hip joint loading during walking and running, measured in two patients', *Journal of Biomechanics*, **26**, 969–90.

Burroughs, B.R. and Blanchet, T.A. (2006) 'The effect of pre-irradiation vacuum storage on the oxidation and wear of radiation sterilized UHMWPE'. *Wear*, **261**, 1277–84.

Christel, P., Meunier, A., Leclercq, S., Bouquet, P. and Buttazzoni, B. (1987) 'Development of a carbon-carbon hip prosthesis'. *Journal of Biomedical Materials Research*, **21**, 191–218.

Des Jardins, J., Aurora, A., Tanner, S.L., Pace, T.B., Acampora, K.B. and LaBerge, M. (2006) 'Increased total knee arthroplasty ultra-high molecular weight polyethylene wear using a clinically relevant hyaluronic acid simulator lubricant'. *Proceedings of the Institution of Mechanical Engineers, Part H: Journal of Engineering in Medicine*, **220**, 609–23.

Fagan, M.J. and Lee, A.J.C. (1986) 'Material selection in the design of the femoral component of cemented total hip replacements'. *Clinical Materials*, **1**, 151–67.

Galvin, A., Kang, L., Tipper, J., Stone, M., Ingham, E., Jin, Z. and Fisher, J. (2006) 'Wear of crosslinked polyethylene under different tribological conditions'. *Journal of Materials Science: Materials in Medicine*, **17**, 235–43.

Herrera, L., Lee, R., Longaray, J., Essner, A. and Wang, A. (2007) 'Hip simulator evaluation of the effect of femoral head size on sequentially cross-linked acetabular liners'. *Wear*, **263**, 1034–7.

Hertzberg, R.W. (1989) *Deformation and Fracture Mechanics of Engineering Materials*. Wiley, New York.

Ingham, E. and Fisher, J. (2005) 'The role of macrophages in osteolysis of total joint replacement'. *Biomaterials*, **26**, 1271–86.

Janssen, M., Zuidema, J. and Wanhill, R. (2002) *Fracture Mechanics*. Spon Press, London, UK.

Jasty, M., Maloney, W.J., Bragdon, C.R., O'Connor, D.O., Haire, T. and Harris, W.H. (1991) 'The initiation of failure in cemented femoral components of hip arthroplasties'. *Journal of Bone and Joint Surgery – Series B*, **73**, 551–8.

Jennings, L.M., Bell, C.J., Ingham, E., Komistek, R.D., Stone, M.H. and Fisher, J. (2007) 'The influence of femoral condylar lift-off on the wear of artificial knee joints'. *Proceedings of the Institution of Mechanical Engineers, Part H: Journal of Engineering in Medicine*, **221**, 305–14.

Jin, Z.M., Stone, M., Ingham, E. and Fisher, J. (2006) 'Biotribology'. *Current Orthopaedics*, **20**, 32–40.

Lindley, T.C. (2004) 'Fretting fatigue in engineering alloys'. *International Journal of Fatigue*, **19**, S39–S49.

McEwen, H.M.J., Barnett, P.I., Bell, C.J., Farrar, R., Auger, D.D., Stone, M.H. and Fisher, J. (2005) 'The influence of design, materials and kinematics on the *in vitro* wear of total knee replacements'. *Journal of Biomechanics*, **38**, 357–65.

Mueller-Rath, R., Kleffner, B., Andereya, S., Mumme, T. and Wirtz, D.C. (2007) 'Measures for reducing ultra-high-molecular-weight polyethylene wear in total knee replacement: A simulator study'. *Biomedizinische Technik*, **52**, 295–300.

Perillo-Marcone, A., Ryd, L., Johnsson, K. and Taylor, M. (2004) 'A combined RSA and FE study of the implanted proximal tibia: Correlation of the post-operative mechanical environment with implant migration'. *Journal of Biomechanics*, **37**, 1205–13.

Pilliar, R.M., Blackwell, R., MacNab, I. and Cameron, H.U. (1976) 'Carbon fibre reinforced bone cement in orthopaedic surgery'. *Journal of Biomedical Materials Research*, **10**, 893–906.

Prendergast, P.J., Monaghan, J. and Taylor, D. (1989) 'Materials selection in the artificial hip joint using finite element stress analysis'. *Clinical Materials*, **4**, 361–76.

Reggiani, M., Tinti, A., Visentin, M., Stea, S., Erani, P. and Fagnano, C. (2007) 'Vibrational spectroscopy study of the oxidation of Hylamer UHMWPE explanted acetabular cups sterilized differently'. *Journal of Molecular Structure*, **834–6**, 129–35.

Rimnac, C.M. and Kurtz, S.M. (2005) 'Ionizing radiation and orthopaedic prostheses'. *Nuclear Instruments and Methods in Physics Research, Section B: Beam Interactions with Materials and Atoms*, **236**, 30–7.

Rohlmann, A., Mossner, U., Bergmann, G., Hees, G. and Kolbelt, R. (1987) 'Effects of stem length and material properties on stresses in hip endoprostheses'. *Journal of Biomedical Engineering*, **9**, 77–83.

Roy Chowdhury, S.K., Mishra, A., Pradhan, B. and Saha, D. (2004) 'Wear characteristic and biocompatibility of some polymer composite acetabular cups'. *Wear*, **256**, 1026–36.

Schwartz, C.J. and Bahadur, S. (2007) 'Development and testing of a novel joint wear simulator and investigation of the viability of an elastomeric polyurethane for total-joint arthroplasty devices'. *Wear*, **262**, 331–9.

Taylor, D. (2007) *The Theory of Critical Distances: A New Perspective in Fracture Mechanics*. Elsevier, Oxford, UK.

Walker, P.S., Blunn, G.W., Broome, D.R., Perry, J., Watkins, A., Sathasivam, S., Dewar, M.E. and Paul, J.P. (1997) 'A knee simulating machine for performance evaluation of total knee replacements'. *Journal of Biomechanics*, **30**, 83–9.

Whalen, R.T., Carter, D.R. and Steele, C.R. (1988) 'Influence of physical activity on the regulation of bone density'. *Journal of Biomechanics*, **21**, 825–37.

Wulpi, D.J. (1985) *Understanding How Components Fail*. ASM, Ohio, USA.

Part III

Clinical applications

13
Using bone repair materials in orthopaedic surgery

A. MEROLLI, The Catholic University in Rome, Italy and P. TRANQUILLI LEALI, University of Sassari, Italy

Abstract: Different classes of materials have been used in orthopaedic surgery, which is one of the fields in medicine where biomaterials have been most applied. In this chapter we will describe the different classes of materials and their applications in orthopaedic surgery, from the perspective of an orthopaedic surgeon. Orthopaedic surgery deals with the treatment of pathological conditions of the musculoskeletal system. Its operative actions may be gathered into the following groups: (1) the geometrical correction of a deformed segment; (2) the replacement of joint components destroyed by a pathological process; (3) the restoration of the anatomical, and possibly mechanical, integrity of a bone defect. A wide range of operative techniques have been developed that can be be grouped in broad categories, the most important of which are osteosynthesis, joint replacement and bone replacement.

Key words: clinical relevance, orthopaedics, traumatology.

13.1 Introduction

Different classes of materials have been used in orthopaedic surgery, which is one of the fields in medicine where biomaterials have been most applied. Description and characterization of these materials forms the bulk of this book and, in this section, we will describe the different classes of materials and their applications in orthopaedic surgery, from the perspective of an orthopaedic surgeon.

Orthopaedic surgery deals with the treatment of pathological conditions of the musculoskeletal system. Its operative actions may be gathered into the following three groups: (1) the geometrical correction of a deformed segment; (2) the replacement of joint components destroyed by a pathological process; (3) the restoration of the anatomical, and possibly mechanical, integrity of a bone defect.

From the point of view of the material scientist, it is important to note that most materials and devices in orthopaedic surgery can be used, without difference, both in orthopaedics and in traumatology.

13.1.1 Orthopaedics and traumatology

Orthopaedics deals with well-defined pre-existent pathological conditions and relies on carefully planned surgical operations which, in most cases, can be carried out with the best choice of options available. Traumatology, in contrast, deals mostly with conditions of sudden on-set, often associated with trauma in areas other than the musculoskeletal system (e.g. brain or abdominal lesions) and in which time for planning the best surgical operation and availability of the best materials and devices, may be limited. Both acquired and congenital conditions may be encountered.

Acquired conditions

Geometrical correction of an acquired deformed segment is required following the traumatic fracture of a bone which is usually associated with a gross alteration in geometry, except in particular cases in which the fractured bone segments maintain their proper reciprocal spatial relationship because of the interlocking of the fracture rims. Sometimes, geometrical correction is required in mal-united fractures; these occur when the healing of a fractured long bone occurs with an abnormal angulation at the fracture site, even after proper treatment has been administered; these mal-united fractures require a successive osteotomy (transection of bone) followed by geometrical correction and new synthesis of the bone ends.

Replacements of joint components destroyed by an acquired degenerative process are common, as exemplified by mechanical-based 'osteoarthrosis' (most often called 'osteoarthritis'), or by the even more common rheumatoid arthritis; these conditions often cause the complete destruction of joint structure.

Restoration of the anatomical, and possibly mechanical, integrity of an acquired bone defect is the goal in the treatment of bone loss which is associated with the removal of a benign or a malignant tumour. It is also the goal in the treatment of a severe condition known as 'non-union', in which the fracture healing process failed to occur at the fracture site and rarefaction and even disappearance of bone tissue follows.

Congenital conditions

Geometrical correction of a congenital deformity may be exemplified by the use of intrapeduncular screws connected by rods that are used to build a frame that straigthens a deformed spine in scoliosis. This is a not uncommon pathological condition which affects adolescents (girls in particular) with progressive severity, during growth, and which can end up, as growth finishes, with severe cosmetic and functional (respiratory) impairments.

Replacement of joint components destroyed by a congenital degenerative process may be exemplified by the total hip joint replacement that is needed in patients born with congenital hip dysplasia. This condition may evolve, in its worst progression, into a painful destruction of the articular surfaces of the acetabulum and of the head of the femur at a relatively young age (before 65 years of age, after which the mechanical-based degenerative affection of osteoarthrosis is more common).

Restoration of the anatomical, and possibly mechanical, integrity of a congenital bone defect is seldom encountered; it is mostly exemplified by the partial development (or lack of development) of a bone segment like in the partial agenesis of ulna, radius, tibia or fibula.

13.2 Operative techniques

A wide range of operative techniques have been developed in orthopaedic surgery. They can be grouped in broad categories, the most important of which are osteosynthesis, joint replacement and bone replacement.

13.2.1 Osteosynthesis

Osteosynthesis is one of the most common operative techniques in orthopaedic surgery, both in elective orthopaedics and in traumatology. It consists of the union of two or more bone fragments, after their proper alignment has been previously gained. The union is mechanically stabilized by a means of screws, nails, plates and several other mechanical devices which are required to remain effective until the biological process of fracture healing has restored the bone segment as a single entity. Materials used in osteosynthesis are, then, required to possess both mechanical properties adequate to take the load in the injured bone segment and, at the same time, biological properties able to keep them in apposition with bone for a period of time during which they must not hamper or interfere with the bone healing process and, if possible, should support and promote it.

Despite several devices being made with materials with a very good biocompatibility or, even, bioactivity, devices used for osteosynthesis should be removed after a period of time, which should not be longer than one year from the implantation, in every patient and not only in growing children (Lovell *et al.*, 1999).

13.2.2 Joint replacement

A joint may be exemplified as a structure which connects two bone segments, allowing them a variable degree of reciprocal motion. Sliding joints are generally enveloped by a fibrous 'joint capsule' which completely seals the joint ends from the other tissues and which contains the 'sinovial fluid', a non-Newtonian fluid that mechanically lubricates the joint ends and biologically feeds their contact surfaces which, in physiological conditions, are not made of bone but of a tissue called 'articular cartilage'.

An increasing number of artificial joint replacements are performed world wide (Crowninshield *et al.*, 2006; Kim, 2008). They are both complete (total) or partial joint replacements, according to whether both joint ends are replaced or only one of them. The most common cause for a joint replacement is the complete destruction and disappearance of the articular cartilage, leading to painful contact with underlying bone, but several pathological conditions may lead to this final condition.

Rheumatoid arthritis is a severe disease which affects several tissues and districts in the body; when there is the involvement of a joint, a total loss of articular cartilage coupled with gross deformity of joint ends (Fig. 13.1), produces a painful and debilitating condition which requires artificial joint replacement. The main mechanism of action of this unfortunately not rare disease is the process of inflammation (hence it is described with the suffix '-itis' in its name).

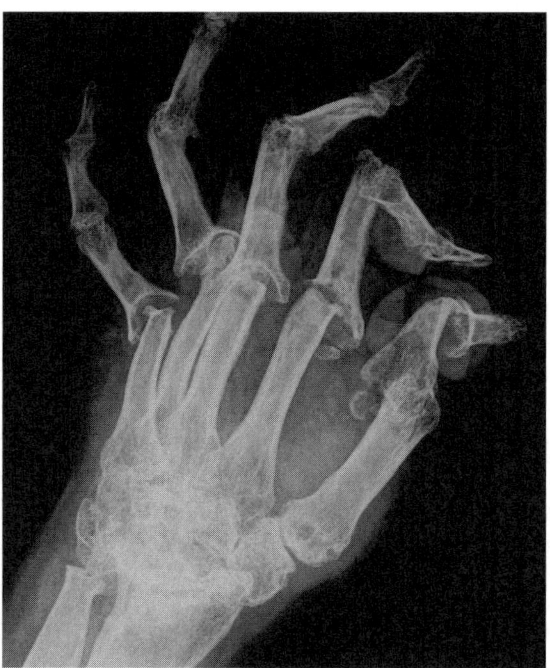

13.1 Rheumatoid arthritis is a severe disease which affects several tissues and districts in the body; a total loss of articular cartilage coupled with gross deformity produce cases like the one shown, where the hand is affected.

Another more common pathological condition, which may end with the complete destruction and disappearance of the articular cartilage and the painful contact of underlying bone, is osteoarthrosis. This is a degenerative chronic non-inflammatory (Dorland's Medical Dictionary, 2007) bone disease (hence the suffix '-osis'), whose mechanism of action is not yet fully understood but where there is a definitive role for excessive and repeated mechanical overload on the joint. It affects all the joints but it is particularly severe in the larger weight-bearing joints of the lower limb, like the hip and the knee. The clinical disturbance in gait, for patients whose lower limb joints are affected, is not different from that associated with inflammatory conditions which were common in the 19th century and which were properly called 'osteoarthritis'; so the names 'osteoarthrosis' and 'osteoarthritis' are both found in broad use with a certain degree of overlap in the orthopaedic literature (Stedman's Medical Dictionary, 2007).

13.2.3 Bone replacement

A bone loss which does not repair spontaneously will require a bone replacement to diminish the risk of fracture in its bone segment. A permanent replacement with an autograft or an artificial material is still commonly applied (Urabe *et al.*, 2007) but a lot of research is directed towards possible replacement with bioactive materials, which could eventually give rise to new bone in the patient until final full recovery of the integrity of the bone segment is achieved.

13.3 Materials

13.3.1 Metals

Stainless steel and titanium alloys are widely used because of their mechanical strength. They are key materials in devices needed for osteosynthesis, in which they must guarantee a mechanical stability in the early phases of fracture healing, prior to the completion of the healing process. They are, also, the main constituents of heavy weight-bearing joint prostheses, like hip and knee.

Designing a metallic device generally achieves the goal of coping with the mechanical performance which is required but problems may arise from the biological response at the metal–bone interface. Several stainless steel alloys promote a fibrous reaction that may end up with a multicellular layer of fibroblasts interposed between the recipient bone and the implant, eventually leading to implant loosening. Titanium alloys proved to be better able to promote integration with bone (Fig. 13.2) and, sometimes, only a tiny non-ossified rim remains between them and the recipient bone, so thin that it can be only characterized by the higher magnification provided by electron microscopy (Fig. 13.3).

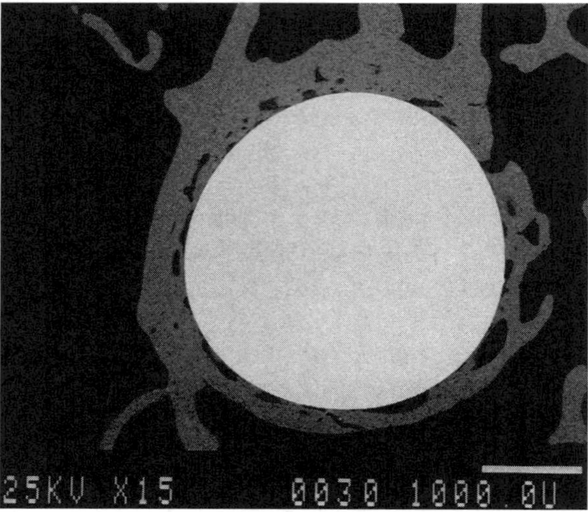

13.2 Titanium alloys proved to be able to promote integration with bone, as shown in this low-magnification (X15) back scattered electron microscopic image; newly formed bone is seen around the transverse section of a Ti6Al4V rod, experimentally implanted into the distal femur of a rabbit.

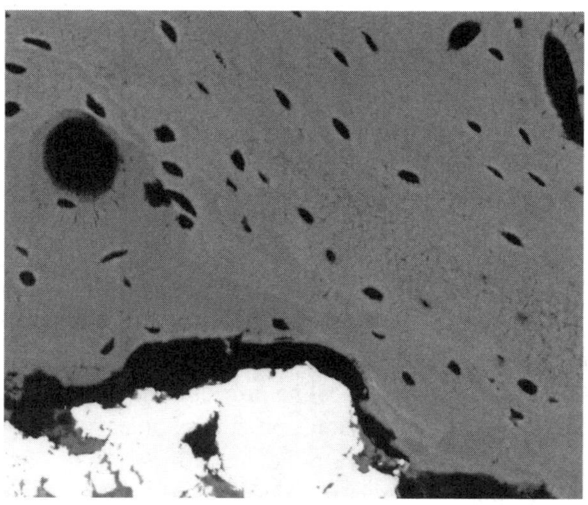

13.3 Higher magnification (X250) back scattered electron microscopy shows that bone is seldom tightly apposed to titanium alloy; a tiny non-ossified rim often remains in between.

In any case, many surface treatment have been developed and applied in designing implants based on metals, to improve their acceptance by the recipient bone or, even, to mask the metal from the bone by processes grouped under the term 'biomimicry'. Hydroxyapatite coating is the most widely applied biomimetic treatment for metallic surfaces but several other methods have been proposed (in some cases reaching clinical application) like a bioactive glass coating or the anodic oxidation of titanium.

Despite composite materials having been studied as a possible replacement for metals in weight-bearing applications, the convenient costs and easier workability of metals support the view that they will keep their predominant role, as long as a material for osteosynthesis or for artificial joint structure has to be selected.

13.3.2 Non-biodegradable polymers

Polymethylmethacrylate (PMMA) and polyethylene (PE) are polymers which have ubiquitous applications in orthopaedic surgery. Despite their physicochemical degradation with time, within the lifespan of an implant inside the body, they are properly considered neither biodegradable nor bioresorbable (meaning by hydrolytic degradation and by cell-mediated degradation, respectively). Their applications in orthopaedic surgery are different and they will be treated separately.

Recently, another non-biodegradable polymer has found a well-defined application in orthopaedic surgery: it is polyether ether-ketone (PEEK). Its main application is in the intersomatic vertebral fusion when a so-called 'cage' is interposed between two vertebral bodies. After the intervertebral disk and the articular cartilage plates have been removed, these 'cages', filled with bone chips, are used to promote bony fusion between the two vertebrae.

Polymethylmethacrylate

PMMA has become the material of reference when a cement is needed to assemble an implant with the recipient bone, in a single unit; cementing the stem of a joint prosthesis is the application of reference. PMMA has been, probably, overused in the sense that sometimes the cement has been required to cope with the mechanical mismatch between the implant and the recipient bone, for example, when stability is needed for a stem too much solicited in torsion, or when an osteoporotic bone, too weak to bear the load transmitted at a joint, receives an implant (Fig. 13.4). Fracture and debris production of the cement, which may occur in these cases, have been considered in the past more a cause than an event in the mechanical mismatch, prompting the possible avoidance of the use of PMMA cement, like it occurs in cementless joint prostheses.

From the surgical point of view, the easy intraoperative workability of PMMA cement favoured several other applications apart from cementing joint stems, like filling large bone cavities produced by the surgical removal of a tumour; in this application, PMMA often assured a long lasting

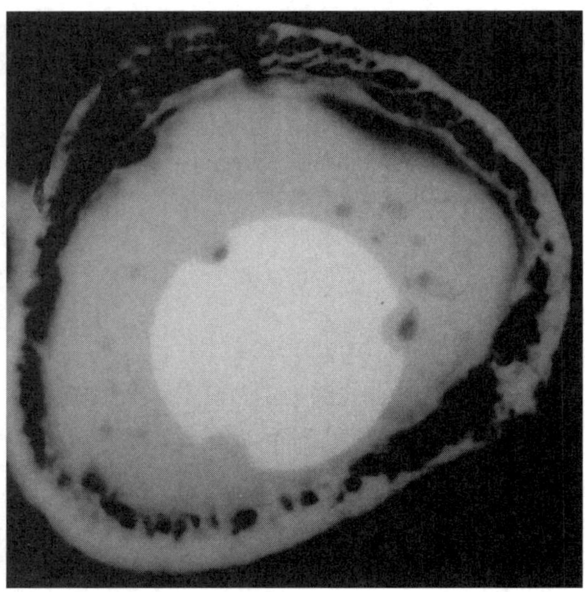

13.4 PMMA cement has been required to cope with the mechanical mismatch between the implant and the recipient bone, as shown in this cadaver explant, which shows an osteoporotic bone too weak to bear the load transmitted at the interface.

mechanical stability and compatibility with the recipient bone (Aboulafia *et al.*, 2007).

Furthermore, PMMA has been applied as *in situ* drug delivery system for antibiotics in cavities produced by osteomyelytis, a severe infectious process which is difficult to eradicate (Kent *et al.*, 2006). It has also been proposed as a drug delivery system for anti-blastic drugs in the *in situ* therapy of tumours affecting the bone (Greco *et al.*, 1992).

More recently, PMMA has been used as a moldable material to cast temporary spacers after the removal of failed joint prostheses which were involved in an infectious process. In this case, PMMA is not required to provide any kinematic performance but just to give a provisional congruence to the joint ends, for the time required by drug therapy to control and possibly eradicate the infection and, then, allow the following implantation of a revision prosthesis.

A new application of PMMA comes from spinal surgery. With the technique of vertebroplasty, a crushed vertebral body can be restored to its original volume and its inner space can be filled with PMMA cement to assure mechanical strength (Pitton *et al.*, 2008).

Polyethylene

PE has experienced a great success in the past because it is easily workable in many different shapes and seemed to be an ideal damper in the coupling with a metallic component in artificial joints. Its character, which is prone to release debris under frictional load, means that when debris are dispersed at the interface between the implant and the recipient bone this can lead to the loosening of the implant. The search for an ever better performing blend was pursued by a constant increase in molecular weight and, recently, in optimizing the crosslinking of the chains.

The main application of PE today remains in coupling with the metallic component of an artificial joint, like the facing of an artificial femural head in artificial hip joints or constituting the tibial plate in artificial knee joints. It has also been proposed as material for temporary multiple-sized joint spacers following the removal of infected artificial joints.

13.3.3 Biodegradable polymers

Performing osteosynthesis by the implantation of a metallic device inside the body sometimes promotes the development of an infectious process which, in the past, has led to amputation of the infected limb. Infection may arise a long time from the end of the healing process, so bearing this in mind, mantaining a metallic device for a longer time, or even for life, is not recommended.

However, the rule that requires removal of an osteosynthesis device after the healing process has ended (and, generally, not longer than 12 months from implantation) is not easy to implement for two main reasons: the first is that in several districts the second operation required to remove the implant may be difficult and risky (think about cervical spine or inner pelvis) and the second is that it is costly.

The idea of having devices made of biodegradable polymers which were able to sustain the mechanical load during the healing process of a fracture but, afterwards, would gradually disapper from the site was welcomed with great enthusiasm in the early 1990s (Fig. 13.5). To summarize in few words the long story of biodegradable materials in orthopaedic surgery (Middleton and Tipton, 2000), the following should be considered.

The mechanical properties of the to-be-substituted metallic devices were seldom matched by the proposed biodegradable materials; the operative techniques with these materials required greater care (Fig. 13.6), and in some ways a different attitude in the sense that greater attention must be taken not to break the implant (while with metallic devices it was more 'not to break the bone').

A reduction in costs, which could be obtained by avoiding a second

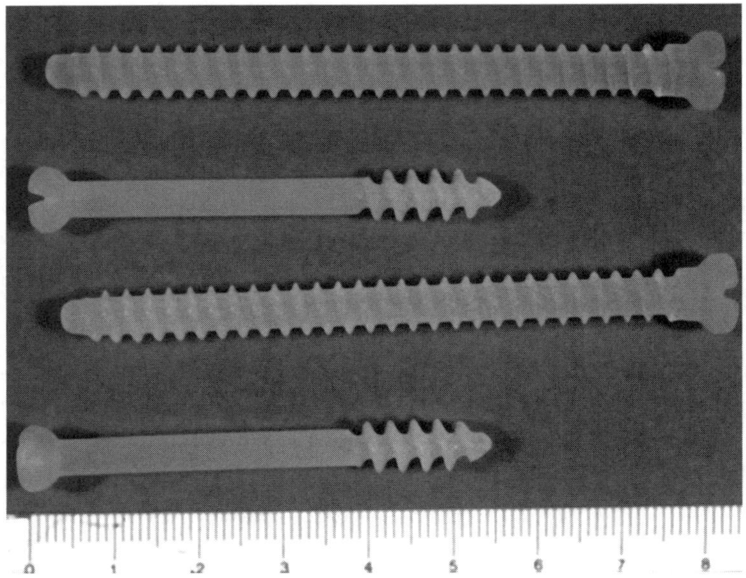

13.5 A set of experimental screws, made of poly-L-lactic acid, tested by the authors in the early 1990s.

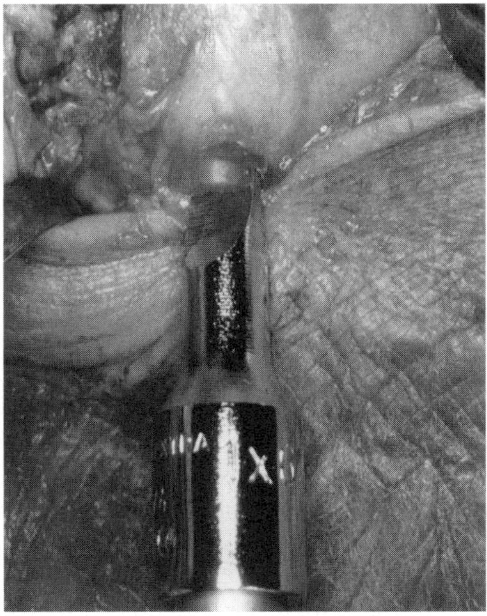

13.6 The first case of a tibial malleolar fracture treated by the authors with a poly-L-lactic acid screw; a dynamometric screw-driver was employed, which stops twisting in the case where a greater-than-set torque is applied.

operation for removal, was hampered by the significantly higher cost of biodegradable implants.

But the biggest disappointment came from the discrepancy which exists between the biological and the clinical idea of 'degradation': as a matter of fact several devices made from biodegradable polymers did not perfom clinically as degradable at all, because of their long degradation time *in vivo* (Merolli *et al.*, 2001).

Discussion of degradability needs to address the discrepancy which exists between what is 'degradable' from a chemical point of view and what can be considered degradable from a clinical point of view. Materials science can describe the degradable behaviour of a material and of an artifact on the basis of its chemical properties. Often, a direct cellular contribution, for example in the form of enzymatic digestion, can further characterize the degradation properties of a material and an artifact and, in this case, the term 'bioresorption' may be even more appropriate. Nevertheless, 'degradation' or 'resorption' of a material and of an artifact should not be considered in terms of the actual time needed for the *in vitro* or *in vivo* processes to occur, but should be correlated with the time required by the healing process in which the material and artifact interact (Fig. 13.7). For example, the real

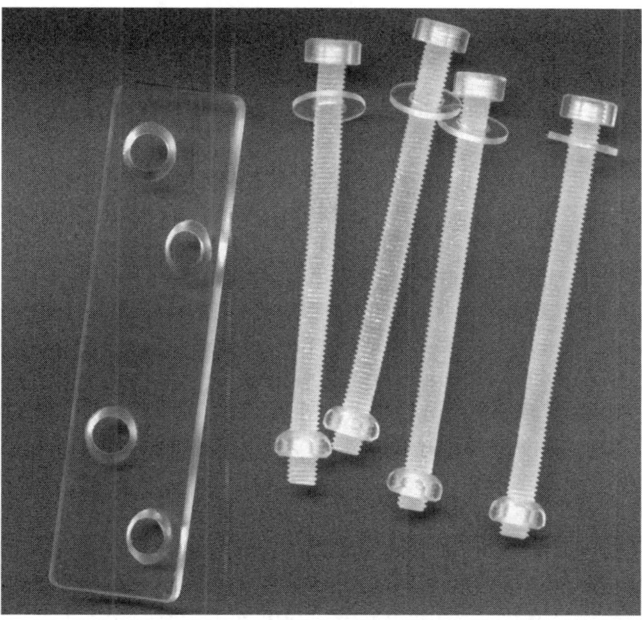

13.7 An experimental fast-degradable plate to be fixed by slow-degradable screws, was designed and tested by the authors; the screws degraded so slowly that, from a biological point of view, they elicited the same morphological response as non-degradable implants.

term of comparison, when defining whether a material or an artifact can be considered permanent or degradable, is the time needed for a bone fracture to consolidate. Any 'degradable' surgical implant should be removed after the healing process in which it is involved is likely to be completed. After that time the degradable implant is no longer needed and could even behave as the unwanted cause of a bone defect.

A strong point against removal of degradable implants is the additional risk, even when minimal, associated with a second surgical procedure in cases when, if everything goes according to expectation, there should be nothing left to be removed. In the opinion of the authors, this is not the right approach for implants where full degradation has not been unmistakably demonstrated; actually, the statement can be reversed by saying that an ensuing damage in failing to remove an implant that may stop or reverse an on-going healing process, far outweighs the risks and the costs associated with a second surgery.

Nowadays, biodegradable implants used in orthopaedic surgery are made mostly from polylactic acid blends and have selected applications like, for example, interference screws for cruciate ligaments surgery in the knee. An ever increasing number of designs has been proposed for less-loaded small implants like those used, for example, in hand surgery.

13.3.4 Ceramics

Inert or bioactive ceramics are used in orthopaedic surgery. Inert non-bioactive ceramics like Al_2O_3 are used in clinical practice as bearings in total joint replacements because of their resistance to wear and their tribological properties (Hamadouche and Sedel, 2000). Bioactive ceramics are employed as coatings to enhance the fixation of a device or as bone-graft substitutes because of their osteoconductive properties. They act as a scaffold to enhance bone formation on their surface.

Hydroxyapatite is the most widely used bioactive ceramic material in orthopaedic surgery. Bone may be defined as a composite tissue with an organic matrix composed primarily of the protein collagen which provides flexibility (about 10% of adult bone mass is collagen) and a mineral phase which is composed of hydroxyapatite, which is an insoluble salt of calcium and phosphorus (about 65% of adult bone mass is hydroxyapatite); water comprises approximately 25% of adult bone mass. Collagen fibres and calcium salts help to strengthen bone. In fact, the collagen fibres in bone have great tensile strength while the calcium salts have great compressional strength. These combined properties, plus the degree of bondage between the collagen fibres and the crystals, provide a bony structure that has both extreme tensile and compressional strength.

The discovery that osteoblasts can grow happily on artificial hydroxyapatite, both as a bulk material and as a plasma-spray coating, significantly improved the possibility of obtaining a favourable response in the implantation of devices which where loaded or coated with industrial-made hydroxyapatite (Fig. 13.8 and 13.9).

Not only are osteoblasts found growing on hydroxyapatite, but osteoclasts seem also able to remove it, in this way reproducing the physiological process

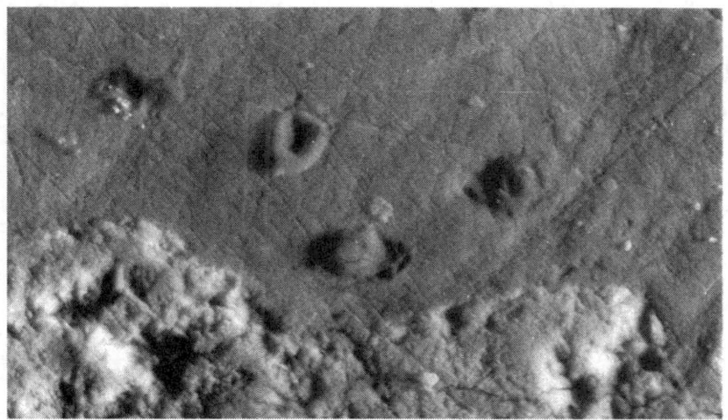

13.8 A scanning electron micrograph (X1200) that shows the surface at the bone-hydroxyapatite coating interface; bone is so tightly apposed to the coating that no gap in between is detectable.

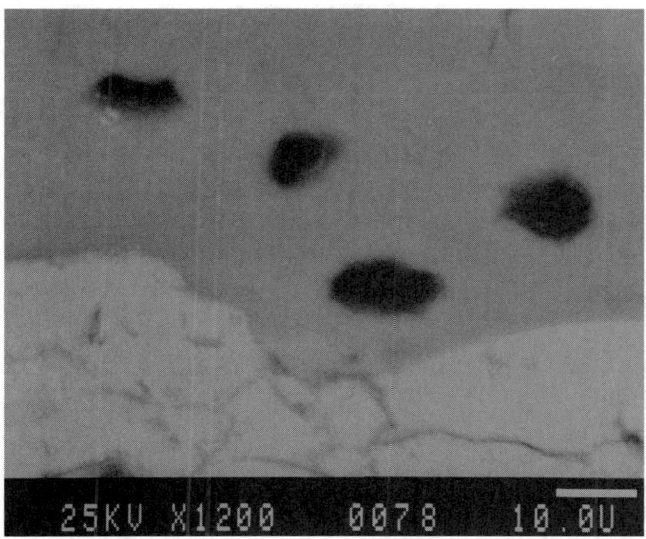

13.9 A back scattered electron micrograph of the same area depicted in Fig. 13.8 clearly shows (X1200) where hydroxyapatite coating (in white), newly formed bone (in grey) and osteocytic lacunae (in black) are located; it confirms the tight apposition between bone and coating.

of apposition and removal that occurs in living bone (Tranquilli Leali *et al.*, 1994). This behaviour well deserves the name 'biomimicry' (Williams, 1995). Then, coating an implant with hydroxyapatite became an effective system for masking the structural material which it is made of, promoting an early favourable response from recipient bone towards the implant (Fig. 13.10).

Hydroxyapatite is also used as bone filler when large cavities are encountered. It must be underlined that, in this role, the complete resorption of the implanted material is not always obtained, even in the long term (Fig. 13.11); furthermore, hydroxyapatite can be used as a filler only when no real mechanical task is required.

Other bioactive ceramic materials, like the calcium phosphates, have been proposed and are now in clinical use, using basically the same principles outlined for hydroxyapatite.

13.3.5 Glasses

In the 1970s, Prof. Larry Hench discovered that a particular range of glass composition could elicit a favourable bone cells growth (Hench *et al.*, 1971). A particular application in orthopaedic surgery came from the deposition of a bioactive glass coating in a similar fashion to hydroxyapatite coating (Merolli *et al.*, 1999). The rationale for a degradable bioactive glass coating

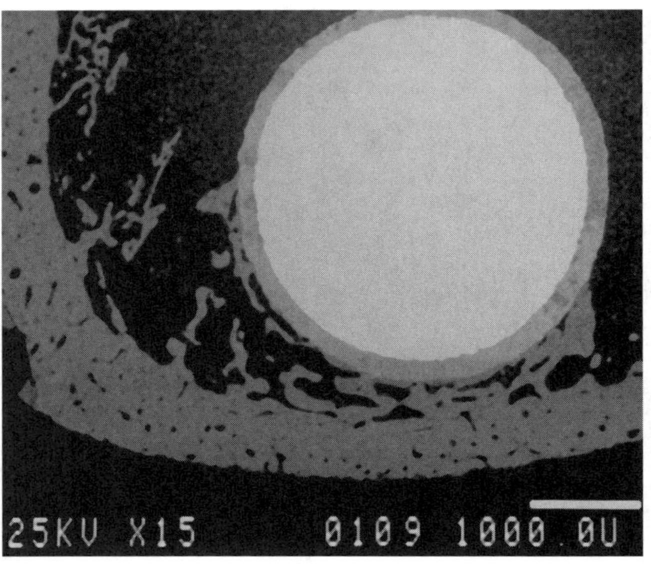

13.10 A low magnification (X15) back scattered electron micrograph which shows trabecular bone growing in apposition to a hydroxyapatite coated metallic rod, in an experimental model in the rabbit.

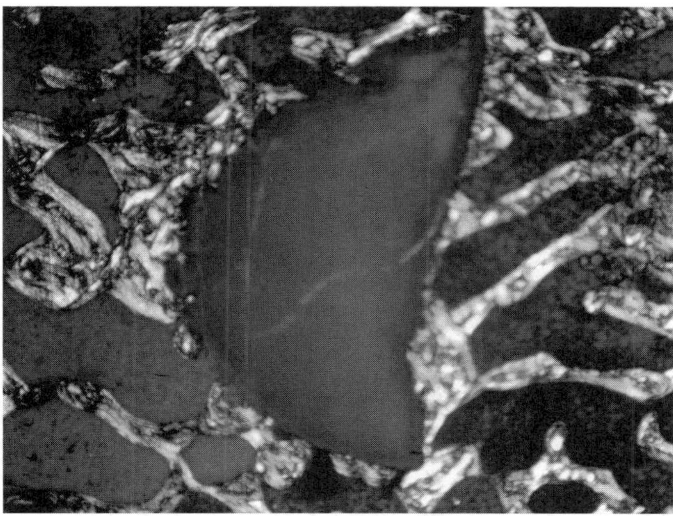

13.11 Despite the excellent apposition and growth of trabecular bone, the complete resorption of a highly crystalline hydroxyapatite granule, experimentally used as bone filler in a cavity, has not been obtained even after two years.

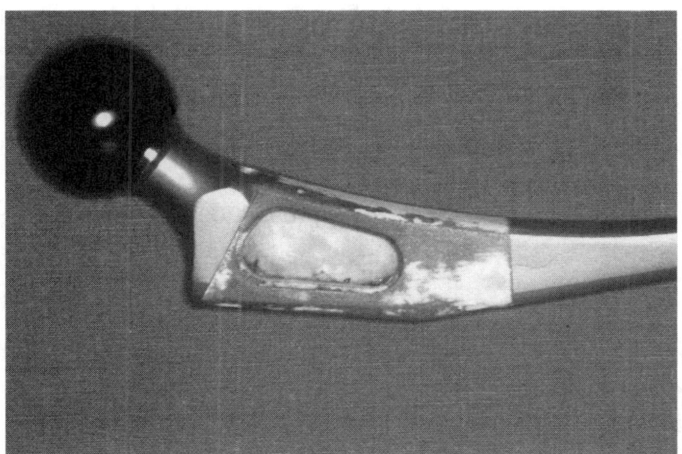

13.12 Deposition of a bioactive glass coating, in a similar fashion to the hydroxyapatite coating, was applied in hip prostheses; in this picture, a coated stem has been retrieved from a patient three months after implantation; the process of resorption of the coating had already started.

is to lead the bone to appose gradually to the metal (Fig. 13.12 and Fig. 13.13); this process should happen without the production, at its end, of bulky non-degradable particles as those observed with the fragmentation of the crystalline phase of hydroxyapatite coatings (Merolli *et al.*, 2004).

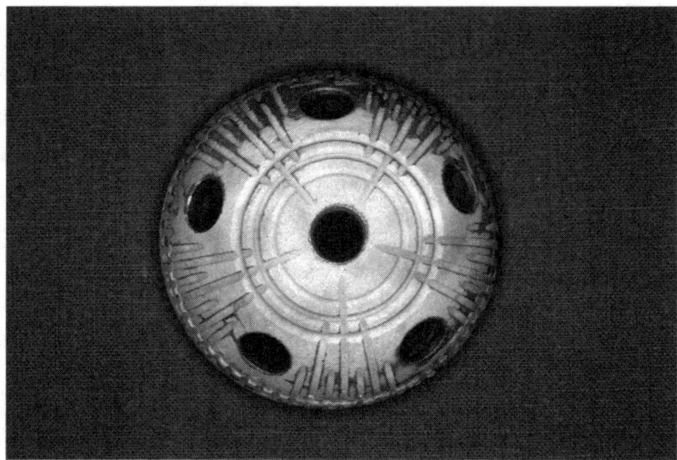

13.13 The metal back of the cup from the same implant in Fig. 13.12; the rationale for a degradable bioactive glass coating is to lead the bone gradually to appose the metal without the production, at the end, of bulky non-degradable particles.

Since the development of the first bioactive glass by Hench, several kinds of glasses and glass–ceramics have been found to interface with living bone. The model in this class of materials is Bioglass 45S5 of which the composition in weight% is: 45% SiO_2, 24.5% CaO, 6% P_2O_5 and 24.5% Na_2O. The bonding mechanism of silicate bioactive glasses to bone has been attributed to a series of surface reactions ultimately leading to the formation of a hydroxycarbonate apatite layer at the glass surface. The critical element necessary for the formation of this is the production of a layer of porous silica gel with a high surface area. The apatite phase is formed when the bioactive material comes into contact with the aqueous component of physiological fluids.

Standardization of hydroxyapatite coating techniques for orthopaedic implants has, probably, limited the exploitation of bioactive glass coatings in orthopaedic surgery, while it is more applied in dental and maxilofacial surgery.

13.3.6 Composites

Composite materials made from carbon fibres and epoxidic resins were proposed for applications in orthopaedic surgery to promote the replacement of metals (Fig. 13.14). This replacement process has happened in other fields, like the aerospace industry, but in orthopaedic surgery the possible unmasking of carbon fibres and their dispersion inside the body was an unacceptable risk (Fig. 13.15). The high costs were also another big concern.

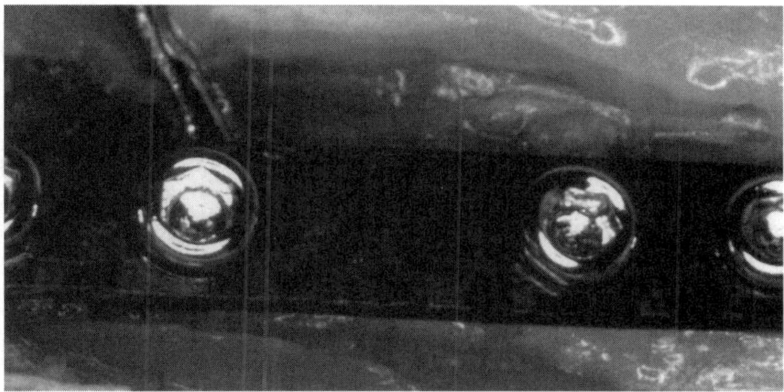

13.14 An experimental plate made from carbon fibres and epoxidic resins, implanted in the rabbit and fixed with stainless-steel screws.

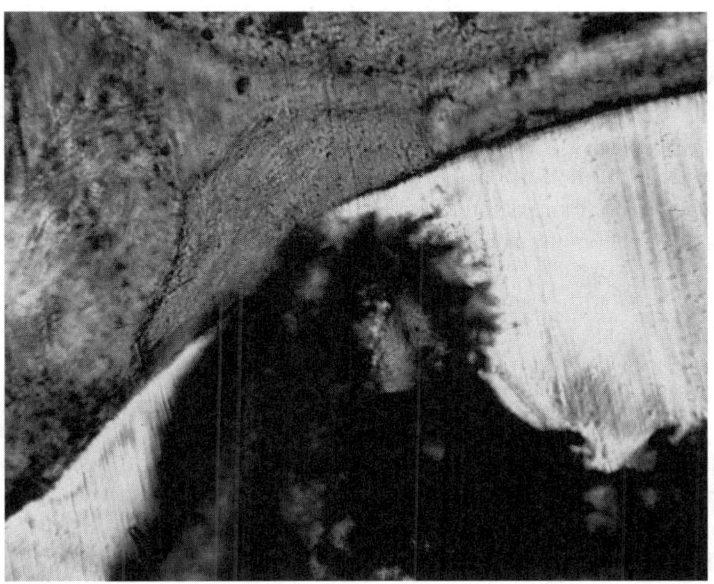

13.15 The unmasking of carbon fibres (in black) from a composite implant is documented in this specimen retrieved from a rabbit femur.

However, composites are trying to find a place in orthopaedic surgey in other preparations (Stein *et al.*, 2005). The two most common families of composites proposed for orthopaedic surgery are the biodegradable material – ceramics (or glass) composite (Boeree *et al.*, 1993; Närhi *et al.*, 2003) – and the PE–HA composite (Di Silvio *et al.*, 1998).

Composites between a biodegradable polymer and a ceramic or a glass material have been developed with the aim of taking advantage of the degradability of the polymer while employing the bioceramic component to try to avoid any excessive inflammatory reaction towards its breakdown products. This should also help in the early stages of interaction with bone.

The same principle applies to the HA–PE composite. These materials have already been applied in fields like inner-ear surgery, dental and maxilofacial surgery. Application in orthopaedic surgery is envisaged for small implants, like those required in hand surgery, for example.

13.4 Devices

Many different devices are used in orthopaedic surgery (Chapman, 1993). From earlier times when devices where often made from a single material, like stainless steel plates to fix long-bone fractures or PE cups for acetabular replacement, it is now possible to assemble different components made of different materials. Examples are HA coated-metallic prosthetic stems or PE-polished metal cups for metal-on-metal joint surfaces. In the near future it has been envisaged that a new 'material' component will be added to the artifact, in the form of cell-loading.

For decription purposes we will present orthopaedic surgery devices according to the main categories of operative techniques addressed in Section 2, namely osteosynthesis, joint replacement and bone replacement.

13.4.1 Devices for osteosynthesis

Screws

Screws are extremely common in the orthopaedic surgery inventory and they are applied as primary internal fixation devices in several instances. Joining two bone fragments by a screw may be a quite straightforward technique. Historically, it has evolved from the 19th century nail transfixtion (where a nail joined the two segments and was 'press-fitted' in place without the help of the screw thread), to the contemporary double-threaded canulated screws. The latter complex devices are screws that have a hollow canal; the two bone segments may be held in place by a tiny nail, termed pin or wire, even without open surgery but percutaneously with the help of intraoperative radioscopy; then the screw is driven through the nail and guided into place with high accuracy (Fig. 13.16). Double-threaded compression screws have a defined pitch in their apex, to grasp the distal segment, and a different pitch in their head, so that while giving the final twists, a further compression between the two bone segments is obtained. A typical application for these screws is the percutaneous osteosynthesis of a carpal scaphoid fracture (Fig. 13.17 and Fig. 13.18), a severe lesion which affects the crucial bone which

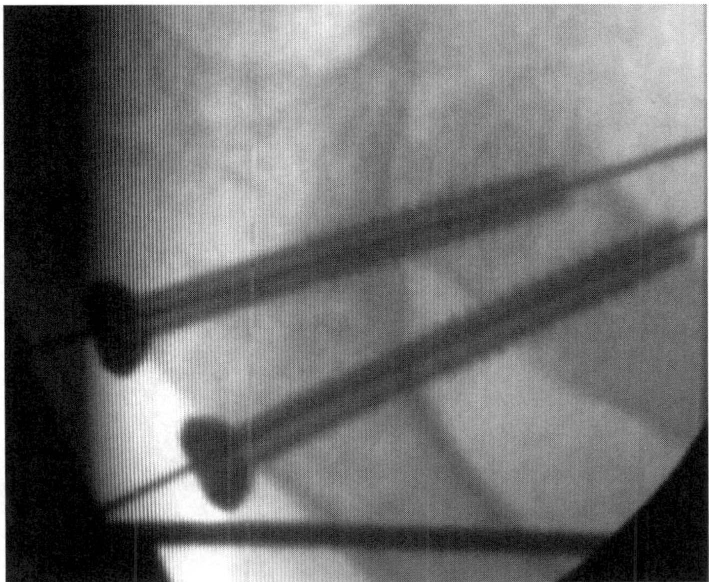

13.16 Double-threaded canulated screws are driven by a tiny nail, percutaneously and with the help of intraoperative radioscopy.

is the biomechanical pivot of the hand and which, not uncommonly, fails to heal, provoking the disability of a deficit of force and a painful condition. In several places in the body screws are now proposed for use with biodegradable materials, particularly when a limited load is required.

But screws are ubiquitously associated with other devices like plates and nails, in which they often constitute the element grasping on to the bone. In these cases, heavy loads are generally required and stainless steel screws are the devices of choice. In these applications, it is important to consider the interaction of the other components from which the plate or the nail are made, since corrosion phenomena may occur owing to a galvanic effect between the different metallic components.

Peculiar screws are those employed in external fixators; these devices have a framework which is mounted outside the body and assures the mechanical performance (Fig. 13.19). The framework is linked to the bony segments by long screws (Fig. 13.20 and Fig. 13.21), historically termed 'pins' or 'nails' because that is what they were in earlier times. External fixators may be loaded cyclically on a daily basis and may be required to stay in place for months. This may lead to the loosening of the screw grasp on the bone. In recent years, a HA coating of stainless steel (Merolli *et al.*, 2003) has been used for external fixator screws and has been introduced into clinical practice (Moroni *et al.*, 2008).

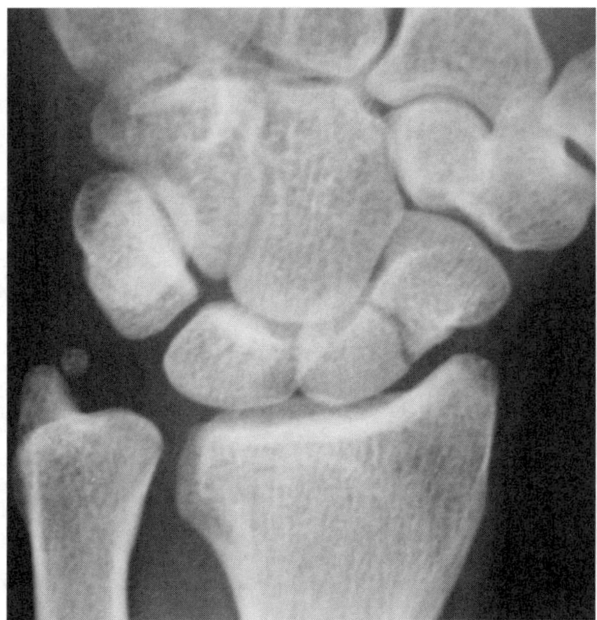

13.17 A carpal scaphoid fracture.

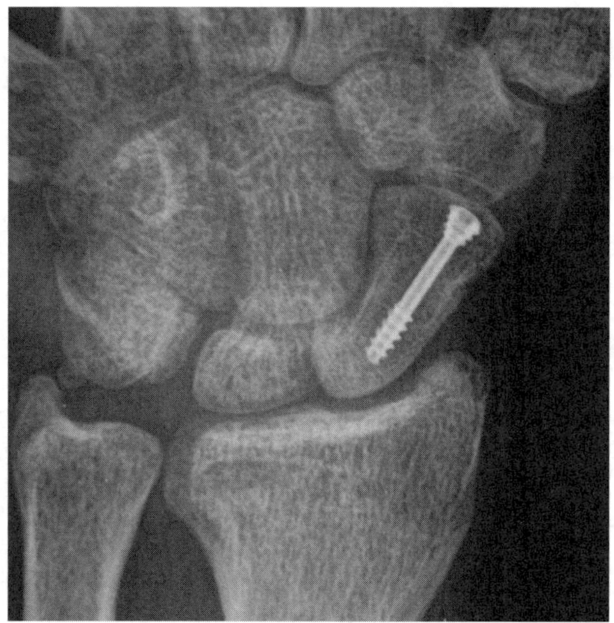

13.18 Healing of the carpal scaphoid fracture in Fig. 13.17, treated by a double-threaded screw (Herbert's screw).

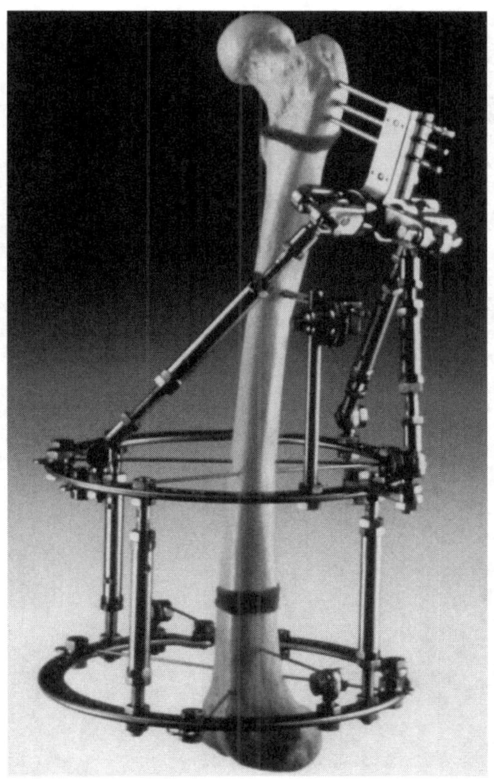

13.19 A picture from the early 1980s shows the first hybrid external fixator which combined rings and bars, for the frame, with wires and screws, for the connection with the bone segment.

Plates

A plate seemed an obvious device to provide an artificial shaft for the alignment of two displaced bone fragments. Also intuitive was the idea of assuring the assembly of the plate and the bone segments by transfixing screws. The treatment of a vast number of fractures relies on this concept but, sometimes, plate fixation may be too rigid and may impair the natural process of bone remodelling (Fig. 13.22). This is a process where bone is deposited in proportion to the compressional load that it must carry and trabeculae follow the lines of stress and can realign if the direction of stress changes (Wolff's law). Without proper loading, bone rarefaction occurs; a too rigid plate–bone assembly may 'shield the stress' from the bone and lead to bone rarefaction beneath the plate (Laftman *et al.*, 1989).

Reflecting what has been stated for the screws, care must be applied in coupling the material of plate and screws to avoid corrosion phenomena.

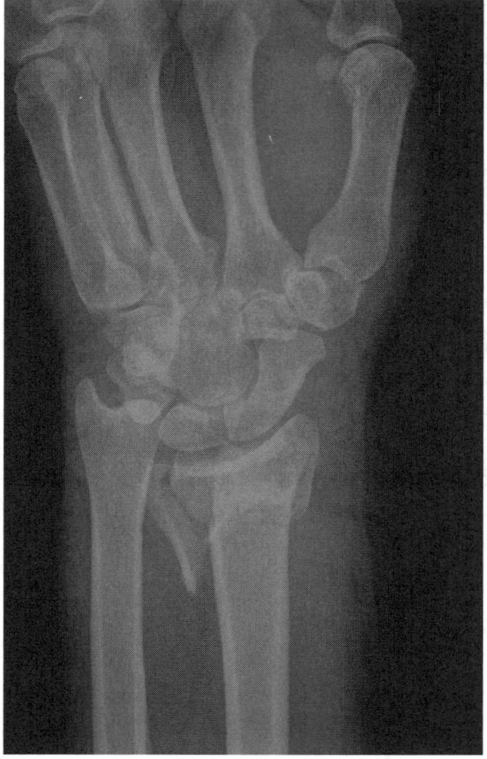

13.20 A severe comminuted fracture in the distal forearm, which produced a lot of bone fragments and a shortening of the radius. See also Fig. 13.21.

Nails

Transfixing nails are still used in orthopaedic surgery, particularly to synthesize percutaneaous small bone segments in the hand or foot. However, the most important application nowadays is intramedullary nailing, which prescribes that a large nail be introduced into the medullary canal of a long bone to restore its axial geometry and support an early load bearing capability (Fig. 13.23 and Fig. 13.24).

Historically, the most successful intramedullary nail was the Kuentscher's nail, which was a press-fit nail developed for fracture of the tibia and femur and which enabled the walking ability of the patient to be restored in a short time. This is because intramedullary nailing is a so-called 'dynamic osteosynthesis' which does not require the rigid fixation of the bone fragments but, quite the opposite, favours a compression–distraction mechanism at the fracture site, a mechanism able to promote bone growth if applied in the proper range (according to Wolff's law).

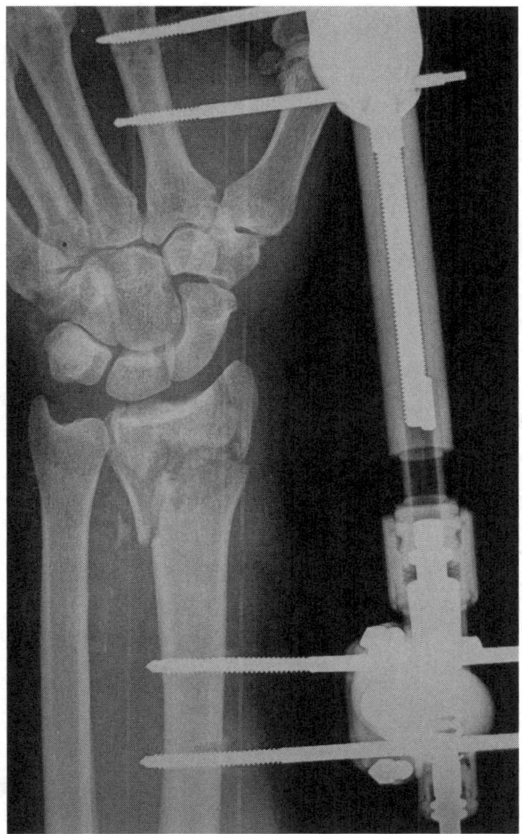

13.21 The appropriate geometry has been restored thanks to an external fixator, connected with screws to the bone segments.

More recently, locked nails have been proposed as systems able to control torsional stresses better at the fracture site. When they are locked only at one end, the dynamic mechanism of the synthesis is preserved; but when both ends are locked, the nail behaves more or less as an internal plate.

13.4.2 Devices for joint replacement

Joint prostheses are experiencing an ever increasing number of applications. Nearly every joint in the body has seen the development of an artificial substitute for its replacement. However, not everything has been successful.

The paradigm for artificial joint replacement is the hip joint. This is a heavy weight-bearing joint which, when affected by a degenerative process, has very little response to any conservative treatment. In fact, both in congenital and in acquired conditions, load bearing worsens the progress of the disease.

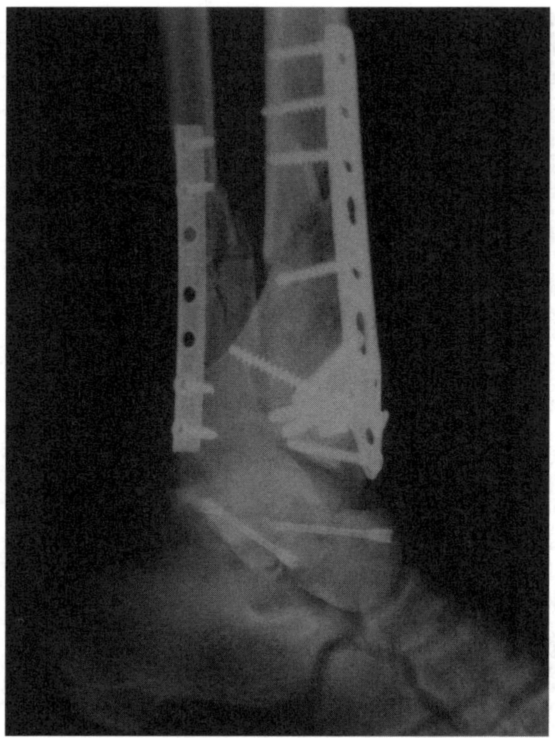

13.22 A case which was received from another hospital, after a delay in healing was evidenced; afterwards, all the plates and screws were removed and an Ilizarov's external fixator was applied, with success.

Avoiding load bearing is impossible on the hip, unless a limitation of daily life activities has already been accepted.

When joint destruction is complete, total joint replacement surgery should take place (and not earlier, as often encountered) which prescibes the reconstruction of the acetabulum (socket) with an artificial cup and the substitution of the femoral head with an artificial counterpart. These two components resemble their anatomical masters but the artificial femoral head transfers the load to the femoral shaft by an 'unnatural' intramedullary stem. This solution is quite sound from a mechanical point of view and it also has an historical basis in the fact that hip relacement followed the tentative treatment of fractures around the femoral neck, which were (and are) treated using 'transfixing' nails and screws; earlier hip prostheses may be described as a transfixing nail with a 'ball' on top.

From the design point of view, the hip prosthesis is mostly oriented to provide the kinematic and mechanical performance required. With this in view, other prostheses stress this concept even further reproducing the

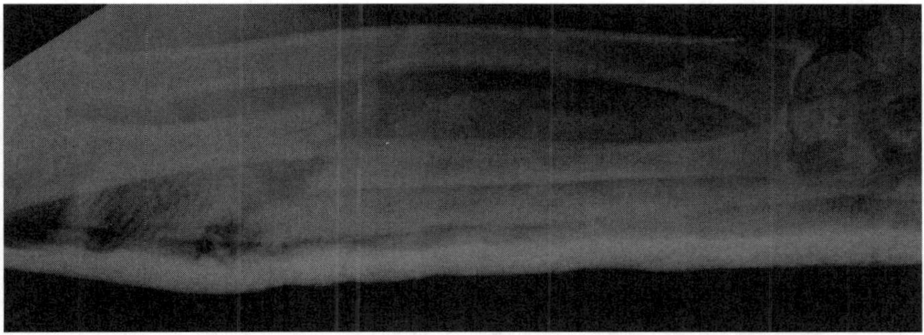

13.23 A dislocation of the head of the radius and a mid-shaft fracture of the ulna, which required surgical treatment.

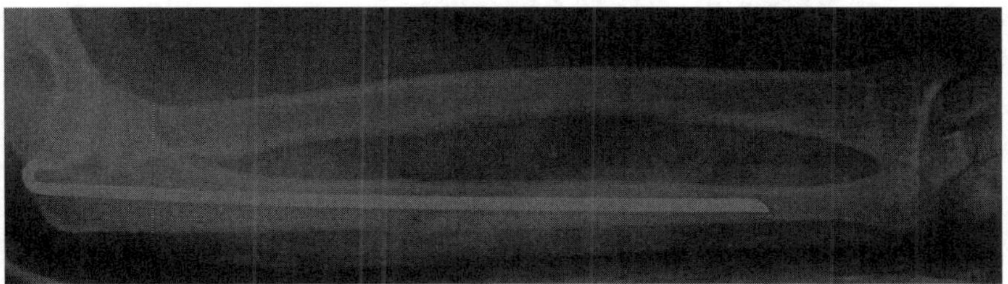

13.24 After reducing the head of the radius in place, appropriate alignment and fixation of the ulna was obtained using an intramedullary nail.

mechanics of a joint in a fashion different from that designed by Nature, like the inverted shoulder prosthesis, for example. In the past, even an inverted hip-prosthesis was proposed (Fig. 13.25) but the vast majority of joint prostheses nowadays reproduce the natural anatomy of a joint. In this way they are 'resurfacing arthroplasty' prostheses, aimed at substituting the worn component of the joint, namely, the articular cartilage. Even with the most sophisticated reproduction of natural geometry, the system does not always work. Joints like the elbow or the metacarpo-phalangeal joint are still far from having an effective artificial substitute able to provide a long-term clinical survival.

The core problem seems to be the appropriate cyclic load transfer between the prosthesis and the recipient bone. Loosening of the artificial joint eventually follows any mismatch in mechanical coupling between the prosthesis and bone. This may be partly circumvented by the best possible biological interface between the prosthesis and the recipient bone but, in the mid- or long-term, no biological integration can counteract the noxious action of an inappropriate load transfer.

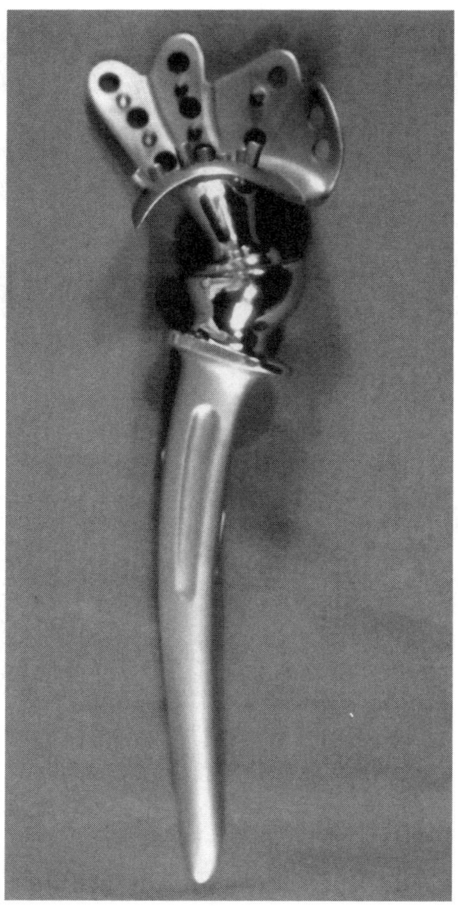

13.25 A past italian design of an inverted hip prosthesis (Picchio MD).

13.4.3 Devices for bone replacement

Until recently there would have been little space for the term 'device' while treating this topic. Actually what was proposed for bone replacement were mostly powders or granules, made of HA or various preparations of calcium phosphates or blends of polylactic acid. More complicated gels and foams and three-dimensional scaffolds have, since then, gradually reached the market. But it is in this field that growth factors and cells will be soon be considered as components of a more complex assembly, together with scaffolds which are proposed in a vast range of degradable new materials, some of them quite exotic, like chitosan-based (Hu *et al.*, 2004) and soybean-based biomaterials (Santin *et al.*, 2007) (Fig. 13.26).

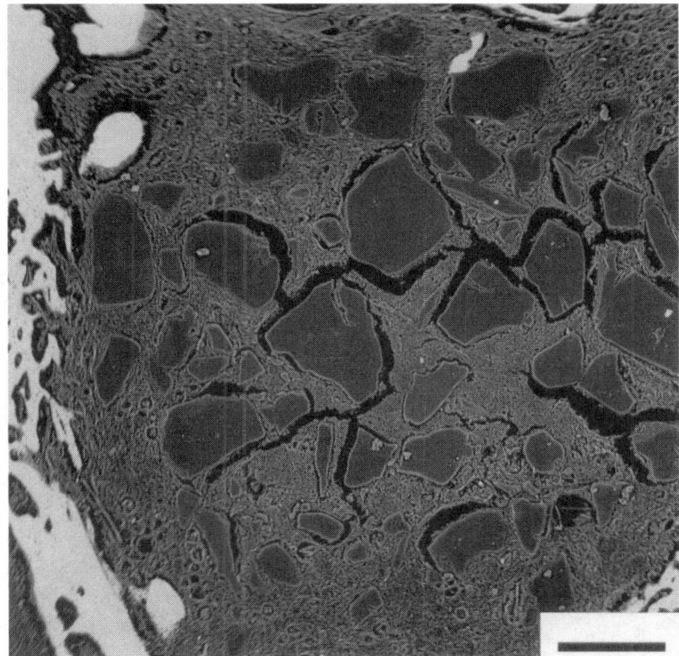

13.26 A back scattered electron micrograph which shows degrading soy-bean-based granules (in dark grey) implanted into a cavity, experimentally produced in the rabbit femur; newly formed trabecular bone starts to repair the wound at the periphery, after one month.

The *in vivo* regeneration of bone at will, particularly in humans and in pathological conditions, is not within easy reach at the moment, but it is the target of intense research carried on in several laboratories around the world.

13.5 Conclusions

The expectations of the orthopaedic surgeon may sometimes differ from those of the material scientist. A biodegradable material may not be considered degradable at all when the clinical requirements, like the duration of the fracture healing process, are taken into consideration; or an osteointegrative surface treatment may be of little help if the implant that should be integrated receives a totally inappropriate load.

It seems quite reasonable to stress that research into bone repair biomaterials should comprehensively assemble all the factors involved. They are not only related to the material properties and to the biological response of recipient tissues, but should also take into consideration the pathophysiology of the clinical condition where their use is proposed, the feasibility of the surgical technique eventually required, sterilization and storage issues, the possibility of an industrial process and the presumptive final cost for the end-user.

13.6 References

Aboulafia AJ, Levine AM, Schmidt D and Aboulafia D (2007) 'Surgical therapy of bone metastases'. *Semin Oncol*, **34**(3), 206–14.

Boeree NR, Dove J, Cooper JJ, Knowles J and Hastings GW (1993) 'Development of a degradable composite for orthopaedic use: mechanical evaluation of an hydroxyapatite-polyhydroxybutyrate composite material'. *Biomaterials*, **14**(10), 793–6.

Chapman MW (1993) *Operative Orthopaedics*, Lippincott, Philadelphia.

Crowninshield RD, Rosenberg AG and Sporer SM (2006) 'Changing demographics of patients with total joint replacement'. *Clin Orthop Relat Res*, **443**, 266–72.

Di Silvio L, Dalby M and Bonfield W (1998) '*In vitro* response of osteoblasts to hydroxyapatite-reinforced polyethylene composites'. *J Mater Sci Mater Med*, **9**(12), 845–8.

Dorland's Medical Dictionary (2007) Elsevier – Saunders, Philadelphia.

Greco F, de Palma L, Specchia N, Jacobelli S and Gaggini C (1992) 'Polymethylmethacrylate-antiblastic drug compounds: an *in vitro* study assessing the cytotoxic effect in cancer cell lines – a new method for local chemotherapy of bone metastasis'. *Orthopedics*, **15**(2), 189–94.

Hamadouche M and Sedel L (2000) 'Ceramics in orthopaedics'. *J Bone Joint Surg Br*, **82B**(8), 1095–9.

Hench LL, Splinter RJ, Allen WC and Greenlee TK (1971) 'Bonding mechanisms at the interface of ceramic prosthetic materials'. *J Biomed Mater Res*, **2**, 117–21.

Hu Q, Li B, Wang M and Shen J (2004) 'Preparation and characterization of biodegradable chitosan/hydroxyapatite nanocomposite rods via *in situ* hybridization: a potential material as internal fixation of bone fracture'. *Biomaterials*, **25**(5), 779–85.

Kent ME, Rapp RP and Smith KM (2006) 'Antibiotic beads and osteomyelitis: here today, what's coming tomorrow? *Orthopedics*, **29**(7), 599–603.

Kim S (2008) 'Changes in surgical loads and economic burden of hip and knee replacements in the US: 1997-2004'. *Arthritis Rheum*, **59**(4), 481–8.

Låftman P, Nilsson OS, Brosjö O and Strömberg L (1989) 'Stress shielding by rigid fixation studied in osteotomized rabbit tibiae'. *Acta Orthop Scand*, **60**(6), 718–22.

Lovell ME, Galasko CS and Wright NB (1999) 'Removal of orthopedic implants in children: morbidity and postoperative radiologic changes'. *J Pediatr Orthop Br*, **8**(2), 144–6.

Merolli A, Guidi PL, Gianotta L and Tranquilli Leali P (1999) 'The clinical outcome of bioactive glass coated hip prostheses'. *Bioceramics 12*, Ohgushi H, Yoshikawa T and Hastings GW (eds). World Scientific, Singapore, 597–600.

Merolli A, Gabbi C, Cacchioni A, Ragionieri L, Caruso L, Giannotta L and Tranquilli Leali P (2001) 'Bone response to polymers based on poly-lactic acid and having different degradation times'. *J Mater Sci Mater Med*, **12**, 775–8.

Merolli A, Moroni A, Faldini C, Tranquilli Leali P and Giannini S (2003) 'Histomorphological study of bone response to hydroxyapatite coating on stainless steel'. *J Mater Sci Mater Med*, **14**, 327–33.

Merolli A, Gabbi C, Santin M, Locardi B and Tranquilli Leali P (2004) 'Bioactive glass coatings on Ti6Al4V promote the tight apposition of newly-formed bone *in-vivo*'. *Key Eng Materials*, **254–6**, 789–92.

Middleton JC and Tipton AJ (2000) 'Synthetic biodegradable polymers as orthopedic devices'. *Biomaterials*, **21**(23), 2335–46.

Moroni A, Cadossi M, Romagnoli M, Faldini C and Giannini S (2008) 'A biomechanical and histological analysis of standard versus hydroxyapatite-coated pins for external fixation'. *J Biomed Mater Res B Appl Biomater*, **86B**(2), 417–21.

Närhi TO, Jansen JA, Jaakkola T, de Ruijter A, Rich J, Seppälä J and Yli-Urpo A (2003) 'Bone response to degradable thermoplastic composite in rabbits'. *Biomaterials*, **24**(10), 1697–704.

Pitton MB, Herber S, Koch U, Oberholzer K, Drees P and Düber C (2008) 'CT-guided vertebroplasty: analysis of technical results, extraosseous cement leakages, and complications in 500 procedures'. *Eur Radiol*, **18**(11), 2568–78.

Santin M, Morris C, Standen G, Nicolais L and Ambrosio L (2007) 'A new class of bioactive and biodegradable soybean-based bone fillers'. *Biomacromolecules*, **8**(9), 2706–11.

Stedman's Medical Dictionary (2007) Lippincott – Raven, Philadelphia.

Stein PS, Sullivan J, Haubenreich JE and Osborne PB (2005) 'Composite resin in medicine and dentistry'. *J Long Term Eff Med Implants*, **15**(6), 641–54.

Tranquilli Leali P, Merolli A, Palmacci O, Gabbi C, Cacchioni A and Gonizzi G (1994) 'Evaluation of different preparations of plasma-spray hydroxyapatite coating on titanium alloy and duplex stainless steel in the rabbit'. *J Mater Sci Mater Med*, **5**, 345–9.

Urabe K, Itoman M, Toyama Y, Yanase Y, Iwamoto Y, Ohgushi H, Ochi M, Takakura Y, Hachiya Y, Matsuzaki H, Matsusue Y and Mori S (2007) 'Current trends in bone grafting and the issue of banked bone allografts based on the fourth nationwide survey of bone grafting status from 2000 to 2004'. *J Orthop Sci*, **12**(6), 520–5.

Williams D (1995) 'Biomimetic surfaces: how man-made becomes man-like'. *Med Device Technol*, **6**(1), 6–8.

14
Bone tissue engineering

M. SANTIN, University of Brighton, UK

Abstract: In the last three decades, tissue engineering has emerged as a new discipline with the aim of addressing serious clinical cases where the spontaneous repair of damaged tissue is impaired. Bone tissue engineering is one of the most investigated areas of application and a large body of data is now available that sheds light on the ideal features of a bone tissue engineering construct. Materials scientists are now able to synthesise biomimetic and bioresponsive biomaterials that fulfil the main requirements for tissue formation *in vitro* or *in vivo*. Biodegradable/bioresorbable polymers, ceramics and composites have been developed which can act as substrates for the adhesion of cells and for the deposition of the calcium phosphate mineral phase of the bony tissues. When engineered into three-dimensional (3D) scaffolds able to host cells (progenitor or differentiated) and bioactive molecules (growth factors, genes and drugs), these biomaterials can constitute an ideal environment to foster the formation of new tissue and to integrate it into the host environment. Although preliminary clinical studies have shown the great potential of bone tissue engineering, the constructs employed still lack an integrated approach where clinical needs are met by a careful design of the construct in all its components and growing conditions. These unmet clinical needs require a coordinated response by scientists, industrialists and policy makers.

Key words: biomaterial engineering, biomaterial scaffolds, bone diseases, bone repair, bone trauma, cell seeding, tissue engineering.

14.1 Introduction

The long clinical history of biomedical implants clearly shows that, while reducing patients' mortality and improving their life quality, they are not able to completely restore the physiology of the damaged tissue. Based on polymeric, metallic and ceramic biomaterials, these implants exert their role, either by replacing the structure and biomechanics of the damaged tissue or by providing a scaffold for its regrowth. In the case of non-degradable biomaterials, the best clinical performance is achieved when good tissue integration is reached. However, the non-degradable biomaterials which are usually employed for the manufacture of permanent devices do not allow the implant to participate in the later remodelling that characterises any tissue.

Conversely, bioresorbable/biodegradable biomaterials offer the opportunity of achieving complete tissue repair, their gradual degradation being accompanied by formation of new tissue. However, unless growth factors or drugs are added to their formulation, this class of biomaterials supports new tissue formation on the mere basis of the surface ability to act as a substrate for cell adhesion and proliferation. This feature may not be sufficient to generate complete tissue repair, especially when implantation is performed to aid tissue repair under pathological conditions. Furthermore, no biodegradable biomaterial can finely tune its degradation rate to that of tissue growth which inevitably varies from patient to patient. As a consequence, biodegradable/bioresorbable biomaterials are not recommended for load-bearing applications.

Nevertheless, the development of biodegradable/bioresorbable biomaterials and their potential to provide full tissue repair has changed the perspective among material scientists and clinicians who now foresee the potential of regenerating a tissue rather than replacing it with a permanent implant.

14.1.1 Definition, brief history and main features of tissue engineering

Since the early 1970s, scientists such as the paediatric orthopaedic surgeon, WT Green at the Children's Hospital, Boston (USA) tried to achieve full cartilage repair by a combination of cultured chondrocytes and scaffolding material constituted by bone spicules (Vacanti, 2006). Although the implantation of such a construct in nude mice was unsuccessful, it probably marked the first attempt at tissue engineering as we define it nowadays, that is 'a therapeutic application, where the tissue is either grown in a patient or outside the patient and transplanted' (Pittsburgh Tissue Engineering definition). Implied in this definition is the combined use of cells (differentiated or stem cells) and biomaterials and, when required, of growth factors able to stimulate cell activity. Indeed, while assessing the outcome of his experiments, Green suggested that future success would have depended on the availability of optimised biomaterials.

In the following years, scientists at the Massachussets General Hospital and Massachussets Institute of Technology (MIT), Boston used a collagen scaffold seeded with fibroblasts to promote skin repair in burn patients. The rationale of using collagen-based scaffolds was obvious as collagen is the main structural protein composing the extracellular matrix of the connective tissues. However, the implantation of collagen-based biomaterials is known to lead to a certain degree of host response and, as a natural polymer, collagen characteristics are not easy to control in a reproducible manner.

A milestone marking the tissue engineering era has been the work performed by Langer and Vacanti at MIT who for the first time published the regeneration of ear cartilage by seeding chondrocytes in a synthetic biodegradable scaffold (Langer and Vacanti, 1993). The seeded scaffold was implanted subcutaneously into nude mice to provide the construct with favourable conditions for new cartilage formation; the final product was an ear that was implanted into a child to treat a congenital malformation.

Regardless of their clinical outcome, these pioneering studies were fundamental in setting the main features required in tissue engineering. These features are still pursued to optimise tissue engineering constructs for different clinical applications. The main components of a tissue engineering construct have been identified and are now widely recognised as indispensable to successful clinical applications. These main constituents and their roles have been presented by the Pittsburgh Tissue Engineering Initiative and by the American NIH as:

1. *Biomaterials* that can direct the adhesion, proliferation and differentiation of cells to produce tissue with the histological properties of the tissue that needs to be repaired.
2. *Cells* that can be reproducibly
   i. isolated either from the same patient (autologous cells) or from a human donor (allogeneic cells) or from an animal source (xenogeneic cells)
   ii. cultured *in vitro* either without losing their original characteristics, as in the case of differentiated cells, or by acquiring the appropriate phenotype as in the case of stem cells.
3. *Biomolecules* such as growth factors, drugs and genes which can stimulate the cells to proliferate and differentiate.
4. *Engineering* that can provide solutions for optimised tissue growth conditions (optimal scaffold morphology and bioreactors) as well as for storage and shipping (packaging suitable for biological materials).

This chapter will present the state-of-the-art of bone tissue engineering by critically assessing the progress made by scientists and industry towards the optimisation of these main four components. The present and future impact of combined multi-disciplinary efforts in clinical practice will be also discussed by using typical examples of clinical applications where bone repair is pursued.

Currently, the success of the surgical procedures for complete bone repair which are not based on the use of permanent artificial implants relies on the use of bone grafts. These are obtained from a different anatomic site of the same patient (e.g. iliac crest) and are considered the gold standard for bone repair in applications such as maxillofacial surgery. However, their use leads to patient's morbidity and discomfort and to surgical procedures relatively more convolute and expensive; two surgical teams have to operate simultaneously on the patient to harvest the graft and to implant it at the site of tissue damage.

14.2 State-of-the-art of biomaterials for bone tissue engineering

The use of biomaterials in tissue engineering has two main functions: (1) temporary support for the cells while they produce new tissue and (2) cell carrier during implantation thus ensuring their appropriate delivery at the site of implantation.

The first function is essential regardless of the tissue engineering strategy. More explicitly, the biomaterial substrate role is essential to the tissue engineering construct, both when a tissue is grown *in vitro*, for example in a bioreactor system, and when the tissue engineering construct is implanted in the body early after its assembly. The second function is important only in those cases where a tissue engineering construct is intended to stimulate tissue repair at the site of implantation. In the last case, the biomaterial has to offer a series of properties which:

- provide an appropriate environment to maximise cell viability
- give ease of handling in the surgical theatre to facilitate the implantation procedure
- provide a mild pro-inflammatory potential to avoid an adverse foreign body response
- give a degradation/resorption rate comparable to that of the host repairing tissue to facilitate complete tissue repair.

Biomaterials for bone tissue engineering will be hereinafter presented taking into account the requirements for both *in vitro* tissue formation and *in vivo* tissue repair. In both cases, the challenge for the material scientists is to produce biomaterials with substrate properties that mimic the natural extracellular matrix of the bony tissue. As these characteristics have to be ideally coupled to degradation/resorption, only biomaterials able to degrade/resorb will be presented. Owing to the bone physicochemical properties to be mimicked, the examples that will be provided will inevitably fall within the categories of polymeric and ceramic materials, and their relative composites.

Furthermore, it has to be observed that extracellular matrix mimicry can target the cell substrate role played by the natural tissue in different phases. More specifically, a biomaterial can favour cell adhesion, either resembling the physicochemical properties of the mature natural tissue (e.g. chemistry, surface topography and surface tension/wettability) or the physicochemical properties and biorecognition processes of the bone tissue during its different phases of formation.

In the case of biomaterials that aim to simulate mature bone, it is obvious that their preponderant feature has to be mimicry of the bone mineral phase. As described early in this book (Part I, Chapter 2), this is composed of calcium phosphate-based hydroxyapatite. Conversely, in those cases where bone formation is mimicked, non-mineralised substrates or substrates with a certain degree of mineralisation have to be considered. When these non-mineralized or partially mineralised substrates are chosen, they should be able to ensure a later complete mineralisation and chemical bonding with the mineral phase of the surrounding bone.

Therefore, the following sections provide a critical assessment of the main ceramic and polymeric materials which have been developed for bone tissue engineering by taking into account their (1) ability to support osteoblast adhesion, proliferation and differentiation and (2) potential to facilitate the deposition of new hydroxyapatite.

These types of *in vitro* studies investigating the growth behaviour of osteoblasts onto biomaterials are important in establishing basic knowledge and screening methods for the development and application of bone tissue engineering scaffolds. Several papers have been published that compare the substrate properties of commercial biomaterials and, therefore, a large database is available that provides a platform for the optimisation of bone tissue engineering constructs (Itthichaisri *et al.*, 2007).

14.2.1 Substrate properties of ceramics for bone tissue engineering

The ceramic biomaterials adopted for bone tissue engineering are mainly those used for the manufacture of traditional implants and they have been exhaustively discussed in Part II, Chapter 7 of this book. In this section, their main substrate properties and limitations will be highlighted and discussed in the light of their ability to participate in the bone formation process.

Synthetic hydroxyapatite

The chemical nature of the synthetic hydroxyapatite (HA) is undoubtedly very similar to mature bone. As a consequence, when compared to other biomaterials, bone cells recognise this substrate as 'natural' and their adhesion and proliferation is thus encouraged (Fig. 14.1).

The HA cell substrate properties are accompanied by the ability of this ceramic material to favour the precipitation of new mineral phase, this leading to complete integration with the repairing bone *in vivo* (Fig. 14.2). Although the bone integration properties of HA when used as an implant have to be considered excellent, this type of ceramic does not perform equally in bone tissue engineering approaches. Two main reasons can be indicated as causes of HA limitations in tissue engineering-driven bone repair:

- New bone tissue formation by osteoblasts may not be optimal on these

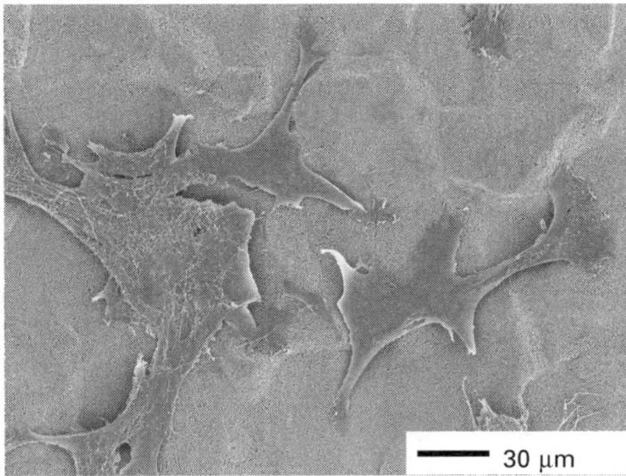

14.1 Scanning electron microscopy of osteoblast adhering onto a HA substrate.

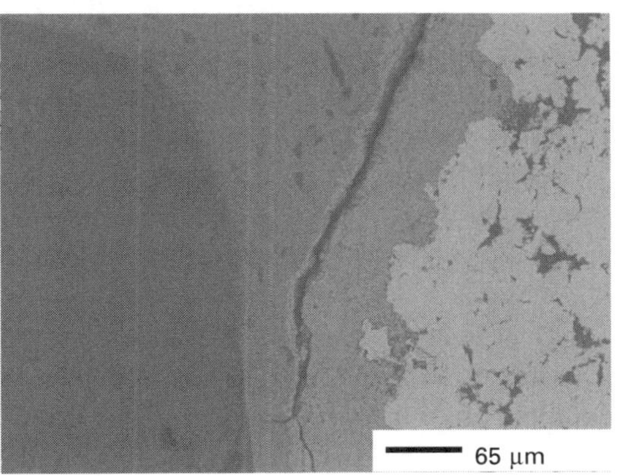

14.2 Backscattering scanning electron microscopy showing the integration of HA with bone.

substrates. The HA physicochemical characteristics are likely to be recognised by the cells as those of a physiological bone where a gradual remodelling rather than a relatively rapid repair is required. This hypothesis seems to be supported by *in vitro* studies that have shown that human osteoblasts adhering on hydroxyapatite (calcium/phosphorus ratio 1.64) have a proliferation rate significantly lower than ceramics with a higher calcium/phosphorus ratio (Santin, unpublished).

- When the crystallinity of HA is relatively high, the degradation of this biomaterial is very slow and it becomes less prone to osteoclast-driven resorption processes and therefore to bone remodelling.

These two limitations, together with the brittle mechanical properties of this type of biomaterial, reduce the potential of HA in bone tissue engineering (Teixeira *et al.*, 2008).

β-tricalcium phosphate and biphasic calcium phosphate

When compared to HA, β-tricalcium phosphate (β-TCP) and biphasic calcium phosphate (BCP, a combination of HA and β-TCP) offer a better alternative in terms of resorption upon bone formation and remodelling. These biomaterials have the same substrate properties as HA, both towards osteoblast adhesion and bone mineral phase deposition. Their advantage is that they are more soluble in a biological environment and more prone to osteoclast-driven resorption (Daculsi, 2006). The setting reaction leading to the formation of these ceramics also results in topographical features more similar to those of the natural tissue and, therefore, more adept at encouraging cell adhesion and activity.

In particular, when BCP composed of HA and β-TCP in a 60/40 ratio was sintered at 1050, 1125 and 1200°C, producing different microporosities, it showed bone repair comparable to that of autologous bone. At 12 weeks after implantation, BCP sintered at 1050°C and BCP processed at 1125°C showed higher degrees of bone apposition, while very little bone formation was observed with the BCP implants treated at 1200°C. These studies clearly demonstrate that bone formation is affected by the physicochemical properties of the ceramics (Fellah *et al.*, 2008).

Bioglasses

Bioactive glasses have a high potential as bone regeneration materials as they stimulate bone cells to produce new tissue, they are degradable in the body and they bind to bone components. The best known bioglass is the Bioglass 45S5 which was discovered by Hench. Bioactive glasses were discovered in 1969 and for the first time provided a biomaterial able to stimulate tissue regeneration and repair using gene activation properties (Hench, 2006).

Recently, an extensive genotypic characterisation of the effect of a commercial bioglass, PerioGlas (US Biomaterials Corp) on cell line human osteosarcoma osteoblast-like cells MG-63 has shown that bone formation by bioglass can be attributable to both osteogenesis (i.e. direct stimulation of osteoblast activity) and osteoconduction (substrate role) (Carinci *et al.*, 2007). By using DNA microarrays containing 20 000 oligonucleotides, several genes were identified in which expression was significantly downregulated. Specifically, this biomaterial seemed to:

- act on signal transduction, especially on the transforming growth factor (TGF-β) paracrine signalling
- inhibit cell apoptosis
- decrease cell adhesion with consequent enhancement of cell mobility and migration
- act on bone marrow stem cell differentiation.

Similar to β-TCP and BCP, the topography of the bioglass also seems to affect cell adhesion and activity. The morphology and activity of human primary osteoblast in response to smooth and roughened bioactive glass of 45S5 has been analysed *in vitro* (Gough *et al.*, 2004). Cell attachment and morphology revealed significant differences between smooth and rough surfaces. Cells adhering to the rough surface were less spread and they showed late organisation of their cytoskeleton when compared to the smooth surface. However, the rough surface induced the formation of a significantly greater number of mineralised bone noduli.

As the use of bioglass in bone tissue engineering is very dependent on the ability to produce porous scaffold (see Section 14.5), this class of biomaterials has been combined with other materials that can improve the engineering of three-dimensional (3D) scaffolds. As a consequence, papers have been published where bioglass has been combined with other elements or biomaterials. For example, a bioactive borate glass was synthesised through normal melting-derived route (Ning *et al.*, 2007). The degradation and bioactivity of this glass when in microsphere formulation showed a degradation rate faster than the silicate-based bioglass, 45S5 glass. HA formed on the borate glass surface, while borate ions inhibited cell proliferation, indicating that the biological performances of the biomaterial are closely dependent on its chemical composition.

Substrate properties of biodegradable polymers for bone tissue engineering

Because of their adaptable chemistry, polymers offer a wide range of choice for mimicking the extracellular matrix of tissues and its composition at different phases of tissue repair. In the case of the bone extracellular matrix, natural and synthetic polymers have also been used because of the possibility of engineering them as 3D scaffolds (see Section 14.5). In this section, as for ceramic materials, the properties of the main polymers in bone tissue engineering will be discussed in the light of their substrate properties for osteoblast adhesion and mineralisation. Furthermore, the potential for the biodegradable polymers and their degradation by-products to trigger a foreign body response will also be evaluated.

Natural polymers (biopolymers)

Bone hydroxyapatite forms and remodels around a collagen type I template (for more details see Part I, Chapter 2 and the biomineralisation section below). As a consequence, collagen type I and its denaturation product gelatine have been widely used as biomaterials for the development of medical devices and bone tissue engineering constructs. The presence of specific bioligands in the collagen structure, such as the amino acid sequences –RGD- (Arg-Gly-Asp) and –DGEA-, favour osteoblast adhesion through their interaction with α(v) β(3) and α(2) β(1) integrins, respectively. However, only recently, more accurate studies have been published that have investigated the effect of these bioligands on osteoblast differentiation. For example, it has been shown that when osteoblast adhering on –RGD- and –DGEA- substrates are stimulated with a growth factor such as the bone morphogenetic protein 9 (pBMP-9) the expression of α(v) integrin subunits in cell membranes increased in presence of –RGD-, but had no effect on β(1) integrin subunits (Marquis *et al.*, 2008). Only on this substratum was osteoblast differentiation induced within 24 hours. These findings show the impact of these adhesion peptides and their biospecificity on the early cell responses to growth factors and they outline how difficult it is to modulate their availability to the cells in collagen-based biomaterials.

The biomimicry potential of collagen has also been enhanced by incorporating other biomacromolecules capable of controlling tissue repair into gels made of this biopolymer. For example, substrate materials such as decorin and biglycan, small leucine-rich proteoglycans which are expressed in bone, have been added to collagen hydrogels. Both these proteoglycans are able to bind to collagen fibrils during fibrillogenesis. These biglycans enhance the formation of human osteoblast focal adhesions on collagen and significantly stimulate their proliferation rate (Douglas *et al.*, 2008).

Bone biomineralisation is a process mediated by collagen and other extracellular matrix proteins (Robey, 1996). However, it is still debated whether collagen is able to induce mineral phase formation directly or through its binding to calcium-binding molecules and structure (e.g. osteopontin, phosphoserine-rich matrix vesicles). The prevailing theories regarding bone tissue mineralisation identify intrafibrillar mineralisation of collagen as the main drive. According to this theory, the growth of the mineral phase is somehow directed by the regular spacing between collagen fibrils that leads to the deposition of uniaxially oriented nanocrystals of hydroxyapatite embedded within and roughly aligned parallel to the long collagen fibril axes. As a consequence, the mineral phase acquires a nanostructured architecture. It is thought that octacalcium phosphate is a precursor of hydroxyapatite, the formation of which is favoured kinetically in supersaturated solutions. However, minor components of the bone organic matrix, such as non-collagenous proteins (NCPs) and the matrix vesicles, are also present and are thought to play an important role in bone mineralisation. To date, there has been no clear understanding of the role of these components, but it is generally assumed that the NCPs regulate crystal growth through some type of 'epitaxial' relationship between specific crystallographic faces and specific protein domains.

Conversely, studies of etched samples of natural bone suggest that the long accepted 'deck of cards' model of bone's nanostructured architecture is not entirely accurate (Olszta *et al.*, 2007). *In vitro* models seem to demonstrate that a highly specific, epitaxial-type interaction with NCPs is not required to induce the nucleation of apatite crystals and to regulate their orientation. These studies would suggest that collagen is the primary template for crystal organisation, but their initial nucleation seems to depend on the infiltration of amorphous precursors in the template structure.

Figure 14.3 shows a typical example of *in vitro* biomineralisation potential in collagen gels. When collagen scaffolds were incubated in a typical simulated body fluid (SBF) no mineralisation was achieved (data not shown). However, collagen scaffolds impregnated with phosphoserine-rich liposomes mimicking the bone matrix vesicles readily mineralised when they were incubated in the same SBF.

For those bone tissue engineering approaches where tissue repair is pursued *in vivo*, the host reaction to collagen has also to be taken into account. It is known that macrophage activation is encouraged by collagen substrates both *in vitro* and *in vivo* (Santin and Cannas, 1999).

Hyaluronan (Hyal) is a biopolymer widely exploited in biomedicine. Hyal plays a predominant role in tissue morphogenesis, cell migration, proliferation and cell differentiation. Studies have shown that Hyal (800 kDa) can induce osteogenic differentiation of bone marrow stromal cells (Zou *et al.*, 2008). In particular, Hyal increased cell proliferation, but it decreased the basal level of bone-related gene expression after 7 days of culture. However, when cells were cultivated in an osteogenic medium, Hyal increased calcium deposit after a longer incubation time (21 days) as well as increasing the expression of

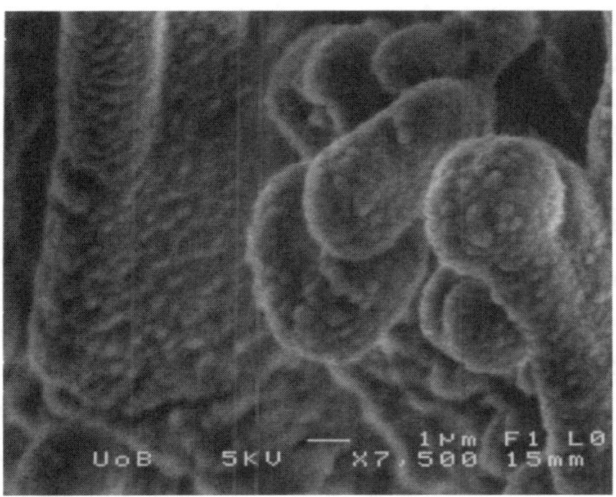

14.3 Cryostat scanning electron microscopy showing the mineralisation of collagen gel entrapping phosphoserine-rich liposomes after 2 days incubation in SBF.

markers of bone formation such as cbfa1, alkaline phosphatase, and type 1 β collagen. At day 21, osteocalcin expression was also significantly upregulated in an osteogenic medium. These results also suggested that exogenous Hyal stimulates the synthesis of endogenous Hyal by the cells, thus playing a synergetic role in osteogenic differentiation. At our knowledge, no reports have shown the mineralisation potential of this biopolymer when incubated in SBF *in vitro*.

Fibrin, the product of polymerisation of fibrinogen, a plasma protein responsible for blood clot formation, is another biopolymer widely used in the biomedical field. The availability of commercial fibrin glues has been exploited in tissue engineering as a matrix to encapsulate cells, among them osteoblasts (Chow *et al.*, 2008).

The inductive effect of the injectable osteoinductive material based on fibrin sealant on the proliferation and differentiation of marrow stromal cells (MSCs) towards osteoblasts has been demonstrated especially when in combination with bone morphogenetic protein spiking (Cui *et al.*, 2007a). MSCs adhering to a fibrin substrate without any growth factor spiking showed a lower degree of MSC differentiation toward osteoblasts and a higher proliferation activity. This behaviour is consistent with the role of fibrin in the early phases of tissue repair when cell proliferation is required.

Human MSC behaviour in eight different formulations of fibrin gels (Tisseel™) prepared with various concentrations of fibrinogen complex and thrombin varied, depending on the gel formulation (Malafaya *et al.*, 2007). In low fibrinogen complex concentration cell proliferation was reduced, while alkaline phosphatase (ALP) activity increased in the formulations containing a high concentration of this complex (Catelas *et al.*, 2006). High fibrinogen complex concentrations also induced the formation of small mineralised bone noduli after 21 and 28 days of culture in hydrogel with high fibrin concentration. This mineralisation process was concomitant with an increase in the bone sialoprotein (BSP) gene expression level, and in ALP and osteopontin levels, although to lesser extent. However, there was no significant increase in the expression of osteocalcin, a late marker of osteogenic differentiation. Therefore, human MSC differentiation in fibrin gels seems to depend on the fibrinogen complex/thrombin ratio, although the cells did not fully differentiate into mature osteoblasts. This cell behaviour in fibrin matrices could be expected if it is considered that in a natural bone repair process, fibrin intervenes in the very early phases of the repair in response to bone fracture.

As fibrin is an ordered organic matrix which has a repeating periodic structure of 230 Å, it could be expected to be a good substrate for HA formation. It has been demonstrated that HA crystallisation in fibrin gels immersed in SBF is a very rapid process (Koutsopoulos and Dalas, 2000). Theoretical calculation seems to show that phosphate is taken up extensively by fibrin and in a manner dependent on the ionic strength and pH of the medium, thus suggesting the establishment of electrostatic forces. The study showed that, surprisingly, calcium ions did not exhibit any detectable adsorption when fibrin gels were incubated in $CaCl_2$/NaCl solutions under physiological conditions (body temperature and pH). Therefore, the data suggested that the initial interaction of the fibrin gels with phosphate was the driver in the HA formation on these types of gels.

Fibroin is another protein-based biopolymer that is extracted from silk. Silk fibroin has been widely used to produce hydrogels by different techniques and their biocompatibility and cell substrate potential clearly demonstrated. It has been shown that this biomaterial can support osteoblast adhesion and that this interaction can be modulated by the method of preparation of the silk fibroin gels. For example, when fibroin hydrogels are prepared either by treating a silk fibroin aqeuous solution at 4°C or by adding glycerol, a higher cell activation and differentiation was found with the substrate formed at low temperature and a faster cell proliferation with the one produced by glycerol mixing (Motta *et al.*, 2004). These different behaviours may be ascribed to the different water content and fibroin conformations.

As for its biocompatibility, the biomineralisation potential of the silk fibroin seems to depend on the protein conformational status. The formation of hydroxyapatite deposits on three types of silk films (water-annealed, methanol-treated and polyaspartic acid (PAA)-mixed) following various cycles of mineralisation has shown that a significant degree of mineralisation could be obtained only on the surface of PAA-mixed silk films, while the water-annealed hydrogels showed the lowest levels (Gupta *et al.*, 2008). The deposits of minerals in the water-annealed films were predominantly flake-like, whereas methanol-treated and PAA-mixed silk films resulted in a densely-packed mineral phase.

In the last few years, a new class of soybean-based biomaterials has been developed. Unlike previous attempts focussing on the manufacture of biomaterials from soybean proteins, this new class is produced from defatted soy flour by thermosetting or extraction procedures and preserves the soy proteins as well as its carbohydrate fraction and isoflavone content (Santin *et al.*, 2007). The combination of these components allows the preparation of different biomaterial formulations suitable for many clinical applications. Above all, this novel class of biomaterials has been shown to induce osteoblast adhesion and differentiation *in vitro* and bone formation *in vivo*, while inhibiting osteoclast activity. Incubation in SBF, clearly shows the relatively rapid formation of a calcium phosphate mineral phase after 2 days incubation.

More detailed information on natural polymers can be found in a review paper published by Malafaya *et al.* (2007). The use of hydrogels made of polysaccharides such as chitosan (the deacetylation product of chitin, the main component of the mollusc shell) and alginate emerges, among others. Chitosan seems to have a poor biomineralisation potential. A significant HA formation could be observed *in vitro* only when chitosan films were immersed in pseudo-SBFs, the ion concentrations of which are doubled in respect to other SBFs (Beppu *et al.*, 2005). Therefore, pseudo-SBFs do not genuinely simulate the ion composition of the *in vivo* bone repair environment. X-ray diffractograms showed that deposits are poorly crystalline (like biological apatites) and a higher crystallinity was shown in those pseudo-SBFs where the phosphorous concentration was higher.

Therefore, chitosan biomineralisation *in vitro* has been pursued through modifications of this polysaccharide. For example, electrospun nanofibrous scaffolds which were prepared by using chitosan/polyvinyl alcohol (CS/PVA) and N-carboxyethyl chitosan/PVA (CECS/PVA) supported the deposition of HA when immersed in a supersaturated $CaCl_2$ and KH_2PO_4 solution (Yang *et al.*, 2008). The presence of poly(acrylic acid) in the ionic solution and the use of matrix with carboxylic acid groups promoted crystal deposition and growth.

Similar substrate potentials for cell adhesion and HA formation were observed in the case of alginate. Satisfactory adhesion, proliferation and differentiation of osteoblasts was found only when gels of this polysaccharide were functionalised with specific bioligands (for more details see Section 14.2.3) (Evangelista *et al.*, 2007).

The effect of soluble sodium alginate on HA crystal growth has been investigated in supersaturated ion solutions (Malkaj *et al.*, 2005). Sodium alginate was found to inhibit HA crystal growth and kinetic studies seem to show that this inhibition is caused by a Langmuir-type adsorption of the alginate on the forming HA surface which may impede HA crystal growth.

Synthetic polymers

As biopolymer physicochemical properties and batch-to-batch variability are difficult to control, biomaterial scientists have tried to develop synthetic polymers able to support tissue repair. As a result, a large number of degradable synthetic polymers has been developed which have been later tested for their potential in tissue engineering and, among the various clinical applications, for bone tissue engineering. The currently available biodegradable synthetic polymers have been optimised for tuneable and safe degradation processes. Conversely, their potential for supporting cell adhesion and biomineralisation relies on the presence of suitable functional groups in their structure rather than in attempting to mimic accurately the features of the extracellular matrix. Only in the last decade, has the importance of their specific functionalisation with biomimetic molecules been considered.

For example, if we consider the cell substrate and mineralisation potential of two biodegradable synthetic polymers, poly(ε-caprolactone) (PCL) and poly(lactic/glycolic acid) (PLA/PGA), approved by the Food and Drug Adminstration (FDA), it is clear that their osteoblast adhesion is not necessarily satisfactory in the case of PCL (Fig. 14.4a) when compared to standard tissue culture plastic (Fig. 14.4b) and no significant mineralisation potential in SBF systems has been reported.

Although the degradation of PLA/PGA co-polymers allows their degradation to be tuned both *in vitro* and *in vivo*, the acidic environment generated by their degradation process may affect cell viability *in vitro* and it has been reported to cause adverse reaction *in vivo* (Hedberg *et al.*, 2005). The osteoblast adhesion properties of this class of copolymers largely employed in manufacturing bone-graft substitutes is also affected by their chemical composition, molecular weight and by the methods of polymerisation and processing (Di Toro *et al.*, 2004). Despite their wide use in clinics, their effects on human osteoblasts *in vitro* have not been accurately investigated.

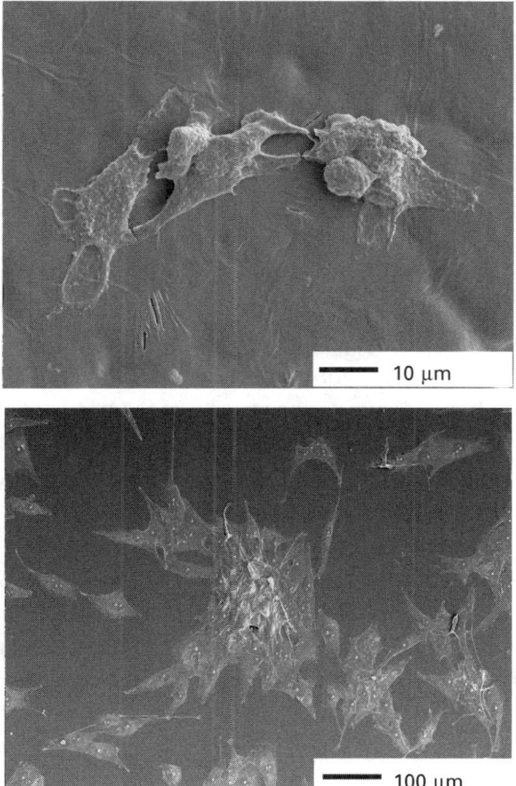

14.4 Osteoblast adhesion on PCL (a) and control tissue culture plate (b).

When typical formulations of these copolymers (75:25 and 50:50 PLA–PGA) were evaluated as substrates for primary human osteoblasts in direct contact tests for 14 days, it was found that there was neither detectable cytotoxicity nor inhibition of cell adhesion and proliferation. The degree of differentiation measured as ALP activity and osteocalcin synthesis was also not affected. Indeed, osteoblast adhesion on these copolymers was found to be mainly β (1)/α(v)/β(1) integrin complex-dependent and only partially dependent on α(v) integrin.

In a similar study, three injectable and biodegradable PLA/PGA 50150 copolymers dispersed in different matrices were tested (Tschon *et al.*, 2007). The PLA/PGA-based bone filler Fisograft-gel (GEL) was dispersed in an aqueous matrix of polyethylglycole (PEG), Slurry2 (SL2) was dispersed in an aqueous matrix of PEG and dextran and Slurry6 (SL6) was dispersed in a 3% agarose matrix. GEL and SL2 induced similar effects on MG-63 osteoblast-like human osteosarcoma cells in terms of viability and differentiation after 7 days in culture, while SL6 caused a higher production of both interleukin-6 and type I collagen. None of these biomaterials showed cytotoxicity. These data were corroborated by *in vivo* studies showing that SL6 was supporting bone repair with more physiological histological features.

Biomineralisation strategies should reproduce the dimension and structural hierarchy of apatite deposits within a demineralised collagen matrix. However, none of the biodegradable synthetic polymers is able to mimic this process. As a consequence, polymers like PLA/PGA, PCL and others have been surface-modified by physical and chemical methods to improve their ability to catalyse the formation of hydroxyapatite crystals.

For example, PLA/PGA (70/30) films and scaffolds have been treated with oxygen plasma to enhance their biomineralisation potential tested in SBF (Qu *et al.*, 2007). It has been hypothesised that the acquired ability of this modified polymer in inducing hydroxyapatite formation was due to the combined effect of the changed surface chemistry and surface topography. It was also observed that the presence of newly formed hydroxyapatite layer enhanced the adhesion and proliferation of OCT-1 osteoblast-like cells, but had no significant effect on their ALP activity after 7 days in culture.

PCL has also been modified to improve its biomineralisation potential. For instance, the polymer surface has been modified by phosphate salts (i.e. NaH_2PO_4, Na_2HPO_4 KH_2PO_4 or K_2HPO_4) (Puska *et al.*, 2008). The results showed that the addition of phosphate salts led to an improvement in the compression strength of PCL as a result of their mineralisation process with a new apatite-like phase.

More information can be found in Chapter 8 of this book and in a comprehensive review paper published by Sokolsky-Papkov *et al.* (2007).

14.2.2 Substrate properties of composites for bone tissue engineering

The sections dedicated to ceramics and polymeric biomaterials have highlighted that, although promising biomaterials for bone tissue engineering have been developed from these two classes, limitations are still present that prevent the complete mimicking of bone extracellular matrix properties (i.e. chemical composition, mechanical properties and biorecognition). Indeed, if analysed from a material viewpoint, bone can be considered to be a composite material, the characteristics of which dynamically change during both repair and remodelling processes. The formation of bone during its repair process involves the synthesis and deposition of a polymeric scaffold (collagen type I) by the osteoblasts which is gradually encased in a HA-based mineral phase. In the remodelling process, the osteoclasts gradually resorb old bone which is replaced by new tissue produced by the oseoblasts; the combination of the activity of these two cell types results in constant changes in the histological features. In both processes, a tissue with a composite nature forms. In the attempt to mimic the composite nature of bone, several polymer/ceramic biomaterials have been developed with the intention of mimicking the collagen template and the HA-based mineral phase.

Here, examples are provided that are based on the use of the ceramics and polymeric materials which were presented in the previous sections. Before providing these examples, it is worth analysing the mechanisms of biomineralisation; understanding them allows us to assess the strategies that have been adopted by researchers to obtain bone biomimicking composites.

Studies on the mechanisms of HA formation in natural systems

The mechanisms of crystal nucleation are very complex and difficult to discern at both the experimental and theoretical level and, as a consequence, understanding the underlying principles leading to the formation of polymeric/matrix composite materials is not always easy. The study and understanding of the mechanisms of crystal nucleation require a profound knowledge of both ion solvation processes (i.e. ion/solvent interactions) and ion–ion interactions. In the case of biocomposites, the study is complicated by the presence of biomolecules and their effect on the crystal growth effect. Special simulation strategies have recently been developed that extend considerably the potential of computational studies in this field. These simulations have been underpinned by experimental studies on the nucleation of biomimetic apatite on gelatine hydrogels during composite preparation processes and they have explained the mechanisms of hierarchical crystal growth at both the micro- and mesoscopic scale. A review paper has been published that outlines future directions and discusses the perspectives of simulation in biomineralisation studies (Zahn *et al.*, 2007).

These studies may soon be fundamental to obtaining highly controlled methods of fabrication of scaffolds for tissue engineering (see Section 14.5). Computational models needs to be underpinned by the background information available in the literature that offers insights into the structure, self-assembly mechanisms and properties of mineralised collagen fibril composites (Robey, 1996, Olszta *et al.*, 2007).

Types of polymer/ceramic composites for bone tissue engineering and their fabrication methods

Thus far, all the polymeric and ceramic materials described in the previous sections have been employed in an attempt to produce composite biomaterials able to mimic bone structures. Above all, collagen/HA composites have been designed because of their close proximity to the bone chemical composition. Investigation and simulation of the collagen fibril structures has presented the knowledge platform for developing bone grafts or for their use as bone biomimetic engineering materials and scaffolds in bone tissue engineering. Indeed, the development of bone grafts based on the mineralisation of self-assembled collagen fibrils *in vivo* and *in vitro* is an active area of research (Cui *et al.*, 2007b).

As a collagen denaturation derivative, gelatin matrix composites reinforced with HA crystals have been investigated for their suitability in bone repair applications (Hillig *et al.*, 2008). At a sufficiently high ratio of HA to gelatin, compressive stiffness and resistance to swelling of these biomaterial suggested their potential in replacing bone structures. However, this was achieved with a degree of porosity not necessarily suitable for tissue engineering scaffolds (see Section 14.5).

Novel composites based on calcium phosphates/collagen doped with other ions (e.g. Zn^{+2}) have been synthesised (Santos *et al.*, 2007). In this approach, type I collagen was added to HA and biphasic hydroxyapatite/β-TCP and the mixture was blended until a homogenous composite was obtained. Doping of the composite was obtained by adding 1.0 wt% Zn^{2+} aqueous solution. The cell substrate properties of the doped composite were compared to those of the non-doped biomaterial. Although both composites were shown to induce osteoblast adhesion and later differentiation, no significant difference was induced by the doped compound.

Collagen/HA composites have also been produced in the form of microparticles (Kim *et al.*, 2007). Because of their physicochemical properties, microparticles are considered among the most suitable candidates for delivering drugs and cells in tissue engineering applications. It has been suggested that microparticles may encourage the recruitment of osteoblasts *in vivo*. Collagen–apatite nanocomposites assembled as microspheres have been obtained in a water-in-oil emulsion condition. Spherical microparticles with diameters ranging from tens to hundreds of micrometres were thus obtained. Morphological studies showed that the nanostructured organisation of HA crystals was evenly distributed in the collagenic matrix. The nanocomposite microspheres supported rat bone stem cell adhesion and growth and expressed a series of genes that indicated their differentiation into osteoblasts. Also, ALP activity on the composite microspheres was higher than on control collagen microspheres.

Antheraea pernyi silk fibroin (Ap-SF) has also been employed to control HA nanocrystal formation (Ren *et al.*, 2007). The mineral phase was formed under relatively mild conditions, that is, incubation in a aqueous solution, pH 7.4 and room temperature. An inorganic phase characterised by small carbonate-HA particles with low crystallinity has been shown to take place. Ultrastructural studies have shown that these nanoparticles interacted with the fibroin to form mineralised rod-like nanofibrils (4–5 nm in diameter). The composites were shown to assemble into mineralised rods 49–74 nm in diameter.

Silk fibroin has been used to prepare HA nanocomposites using other protocols. For example, silk fibroin can be used to produce HA-based composites by a previous chemical modification of the protein with alkali solution or enzyme digestion in an attempt to improve the interface between the mineral and the organic matrix (Wang *et al.*, 2007). Both pretreatments favoured the formation of a highly ordered 3D porous network promoting the preferential growth of HA crystallites along the *c*-axis. In particular, in the case of the enzyme treatment, the composite acquired a hierarchical microstructure with higher degree of organization and more uniform pore size distribution, where HA crystallites underwent morphological transformation from rod-like to whisker-like structures growing along the *c*-axis. The alkali pretreatment induced more stable interactions between the biopolymer and the forming HA.

Alternatively, fibroin/HA composites were manufactured by alternating film deposition in a lamination method where temperature and compression times were varied (Kino *et al.*, 2007). HA was deposited on fibroin films by soaking methanol-treated fibroin films containing > 5 wt% $CaCl_2$ in SBF with an ion concentration 1.5-fold higher than standard SBF. In the multilayered fibroin/HA films obtained in this reiterated process, HA layers of an approximate thicknesses of 3–5 μm were obtained. The bonding strength between the fibroin and the HA layers was significantly affected by temperature and compression time under the lamination method. The optimal conditions for achieving the maximum T-peel strength and protein β-sheet contents were determined to be 130°C for 4 min. The biocompatibility of the composites when they were tested with cell line osteoblasts (MC3T3-E1) indicated good substrate properties for the cells that were able to differentiate.

HA-based composites have also been pursued with the use of synthetic polymers. Among the biodegradable synthetic polymers that have been presented above, PLA/PGA co-polymers have been considered. In particular, apatite-coating has been integrated on poly(L-lactide) (PLLA) surfaces (Jao *et al.*, 2007). This study focussed on the effect of the hydrolysis of PLLA surfaces on the formation ability of bone-like HA. PLLA films and porous PLLA scaffolds were hydrolysed for different time periods in alkaline solution. The rationale of using a hydrolysis process is to enrich the polymer surface with carboxylic and hydroxyl groups as well as to increase its roughness, features which are known to be able to catalyse HA formation. The HA coating was formed by mineralising the hydrolysed PLLA in SBF for 3 weeks and then characterising it. Indeed, this hydrolysis process increased HA formation on PLLA when compared with the pure PLLA and this increase was more evident with longer hydrolysis times.

In a different method, PLA/HA composites using high-modulus polylactic acid fibres were prepared using a cyclic precipitation technique (Kothapalli *et al.*, 2008). Small calcium phosphate crystal nuclei formed after the first soaking cycle, while large quantities of mineral particles were observed after six cycles (35%). The amount of mineral phase deposited on the polymer yarn increased with deposition time in the calcium and phosphorous-rich solutions and with the number of cycles, but it decreased with stirring rate during washing cycles. The composites were then encased in a PCL matrix to exhibit flexural moduli within the range of that of the cortical bone.

14.2.3 Substrate properties of functionalisation molecules

The sections above have shown that the ability of collagen to act as a substrate for cell adhesion and mineralisation during bone formation depends on the presence of specific functional groups in this protein. Specific amino acid sequences act as bioligands for cell receptors (i.e. cell membrane integrins), while other functionalities or collagen-bound NCPs work as nucleation points for the formation of HA crystals. Biomaterial surface functionalisation strategies have been designed that allow the biomimicking of the chemical, conformational and architectural features of these macromolecules.

These functionalisation strategies have made available a new generation of biomaterials ready for use as synthetic 3D biocompetent extracellular microenvironments (see Section 14.5) able to mimic the regulatory characteristics of natural extracellular matrices (ECM) and ECM-bound growth factors (see Section 14.4). This new generation of bioinstructive biomaterials include self-assembling macromolecules and peptide-conjugated synthetic polymers that present bioactive ligands and that are able to respond to secreted cellular signals participating in the tissue repair process (Ehrbar *et al.*, 2008; Hubbell, 1998; Lutolf and Hubbell, 2005).

Surface functionalisation with adhesion and bioresponsive peptides

Ultimately, reproducing the ECM bioadhesive character, susceptibility to enzymatic degradation and ability to bind growth factors will have a role in maintaining homeostasis and, as a consequence, will contribute to control tissue repair. The biospecific adhesion of cells to the ECM stimulates intracellular pathways, ultimately leading to gene regulation and cell proliferation or differentiation as well as protease secretion that modulates cell migration (Hubbell, 2003).

Work that has been produced over the last decade by J Hubbell and collaborators has certainly opened a new route to obtaining such an accurate level of biomimicry. In his best known approach, Hubbell has functionalised synthetic hydrogels with specific peptides able to confer a bioresponsive character to the synthetic polymer during the tissue repair process. These amino acid sequences are naturally contained in ECM structural proteins; the relative peptides can be synthesised in a relatively easy manner by conventional peptide synthetic methods.

In particular, synthetic hydrogels have been engineered with biomolecules able to make them responsive to cell adhesion and migration (Lutolf *et al.*, 2003a). Poly(ethylene glycol) (PEG) hydrogels were functionalised by a combination of integrin-binding sites and substrates for matrix metalloproteinases (MMP). The former ensured cell adhesion, while the latter made the hydrogel mesh controllable by the secretion of MMP, thus facilitating cell migration. In particular, these networks contain a combination of pendant oligopeptide ligands for cell adhesion (RGDSP) and substrates for MMP as linkers between PEG chains. Cell culture experiments demonstrated that proteolytic sensitivity and suitable mechanical properties were critical for 3D cell migration inside these synthetic matrixes (Lutolf *et al.*, 2003b). These new properties were optimised by studying the enzyme kinetics of the soluble substrate and, then, of its polymer-grafted form. The infiltration of cells in these matrices was also proven and showed to depend on MMP substrate activity, adhesion ligand concentration and network crosslinking density. When these gels were loaded with recombinant human bone morphogenetic protein-2 (BMP-2), they showed complete cell infilatration in rat bone critical defects and the tissue was found to repair within 4 weeks. Bone regeneration was also shown to depend on the proteolytic sensitivity of the matrices.

In a step forward, additional biocompetent molecules were integrated in PEG gels with the purpose of biomimicking other properties of the ECM, such as those of retaining important growth factors and responding to cell activity. PEG-bis-vinylsulfone has been crosslinked by a Michael-type addition reaction with a peptide containing three cysteine residues (Pratt *et al.*, 2004). The presence of these cysteine residues makes the peptide susceptible to cleavage by cell-associated plasmin, a protease able to digest ECM protein components. As a consequence, cells contacting this type of hydrogel were able to invade its network where they interact with grafted adhesion peptides which were linked to main polymer backbone through plasmin resistant peptides. When BMP-2 was loaded in these bioresponsive hydrogels, they were able to induce bone repair *in vivo* in a rat model. This bone repair potential was improved by the integration of grafted heparin in the PEG structure, this molecule possessing affinity for the BMP-2. It can be argued that by introducing BMP-2 binding domains, the ability of the ECM to bind growth factor was successfully mimicked, creating microenvironments with relatively high BMP-2 bioavailability. This work confirms the feasibility of attaining desired biological responses *in vivo* using engineering material properties through the design of single components at the molecular level. In these studies, human recombinant BMP-2 was used, providing a very good example of the technological potential that can be achieved by combining polymer science with recombinant DNA technology (Rizzi *et al.*, 2006).

In a similar approach, RGD- was coupled in a binary (low and high molecular weight) injectable alginate composition in order to influence bone cell differentiation in a 3D structure (Evangelista *et al.*, 2007). Cells within RGD-modified alginate microspheres were shown to establish more interactions with the biomimetic matrix and to express higher levels of differentiation markers.

Importantly, these studies highlight the importance of the grafting strategy for these types of bioligands; grafting is engineered to provide resistant or protease-sensitive linkage as well as adequate exposure to the cell receptors. To achieve this, several chemical strategies have been developed. A review paper by Hersel *et al.* (2003) offers a very comprehensive overview of the different grafting methods and highlights the importance of the degree of exposure of RGD-peptides to cells. Indeed, the synthesis of loop-shaped RGD peptides maximising the exposure of the relevant amino acid sequence has been shown to support higher levels of cell biorecognition.

It has to be outlined that, although the –RGD- sequence has been the most investigated, other amino acid sequences are able to support cell adhesion and migration and, in particular, biospecific interactions with osteoblasts. Among them the –FHRRIKA- sequence has been shown to favour osteoblast migration (Rezania and Healy, 1999) and the –KRSR- which promotes osteoblast adhesion. FHRRIKA and KRSR have in common their ability to bind proteoglycans (Sawyer *et al.*, 2007).

The use of these peptides has to be evaluated in different scenarios as their active role in cell biorecognition processes may be affected by the biomaterial surface to which they are grafted. A study aiming at verifying the reported ability of the –RGD- sequence to favour MSCs adhesion, showed that RGD peptides bound to HA surfaces increased the attachment of MSCs to the ceramic, but did not promote their spread. To improve MSC spreading, –KRSR- and –FHRRIKA- were combined with RGD onto HA surfaces. The peptide combinations did not achieve the goal of enhancing MSCs spreading. Similar results were obtained when the proteoglycan-binding peptides were modified with a heptaglutamate domain, a motif that is known to improve peptide binding onto HA surfaces. This study also verified the potential bioadhesive properties of HA functionalised with these peptides after surface conditioning with serum showing no significant effect by the peptides.

Osteoblast adhesion assays on acellular bone matrix using a novel peptide, carrying the X-B-B-B-X-B-B-X motif (where B is a basic amino acid and X is a non-basic residue), were shown to promote proteoglycan-mediated osteoblast adhesion more efficiently than the –KRSR- sequence that is considered to be a heparan sulfate-binding peptide (Dettin *et al.*, 2002).

Therefore, the studies so far performed seem to demonstrate that, although effective in many situations, the use of these peptides for improving cell biorecognition may not always be suitable in bone tissue engineering. It may be suggested that the use of these bioligands is more promising in those applications where bone formation has to be achieved *in vitro*. The implantation of tissue engineering constructs aiming to promote bone formation *in vivo* may not always benefit from the presence of these functionalisation peptides. Finally, the costs of synthesis and storage of these relatively unstable peptides need to be taken into account. The real benefits of the use of these expensive and relatively unstable molecules need also to be assessed in the light of other effective and cost competitive technologies and, moreover, in terms of a significantly improved clinical outcome.

Biomineralisation molecules

Mimicry of the bone organic matrix has not been limited to the structure of collagen. NCPs, proteins playing a key role in the biomineralisation process, have also been mimicked in the structure of biomaterials for bone applications. Interpenetrating nanostructured architecture, using relatively simple anionic polypeptides that mimic the polyanionic character of the NCPs has been used for this purpose (Olszta *et al.*, 2007). The system was prepared by combining an amorphous liquid-phase mineral precursor to the polymer to generate hydroxyapatite and to facilitate intrafibrillar mineralisation of type-I collagen. The fluidic character of the amorphous precursor phase enables it to penetrate into the nanoscopic gaps and grooves of collagen fibrils by capillary action thus providing diffuse and regularly spaced apatite nucleation loci with a mechanism mimicking that of collagen mineralisation *in vivo*.

Electron diffraction patterns of these highly mineralised collagen fibrils were similar to those of natural bone, HA crystallites being preferentially aligned with [0 0 1] orientation along the collagen fibril axes.

A novel class of nanostructured, semidendrimeric polymers has been recently designed to induce biomineralisation on biomaterial surfaces (Santin *et al.*, 2006). Dendrimers are hyperbranched polymers obtained by liquid-phase synthesis from a core molecule. These molecules have been used as gene delivery carriers in cell transfection techniques. Their use as drug carriers has also been postulated. Dendrimers with different branching generations can be synthesised to form spherical structures. However, when solid-phase synthesis is adopted, semidendrimers are obtained. The advantages of semidendrimers in the biomaterial and tissue engineering fields include the possibility of synthesising molecules with a dual functionality (Fig. 14.5 a). The root of

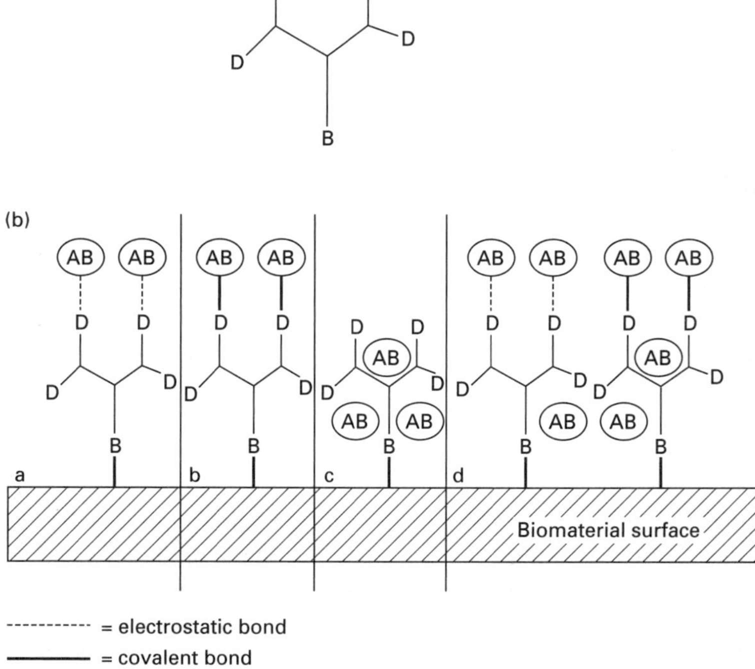

14.5 Schematic representation of dual functional, biocompetent semidendrimers. (a) Single molecule showing different functional groups at the root and branches of the nano-tree and (b) surface functionalisation strategies of this class of nanostructured biomaterials. D indicates a functional group able to bind a biomaterial surface or another type of semidendrimer. AB indicates an active biomolecule covalently or physically bound to semi-denderimers.

the nano-tree can be designed to expose functionalities able to recognise the biomaterial surface or another semidendrimer root, while the branches can be tethered with biospecific moieties. Poly(ε-lysine) and poly(amido amine) semidendrimers have been synthesised following this strategy to obtain uppermost branching generations functionalised with phosphoserine, one of the most potent biomineralisation agents. These phosphoserine-tethered semidendrimers can be grafted on the surface of biomaterials or interact with each other to induce apatite formation. Furthermore, the mesh of the nanogel created by the close apposition of these nanostructured molecules provides an opportunity for the entrapment of growth factors and drugs able to stimulate bone repair (Fig. 14.5 b).

14.3 Cells for bone tissue engineering

Scientific knowledge acquired in the last three decades in biomaterial science has recently been translated into advanced tissue engineering products that can combine the use of such materials with cells and their ability to repair tissues. However, the clinical use of tissue engineering constructs hosting either cells or *in vitro*-formed tissues depends on a thorough understanding and standardisation of cell sourcing and bioactive stimuli. Basically, orthopaedic tissue engineering relies on a strategy (or combination of strategies) aiming at enhancing the activity of bone-forming cells. To this end, scientists have been pursuing the incorporation of differentiated osteobasts or stem cells into tissue engineering scaffolds. These cells can be sourced either from the same patient (autologous cells) or from human donors (allogeneic cells), the latter being either primary cells or immortalised cell lines. However, the use of differentiated cells suffers major drawbacks:

- The availability of autologous cells is limited and their expansion is time consuming.
- Allogeneic primary cells bear the risk of immunogenic reaction and transmittable diseases. When immortalised, these cells can lose their phenotype and their use is shadowed by an intrinsic carcinogenic potential in their unlimited ability to proliferate.

The indefinite proliferation and differentiation potential of embryonic and adult mesenchymal stem cells, as well as the absence of any ascertained host immunoreaction towards them, make these two types of cell an attractive alternative in bone tissue engineering (Caplan, 1991; Gerecht-Nir and Itskoviz-Eldor, 2004). Human embryonic stem cells, which are derived from the inner cell mass of the embryo blastocyst, have been for years considered to be pluripotent cells. However, more recently it has been shown that these cells have the ability to proliferate perpetually, while retaining an undifferentiated phenotype, but they are also able to differentiate into several specific phenotypes, thus suggesting their totipotency which has been defined as the ability of a cell to form both the embryo and extra-embryonic membranes and tissues. Therefore, pluripotent stem cells, which are able to transform into cells from all three germ lineages, seem to be the most ideal candidates for cell therapy-based bone repair. However, since the embryonic source of pluripotent stem cells for potential therapeutic purposes remains controversial, researchers have been focussing on the isolation of stem cells from adult tissues (Ratajczak *et al.*, 2008).

Connective tissue progenitors are those heterogeneous populations of stem and progenitor cells that are found in native tissue and that are capable of differentiating into one or more connective tissue phenotypes. These mesenchymal stem or progenitor cells are found in various tissues and show varying ability to differentiate into specific cell lineages. Indeed, MSCs are multipotent cells that arise from the mesenchyme during development. They reside in the bone marrow close to the hematopoietic stem cell niches and are responsible for maintaining bone marrow homeostasis and for regulating the maturation of both hematopoietic and non-hematopoietic cells. Although it has been ascertained that MSCs possess an extensive potential to proliferate and differentiate into osteoblasts and osteocytes, the complete pathway(s) leading to their differentiation has not yet been clarified. For these reasons, MSCs are of interest in clinical applications, since they can be easily isolated from bone marrow aspirates and expanded *in vitro*. When the source of osteoprogenitors is compromised, cell-based therapies could provide a novel way to repair bone defects (Heino and Hentunen, 2008). Indeed, most of the available cell-based strategies target the differentiation and tissue regeneration potential of either local cells or transplanted autologous connective tissue progenitor cells derived from bone marrow or other tissues (with or without their expansion in culture) (Patterson *et al.*, 2008).

A discrepancy between the data obtained from research studies and clinical trials highlights the need to identify the type of cells to be used in bone tissue engineering. Most scientific publications focus on the use of isolated MSCs. However, many clinical studies have demonstrated the strong osteogenic potential of fresh harvested total bone marrow. There has been, nevertheless, little research work on the use of total bone marrow as a source of cells for bone tissue engineering.

Recent advances in the isolation, expansion and characterisation of human MSCs have raised the possibility of using them in cell therapies and tissue engineering for bone reconstruction. It has been demonstrated that hMSCs, isolated from the bone marrow of healthy adult donors, were minimally expanded *ex vivo* and pulsed twice toward osteogenic lineage (Trombi *et al.*, 2008). However, when the cells were then included into autologous plasma-derived clots, cell proliferation was sustained under appropriate cell culture conditions.

The main limitations to be faced in achieving a widespread therapeutic use of MSCs include both their scarcity in adult tissues and the current lack of simple unambiguous identifying markers. These are major issues contributing towards the cost effectiveness and standardisation of their use. On the other hand, evidence suggesting wider MSC tissue distribution and greater plasticity stimulates research in this field (Godara *et al.*, 2008a). Therefore, advances in stem cell biology research are fundamental steps to understanding fully the role of these cells in tissue regeneration and to optimising their exploitation in a therapeutic context (Dawson and Oreffo, 2008).

In the past few years, intensive research into understanding the biological characteristics of MSCs has already shed light on some of their phenotypic markers, their immunosuppressive–non-immunogenic properties and their role in the treatment of graft-versus-host disease, in the acceleration of haematopoietic recovery and in the treatment of selected inherited diseases (Pelagiadis *et al.*, 2008).

Although autologous bone marrow represents the main source of MSCs for both experimental and clinical studies, their clinical use may be limited by both their number and their declined differentiation potential in relatively elderly patients. For this reason, alternative sources of MSCs have been investigated that include adipose tissue obtained by lipoaspiration and umbilical cord blood, the latter containing high precursor frequencies and youngest cells. The yields when isolating these cells from each of these tissues, as well as their expansion and differentiation potentials, have been analysed (Bieback *et al.*, 2008).

Adipose tissue-derived mesenchymal stem cells (ATMSCs) have been shown to differentiate into bone, cartilage, fat or muscle. However, it is not certain that ATMSCs are equal to bone marrow-derived mesenchymal MSCs for their bone and cartilage forming potential. For this purpose, studies have been performed where MSCs from adipose and bone marrow tissues have been compared for their ability to express typical MSC markers such as STRO-1 and CD34 and for their osteogenic potential in typical osteogenic cell culture media (Im *et al.*, 2005). The results showed that both bone-derived MSCs and ATMSCs were STRO-1 positive and CD34 negative, but osteoblastic differentiation of ATMSCs was significantly lower than in cells derived from bone marrow, suggesting that ATMSCs may have an osteogenic potential inferior to the cells derived from bone marrow.

In a similar study, ATMSCs osteogenic potential was compared to that of cells deriving from bone marrow and periosteum (PMSCs) in *in vitro* and *in vivo* tests (Hayashi *et al.*, 2008). Colony-forming unit frequency in bone marrow-derived cells in this type of MSCs, together with the PMSCs, showed the highest osteogenic activity both in culture and upon subcutaneous implantation in rats by hydroxyapatite scaffolds.

The pluripotent nature and self-renewal capability of hematopoietic stem cells (HSCs) has also been considered as a potential stem cell source for tissue engineering. However, their potential as a source for cell-based therapy has not yet been fulfilled because these cells are difficult to expand *in vitro* in clinically relevant numbers. One of the reasons for this poor yield is the absence of a single cell surface antigen which may allow their identification and optimal culturing conditions. However, studies in this direction are now providing important information for their use in clinics (Hines *et al.*, 2008).

In a different approach, human dental germ pulp has also been used as a source of haematopoietic $CD34^+$ stem cell population capable of differentiating into pre-osteoblasts (Graziano *et al.*, 2008). These cells were allowed to adhere to PLA/PGA scaffolds without pre-expansion in culture and then transplanted into immunocompromised rats, subcutaneously. Histology showed ectopic bone noduli formation after 60 days. In addition, the presence of platelet endothelial cell adhesion molecules and von Willebrand factor immunoreactivity suggested neo-angiogenesis within nodules. Importantly, these vessels were $HLA\text{-}1^+$ and, thus, clearly human in origin. This study suggests that $CD34^+$ cells obtained from dental pulp may be used for engineering bone without the need for prior culture expanding procedures, offering the advantage of angiogenesis, a key factor in the long-term survival of newly formed bone.

Indeed, the vascularisation of bone tissue engineering constructs is a key factor in ensuring their integration in large bone defects with no risk of ischaemia. Angiogenesis could be promoted by seeding tissue engineering scaffolds with a co-culture of osteoblasts and endothelial cells. However, as discussed for osteoblasts, the use of differentiated endothelial cells suffers from limitations such as their limited availability and proliferation capability. Advances in stem cell technology have enabled researchers to derive endothelial or endothelial-like cells from stem cells or other precursor populations (Kim and Von Recum, 2008).

From the analysis of all these aspects linked to the use of stem cells, it emerges that the future of bone tissue engineering may depend on the ability to regulate the pathways of cell proliferation and differentiation in a biochemically, spatially and chronologically tuned manner. This tuning may include technological strategies for:

- homing circulating connective tissue progenitor cells by stimulation with growth factors, drugs and other bioactive molecules
- modifying the biological performance of connective tissue progenitor cells by means of genetic modifications.

Cell engineering is therefore likely to become a fundamental tool in delivering clinically performing tissue engineering constructs. In addition to genetic engineering, a discipline in an advanced stage of development, other forms of cell engineering have been recently emerging. For example, it has been shown that, by binding magnetic nanoparticles to the surface of cells, it is possible to manipulate and control cell function with an external magnetic field. The technique of activating cells with magnetic nanoparticles offers a means of isolating and exploiting cellular mechanics to drive cell delivery *in vivo* and to tune their functions and processes (Dobson, 2008). Finally, the optimisation/standardisation and monitoring of *in vitro* procedures (e.g. cell density within the scaffold) for the construction of biohybrid scaffolds requires more emphasis in order to make the cell-based approach a reliable treatment option in tissue engineering (Materna *et al.*, 2008). For these reasons, alongside the substrate properties of biomaterials, bone tissue engineering constructs need to integrate the biochemical signalling and 3D environment which are required for the cell to deposit new mineralised tissue.

14.4 Bioactive molecules for tissue engineering

Morphogenesis in tissue repair is guided by a variety of signals from the extracellular milieu, including growth factors that are sequestered in the extracellular matrix. Since its dawn, the field of tissue engineering has been developing systems able to simulate target cells (Hubbell, 2006).

Tissue repair is governed by the regulatory role exerted by cytokines and growth factors on cell activity through gene expression. As a consequence, research in tissue engineering has explored the potential of modulating cell processes and functions by growth factor stimulation and gene delivery. The following sections provide an overview of the use of these two strategies in bone tissue engineering.

14.4.1 Growth factors

Several types of growth factor have been shown to stimulate bone repair, either through a direct effect on bone cells (i.e. osteoblasts and osteoclasts) or through an indirect effect on other cell phenotypes participating in the formation of tissues indispensable to bone metabolism (e.g. endothelial cells in angiogenesis) (Lee and Shin, 2007).

The most important class of growth factors used in bone tissue engineering is the TGF-β superfamily which includes the TGF-β 1 and the bone morophogenetic proteins (BMPs). In particular, BMPs have been the most used as they are key factors in a variety of bone processes. BMPs act as a stimulating factor for stem cell differentiation into osteoblasts and direct osteochondral calcification. The insulin-like growth factor (IGF) is another growth factor that has been carefully investigated in relation to bone repair and found to stimulate the migration and proliferation of several cell types relevant to osteogenesis. However, the mechanism of action of IGF in bone healing seems to differ from that of BMPs. The role of the fibroblast growth factor-2 (FGF-2) in stimulating bone repair has also been investigated, but conflicting evidence has emerged. Conversely, it is widely recognised that the vascular endothelial growth factor (VEGF) plays an important role as it is able to improve vascularisation of newly formed bone. In addition, it has been demonstrated that VEGF is also a mediator of various osteoinductive factors such as TGF-β 1, thus providing an indirect stimulus for osteogenesis.

In therapeutic applications, the use of these growth factors is limited by their known instability under storage and short lifespan under physiological conditions. Furthermore, their ability to stimulate cells closely depends on their bioavailability. Therefore, it is important to engineer delivery systems which are able to preserve the native conformation of these growth factors and to provide appropriate concentrations and gradients in extracellular space. In most studies, growth factors for bone repair have been delivered from polymeric, ceramic and composite biomaterials on the basis of their diffusion in a physiological environment. The review papers by Lee and Shin (2007) and by Seeherman and Wozney (2005) offer an overview of the various combinations of biomaterial and growth factors employed. However, these are relatively simplistic approaches and do not fulfil the requirements for enhancing stability and bioresponsive release of these growth factors.

To fulfil these requirements, nature has developed fine interactions between the growth factors and components of the extracellular matrix; this reversible binding enables the ECM to retain these factors until they are locally mobilized by cells. Fibrin-based biomaterials for bone tissue engineering have been developed which are able to bind an engineered bone morphogenetic protein-2 (BMP-2) fusion protein and release it under the action of proteases associated with the cell surface (Schomoekel *et al.*, 2005). An N-terminal transglutaminase substrate domain provides covalent attachment for fibrin during the polymerization process by the activity of the blood transglutaminase factor XIIIa. A central plasmin substrate domain provides a cleavage site for proteases and allows the localised release of the attached growth factor. An enhanced bone repair process was observed when these biomaterials were implanted *in vivo*, suggesting that the stability and controlled delivery of the growth factor had been optimised.

In a similar approach, the reversible binding of BMP-2 was pursued by a heparin-conjugated poly(L-lactic-co-glycolic acid) (HP-PLGA) scaffold (Jeon *et al.*, 2007). Heparin conjugation to PLGA was found to be enhanced when star-shaped PLGA were used and the release of BMP-2 from the HP-PLGA scaffold was sustained for at least 14 days *in vitro*. BMP-2 release induced osteoblast differentiation *in vitro* over 14 days, while non-heparinised PLGA was shown to induce osteoblast differentiation only during the early incubation times (up to day 3). *In vivo* bone formation by the BMP-2-loaded HP-PLGA scaffolds was four-fold greater than the BMP-2-loaded unmodified PLGA scaffold group.

Site-specific delivery of FGF-1, entrapped in a fibrin/hydroxyapatite composite, has also been evaluated. Kinetic analysis *in vivo* revealed that the biocomposite was capable of delivering biologically active FGF-1 and that FGF-1-containing implants induced increased angiogenesis and infiltration of cells expressing osteogenic related markers (i.e. osteopontin, osteocalcin) (Kelpke *et al.*, 2004,).

FGF-2 release from p(HEMA-co-VP) showed that FGF-2 was able to enhance bone formation by increasing bone volume. However, the effect appeared to vanish rapidly soon after surgery (Mabilleau *et al.*, 2008).

14.4.2 Genes

Gene delivery offers an alternative to the use of unstable growth factors. However, to reduce the risks associated with the genetic manipulation of cells, this approach is believed to be more suitable for *ex vivo* bone regeneration such as that pursued in bioreactor systems. In general, cells can be transfected to enhance their ability to express a particular gene encoding the synthesis of growth factors relevant to bone formation such as BMPs and VEGF (Partridge, 2007). Cell transfection *in vitro* is a well-established process that relies on viral and non-viral gene delivery systems. Among the viral delivery systems, it is worth recalling the adenovirus and retrovirus systems that have been applied for the transduction of BMP-2 expressing MSCs seeded in PLGA and PEG scaffolds. A comprehensive review of gene delivery in tissue engineering has been published by De Laporte and Shea (2007). Here, typical examples are provided in relation to bone tissue engineering.

Bone marrow-derived MSCs have also been transduced with E1-deleted adenoviral vectors containing either human BMP-2 or BMP-6 coding sequence under cytomegalovirus (CMV) promoter control and either sustained in a monolayer or suspended in 1.2% alginate beads for 22 days (Zachos *et al.*, 2006). The enhanced gene expression led to higher levels of osteoblast differentiation and mineralised bone noduli formation.

Enhanced expression of plasmid DNA in MSCs has also been attempted in 3D scaffolds by non-viral gene carriers (Hosseinkhani *et al.*, 2008). Acetylated polyethylenimine (PEI) was shown to enhance gene delivery from collagen sponges reinforced by PGA fibres. DNA nanoparticles formed through simple mixing of plasmid DNA encoding bone BMP-2 and acetylated PEI solutions were encapsulated within these scaffolds. Within these scaffolds, the level of BMP-2 expression by transfected MSCs was significantly enhanced compared to MSCs transfected by DNA nanoparticles in solution. Homogeneous bone formation was shown when the scaffolds were analysed histologically.

The reported death of a patient who underwent gene therapy as well as the high risks of leukaemias raise concerns about gene delivery mediated by viral vectors. Conversely, non-viral vectors do not ensure the required transfection efficiency. Furthermore, gene carriers can exacerbate the host response already elicited by biomaterials. Therefore, the future of gene delivery in bone tissue engineering is very uncertain.

14.5 Scaffolds for bone repair

The favourable cell and mineralisation substrate offered by ceramics, polymers and composites as well as the stimulation by specific growth factor needs to be accompanied by architectural features similar to those of bone. Natural bone consists of cortical and trabecular morphologies, the latter having variable pore sizes. Most of the studies performed so far have focussed on mimicking this structure through engineering 3D macroporous scaffolds with the aim of providing the growing bone with an architectural structure where cells can proliferate and deposit a new extracellular matrix. In addition, to allow the integration of the tissue engineering construct, scaffolds have to favour the in-growth of the surrounding tissues (i.e. bone and vessels). This can be achieved through suitable porosity (range 100–300 μm diameter pores), degradation rate and remodelling potential. Various techniques are currently available to produce 3D scaffolds bearing these properties. Almost all the materials discussed in Section 14.2 can be processed into 3D porous structures.

14.5.1 Three-dimensional scaffold fabrication techniques

The most used methods for processing biodegradable biomaterials into 3D porous scaffolds are (Chung and Park, 2007):

1. *Fibre bonding*. In this technique fibres of polymers can be assembled by generating crosspoints with a second polymer in the solution in which the first polymer is embedded. This technique suffers from relatively poor control of the porosity.
2. *Emulsion freeze drying*. This method consists in freeze drying an emulsion solution where the organic polymeric phase is dispersed in a aqueous phase. Sublimation of the water phase leads to the formation of a polymeric structure with interconnected pores up to 200 μm.
3. *Solvent casting/particulate leaching*. This can be considered one of the most suitable methods for producing scaffolds. It consists of adding a given amount of salt granules to a polymer solution in organic solvent. After solvent evaporation, the salt granules are removed from the matrix by immersion in an aqueous solution, obtaining a porosity up to 90%.

However, leaching of the salt particles is limited by the thickness of the scaffold and, therefore, only relatively thin porous membranes can be obtained.

4. *High pressure processing*. This technique is best known as supercritical fluid technology. It is performed by applying a gas, such as supercritical carbon dioxide, to the dry polymer to form a single phase polymer/gas solution. When the pressure is released, the expansion of the dissolved carbon dioxide leads to the formation of gas bubbles that generate porosity within the polymeric matrix. One of the main advantages of this method is the uniform distribution and size of the formed pores, but its disadvantage is the poor interconnectivity between them; this is a major limitation in tissue engineering where cells and tissue have to penetrate throughout the scaffold and communicate with each other.
5. *Gas foaming/particulate leaching*. In this method, pores are produced using effervescent salt particles. The dissolution of the salt and the simultaneous effervescence lead to the formation of interconnected pores with a diameter ranging from 100 to 200 μm.
6. *Thermally induced phase separation*. The porosity obtained by this procedure is obtained by thermodynamic demixing of a homogeneous polymer–solvent solution. The demixing leads to the formation of two phases; a polymer-rich phase and a polymer-poor phase. This demixing is obtained either by cooling to below the bimodal solubility curve or by addition of an immiscible solvent. Although the technique does not lead to the formation of large pores (max 10 μm), a coarsening step has been shown to enlarge the interconnected pores up to 100 μm.
7. *Electrospinning*. This method provides non-woven nanofibre matrices. A polymer solution or a molten polymer is drawn from a nozzle by gravity or mechanical pressure. This action is combined with an electric field of high voltage (from 10 to 20 kV) which enables the electric charge to overcome the surface tension of the polymer solution, transforming the polymer solution droplets into a polymer jet yielding solid nanofibres upon solvent evaporation. With this method, scaffolds with an interconnected porosity can be obtained.
8. *Rapid prototyping*. This process is based on a computer-driven equipment able to construct 3D scaffolds by a melt–dissolution deposition process relying either on fused deposition modelling, on 3D fibre deposition or on particle bonding techniques (e.g. melt deposition) (Boland *et al.*, 2007).

Other different approaches, applications and biological performances of scaffolds can be found in the review paper by Jones *et al.* (2007) and by Lee *et al.* (2008).

Below, a few examples of 3D scaffold productions are presented that focus on the types of biomaterials discussed in Section 14.2.

14.5.2 Examples of three-dimensional scaffolds for bone tissue engineering

Bioglass foams for bone tissue engineering have been prepared by a process based on bioglass-loaded polyurethane foam. This *in situ* foaming method provides a bioglass porous monolith, starting from sol–gel synthesised bioglass powders (Rainer *et al.*, 2008).

Interconnected porous chitosan scaffolds have been prepared by a freeze-drying method and mineralised by calcium and phosphate solution using a double-diffusion method to induce nanoapatite deposition. Studies with osteoblasts demonstrated that the presence of apatite nanocrystals in chitosan scaffolds does not significantly influence the growth of cells, but does induce the formation of an extracellular matrix and therefore has the potential to serve in bone tissue engineering (Manjubala *et al.*, 2008).

Biodegradable scaffolds reinforced with a frame have been obtained by mixing synthesised carbonate apatite with neutralised collagen gel (Hirata *et al.*, 2007). The mixture was lyophilised into sponges to form a porous hydroxyapatite frame. The scaffold was completed by the encapsulation of recombinant human BMP-2 providing significant new bone formation at the surface of the periosteum cranii after 4 weeks of implantation.

Similarly, porous hydroxyapatite/collagen scaffolds for bone tissue engineering were obtained by mixing a self-organised HA/collagen nanocomposite and sodium phosphate buffer in neutral conditions at 37°C, resulting in gelation of the mixture (Yunoki *et al.*, 2007). The porous composites with and without the incubation were obtained by a freeze-drying technique, in which macroscopic open pores were formed. *In vivo* implantations of the porous composites treated with a dehydrothermal treatment in bone defects showed a relationship between the rate of resorption and the presence of collagen fibrils.

The ability of silk fibroin scaffolds combining pores with different sizes (112–224 and 400–500 μm) to support MSCs has been tested in static and dynamic conditions (Hofmann *et al.*, 2007). Dynamic cell seeding resulted in equal cell viability and proliferation, but it led to a better cell distribution throughout the scaffolds. The dynamic conditions improved the levels of MSC differentiation and mineralised bone noduli formation in an osteogenic medium.

Several investigations have also pointed out the importance of angiogenesis in bone repair. Indeed, although the repair of bone is driven by osteoblasts, its long-term survival is determined by its degree of vascularisation. However, the mechanisms involved in the context of the complex healing microenvironment are poorly understood and, as a consequence, it is difficult to optimise biomaterials that can tune this process.

In a typical investigation, angiogenesis was assessed in different 3D scaffolds using most of the biomaterials presented in Section 14.2; porous hydroxyapatite, porous calcium phosphate and silk fibroin nets (Unger *et al.*, 2007). The vascularisation potential of these biomaterials for bone repair was tested in the presence of angiogenic stimuli by cell culture systems including human dermal microvascular endothelial cells (HDMEC). HDMEC did not migrate to form microcapillary-like structures as they did on cell culture plastic. In co-cultures of HDMEC and primary human osteoblast cells or the human osteoblast-like cell line MG-63 on these biomaterials, cells assembled into an organised tissue-like structure, the endothelial cells forming microcapillary-like structures containing a lumen and giving strong PECAM-1 expression. These microcapillary-like structures infiltrated osteoblast cell layers and did not form when exogenous angiogenic stimuli were added to these co-cultures. The life span of HDMEC was also significantly enhanced by the co-culture. These data raise important questions concerning the exact nature of pro-angiogenic drug- or gene-delivery systems to be incorporated into scaffolds which has to take into account the production of growth factors by invading mesenchymal cells.

Despite the wide choice of biomaterials and techniques to engineer 3D scaffolds, two main limitations have not yet been overcome:

- In most of the cases, uniform cell seeding throughout the scaffold is difficult to achieve and, in the majority of the cases, cells sitting at the periphery of the scaffold proliferate more quickly, generating a layer of tissue that impedes the diffusion of nutrients and gases as well as the elimination of cell activity by-products. As a consequence, the viability of the cells which are located in the core of the material is impaired. Dynamic methods such as that indicated above may improve cell distribution throughout the material mesh, but not necessarily improve the viability of the cells at the scaffold core.
- The need for a macroporous structure that can facilitate tissue in-growth may not offer the ideal microenvironment for the cells. Indeed, cells adhering to the surface of a macropore recognise that surface as two-dimensional (2D) rather than 3D. This situation does not reflect the true ECM environment which surrounds cells in a natural tissue. For this reason, it is envisaged that although macroporous scaffolds are required to favour tissue deposition at macroscopic scale, the early phases of the tissue repair process need to be induced by the optimisation of cell encapsulation milieus. The development of bioresponsive hydrogels like those described in the section entitled 'Biomineralisation molecules' are a significant step forward in this direction and their combination with macroporous scaffolds may result in optimal conditions for tissue formation.

For those applications where bone repair is pursued by *in vitro* tissue engineering, closer mimicking of the physiological environment is required and needs to include control of parameters such as the turnover of nutrients, the regulation of pH and gas partial pressures and biomechanical stimuli. All these different parameters have been taken into account and integrated in the development of bioreactors.

14.6 Bioreactors

The future development of tissue engineered products depends on scalable production processes with standards of safety and efficacy similar to those established for the pharmaceutical industry. Many of the bioreactor design principles established for production of biopharmaceuticals can be applied to production of tissue engineering products. Bioreactors integrating dynamic conditions such as stirrings, perfusion or microfluidic bioreactors have the potential to address efficiently the clinical need for the production of tissue engineering products (Godara *et al.*, 2008b).

It is widely accepted that the behaviour of cells is significantly affected by the hydrodynamic environment and mechanical stimuli. To this purpose, computer modelling and bioreactor systems have been developed to set the appropriate conditions in bioreactors for tissue engineering.

Computational fluid dynamic (CFD) studies have been performed to provide the scientific community with a more detailed description of fluid mechanics and nutrient transport within bioreactor equipments (Hutmacher and Singh, 2008). The definitions of CFD parameters will certainly have an impact on the understanding of the cellular response to fluid flow processes.

The study of the parameters affecting tissue repair at the cellular level should also be accompanied by investigations satisfying the requirements for engineering customised, anatomically shaped and histologically differentiated (e.g. osteochondral tissue including bony and cartilagineous layers) grafts. The design of these grafts should take into account the need for an immediate functionality (e.g. load bearing, structural support) and long-term regeneration (i.e. graft formation, integration and remodeling) (Grayson *et al.*, 2008).

MSCs and differentiated bone cells (osteoblasts and osteocytes) are able to sense mechanical stimuli deriving from the surrounding environment. The importance of mechanical stimuli has been observed in both bone homeostasis and osteogenesis, but the mechanisms responsible for osteogenic induction in response to mechanical signals are still poorly understood. Studies have tried to discern the effect of biomechanical stimuli on osteoblasts in 3D scaffolds. Electrospun PCL scaffolds were seeded with osteoblasts and subjected to different levels of externally applied compressive force (Rath *et al.*, 2008). The study showed that progenitor cells adhered, proliferated and differentiated in the scaffolds and deposited new ECM. The biochemical stimuli led to an enhanced expression of genes and proteins required for the synthesis of a mineralised ECM. However, the biomechanical stimuli were not effective when the constructs were exposed to 20% compressive strain (30.96 +/– 2.82 kPa) demonstrating that these signals were not osteogenic. Overall, the study indicates that appropriate physical activities or microscale compressive loading can enhance fracture healing partially involving anabolic osteogenic effects on bone cells.

However, a complete knowledge of the deformation sensed by cells at a microscopic level when mechanical loads are applied is still missing. Studies have been performed on ceramic scaffolds to characterise stress and strain distributions in the solid material phase and fluid velocity, fluid pressure and fluid shear stress distributions in the pores filled with fluid. This investigation has demonstrated that different levels of mechanical stimuli can be generated within the samples according to the morphology of the materials under mechanical load and fluid flow (Sandino *et al.*, 2008).

Despite these attempts, the body of published data is still too scattered, lacks protocol standardisation and is mostly limited to specific biomaterials. A significant step forward towards standardisation of growth conditions has been made by the commercialisation of a new type of equipment by the Bose Electroforce group. New equipment able finely to control and monitor the hydrodynamic and mechanical conditions in 3D cell culture systems has been made available on the market and is applicable to bone tissue engineering products as well as to the testing of other types of constructs (http://www.bose-electroforce.com/home.cfm).

14.7 Clinical applications

Bone has an intrinsic ability to repair when traumatic, pathological and surgical defects are smaller than what has been defined as critical size defects (>5 cm). Larger gaps can still be healed with the support of biodegradable biomaterials with osteoconductive or osteogenic properties. However, when pathological conditions and/or larger areas of damage are predominant, a tissue engineering aid is required. In most of these cases, a vascularised tissue integrated with the surrounding circulatory system is required to ensure the long-term viability of the tissue. In the case of the use of autologous bone grafts, this is achieved by harvesting bone grafts bearing vascular structures. Bone tissue engineering products able fully to reproduce the graft features will significantly reduce the patient's discomfort/morbidity. In this section, three typical surgical scenarios will be presented where the extent of the damage or the pathological conditions of the host bony tissue have prompted the development of bone tissue engineering products and their clinical validation. The efficiency of the implanted tissue engineering constructs will be discussed by taking into account their use of the technology available in the field.

14.7.1 Maxillofacial defects and their treatment by bone tissue engineering constructs

Among the different types of maxillofacial surgeries, those mostly benefiting from bone tissue engineering products are:

- Surgical removal of soft tissue and bony tumours of odontogenic and other origins.
- Reconstruction of critical size congenital, developmental, post-trauma, post-tumour, or ageing-related defects in orofacial tissues. These include, for example, forehead-temporal regions and more anterior and inferior facial structures.
- Trauma surgery for trauma of the head, neck and facial areas.

In a typical bone tissue engineering approach, a construct was tested in six patients to reconstruct jaw defects (Meijer *et al*., 2008). A bone marrow aspirate was harvested, stem cells were cultured, expanded and grown for 7 days on a biomaterial scaffold in osteogenic culture conditions until it formed a layer of extracellular bone matrix. At the end of the procedure, construct specimens were reimplanted in the patient and, simultaneously, subcutaneously implanted in mice to prove its osteogenic potential. The constructs clearly showed osteogenic activity in mice as they induced ectopic bone formation. However, the bone tissue engineering constructs did not lead to any significant bone repair in patients with intra-oral osseous defects (orthotopic bone formation). Biopsies at month 4 showed that only one patient had bone formation induced by the tissue-engineered construct. This study clearly shows that testing bone tissue engineering constructs in animal models does not necessarily reflect its clinical potential.

When this type of defect is treated with autologous bone graft, elements of the vasculature are also harvested and implanted together with the bone graft. This is a fundamental aspect of the surgical procedure that allows the long-term survival of the bone. The poor clinical outcome of this study may well be due to the absence of any engineered vascularisation within the construct.

14.7.2 Osteochondral defects and their treatment by bone tissue engineering constructs

Osteochondral defects (OCD) are localised areas of joint damage. These conditions usually occur in anatomical districts when both the cartilage and the underlying bone have been disrupted. The extent of damage of the tissue layers varies from 'bruising' to a deep defect on the surface of the joint, which lacks both the underlying bone as well as cartilage.

Until recently, it was agreed that osteochondral defects have been thought to occur as a result of repetitive trauma within the joint. However, more recent studies suggest the possibility of a metabolic or genetic origin that may cause alteration of bone architecture.

These types of injury may cause a shearing of the cartilage or a focal bone and cartilage injury with a saucer-shaped defect. Whereas, in the case of defects without a history of trauma where bone injury occurs, the vascularised bone scaffold is lost through formation of a cystic lesion that gradually fails to support the overlying cartilage thus leading to its collapse.

Spontaneous OCD is only partial and transient and relies on the invasion of the defect by chondroprogenitor cells (Cancedda *et al.*, 2003). Thus far, surgical approaches based on tissue engineering strategies have targeted the regeneration of the cartilage while failing to address the underlying bone failure. More importantly, the techniques of choice are autologous chondrocyte implantation (ACI) and mosaicplasty where cells are not used in conjunction with biomaterials.

A multi-centre trial at orthopedic clinics and university hospitals was conducted from 1997 to 2000 on 47 patients who were randomly assigned to ACI or mosaicplasty and subjected to arthroscopic debridement of the lesion at the time of enrollment. They were called for surgery 6 months after the initial debridement (Dozin *et al.*, 2005).

ACI and mosaicplasty showed similar clinical performance. The high percentage of spontaneous improvement observed after simple debridement questions the need for reconstructive surgery in patients with lesions similar to those included in this clinical trial.

14.7.3 Long bone diaphysis defects and their treatment with bone tissue engineering constructs

Bone tissue engineering was used to treat four patients with large bone diaphysis defects and poor therapeutic alternatives (Marcacci *et al.*, 2007). The study was assessed after 7 years follow up. Progenitor cells isolated from the patients' bone marrow stroma were expanded in culture and seeded onto porous HA scaffolds designed to match the bone deficit in terms of size and shape. Implantation of the bone tissue engineering construct was supported by either an Ilizarov apparatus or a monoaxial external fixator that was positioned on the patient's affected limb. Patients were evaluated at different post-surgery time intervals by conventional radiographs and computed tomography scans. In one patient, an angiographic evaluation was also performed after 6.5 years. No major complications occurred in the early or late post-operative periods and a complete fusion between the implant and the host bone was observed from 5 to 7 months after surgery. The latest follow-up (6 to 7 years post-surgery) showed good integration of the implants and no late fractures in the implant area. It has to be observed that, although showing a positive clinical outcome, the bone tissue engineering construct of this study only partially exploited the ideal features of a tissue engineering construct as described in this chapter.

14.8 Conclusions

The impressive progress in knowledge that has been made in the last few decades in the field of biomaterials and cell biology has created a unique technological platform for the development of bone tissue engineering constructs able to aid bone repair in critical clinical scenarios. However, despite the efforts made by members of the scientific community to highlight the characteristics of an ideal bone tissue engineering construct, information contained in the vast literature body is still relatively scattered and only partially addresses the clinical problems. Although most of the research is conducted using a multi-disciplinary approach, only the major components required in bone repair are taken into account and other key elements of this complex pattern are neglected or not fully integrated. It is time for scientists and policy makers to produce coordinated projects where biological, pathological and procedural requirements are addressed by the combined effort of scientists, industrialists and clinicians.

14.9 References

Beppu MM, Torres MA, Aimoli CG, Goulart GAS and Santana CC (2005). '*In vitro* mineralization on chitosan using solutions with excess of calcium and phosphate ions'. *J Mat Res*, **20**(12), 3303–11.

Bieback K, Kern S, Kocaomer A, Ferlik K and Bugert P (2008). 'Comparing mesenchymal stromal cells from different human tissues: bone marrow, adipose tissue and umbilical cord blood'. *Biomed Mater Eng*, **18**(1), S71–6.

Boland T, Ovsianikov A, Chickov BN, Doraiswamy A, Narayan RJ, Yeong WY, Leong KF and Chua CK (2007). 'Rapid prototyping of artificial tissues and medical devices'. *Adv Mater Processes*, **165**(4), 51–3.

Cancedda R, Dozin B, Giannoni P and Quarto R (2003). 'Tissue engineering and cell therapy of cartilage and bone'. *Matrix Biol*, **22**, 81–91.

Caplan AI (1991). 'Mesenchymal stem cells'. *J Orthop Res*, **9**, 641–50.

Carinci F, Palmieri A, Martinelli M, Perrotti V, Piattelli A, Brunelli G, Arlotti M and Pezzetti F (2007). 'Genetic portrait of osteoblast-like cells cultured on PerioGlas'. *J Oral Implantol*, **33**(6), 327–33.

Catelas I, Sese N, Wu BM, Dunn JCY, Helgerson S and Tawil B (2006). 'Human mesenchymal stem cell proliferation and osteogenic differentiation in fibrin gels *in vitro*'. *Tissue Eng*, **12**(8), 2385–96.

Chow M, Duong H, Wu B and Tawil B (2008). 'Mesenchymal stem cells differentiation into osteoblasts on 2D and in 3D fibrin scaffolds'. *Wound Rep Reg*, **16**(2), A10–A58.

Chung HJ and Park TG (2007). 'Surface engineered and drug releasing pre-fabricated scaffolds for tissue engineering'. *Adv Drug Del Res*, **59**, 249–62.

Cui G, Li J and Lei W (2007a). 'Effect of injectable fibrin sealant compounded with bone morphogenetic protein on proliferation and differentiation of marrow stromal cells towards osteoblasts in rabbits'. *Zhongguo Xiu Fu Chong Jian Wai Ke Za Zhi*, **21**(1), 70–5.

Cui FZ, Li Y and Ge J (2007b). 'Self-assembly of mineralized collagen composites'. *Mater Sci Eng R*, **57**(1–6), 1–27.

Daculsi G (2006). 'High performance of micro macroporous biphasic calcium phosphate matrices for bone tissue engineering'. *Biomaterialen*, **7**, 21.

Dawson JI and Oreffo ROC (2008). 'Bridging the regeneration gap: stem cells, biomaterials and clinical translation in bone tissue engineering'. *Arch Biochem Biophys*, **473**(2), 124–31.

De Laporte L and Shea LD (2007). 'Matrices and scaffolds for DNA delivery in tissue engineering'. *Adv Drug Del Rev*, **59**, 292–307.

Dettin M, Conconi MT, Gambaretto R, Pasquato A, Folin M, Di Bello C and Parnigotto PP (2002). 'Novel osteoblast-adhesive peptides for dental/orthopedic biomaterials'. *J Biomed Mater Res*, **60**(3), 466–71.

Di Toro R, Betti V and Spampinato S (2004). 'Biocompatibility and integrin-mediated adhesion of human osteoblasts to poly(DL-lactide-co-glycolide) copolymers'. *Eur J Pharmacol Sci*. **21**(2–3), 161–9.

Dobson J (2008). 'Remote control of cellular behaviour with magnetic nanoparticles'. *Nature Technol*, **3**(3), 139–43.

Douglas T, Hempel U, Mietrach C, Viola M, Vigetti D, Heinemann S, Bierbaum S, Scharnweber D and Worch H (2008). 'Influence of collagen-fibril-based coatings containing decorin and biglycan on osteoblast behaviour'. *J Biomed Mater Res A*, **84A**(3), 805–16.

Dozin B, Malpeli M, Cancedda R, Bruzzi P, Calcagno S, Molfetta L, Priano F, Kon E and Marcacci M (2005). 'Comparative evaluation of autologous chondrocyte implantation and mosaicplasty – A multicentered randomized clinical trial'. *Clin J Sport Med*, **15**(4), 218–24.

Ehrbar M, Lutolf MP, Rizzi SC, Hubbell JA and Weber FE (2008). 'Artificial extracellular matrices for bone tissue engineering'. *Bone*, **42**, (Supp. 1) S72–S72.

Evangelista MB, Hsiong SX, Fernandes R, Sampaio P, Kong HJ, Barrias CC, Salema R, Barbosa MA, Mooney DJ and Granja PL (2007). 'Upregulation of bone cell differentiation through immobilization within a synthetic extracellular matrix'. *Biomaterials*, **28**(25), 3644–55.

Fellah BH, Gauthier O, Weiss P, Chappard D and Layrolle P (2008). 'Osteogenicity of biphasic calcium phosphate ceramics and bone autograft in a goat model'. *Biomaterials*, **29**(9), 1177–88.

Gerecht-Nir S and Itskoviz-Eldor J (2004). 'Cell therapy using human embryonic stem cells'. *Transplant Immunol*, **12**, 203–9.

Godara P, Nordon RE and McFarland CD (2008a). 'Mesenchymal stem cells in tissue engineering'. *J Chem Technol Biotechnol*, **83**(4), 397–407.

Godara P, McFarland CD and Nordon RE (2008b). 'Design of bioreactors for mesenchymal stem cell tissue engineering'. *J Chem Technol Biotechnol*, **83**(4), 408–20.

Gough JE, Notingher I and Hench LL (2004). 'Osteoblast attachment and mineralized nodule formation on rough and smooth 45S5 bioactive glass monoliths'. *J Biomed Mater Res A*, **68A**(4), 640–50.

Grayson WL, Chao PHG, Marolt D, Kaplan DL and Vunjak-Novakovic G (2008). 'Engineering custom-designed osteochondral tissue grafts'. *Trends Biotechnol*, **26**(4), 181–9.

Graziano A, d'Aquino R, Laino G, Proto A, Giuliano MT, Pirozzi G, De Rosa A, Di Napoli D and Papaccio G (2008). 'Human CD34(+) stem cells produce bone nodules *in vivo*. *Cell Prolif*, **41**(1), 1–11.

Gupta S, Hunter M, Cebe P, Levitt JM, Kaplan DL and Georgakoudi I (2008). 'Non-invasive optical characterization of biomaterial mineralization'. *Biomaterials*, **29**(15), 2359–69.

Hayashi O, Katsube Y, Hirose M, Ohgushi H and Ito H (2008). 'Comparison of osteogenic ability of rat mesenchymal stem cells from bone marrow, periosteum, and adipose tissue'. *Calcif Tissue Int*, **82**(3), 238–47.

Hedberg EL, Kroese-Deutman HC, Shih CK, Crowther RS, Carney DH, Mikos AG and Jansen JA (2005). '*In vivo* degradation of porous poly(propylene fumarate)/poly(DL-lactic-co-glycolic acid) composite scaffolds'. *Biomaterials*, **26**(22), 4616–23.

Heino TJ and Hentunen TA (2008). 'Differentiation of osteoblasts and osteocytes from mesenchymal stem cells'. *Curr Stem Cell Res Ther*, **3**(2), 131–45.

Hench LL (2006). 'The story of bioglass®'. *J Mater Sci Mater Med*, **17**(11), 967–78.

Hersel U, Dahmen C and Kessler H (2003). 'RGD modified polymers: biomaterials for stimulated cell adhesion and beyond'. *Biomaterials*, **24**, 4385–15.

Hillig WB, Choi Y, Murtha S, Natravali N and Ajayan P (2008). 'Open-pored gelatin/hydroxyapatite composite as a potential bone substitute'. *J Mater Sci Mater Med*, **19**(1), 11–17.

Hines M, Nielsen L and Cooper-White J (2008). 'The hematopoietic stem cell niche: what are we trying to replicate?' *J Chem Technol Biotechnol*, **83**(4), 421–43.

Hirata I, Nomura Y, Ito M, Shimazu A and Okazaki M (2007). 'Acceleration of bone formation with BMP2 in frame-reinforced carbonate apatite-collagen sponge scaffolds'. *J Artif Org*, **10**(4), 212–17.

Hofmann S, Hagenmuller H, Koch AM, Muller R, Vunjak-Novakovic G, Kaplan DL, Merkle HP and Meinel L (2007). 'Control of *in vitro* tissue-engineered bone-like structures using human mesenchymal stem cells and porous silk scaffolds'. *Biomaterials*, **28**(6), 1152–62.

Hosseinkhani H, Hosseinkhani M, Gabrielson NP, Pack DW, Khademhosseini A and Kobayashi H (2008). 'DNA nanoparticles encapsulated in 3D tissue-engineered scaffolds enhance osteogenic differentiation of mesenchymal stem cells'. *J Biomed Mater Res A*, **85A**(1), 47–60.

Hubbell JA (1998). 'Synthetic biodegradable polymers for tissue engineering and drug delivery'. *Curr Opin Solid State Mater Sci*, **3**(3), 246–51.

Hubbell JA (2003). 'Materials as morphogenetic guides in tissue engineering'. *Curr Opin Biotechnol*, **14**(5), 551–8.

Hubbell JA (2006). 'Matrix-bound growth factors in tissue repair'. *Swiss Med Weekly*, **136**(25–6), 387–91.

Hutmacher DW and Singh H (2008). 'Computational fluid dynamics for improved bioreactor design and 3D culture'. *Trends Biotechnol*, **26**(4), 166–72.

Im GI, Shin YW and Lee KB (2005). 'Do adipose tissue-derived mesenchymal stem cells have the same osteogenic and chondrogenic potential as bone marrow-derived cells?' *Osteoarth Cartilage*, **13**(10), 845–53.

Itthichaisri C, Wiedmann-Al-Ahmad M, Huebner U, Al-Ahmad A, Schoen R, Schmelzeisen R and Gellrich NC (2007). 'Comparative *in vitro* study of of human osteoblast-like cells the proliferation and growth on various biomaterials'. *J Biomed Mater Res A*, **82A**(4), 777–87.

Jao YP, Liu ZH, Cui FZ and Zhou CR (2007). 'Effect of hydrolysis pretreatment on the formation of bone-like apatite on poly(L-lactide) by mineralization in simulated body fluids'. *J Bioactive Compable Polyn*, **22**(5), 492–507.

Jeon O, Song SJ, Kang SW, Putnam AJ and Kim BS (2007). 'Enhancement of ectopic bone formation by bone morphogenetic protein-2 released from a heparin-conjugated poly(L-lactic-co-glycolic acid) scaffold'. *Biomaterials*, **28**(17), 2763–71.

Jones JR, Gentleman E and Polak J (2007). 'Bioactive glass scaffolds for bone regeneration'. *Elements*, **3**(6), 393–9.

Kelpke SS, Zinn KR, Rue LW and Thompson JA (2004). 'Site-specific delivery of acidic fibroblast growth factor stimulates angiogenic and osteogenic responses *in vivo*'. *J Biomed Mater Res A*, **71A**(2), 316–25.

Kim HW, Gu HJ and Lee HH (2007). 'Microspheres of collagen-apatite nanocomposites with osteogenic potential for tissue engineering'. *Tissue Eng*, **13**(5), 965–73.

Kim S and Von Recum H (2008). 'Endothelial stem cells and precursors for tissue engineering: Cell source, differentiation, selection, and application'. *Tissue Eng Part B-Rev*, **14**(1), 133–47.

Kino R, Ikorna T, Yunoki S, Nagai N, Tanaka J, Asakura T and Munekata M (2007). 'Preparation and characterization of multilayered hydroxyapatite/silk fibroin film'. *J Biosci Bioeng*, **103**(6), 514–20.

Kothapalli CR, Shaw MT, Olson JR and Wei M (2008). 'Fabrication of novel calcium phosphate/poly(lactic acid) fiber composites'. *J Biomed Mater Res B-Appl Biomater*, **84B**(1), 89–97.

Koutsopoulos S and Dalas E (2000). 'The calcification of fibrin *in vitro*'. *J Crystal Growth*, **216**(1–4), 450–8.

Langer R and Vacanti JP (1993). 'Tissue engineering'. *Science*, **260**, 920–6.

Lee SH and Shin H (2007). 'Matrices and scaffolds for delivery of bioactive molecules in bone and cartilage tissue engineering'. *Adv Drug Del Rev*, **59**, 339–59.

Lee J, Cuddihy MJ and Kotov NA (2008). 'Three-dimensional cell culture matrices: State of the art'. *Tissue Eng Part B-Rev*, **14**(1), 61–86.

Lutolf MP and Hubbell JA (2005). 'Synthetic biomaterials as instructive extracellular microenvironments for morphogenesis in tissue engineering'. *Nature Biothechnol*, **23**(1), 47–55.

Lutolf MP, Weber FE, Schmoekel HG, Schense JC, Kohler T, Muller R and Hubbell JA (2003a). 'Repair of bone defects using synthetic mimetics of collagenous extracellular matrices'. *Nature Biotechnol*, **21**(5), 513–18.

Lutolf MP, Lauer-Fields JL, Schmoekel HG, Metters AT, Weber FE, Fields GB and Hubbell JA (2003b). 'Synthetic matrix metalloproteinase-sensitive hydrogels for the conduction of tissue regeneration: Engineering cell-invasion characteristics'. *Proc Natl Acad Sci, USA*, **100**(9), 5413–18.

Mabilleau G, Aguado E, Stancu IC, Cincu C, Basle ME and Chappard D (2008). 'Effects of FGF-2 release from a hydrogel polymer on bone mass and microarchitecture'. *Biomaterials*, **29**(11), 1593–600.

Malafaya PB, Silva GA and Reis RL. (2007) 'Natural-origin polymers as carriers and scaffolds for biomolecules and cell delivery in tissue engineering applications'. *Adv Drug Del Rev*, **59**(4–5), 207–33.

Malkaj P, Pierri E and Dalas E (2005). 'The crystallization of Hydroxyapatite in the presence of sodium alginate'. *J Mater Sci Mater Med*, **16**(8), 733–7.

Manjubala I, Ponomarev I, Wilke I, Jandt KD and Klaus D (2008). 'Growth of osteoblast-like cells on biomimetic apatite-coated chitosan scaffolds'. *J Biomed Mater Res B – Appl Biomater*, **84B**(1), 7–16.

Marcacci M, Kon E, Moukhachev V, Lavroukov A, Kutepov S, Quarto R, Mastrogiacomo M and Cancedda R (2007). 'Stem cells associated with macroporous bioceramics for long bone repair: 6-to 7-year outcome of a pilot clinical study'. *Tissue Engineering*, **13**(5), 947–55.

Marquis ME, Lord E, Bergeron E, Bourgoin L and Faucheux N (2008). 'Short-term effects of adhesion peptides on the responses of preosteoblasts to pBMP-9'. *Biomaterials*, **29**(8), 1005–16.

Materna T, Rolf HJ, Napp J, Schulz J, Gelinsky M and Schliephake H (2008). '*In vitro* characterization of three-dimensional scaffolds seeded with human bone marrow stromal cells for tissue engineered growth of bone: mission impossible? A methodological approach'. *Clin Oral Implant Res*, **19**(4), 379–86.

Meijer GJ, de Bruijn JD, Koole R and van Blitterswijk C (2008). 'A Cell based bone tissue engineering in jaw defects'. *Biomaterials*, **29**(21), 3053–61.

Motta A, Migliaresi C, Faccioni F, Torricelli P, Fini M and Giardino R (2004). 'Fibroin hydrogels for biomedical applications: preparation, characterization and *in vitro* cell culture studies'. *J Biomater Sci – Polym Ed*, **15**(7), 851–64.

Ning J, Yao A, Wang DP, Huang WH, Fu HL, Liu X, Jiang XQ and Zhang XL (2007). 'Synthesis and *in vitro* bioactivity of a borate-based bioglass'. *Mater Lett*, **61**(30), 5223–6.

Olszta MJ, Cheng XG, Jee SS, Kumar R, Kim YY, Kaufman MJ, Michael J, Douglas EP and Gower LB (2007). 'Bone structure and formation: A new perspective'. *Mater Sci Eng R*, **58**(3–5), 77–16.

Partridge K (2007). 'In the bone'. *Biochemist*, **29**(1), 8–11.

Patterson TE, Kumagai K, Griffith L and Muschler GF (2008). 'Cellular strategies for enhancement of fracture repair'. *J Bone Joint Surg*, **90A**(Suppl. 1), 111–19.

Pelagiadis I, Dimitriou H and Kalmanti M (2008). 'Biologic characteristics of mesenchymal stromal cells and their clinical applications in pediatric patients'. *J Pediatric Hematol Oncol*, **30**(4), 301–9.

Pratt AB, Weber FE, Schmoekel HG, Muller R and Hubbell JA (2004). 'Synthetic extracellular matrices for in situ tissue engineering'. *Biotechnol Bioeng*, **86**(1), 27–36.

Puska M, Korventausta J, Aho A and Seppala J (2008). 'Modified poly-epsilon-caprolactone (PCL) with phosphorus containing compounds for biomineralization'. *Key Eng Mater*, **361–3**, 451–4.

Qu X, Cui WJ, Yang F, Min CC, Shen H, Bei JZ and Wang SG (2007). 'The effect of oxygen plasma pretreatment and incubation in modified simulated body fluids on the formation of bone-like apatite on poly(lactide-co-glycolide) (70/30)'. *Biomaterials*, **28**(1), 9–18.

Rainer A, Giannitelli SM, Abbruzzese F, Traversa E, Licoccia S and Trombetta M (2008). 'Fabrication of bioactive glass-ceramic foams mimicking human bone portions for regenerative medicine'. *Acta Biomater*, **4**(2), 362–9.

Ratajczak MZ, Zuba-Surma EK, Wysoczynski M, Wan W, Ratajczak J, Wojakowski W and Kucia M (2008). 'Hunt for pluripotent stem cell – Regenerative medicine search for almighty cell'. *J Autoimmun*, **30**(3), 151–62.

Rath B, Nam J, Knobloch TJ, Lannutti JJ and Agarwal S (2008). 'Compressive forces induce osteogenic gene expression in calvarial osteoblasts'. *J Biomech*, **41**(5), 1095–103.

Ren YJ, Sun XD, Cui FZ, Wei YT, Cheng ZJ and Kong XD (2007). 'Preparation and characterization of Antheraea pernyi silk fibroin based nanohydroxyapatite composites'. *J Bioactive Compible Polyn*, **22**(5), 465–74.

Rezania A and Healy KE (1999). 'Biomimetic peptide surfaces that regulate adhesion, spreading, cytoskeletal organization, and mineralization of the matrix deposited by osteoblast-like cells'. *Biotechnol Prog*, **15**, 19–32.

Rizzi SC, Ehrbar M, Halstenberg S, Raeber GP, Schmoekel HG, Hugo G, Hagenmuller H, Muller R, Weber FE and Hubbell JA (2006). 'Recombinant protein-co-PEG networks as cell-adhesive and proteolytically degradable hydrogel matrixes. Part II: Biofunctional characteristics'. *Biomacromolecules*, **7**(11), 3019–29.

Robey PG (1996). 'Vertebrate mineralized matrix proteins: structure and function'. *Connect Tissue Res*, **35**(1–4), 131–6.

Sandino C, Planell JA and Lacroix D (2008). 'A finite element study of mechanical stimuli in scaffolds for bone tissue engineering'. *J Biomech*, **41**(5), 1005–14.

Santin M and Cannas M (1999). 'Collagen-bound α1-microglobulin in normal and healed tissues and its effect on immunocompetent cells'. *Scand J Immunol*, **50**, 289–95.

Santin M, Standen G, Meikle S, Oliver G and Lloyd A (2006). *Biomaterial Surface Functionalisation*. Patent application, GB0624423.0.

Santin M, Morris C, Standen G, Nicolais L and Arnbrosio L (2007). 'A new class of bioactive and biodegradable soybean-based bone fillers'. *Biomacromolecules*, **8**(9), 2706–11.

Santos MH, Valerio P, Goes AM, Leite MF, Heneine LGD and Mansur HS (2007). 'Biocompatibility evaluation of hydroxyapatite/collagen nanocomposites doped with Zn^{+2}'. *Biomed Mater*, **2**(2), 135–41.

Sawyer AA, Hennessy KM and Bellis SL (2007). 'The effect of adsorbed serum proteins, RGD and proteoglycan-binding peptides on the adhesion of mesenchymal stem cells to hydroxyapatite'. *Biomaterials*, **28**(3), 383–92.

Schmoekel HG, Weber FE, Schense JC, Gratz KW, Schawalder P and Hubbell JA (2005). 'Bone repair with a form of BMP-2 engineered for incorporation into fibrin cell ingrowth matrices'. *Biotechnol Bioeng*, **89**(3), 253–62.

Seeherman H and Wozney JM (2005). 'Delivery of bone morphogenetic proteins for orthopedic tissue regeneration'. *Cytokine Growth Factor Rev*, **16**, 329–45.

Sokolsky-Papkov M, Agashi K, Olaye A, Shakesheff K and Domb AJ (2007). 'Polymer carriers for drug delivery in tissue engineering'. *Adv Drug Del Rev*, **59**, 187–206.

Teixeira S, Oliveira S, Ferraz MP and Monteiro FJ (2008). 'Three dimensional macroporous calcium phosphate scaffolds for bone tissue engineering'. International society for Ceramics in Medicine, *Bioceramics 20*, Daculsi G and Layrolle P (eds). Book Series: Key Engineering Materials, Vol 361–363: Part 1-2, 947–50.

Trombi L, Mattii L, Pacini S, D'Alessandro D, Battolla B, Orciuolo E, Buda G, Fazzi R, Galimberti S and Petrini M (2008). 'Human autologous plasma-derived clot as a biological scaffold for mesenchymal stem cells in treatment of orthopedic healing'. *J Orthop Res*, **26**(2), 176–83.

Tschon M, Fini M, Giavaresi G, Torricelli P, Rimondini L, Ambrosio L and Giardino R (2007). '*In vitro* and *in vivo* behaviour of biodegradable and injectable PLA/PGA copolymers related to different matrices'. *Int J Artificial Organs*, **30**(4), 352–62.

Unger RE, Sartoris A, Peters K, Motta A, Migliaresi C, Kunkel M, Bulnheim U, Rychly J and Kirkpatrick CJ (2007). 'Tissue-like self-assembly in cocultures of endothelial cells and osteoblasts and the formation of microcapillary-like structures on three-dimensional porous biomaterials'. *Biomaterials*, **28**(27), 3965–76.

Vacanti C (2006). 'The history of tissue engineering'. *J Cell Mol Med*, **10**(3), 569–76.

Wang L, Li CZ and Senna M (2007). 'High-affinity integration of hydroxyapatite nanoparticles with chemically modified silk fibroin'. *J Nanopart Res*, **9**(5), 919–29.

Yang DZ, Jin Y, Zhou YS, Ma GP, Chen XM and Lu FM (2008). '*In situ* mineralization of hydroxyapatite on electrospun chitosan-based nanofibrous scaffolds'. *Macromol Biosci*, **8**(3), 239–46.

Yunoki S, Marukawa E, Ikoma T, Sotome S, Fan HS, Zhang XD, Shinomiya K and Tanaka J (2007). 'Effect of collagen fibril formation on bioresorbability of hydroxyapatite/collagen composites'. *J Mater Sci Mater Med*, **18**(11), 2179–83

Zachos TA, Shields KM and Bertone AL (2006). 'Gene-mediated osteogenic differentiation of stem cells by bone morphogenetic proteins-2 or-6'. *J Orthop Res*, **24**(6), 1279–91.

Zahn D, Hochrein O, Kawska A, Brickmann J and Kniep R (2007). 'Towards an atomistic understanding of apatite-collagen biomaterials: linking molecular simulation studies of complex-, crystal- and composite-formation to experimental findings'. *J Mater Sci*, **42**(21), 8966–73.

Zou LJ, Zou XN, Chen L, Li HS, Mygind T, Kassem M and Bunger C (2008). 'Effect of hyaluronan on osteogenic differentiation of porcine bone marrow stromal cells *in vitro*'. *J Orthop Res*, **26**(5), 713–20.

15
Retrieval and analysis of orthopaedic implants

A. PALMQUIST, P. THOMSEN, R. BRÅNEMARK, Sahlgrenska Academy at University of Gothenburg, Sweden, H. ENGQVIST, Uppsala University, Sweden and J. LAUSMAA, SP Technical Research Institute of Sweden, Sweden

Abstract: Implants and prostheses inserted *in vivo* may be removed/retrieved for analysis of material properties and tissue reactions. In humans, the retrieval procedure is commonly part of a clinical study and usually performed in association with revision surgery and post-mortem examination. A significant amount of information on material–tissue interactions is gained from systematic studies on retrieved implant–tissue specimens. Although a major interest is focussed on the structural correlation to the functional performance of the device, modern tools of cell and molecular biology provide important means of acquiring additional information about biological events which occur adjacent to an implant *in vivo*. The chapter provides an introduction to the field of retrieval analysis by discussing some of the opportunities for characterization of the bone response to implanted devices in the human. Techniques like focused ion beam microscopy (FIB) provide new possibilities for obtaining intact material–tissue specimens. Light microscopy, scanning electron microscopy and transmission electron microscopy are techniques which allow quantitative information and ultrastructural details of the composition of the bone–material interface to be gathered.

Key words: bone, FIB, histology, implant, interface, retrieval, sample preparation, SEM, TEM, ultrastructure.

15.1 Introduction

Biomaterials are increasingly used for the restoration of function in different parts of the body. Medical devices for the repair of musculoskeletal tissues are manufactured from a range of materials, including ceramics, metals, polymers or combinations thereof (see Chapters 6, 7, 8 and 9). The material properties, both intrinsic ones, such as mechanical and corrosion properties, and the extrinsic ones, such as the biocompatibility and the performance under functional loading, are important for clinical success.

Different methods for evaluation of clinical implants exist, including X-ray imaging, stability measurements and evaluation of functional performance. However, the retrieval and analysis of the implant and associated tissues is useful for a more thorough understanding of the implant performance. Obviously, a major incentive for performing an analysis of the material–tissue interface in humans is the need to obtain the structural correlation to the function of the device in the patient. Such knowledge provides a logical extension of the pre-clinical studies where almost all aspects of the systemic and local tissue response may have been evaluated in animal models. Data obtained from studies in humans are therefore extremely important in a feed-back loop where new materials, surfaces and designs can be improved.

It is the authors' experience that significant information is generally missing about the tissue response adjacent to successfully performing implants placed in the musculoskeletal system of humans. Instead, the objective of the analysis of retrieved implant–tissue specimens is usually to establish the mechanisms of failure of a device. Understanding the mechanisms and causes of clinical failure, such as implant loosening, infection and material failure, provide important steps in the design and manufacture of implants and prostheses, as well as establishing which patient groups are to be treated and the optimal clinical treatment protocol. However, test implants placed in humans could also serve as important steps in the evaluation of implant materials and designs. By using a variety of techniques, different features can be analysed, such as the general histological response to a material, the identity and behaviour of cells, their activity as well as the distribution of proteins and factors important for analysing the processes of inflammation, repair and regeneration.

Important aspects of a thorough, high quality implant retrieval programme have been recognized. For example, Schoen has identified essential features of heart valve retrieval and analysis, of which several are generic prerequisites for a successful retrieval analysis.[1] These include knowledge of the clinical data and experience and knowledge of known and potential failure modes of specific materials, their modifications and entire devices. In general, this effort requires a systematic approach, with the pathologist and scientists working in close collaboration with a network of clinicians. On the laboratory side, it is also of great importance that basic information, for example histological analyses, can be supplemented by additional, specialized analyses whenever needed and motivated from the perspectives of the patient, the clinician and the sponsor/manufacturer. This requires an extremely good technical set-up and experience, either in a single unit or in a network of specialized laboratories. It is our belief that it is possible to obtain a significant wealth of information, preferably from clinical studies where retrieval analysis is already incorporated at the planning stage.

This chapter will not attempt to summarize the available information from retrieved implants and tissues in experimental animal and human studies. Reviews and book chapters have been published on the analysis of failure mechanisms of implants and arthroplasties in the musculoskeletal system of humans. Several excellent summaries have been presented elsewhere on specific topics, such as the mechanisms of failure of certain arthroplasties, the interactions between titanium and bone, and so on. The interested reader is referred, for example, to Pappas and co-workers,[2] Morlock and co-workers,[3] al-Saffar and co-workers,[4, 5] Jones and co-workers,[6] Revell,[7] Jacobs and co-workers,[8] and Goodman,[9] for different aspects (loosening, wear particles and more) of retrieved hip components, Steflik and co-workers,[10] Sennerby and co-workers,[11] and Bolind and co-workers,[12, 13] for retrieved dental implants, Bolind and co-workers,[14] and Granström,[15] for retrieved maxillofacial implants and Collier,[16] for retrieval analysis of spine components, and references therein.

The aim of this chapter is to discuss some of the key factors for obtaining information about the intact material–tissue interface in human bone. This will include different methods of fixation and sample preparation. Further, some different analytical techniques and examples of new techniques for studies of the structure between bone and retrieved implants are presented.

15.2 Retrieval

Clinically used implants are retrieved for different reasons. Some of the most common causes are implant loosening, material failure, pain and post-mortem examination. Investigations of retrieved clinical implants are useful for understanding the mechanisms of success and failure under clinical conditions, information that may not be possible to achieve in experimental models. The implants should preferably be removed with surrounding tissue, allowing histological analysis. Furthermore, the proper handling of the tissue is of utmost importance as the tissue rapidly starts to degenerate owing to loss of blood and nutrition supply. Further, the need to categorize the harvested implants is of utmost importance for back-tracking individual implants with the complete medical history of the patients with radiographs. A brief introduction to such programmes can be found elsewhere.[17]

15.3 Tissue preservation

Tissue is a living material and deterioration will rapidly occur after cessation of blood flow owing to insufficient blood/nutrition supply. Therefore the tissue must be preserved and different formulations have been optimized depending on the type of tissue and analysis intended.[18] Key factors to preserve are the areas of interest, for example the general histology, the cellular details, the RNA, the mineral content and more. As any modification will alter the tissue and its content, the choice of fixative is important. For histology and histomorphometry, aldehyde fixation allows long storage, however the RNA content and certain details of the tissue are altered. To keep the RNA intact, freezing or fixation in alcohol render higher quality RNA left in the sample. Further, for sample handling, as the area of interest is usually close to the implant surface and requires cutting or sawing and grinding, stabilization with embedding techniques is required. Different plastic resins which easily penetrate the tissue are commercially available. These give rise to differences in volume changes and temperature during curing and the adhesion to the implant surface varies as well as preserving the antigenicity of the tissue.[19] Prior to infiltration and embedding, the tissue undergoes a dehydration where water is removed with the help of alcohol in a graded series of baths.

15.4 Analysis

A variety of different analytical techniques exist, ranging from static imaging at different resolution levels to microbiological, chemical, biochemical, immunological and molecular techniques to identify different components in the tissue in close proximity to the medical device.

15.4.1 Histology/histomorphometry

Qualitative (histology) and quantitative (histomorphometry) morphological evaluations are mainly based on fixated and resin-embedded ground sections. The methodology for un-decalcified ground sections of implant and tissue blocks was first described in the early 1980s and is today the most commonly used method for histological examination of the tissue response adjacent to implants in bone. The method consists of tissue fixation, with either formalin or glutaraldehyde, dehydration with ethanol, resin infiltration and polymerization. The resin embedded block is then divided along the long axis of the implant prior to sawing a thin section which is later ground to a thin section prior to staining.[20, 21] Important parameters are the sawing direction and the final thickness of the ground sections.[22, 23]

Subsequent analyses of the stained ground sections are performed in transmission light microscopy enabling qualitative and quantitative analysis of the tissue response around the implant. Different polymer resins for embedding have been used and evaluated such as epoxy, methyl methacrylate and polyester.[24–26] The polymerization, which most often is performed by heat treatment, UV-light treatment or by adding an accelerator to the resin, will result in a hardened block. The hardness will differ between different polymers and different polymerization methods as well as the degree of polymerized monomers. An important factor is the viscosity of the resin, where lower viscosities penetrate the tissue more easily. Using an image analysis software program, different structures may be quantified.

Today, in routine studies, most laboratories have developed techniques for assaying the relative amounts/volumes of tissues adjacent to, inside and in contact with the surface of the implanted device. For example, such measurements may include the amount of bone tissue in direct contact with the implant and the bone area occupying the space between the threads (Fig. 15.1).

15.4.2 Scanning electron microscopy

Scanning electron microscopy (SEM) allows the analysis of different features of retrieved specimens and could be performed in two different modes.

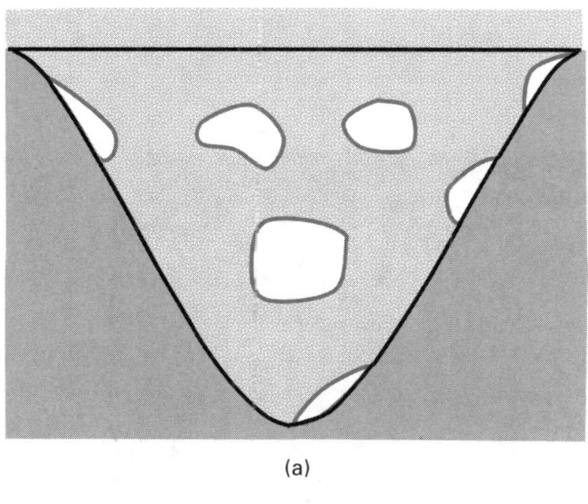

(a)

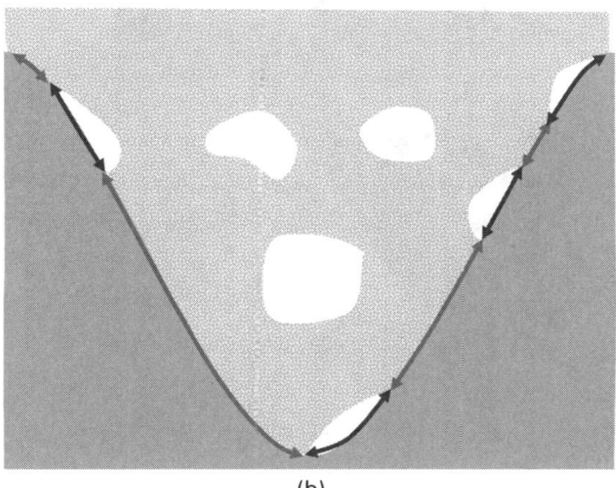

(b)

15.1 Schematics of routine light microscopic histomorphometry of tissue adjacent to the surface of a threaded implant in ground sections. (a) The bone area within the threads is measured by the area of bone tissue (black triangle minus white islands) divided by the total area (black triangle). (b) The bone implant contact is measured by the length of bone contact (grey arrows) divided by the total length (black plus grey arrows).

Low energy electrons (secondary electrons) or high energy electrons (back-scattered electrons) could be used to image the specimen. The difference between the modes is the amount of contrast between different elements and topographical information, where the back-scattered electrons give larger contrast differences between metal and bone compared to secondary electrons, which provide more topographical features (Fig. 15.2). SEM is a very useful technique for analysis of bone in association with implanted materials.[27–29] The technique is also valuable for the identification of relevant areas which may be selected for further analysis, using, for example, the new focused ion beam microscopy (FIB) technique.

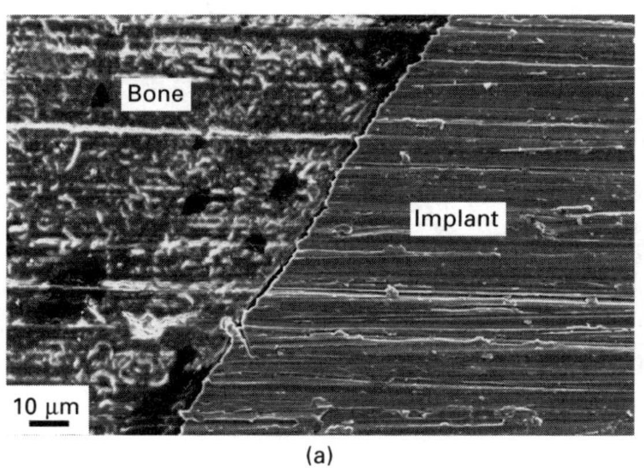

(a)

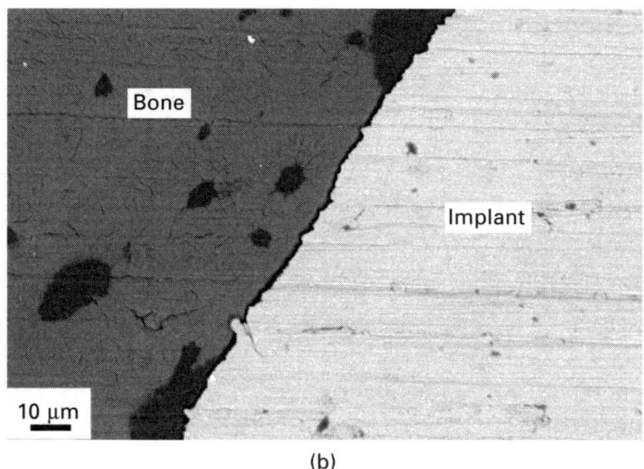

(b)

15.2 Scanning electron micrographs of titanium alloy implant in rabbit tibia after 8 weeks of healing. (a) Secondary electron image. (b) Back-scatter electron image.

15.4.3 Ultrastructural interface analysis

For ultrastructural analysis using transmission electron microscopy (TEM), sample preparation is cumbersome owing to several factors, including the difference in mechanical properties between the tissue and implant and the limited thickness (<100 nm) required for the final sample. Some different techniques have been introduced in order to circumvent the difficulty in cutting the implant material with the ultramicrotome. A common approach found in the literature is the separation of the tissue from the implant before or after embedding in resin but prior to sectioning[30] or using plastic implant replicas coated with a thin layer of metal.[31] The latter is restricted to animal experimental studies owing to the lack of relevant bulk properties of the implant. Other methods are based on removal of the bulk metal prior to sectioning, leaving the outermost oxide layer intact and therefore a true oxide–tissue interface. This could be performed by electrochemical dissolution[11, 32] or by mechanically removing the bulk.[33] Electrochemical dissolution induced artefactual demineralization of the interface zone while the latter is restricted to thicker oxide layers or plasma-coated implants.

The only sample preparation method known today where both the implant and tissue could be present in the section is FIB microscopy.[34] This method allows analysis of the intact interface zone as well as the surface properties of the implant and the tissue at a limited distance from the implant surface. The basics of FIB is that a focused gallium ion beam sputters material from the sample surface and, by protecting an area of interest, a thin lamella can be cut (Fig. 15.3). Different sample lift-out techniques are available depending on the instrument used.[35, 36] Possible analyses in transmission electron microscopy are elemental and structural analysis at a resolution down to the sub-nanometer level revealing information which could not be assessed by light microscopy.

15.4.4 Implant material characterization

Characterization of the retrieved implant can be useful for investigating changes that have occurred in the implant as a result of the interaction with the host tissue. In the case of material failures (e.g. implant fractures), the analysis of the fractured surfaces can also provide information about the type of fracture. Numerous methods are available for the material analysis, among which scanning electron microscopy (SEM) combined with X-ray fluorescence spectroscopy (EDX), Fourier transform infrared spectroscopy (FT-IR), and surface spectroscopic techniques (e.g. Auger electron spectroscopy–AES, X-ray photoelectron spectroscopy–XPS/electron spectroscopy for chemical analysis–ESCA and time of flight secondary ion mass spectroscopy–TOF-SIMS) are the most useful.

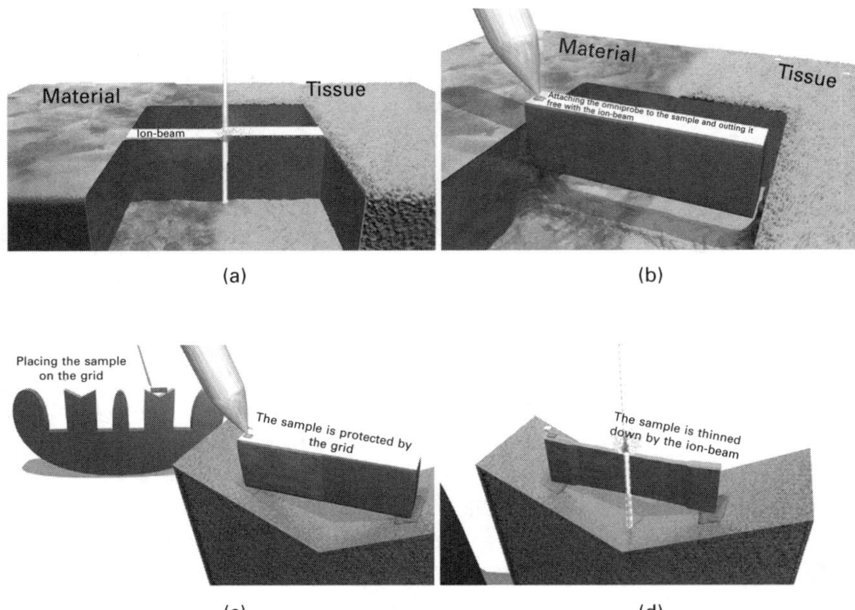

15.3 Schematic presentation of the FIB sample preparation for TEM analysis using *in situ* lift-out. (a) Trenches are cut on either side of the protected area of interest. (b) The lamella is attached to a micromanipulator. (c) The lamella is transferred and attached to a TEM grid. (d) Finally the sample is thinned until it reaches electron transparency (~100 nm).

15.5 Examples of results

15.5.1 Arthroplasty

Excessive wear of the articulating surfaces of joint implants leads to particulate generation which may eventually cause implant loosening and clinical failure in arthroplasties. For example, Lausmaa and co-workers[37] studied hip arthroplasties that had been retrieved owing to displacement, which in turn was caused by excessive wear of the plastic acetabular lining. By using different methods of materials analysis, it could be concluded that different factors had contributed to the wear. FT-IR-analysis of unused and retrieved acetabular cups revealed a surface zone that was degraded by oxidation, probably caused by the sterilization method used (gamma irradiation). SEM/EDX analysis of the worn plastic surfaces also showed the presence of calcium phosphate particles embedded in the plastic. Apparently, this material originated from the metallic backing of the acetabular component, which was coated with plasma sprayed hydroxyapatite. Plasma sprayed coatings are often associated with poor integrity, causing release of particles either by cracking or adhesion failure. In summary, the analysis of the failed components pointed towards two materials-related causes of the clinical failures, one being improper sterilization process parameters, the other being a design that led to generation of hard particles that could enter the articulating surfaces, where they acted as an abrasive agent.

15.5.2 Bone anchored amputation prosthesis

An example of another application of osseointegration where retrieval analysis has been performed is the bone anchored amputation prosthesis. The treatment of amputees with this technology was introduced in the early 1990s, when the first surgery was performed on a bilateral trans-femoral amputee. The surgery is performed in two stages where first a titanium fixture is placed in the remaining bone and, after about 6 months of healing, a percutanous abutment is installed.[38] Implant installations have been performed on both upper and lower limb (Fig. 15.4) amputations.[39] In clinical studies it has been demonstrated that the treatment increases the quality of life[40, 41] of the patients as well as increases the perception of the environment through a phenomenon called osseoperception.[42]

A forearm bone anchored amputation prosthesis which had suffered a fatigue fracture after 11 years of use was removed with a threphine together with the surrounding bone tissue (Fig. 15.5), a removal method which allows installation of a new implant.[43]

The removed implant–tissue block was immersed in buffered formalin prior to dehydration in a graded series of ethanol baths. A stepwise infiltration of plastic resin was performed in order to fill out all voids in the bone tissue prior to curing with an accelerator (LR White, London Resin Company). The cured embedded block was divided along the long axis by band saw (EXAKT Apparatebau GmbH&Co, Norderstedt, Germany). A ground section was prepared according to Fig. 15.6 and subsequently contrasted with toluidine blue.

The final section thickness was 50 μm containing the whole cross-section of the implant and the surrounding bone tissue (Fig. 15.7). The counterpart was gently cut with a slow rotating diamond saw and gently polished prior to gold sputtering for electron conductivity. The specimen was then mounted in the vacuum chamber of the FIB system (FEI strata 235 DB FIB/SEM) and a 100 nm thick sample in cross-section was prepared containing both bone tissue and implant (Figu. 15.7). TEM analysis was performed using different analytical tools such as electron energy loss spectroscopy (EELS), high resolution and energy filtered and transmission electron microscopy (HRTEM and EFTEM).

The results of the histomorphometrical evaluation showed a large amount of mineralized bone in direct contact with the implant (85%) and large

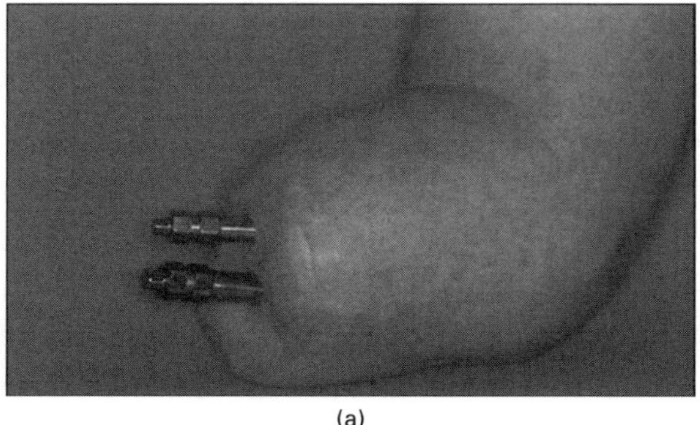

(a)

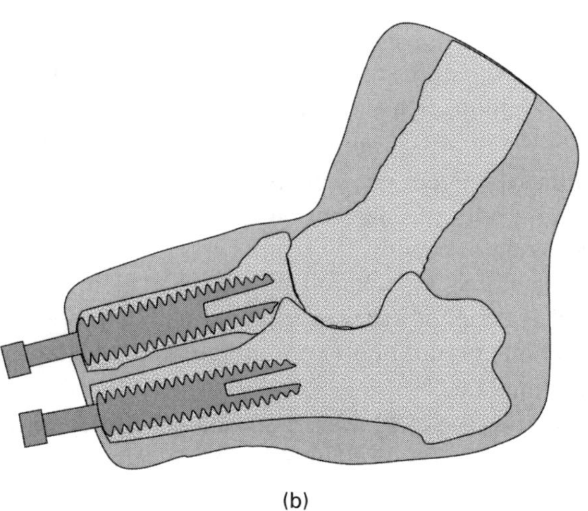

(b)

15.4 Photograph of a forearm bone anchored amputation prosthesis (a) and a schematic image of the implants and abutments (b).

amount of bone tissue within the threads (75%), with values comparable to retrieved oral implants.[11] Both cortical bone and trabecular bone surrounded the implant, where the threaded outer surface of the implant was dominated by cortical bone with Haversian systems, while the inner hollow compartment at the apical end was dominated by trabecular bone with a thickness of an average 200 μm (Figs 15.7 and 15.8).

At the electron microscopy level, it was observed that an artefactual separation filled by plastic resin was present at the interface between bone and implant, a possible artefact created during the dehydration and plastic embedding where volume changes occur.[44, 45] Collagen banding could be observed close to the artefact, together with scattered apatite crystals indicating mineralized bone (Fig. 15.9). Using energy filtered TEM, calcium could be detected at the immediate surface of the implant which was further

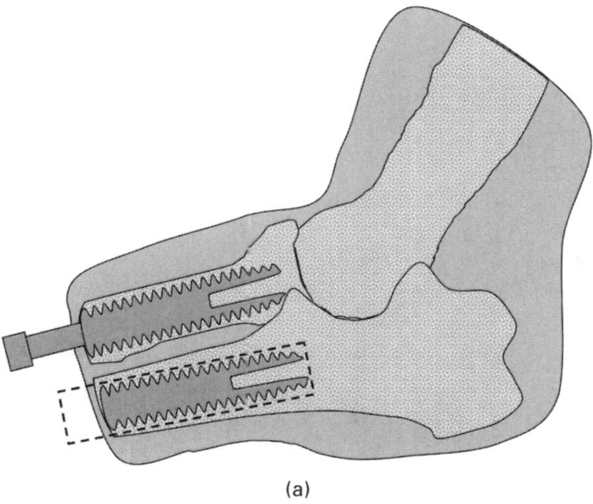

(a)

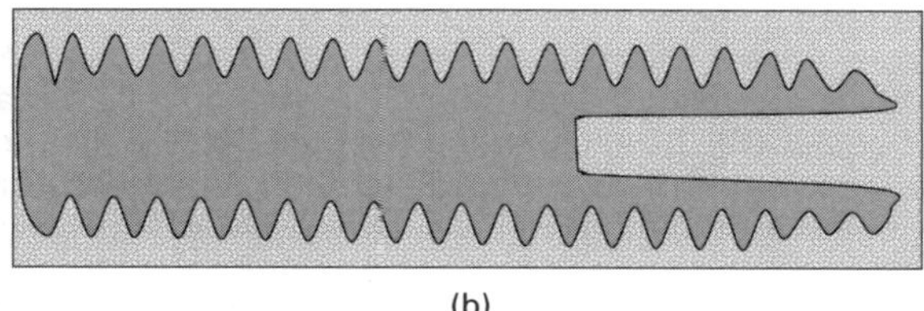

(b)

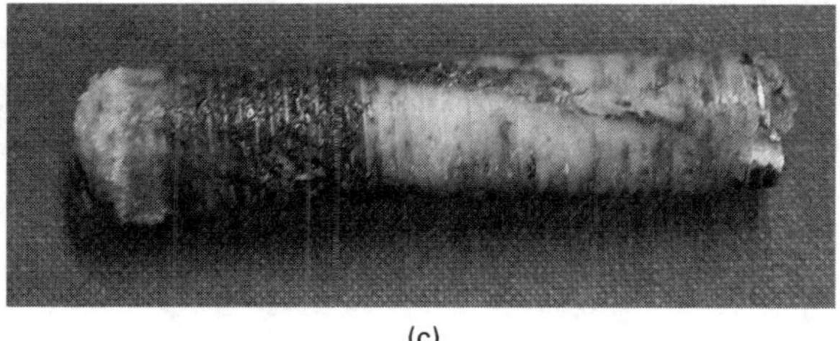

(c)

15.5 (a) The dotted line represents the trephine during retrieval of the implant with surrounding tissue from the ulnar bone. A schematic image (b) and photograph (c) of the retrieved implant–tissue block.

analysed by high resolution TEM and identified as hydroxyapatite via lattice parameters (Fig. 15.10). Hence the artefact is created in the bone tissue rather than at the immediate implant surface. Further, the closest nanometers to the implant surface is mineralized in contrast to results from other researchers using different sample preparation techniques in animal experiments and clinically retrieved oral implants.[11, 31, 46, 47]

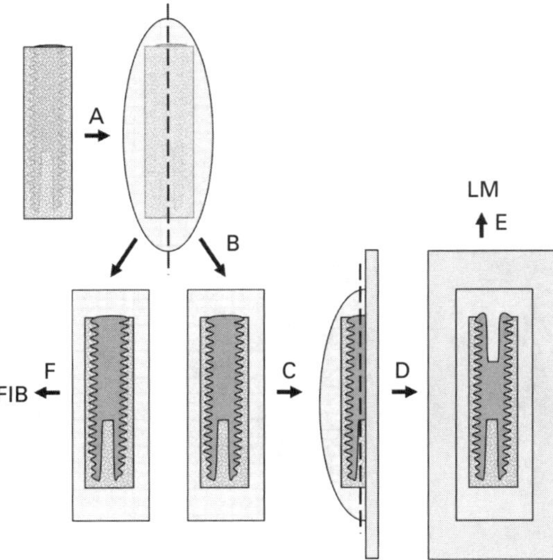

15.6 Schematic presentation of the sample preparation chain. (A) Fixation, dehydration and plastic embedding. (B) Dividing the embedded tissue–implant block in half. (C) Mounting on a plastic slide and sawing. (D) Grinding until a final thickness of 50 μm. (E) Staining prior to light microscopic analysis. (F) Sputter coating with gold prior to FIB sectioning for TEM analysis. LM is light microscopy.

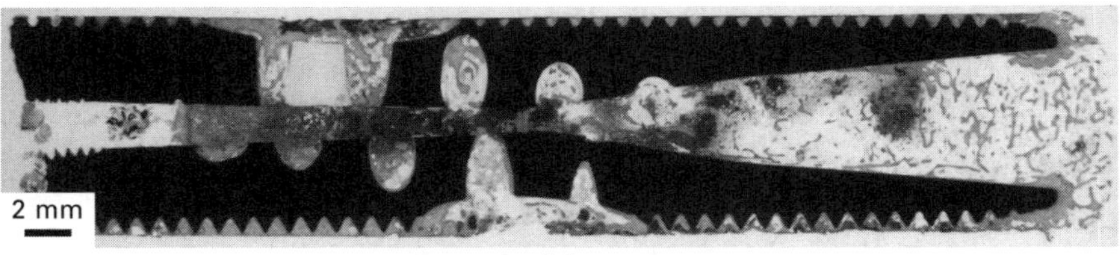

(a)

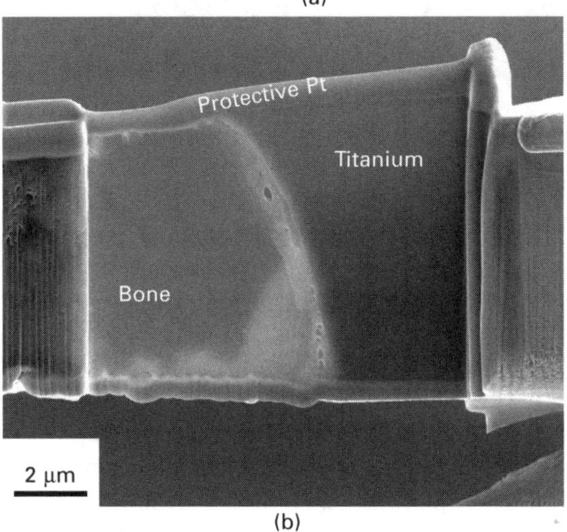

(b)

15.7 (a) Light micrograph of the stained ground section. (b) SEM micrograph of the FIB prepared TEM sample.

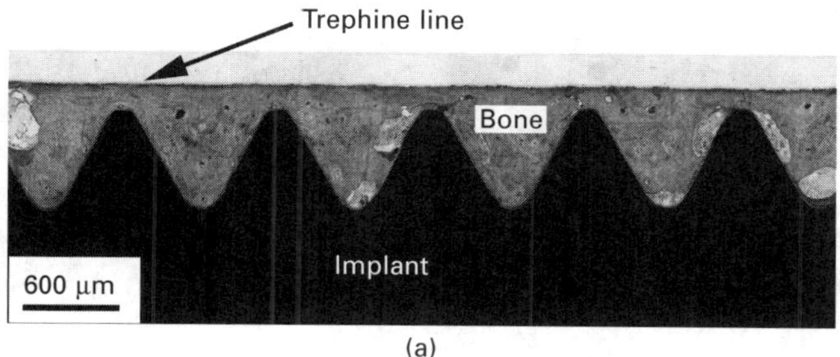

(a)

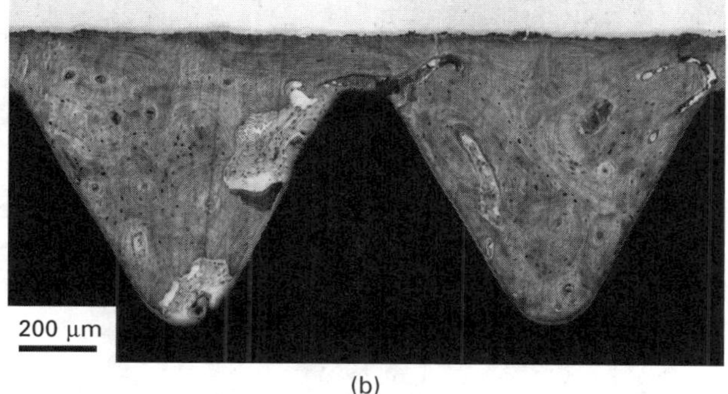

(b)

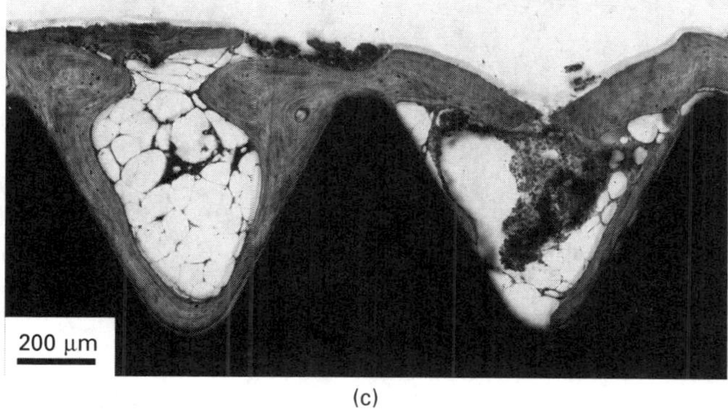

(c)

15.8 Light optical micrographs of the ground section. Most threads are surrounded by mature cortical bone tissue with organized Haversian systems (a) (b) while other threads are dominated by trabecular bone and bone marrow (c).

15.5.3 Surface analysis of retrieved titanium implants

Several studies[48–51] have been made on retrieved titanium implants, attempting to elucidate the changes that may occur at the implant surface under *in vivo* conditions. Early studies of experimental implants by Sundgren and co-workers

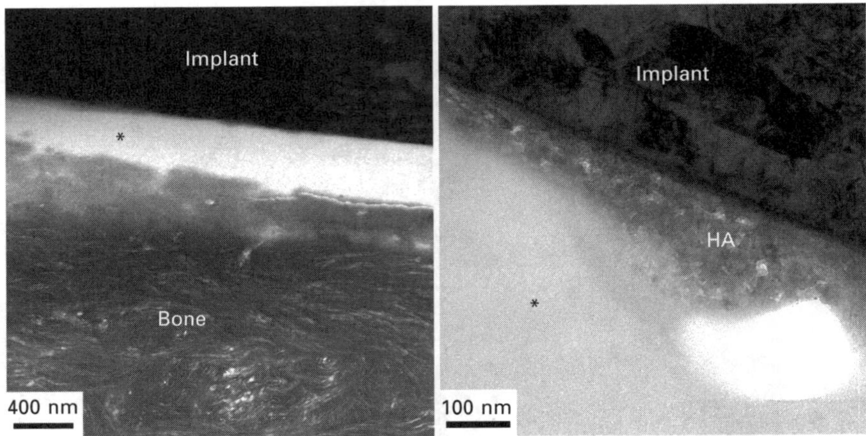

15.9 Electron micrographs of the ultrathin section prepared by FIB. Characteristic collagen banding is present close to the artefact (*) while apatite formation is present at the implant surface.

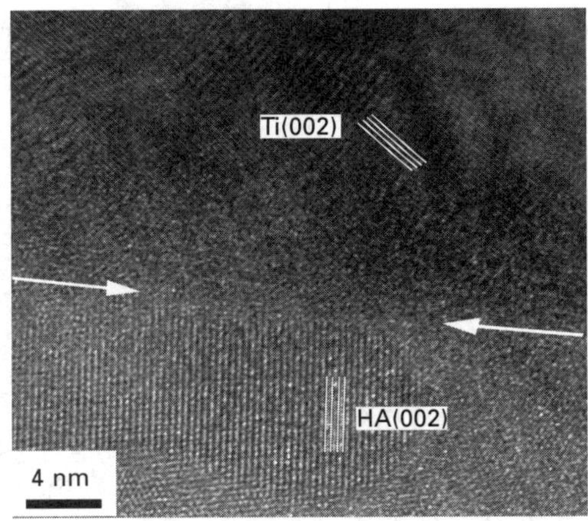

15.10 High resolution electron micrograph of the interface zone, showing the lattice parameters for alpha-titanium and hydroxyapatite. Arrows show the implant–bone interface.

indicated that the oxide layer of titanium may grow with time *in vivo*, and that foreign elements (calcium, phosphorus and sulphur, depending on host tissue) become incorporated in the growing oxide layer.[51] However, later studies on human and animal experimental implants by surface spectroscopic methods[48, 50] and FIB–TEM[43, 52] have shown no such oxide growth to any significant extent. Current findings thus indicate that the oxide layer on titanium implants can be regarded as stable during normal *in vivo* conditions, unless wear is present.

15.6 Acknowledgements

Support from the VINNOVA Forska&Väx((2006-02247), the VINNOVA VinnVäxt Program Biomedical Development in Western Sweden, the BIOMATCELL VINN Excellence Center, the Swedish Research Council (grant K2006-73X-09495-16-3), LUA project (ALFGBG-11128) and Integrum AB is gratefully acknowledged.

15.7 References

1. Schoen FJ. 'Role of device retrieval and analysis in the evaluation of substitute heart valves', *Clinical Evaluation of Medical Devices: Principles and Case Studies*. Witkin KB (ed.), Humana Press, Totowa, NJ, USA, 1998, 209–31.
2. Pappas MA, Schmidt CC, Shanbhag AS, Whiteside TA, Rubash HE and Herndon JH. 'Biological response to particulate debris from nonmetallic orthopedic implants', *Human Biomaterials Applications*, Wise DL, Trantolo DJ, Altobelli DE, Yaszemski MJ and Gresser JD (eds). Humana Press, Totowa, NJ, USA, 1996, 115–35.
3. Morlock MM, Bishop N, Zustin J, Hahn M, Ruther W and Amling M. 'Modes of implant failure after hip resurfacing: morphological and wear analysis of 267 retrieval specimens', *J Bone Joint Surg Am*, 2008, **90**(Suppl 3), 89–95.
4. Al-Saffar N and Revell PA. 'Pathology of the bone-implant interfaces', *J Long Term Eff Med Implants*, 1999, **9**(4), 319–47.
5. Al-Saffar N and Revell PA. 'Differential expression of transforming growth factor-alpha and macrophage colony-stimulating factor/colony-stimulating factor-1R (c-fins) by multinucleated giant cells involved in pathological bone resorption at the site of orthopaedic implants', *J Orthop Res*, 2000, **18**(5), 800–7.
6. Jones RE, Willie BM, Hayes H and Bloebaum RD. 'Analysis of 16 retrieved proximally cemented femoral stems', *J Arthroplasty*, 2005, **20**(1), 84–93.
7. Revell PA. 'The combined role of wear particles, macrophages and lymphocytes in the loosening of total joint prostheses', *J Roy Soc Interface*, 2008, **5**(28), 1263–78.
8. Jacobs JJ, Patterson LM, Skipor AK, Hall DJ, Urban RM, Black J *et al.* 'Postmortem retrieval of total joint replacement components', *J Biomed Mater Res*, 1999, **48**(3), 385–91.
9. Goodman SB. 'Wear particles, periprosthetic osteolysis and the immune system', *Biomaterials* 2007, **28**(34), 5044–8.
10. Steflik DE, Corpe RS, Young TR, Parr GR, Tucker M, Sims M *et al.* 'Light microscopic and scanning electron microscopic retrieval analyses of implanted biomaterials retrieved from humans and experimental animals', *J Oral Implantol*, 2001, **27**(1), 5–15.
11. Sennerby L, Ericson LE, Thomsen P, Lekholm U and Astrand P. 'Structure of the bone-titanium interface in retrieved clinical oral implants', *Clin Oral Implants Res*, 1991, **2**(3), 103–11.
12. Bolind P, Johansson CB, Balshi TJ, Langer B and Albrektsson T. 'A study of 275 retrieved Branemark oral implants', *Int J Periodontics Restorative Dent*, 2005, **25**(5), 425–37.
13. Bolind PK, Johansson CB, Becker W, Langer L, Sevetz EB Jr. and Albrektsson TO. 'A descriptive study on retrieved non-threaded and threaded implant designs', *Clin Oral Implants Res*, 2005, **16**(4), 447–55.

14. Bolind P, Acton C, Albrektsson T, Bonding P, Granstrom G, Johansson C, Lindeman P, Mühlbauer W and Tjellström A. 'Histologic evaluation of retrieved craniofacial implants', *Otolaryngol Head Neck Surg*, 2000, **123**(1 Pt 1), 140–6.
15. Granström G. 'Measurement of bone metal contact (BMC) in retrieved maxillofacial osseointegrated implants', *Acta Otolaryngol Suppl*, 2000, **543**, 114–17.
16. Collier JP. 'The value of spine implant retrieval analysis', *Spine*, 2008, **33**(5), 457.
17. Anderson JM. 'Implant retrieval and evaluation', *Biomaterials Science : an Introduction to Materials in Medicine*. Ratner BD, (ed). 2nd edition Elsevier, Amsterdam, 2004, xii, 851 s.
18. Moran DT and Rowley JC. 'Biological specimen preparation for correlative light and electron microscopy', *Correlative Microscopy in Biology: Instrumentation and Methods*. Hayat MA (ed). Academic Press, Orlando, FL, USA, 1987, 1–22.
19. Knabe C, Kraska B, Koch C, Gross U, Zreiqat H and Stiller M. 'A method for immunohistochemical detection of osteogenic markers in undecalcified bone sections', *Biotech Histochem*, 2006, **81**(1), 31–9.
20. Donath K and Breuner G. 'A method for the study of undecalcified bones and teeth with attached soft tissues. The Sage-Schliff (sawing and grinding) technique', *J Oral Pathol*, 1982, **11**(4), 318–26.
21. Donath K. 'Die Trenn-Dunnscliff-Technik zur Herstellung histologischer Präparaten von nicht schneidbaren Geweben und Materialen', *Der Präparator*, 1988, **34**, 318–25.
22. Johansson CB and Morberg P. 'Importance of ground section thickness for reliable histomorphometrical results', *Biomaterials*, 1995, **16**(2), 91–5.
23. Johansson CB and Morberg P. 'Cutting directions of bone with biomaterials in situ does influence the outcome of histomorphometrical quantifications', *Biomaterials*, 1995, **16**(13), 1037–9.
24. Hipp JA, Brunski JB and Cochran GV. 'Method for histological preparation of bone sections containing titanium implants', *Stain Technol*, 1987, **62**(4), 247–52.
25. Kihara A, Morimoto K and Suetsugu T. 'Improved method using a bubble-free adhesion technique for the preparation of semi-serial undecalcified histologic sections containing dental implants', *J Oral Implantol*, 1989, **15**(2), 87–94.
26. Pasyk KA and Hassett CA. 'Modified hematoxylin and eosin staining method for epoxy-embedded tissue sections', *Pathol Res Pract*, 1989, **184**(6), 635–8.
27. Bloebaum RD, Bachus KN, Jensen JW and Hofmann AA. 'Postmortem analysis of consecutively retrieved asymmetric porous-coated tibial components', *J Arthroplasty*, 1997, **12**(8), 920–9.
28. Bloebaum RD, Skedros JG, Vajda EG, Bachus KN and Constantz BR. 'Determining mineral content variations in bone using backscattered electron imaging', *Bone*, 1997, **20**(5), 485–90.
29. Vajda EG, Humphrey S, Skedros JG and Bloebaum RD. 'Influence of topography and specimen preparation on backscattered electron images of bone', *Scanning*, 1999, **21**(6), 379–87.
30. Thomsen P and Ericson LE. 'Light and transmission electron microscopy used to study the tissue morphology close to implants', *Biomaterials*, 1985, **6**(6), 421–4.
31. Albrektsson T, Brånemark PI, Hansson HA, Ivarsson B and Jönsson U. 'Ultrastructural analysis of the interface zone of titanium and gold implants', *Advances in Biomaterials*. Albrektsson T, Lee AJC, Brånemark PI (ed). Wiley, Chichester, 1982, 167–77.
32. Bjursten LM, Emanuelsson L, Ericson LE, Thomsen P, Lausmaa J, Mattsson

L, Rolander U and Kasemo B. 'Method for ultrastructural studies of the intact tissue–metal interface', *Biomaterials*, 1990, **11**(8), 596–601.

33. Leize EM, Hemmerle J and Leize M. 'Characterization, at the bone crystal level, of the titanium-coating/bone interfacial zone', *Clin Oral Implants Res*, 2000, **11**(4), 279–88.
34. Engqvist H, Botton GA, Couillard M, Mohammadi S, Malmstrom J, Emanuelsson L *et al.* 'A novel tool for high-resolution transmission electron microscopy of intact interfaces between bone and metallic implants', *J Biomed Mater Res A*, 2006, **78**(1), 20–4.
35. Jarmar T, Palmquist A, Branemark R, Hermansson L, Engqvist H and Thomsen P. 'Technique for preparation and characterization in cross-section of oral titanium implant surfaces using focused ion beam and transmission electron microscopy', *J Biomed Mater Res A*, 2008, **87**(4), 1003–9.
36. Phaneuf MW. 'FIB for materials science applications – a review', *Introduction to Focused Ion Beams: Instrumentation, Theory, Techniques and Practice*. Giannuzzi LA and Stevie FA (eds). Springer, Boston, 2005.
37. Lausmaa J, Carlsson L, Möller K and Rökkum M, 'Analysis of abnormal wear in UHMWPE acetabular cups,' 14th European Biomaterials Conference, The Hague, Netherlands, 1998.
38. Robinson K, Brånemark R and Ward D. 'Future developments: osseointegration in transfemoral amputees', *Atlas of Amputations and Limb Deficiencies: Surgical, Prosthetic and Rehabilitation Principles*. Smith D, Michael J and Bowker J (eds). 3rd edition, 2004, 673–81.
39. Rydevik B. 'Amputation prostheses and osseoperception in the lower and upper extremity', *Osseointegration in Skeletal Reconstruction and Joint Replacement*. Brånemark P-I, Rydevik B and Skalak R (eds). Guintessence Books, London, 1997, 175–82.
40. Hagberg K, Brånemark R, Gunterberg B and Rydevik B. 'Osseointegrated trans-femoral amputation prostheses: Prospective results of general and condition-specific quality of life in 18 patients at 2-year follow-up', *Prosthet Orthot Int*, 2008, **32**(1), 29–41.
41. Hagberg K, Haggstrom E, Uden M and Branemark R. 'Socket versus bone-anchored trans-femoral prostheses: hip range of motion and sitting comfort', *Prosthet Orthot Int*, 2005, **29**(2), 153–63.
42. Jacobs R, Branemark R, Olmarker K, Rydevik B, Van Steenberghe D and Branemark PI. 'Evaluation of the psychophysical detection threshold level for vibrotactile and pressure stimulation of prosthetic limbs using bone anchorage or soft tissue support', *Prosthet Orthot Int*, 2000, **24**(2), 133–42.
43. Palmquist A, Jarmar T, Emanuelsson L, Branemark R, Engqvist H and Thomsen P. 'Forearm bone anchored amputation prosthesis: a case study on the osseointegration', *Acta Orthopaedica*, 2008, **79**(1), 78–85.
44. Lawton DM, Oswald WB and McClure J. 'The biological reality of the interlacunar network in the embryonic, cartilaginous, skeleton: a thiazine dye/absolute ethanol/LR White resin protocol for visualizing the network with minimal tissue shrinkage', *J Microsc*, 1995, **178**(Pt 1), 66–85.
45. Palmquist A, Jarmar T, Emanuelsson L, Brånemark R, Engqvist H and Thomsen P. 'Comparison of embedding resins with regards to implant surface adhesion, an important factor for ultrastructural analysis', *8th World Biomaterials Congress*, Amsterdam, Netherlands, 2008.

46. Albrektsson T and Hansson HA. 'An ultrastructural characterization of the interface between bone and sputtered titanium or stainless steel surfaces', *Biomaterials*, 1986, **7**(3), 201–5.
47. Albrektsson T, Hansson HA and Ivarsson B. 'Interface analysis of titanium and zirconium bone implants', *Biomaterials*, 1985, **6**(2), 97–101.
48. Arys A, Philippart C, Dourov N, He Y, Le QT and Pireaux JJ. 'Analysis of titanium dental implants after failure of osseointegration: combined histological, electron microscopy, and X-ray photoelectron spectroscopy approach', *J Biomed Mater Res*, 1998, **43**(3), 300–12.
49. Aparicio C and Olive J. 'Comparative surface microanalysis of failed Branemark implants', *Int J Oral Maxillofac Implants*, 1992, **7**(1), 94–103.
50. Esposito M, Lausmaa J, Hirsch JM and Thomsen P. 'Surface analysis of failed oral titanium implants', *J Biomed Mater Res*, 1999, **48**(4), 559–68.
51. Sundgren JE, Bodo P, Lundstrom I, Berggren A and Hellem S. 'Auger electron spectroscopic studies of stainless-steel implants', *J Biomed Mater Res*, 1985, **19**(6), 663–71.
52. Palmquist A, Lindberg F, Brånemark R, Engqvist H and Thomsen P. 'Biomechanical, histological and ultrastructural analysis of micro- and nano-structured titanium alloy implants: a study in rabbit', *J Biomed Mater Res*, 2009, in press.

16
Ethical issues in bone repair and bone tissue engineering

L. TROMMELMANS, J. SELLING and K. DIERICKX,
Katholieke Universiteit Leuven, Belgium

Abstract: Of the approaches toward bone repair, bone tissue engineering elicits some of the more complex ethical questions, owing to the incorporation of living, considerably altered cells in the product. We discuss three areas where ethical issues occur: cell sourcing, clinical trials and therapy. Cells are key components of all bone tissue engineered products. Embryonic stem cells may be used in the future, but this remains ethically controversial. Non-embryonic cells are not controversial but cell donation and the informed consent procedure accompanying it raises questions: both the cells' material value and their informational value for the donor need to be examined when deciding on the conditions of cell donation for tissue engineering purposes. Regeneration through the creation and implantation of metabolically active constructs is a new medical approach which requires a profound analysis of the implications of the new approach for the design of clinical trials and of therapy to protect the safety and autonomy of vulnerable persons. This includes assessments of efficacy, risks and safety. It also requires an evaluation of informed consent procedures. This may not only benefit bone tissue engineering, but other bone repair interventions as well. A third issue is safeguarding the access of patients. The economic thresholds for this therapy will be considerable. However, the presence of living cells may also create a biological threshold owing to immunological requirements. Tissue engineered products may be unavailable for some persons, unless biological diversity is taken into account from the design of bone tissue engineered products and through accurate cell sourcing strategies.

Key words: bone, cell donation, clinical trials, ethics, informed consent, patient follow-up, regenerative medicine, stem cells, therapy, tissue engineering.

16.1 Introduction: the ethical analysis of bone repair

The notion of good science and good medicine has an ethical undertone: the pursuit of human enrichment through science, engineering and medicine is an unquestionable good and should be encouraged. Most persons would also claim that this end does not justify any means. Science and medicine conducted at the expense of human dignity or causing needless suffering is considered to be bad science and bad medicine and is therefore widely and rightly condemned.

The scientific and medical community is increasingly aware that fundamental ethical principles should govern research and medicine. Nearly every person engages in ethical discourse, but the ethical analysis of complex biomedical events, like regenerative medicine and the development of appropriate ethical guidance, is usually considered to be the province of (bio)ethicists. While ethicists are addressing these issues, it is unrealistic to expect that they will provide simple answers to complex questions, or that they will present the community with clear and prohibitive rules for shaping human conduct. Moreover, ethicists do not operate in a vacuum, but work within particular paradigms and narratives that influence their analyses and conclusions. Therefore ethicists will seldom be able to 'solve' ethical problems, such as the use of human embryonic stem cells, in the same way that scientists, engineers or physicians are able to solve the challenges they face. What ethicists do is analyse the ethical relevance of a medical/scientific innovation, of the circumstances under which it is applied and of its ends and ramifications. They argue their position and advise those who must eventually make their own decisions. Sometimes this advice may gather a consensus and be formalised later in guidelines, codes of conduct, conventions or legislation at national or supranational level.

In this chapter we will focus exclusively on the ethical issues generated by the development of bone tissue engineering as an example of regenerative medicine because the inclusion of human cells in a tissue engineered product entails a number of specific ethical issues that are not present in other applications of bone repair (Trommelmans *et al.*, 2007a). However, many of the issues covered here are also relevant for other bone repair therapies, such as the conduct of clinical trials and the difficulties of obtaining informed consent.

Two questions come to mind: are there fundamental arguments for rejecting regenerative medicine on ethical grounds? If not, what would be the ethical requirements for the development and application of this new technology?

Does the concept of regeneration itself raise fundamental ethical objections that would compel us to reject this paradigm altogether? We argue that this is not the case.

Regenerative medicine contrasts with other medical approaches in that it explicitly intends to regenerate the body into full physiological capacity. The *ex vivo* construction of a bone tissue engineered product (BTEP), its implantation and integration in the recipient's body is but one application of regenerative medicine. Regeneration occurs continuously in the human body, although some tissues have an extremely limited spontaneous regenerative capacity. Regeneration of bone with the aid of a BTEP therefore does not seem to alter any fundamental quality of the human body or person, unless one finds every intervention in the body ethically unacceptable *per se*. Enabling tissue regeneration through a medical intervention is not altogether new, even if the science behind regenerative medicine and the applied methodology are. Casts have routinely been used to enable the body to heal a fracture. Implanted tissue engineered bone may similarly enable the body to close large bone defects. From this point of view there is no fundamental reason to reject regenerative medicine.

Another fundamental objection to regenerative medicine might be that it would inevitably lead to undesirable ends such as the creation of 'post-humans', either by enhancing their physical capacities through the implantation of enhanced tissues or organs or by lengthening their life span considerably through a succession of interventions targeted at various degenerating tissues (Gordijn, 2004). While it might become possible to achieve this goal, it would not be the inevitable consequence of regenerative medicine. These objections do not stem from the principle of regeneration, but from the construction and application of particular products under specific circumstances. While such 'slippery slope' arguments may sound attractive, they do not carry much ethical weight (Launis, 2002).

However, while the concept of regenerative medicine in general and of bone tissue engineering in particular seems to be ethically acceptable, the development and application of these technologies may raise poignant ethical questions. We discuss in this chapter three areas where such ethical pitfalls might occur in bone tissue engineering: cell sourcing, clinical trials and therapy.

16.2 Cells in bone tissue engineered products (BTEPs)

16.2.1 Introduction

Whenever ethical concerns have so far been raised with regard to the development of human tissue engineered products, they were usually related to the use of specific cell types such as human embryonic stem cells or xenogeneic cells.

Cells have only recently become the object of ethical scrutiny. Until the work of Harrison in 1907 and Carrel in 1912, it was presumed that cells could not exist outside the '*milieu intérieur*' of the body. Cell culturing has since demonstrated the remarkable autonomy and plasticity of cells. We have 'liberated' cells from the constraints of the body, immortalised and hybridised them. We have learned to manipulate their fate by exposing them to various media. We have made them into factories that produce the products we want and that can be patented and traded (Landecker, 2007). Now we are learning how to alter them considerably, incorporate them in *ex vivo* structures and reintegrate them in the dynamic environment of bodies other than the ones they originally belonged to. These developments have not only resulted in enormous scientific advances, they have also generated new ways of interpreting the relationships between cells, bodies and human persons. It is because of these new or altered relationships that human cells and the products in which they are incorporated obtain their ethical relevance.

As a biological entity, cells have become the focus of tissue engineering. Using them efficiently and safely are prime concerns for tissue engineers (European Commission, 2002). However, cells remain the building blocks of (potential) living entities from which they are derived. But cells are also repositories of information that connect them to the organism from which they have been isolated. Cells have become discrete entities that can be donated or sold, placing them firmly in the tissue economies that are increasingly influencing the development of research, medicine and health care (Waldby and Mitchell, 2006).

In all of these qualities, cells link diverse stakeholders with each other, establishing new forms of relationships. Various stakeholders may well have widely differing and sometimes conflicting views and interests about these subjects, often based on strong ethical convictions and sensitivities. These will influence, amongst others, the acceptability of the use of certain cell types for BTEPs and the modalities for their procurement.

16.2.2 Use of specific cell types in bone tissue engineering

Various cell types have been put forward for incorporation in BTEPs. Two cell types are frequently mentioned in bone tissue engineering and should therefore also be analysed for their moral relevance: embryonic stem cells (ES) and multipotent stem cells. Of this last cell type, mesenchymal stem cells (MSC) are predominant in bone tissue engineering research (Salgado *et al.*, 2004). Owing to our presently very limited ability to consistently and reliably control and direct the developmental pathways of ES, and the more reliable results already obtained with differentiated cells, the present choice for bone tissue engineering is predominantely a choice for differentiated cells.

Embryonic stem cells

ES are the most controversial of all cell types that qualify for application in BTEPs because it is – for the moment – still necessary to destroy the early embryo in order to retrieve the ES. The question whether the use of ES is acceptable must therefore be retraced to the status of the embryo. There are various opinions concerning this status (UNESCO, 2001). These convictions are rooted in religious, philosophical and/or moral systems and are profoundly influenced by anthropological concepts and by historic events that have greatly influenced the evaluation of scientific and medical conduct (Lenoir, 2008).

Many people argue that embryos have the same status and moral worth as human persons because they have the potentiality to become human persons and should consequently be protected from harm (including destruction) in the same way any human person should be. In this view, the destruction of embryos to retrieve ES and, by extension, research using these ES, is unacceptable under any circumstance or for any purpose. From this perspective, weighing the various advantageous and disadvantageous consequences of destroying the embryo is totally out of order because the destruction of the embryo is in itself morally wrong (Pontifical Academy for Life, 2000). Consequently the proponents of this view will not change their conviction as a result of any breakthroughs that this research may deliver.

Others hold the more gradualistic position that, while the embryo has moral worth and deserves respect, its moral worth increases gradually throughout the development of the embryo and the foetus. The degree of the embryo's protectability is linked to its developmental stage. Destroying the embryo and using its ES can from this perspective not be categorically forbidden, although there are constraints on the age until which it is allowed to destroy the embryo and/or to the specific use of the derived ES (Nuffield Council on Bioethics, 2001). This approach lies at the basis of the Human Fertilisation and Embryology Act in the UK.

A final position does not attribute any moral worth to the blastocyst because it lacks the essential characteristics associated with the human person and can therefore not be treated at the same level. Therefore the blastocyst can be destroyed and its cells used for research. Proponents of this position will advocate that it is actually morally wrong not to continue with ES research because it may eventually result in therapies that could benefit a large number of persons, while not harming anybody (Devolder and Savulescu, 2006). This approach tends to be utilitarian. Hutcheson defines the principle of utility as 'that action is best, which procures the greatest happiness for the greatest numbers; and that, worst, which, in like manner, occasions misery' (Rawls, 1971). The aggregated happiness that results from ES research may indeed be enormous, while the misery (the destruction of the embryo) is in this view extremely limited.

Because of the completely different starting positions and analyses, these three approaches are not likely to converge to any kind of a consensus or compromise. It is therefore not to be expected that the eventual production and use of BTEPs based on ES will be legally approved throughout the European Union in the short term (Trommelmans *et al.*, 2007b). The gradualistic approach of the embryo's protectability as it is taken in the UK continues nonetheless to have a large impact on the debate in Europe, especially in the scientific community which is one of the main interested parties. The main reasons for this impact are the early introduction of legislation by the UK government and the establishment of a national stem cell bank, providing both a legal and a practical framework for the development of research which is attractive to many scientists (Healy *et al.*, 2005).

Another issue arises in ES research. Where do these embryos come from? It is probable that existing ES cell lines will not be sufficient to allow for equitable access (Faden *et al.*, 2003) or that supernumerary oocytes are not the best choice from a qualitative point of view. Should we allow the deliberate creation of embryos for tissue engineering or should we only be allowed to use supernumerary embryos that were created during an *in vitro* fertilisation procedure (IVF) and later donated for research purposes? To some, the premeditated creation of an embryo with the explicit aim to destroy it subsequently is unpalatable. Using an embryo for ES derivation that has become supernumerary after successful IVF treatment and that will sooner or later be destroyed anyway, is acceptable to some who take the viewpoint that under these circumstances 'nothing goes to waste' (Outka, 2002). However this argument is not valid when one creates an embryo in the full awareness of its imminent destruction, because it instrumentalises the embryo and reduces it to a mere means and does not regard it as an end in itself when bringing it into existence.

Creating embryos also requires the willingness of women to donate oocytes, a burdening, time consuming and not risk-free intervention (Delvigne and Rozenberg, 2002). One could ask women to allow more oocytes to be 'harvested' and fertilised during an IVF procedure than are strictly necessary for a successful pregnancy and to donate the resulting embryos for research purposes, or even give them incentives to do so, such as a reduction in the fee for the IVF treatment (Anon., 2006). This approach has been criticised because it could easily lead to the inducement of women, which could turn into outright exploitation if women were 'invited' to donate oocytes in countries or social environments where women can exert very little control over their bodies, lives and choices, or where a 'modest' compensation for the discomforts of the donation may amount to a substantial increase in the family's income (Check, 2006).

The sobering outcome of a US campaign to recruit unpaid egg donors for research purposes has demonstrated that an appeal to purely altruistic motives will probably not result in the availability of a large number of oocytes for ES research (Dizikes, 2007). As payment of oocyte or embryo donors is currently prohibited in Europe, even though financial compensation can be provided for expenses and the inconvenience related to the donation procedure (The European Parliament and Council, 2004), a shortage of eggs and embryos for research is not unthinkable and the criteria for the allocation of oocytes, embryos or cell lines to research projects will have to be refined.

Whether ES cells for bone tissue engineering research will rank highest in the pecking order of medical priorities is arguable.

Multipotent stem cells

Multipotent stem cells, in particular mesenchymal stem cells (MSC), are the subject of intense research in bone tissue engineering (Salgado *et al.*, 2004; Caplan, 2007). MSC do not face the ethical objections attached to ES because they can be isolated comparatively easily from the donor without seriously harming him or her. The number of sources from which MSC can be derived is expanding, including bone marrow, umbilical cord blood, adipose tissue, peripheral blood and others (Krampera *et al.*, 2006). The easier access and the better understanding of their developmental pathways make MSC in many cases the preferred stem cells for most researchers in bone tissue engineering.

While the use of MSC is not ethically controversial, the derivation of these cells for allogeneic use gives rise to some challenges because these cells will be transferred between two parties. This transfer will, however, not be a direct transfer as it is in whole blood or organ donation, where a donor gives his/her blood/organs to a recipent who receives this minimally altered blood/organ. Donation of MSC or other multipotent stem cells for tissue engineering will, on the contrary, be a mediated transfer in which the intermediaries, be they a cell bank, a tissue engineering company or any other appropriate organisation, will take on a number of new roles. They will not only be the primary recipients of the cells but will equally be the custodians of the cells, guaranteeing their safe manipulation, storage and distribution. They will most probably also be active in research, altering cells substantially to reach specific goals and will in some cases become the producers of the BTEPs themselves, presenting them to surgeons who will eventually implant them in the final recipient. These intermediaries will also be able to hold intellectual property rights on cell lines and/or production processes, thus protecting their commercial interests and being able to steer research one way or another. Cells are therefore not purely a biological matter; they are also exchangeable entities and carriers of transmittable information. If we look at them from this perspective, these 'ethically naïve cells' gain ethical relevance because they establish new relationships.

16.2.3 Cells as exchangeable entities

The status of exchanged cells

No BTEP can be produced without cells. Those who provide these cells are generally referred to as donors and we will use this term here as well.

However, the term 'donor' in common language implies that the cells have been freely given without payment. Donation has always been considered as the etablishment of a gift relationship, as an expression of social virtues such as altruism and citizenship and as a way to reinforce the social contract between the individual and society (Titmuss, 1997). This perception is philosophically based on the Kantian view that there is an oppositon between dignity and price, or between absolute and relative value. For Kant, and in civil law, the human body and its parts are the locus of absolute value and dignity. Commercialising the body and its parts is assigning a market value to it and consequently destroying its dignity. Countries applying common law come to a similar prohibition of the sale of body parts, but use different arguments. In common law one has no property rights in and cannot exert ownership over his/her body, or over its parts. Consequently body parts that have been donated are considered as '*res nullius*' or abandoned material (Dickenson, 2007). These arguments both from common and civil law lie at the basis of the current ubiquitous prohibition on the sale of bodily material in Europe (The European Parliament and Council, 2004).

Yet despite current legislation and several court rulings, we are faced with the fact that scientific advances have rendered the body into an 'open source of free biological material for commercial use' and whose 'products' can be transacted and sold in a global economy that is governed by the laws and customs of the neoliberal economies (Andrews and Nelkin, 2001; Waldby and Mitchell, 2006). There is a felt discrepancy between the prohibition on selling one's own cells, based on a high morality of altruism and citizenship on the one hand and the incorporation of these cells, once they have been altruistically donated, in a system that adheres to rather different morals. A new and refined ethical evaluation is necessary concerning the meaning and implications of the concepts of property, of selling and donating, of commodity and gift in relation to cells and of the repercussions these concepts have for the development of tissue engineering (Dickenson, 2007).

Informed consent in cell exchanges

In the absence of a clear and useful conceptual framework of bodily material as a gift and/or commodity, the only element that orders the relationships between the two parties in the cell exchange is the informed consent of the donor that is obtained before the prelevation of these cells (Dickenson, 2007). The informed consent procedure must inform the donor of the procedure and the risks of the intervention. Whenever the procurement of the cells is accompanied by the collection of personal data of the donor, it is evident that this data collection is equally addressed and that donors also consent to the collection and management of the data (The European Parliament and Council, 2004).

We argue that the informed consent procedure should also inform the donor about what will happen to the cells after donation. Informed consent procedures will have to address the issues related to the material value of the cells and the donor's interests in them (financial and otherwise). If the donation entails the donor having no say whatsoever in what is going to be done with the cells he/she donates, then the informed consent form can be regarded as a blanket consent, as an 'act of abandonement' or an 'act of renunciation'. If however the donor retains certain rights, such as the right to determine how others should use these cells or to define the conditions for further transfer of these cells (e.g. solely for clinical purposes), the informed consent form will have to stipulate these specific conditions. (Dickenson, 2007)

16.2.4 Cells as carriers of information

Donated cells have two very distinct kinds of value. Cells have material value, that is their capacity for metabolical, replicative and regenerative activity which lies at the basis of their usefullness in tissue engineering. But cells also carry genetic information that is valuable to the donor, the tissue engineer and the future recipient of the tissue engineered product. This informational value is retained whenever a cell is transferred from donor to intermediary/ies and on to the final recipient. The consequence of this persistent presence of informational value is that there is an incomplete 'disentanglement' between the donor, his or her cells, the tissue engineering community, the BTEP that is derived from them and the patient receiving the BTEP.

If we add to this incomplete disentanglement the required traceability of BTEPs and their components both upstream and downstream (European Parliament, 2007), it is clear that the donor continues to have interests throughout the entire process of donation, cell storage, tissue engineering and the final application of the BTEP. The informational value associated with the cells thus remains important even when donating is an 'act of abandonment' of the material value of the cells by the donor. Informed consent procedures will have to address how the persistent informational value of the BTEP will be treated and what its consequences are for donors and the exertion of their rights.

Although retracing donors and informing them of relevant findings may be an extra burden for tissue engineers, it is advisable that this possibility is considered. Showing respect for the person who contributed to your research by giving him or her crucial information is a recommendable mode of action, if not a moral duty. It would, after all, not be very consistent to aspire to the healing of one person through the application of a BTEP while on the other hand withholding information that could be crucial for the donor, who has significantly contributed to your research (CCNE and Nationaler Ethikrat, 2003).

16.3 Clinical trials with bone tissue engineered products

16.3.1 Introduction

Innovative research on human volunteers through clinical trials is both necessary and risky, given the possible negative (side) effects for the participants. To avoid exploitation, general guidance for trials has been developed and incorporated in a number of conventions and guidelines (National Commission for the Protection of Human Subjects of Biomedical and Behavioral Research, 1979; World Medical Association, 1997; EMEA, 2002; Council of Europe, 2005). These have to be adapted to the context of particular innovations such as bone tissue engineering. In this way research subjects are not merely used but treated with respect, while at the same time contributing to generalisable biological knowledge and/or the improvement of health. Emanuel *et al.* (2000) discern seven ethical requirements for every clinical trial: (1) value, that is a better understanding of health or knowledge as a result of the research; (2) scientific validity, i.e. the research should be methodologically rigorous in order to make the results valid outside of the trial conditions; (3) fair subject selection; (4) favourable risk–benefit ratio; (5) independent review; (6) informed consent and (7) respect for enrolled subjects.

Testing BTEPs under the controlled circumstances of clinical trials following these seven criteria will advance the development of BTEPs, while simultaneously showing respect for participants. Appropriate regulation is therefore being developed both in the USA (Halme and Kessler, 2006) and in Europe (EMEA, 2007).

16.3.2 Preclinical testing

The fundamental requirement for the initiation of clinical trials is that sufficient evidence about the expected efficacy, possible benefits and foreseeable risks of the product or intervention under consideration is collected through preclinical tests and animal trials. The value of animal trials depends on the relevant knowledge that they provide. The limited relevance of animal models in tissue engineering is a serious hindrance (Tawqeer *et al.*, 2004; Giannoni *et al.*, 2005). Furthermore, the application of BTEPs on healthy volunteers is problematic. These two elements may have as a consequence that a number of issues pertaining to the efficacy, the safety and risks of the BTEP will remain unanswered before clinical trials are initiated.

16.3.3 Complexity of bone tissue engineered products

It would be inaccurate to think of BTEPs as highly sophisticated medical devices that happen to contain human or animal derived cells. The incorporation of substantially modified and active cells was a key argument in defining tissue engineered products as advanced therapy medicinal products, a new category of health care products in European regulation (European Parliament, 2007). The bare fact that these products contain altered human or animal derived material brings new elements into the ethical reflection on clinical trials.

It is the incorporation of living cells in the BTEPs that generates perhaps their most distinctive feature: the complexity of the process and the product. This complexity is not present as extensively in other medical interventions such as the implantation of prostheses. There are three closely related aspects to this complexity: (1) BTEPs are inherently variable constructs because they contain metabolically active cells in a dynamic extracellular environment. Consequently, BTEPs cannot be constructed in uniform batches according to well-defined standards to the same extent as medical devices or medicinal products (European Commission, 2002).

(2) When a BTEP is implanted, we create a threefold dynamic to achieve regeneration; (a) the dynamic within the BTEP itself, (b) the dynamic in the recipient's body which may influence the incorporation of the BTEP (Stocum, 1998) and (c) the interaction of the recipient's body with the BTEP (Ahsan and Nerem, 2005; Caplan, 2007). A mismatch between the dynamics in BTEPs and the body can render the product at best inefficacious, at worst unsafe. For instance, the ideal implantation time for the BTEP may be dependent on its developmental stage. If it is too 'green', or by contrast too far developed, it may not integrate with the surrounding tissue. Understanding the interactions between product and recipient is therefore essential for the successful development of BTEPs. To assess these challenges and to respond to them accurately, a profound understanding of the biological processes of tissue formation and regeneration, both in healthy and diseased tissues, is essential, as is the ability to control cell phenotype and tissue formation (Hollander *et al.*, 2006).

(3) Once the process of regeneration is initiated, it is impossible to reverse it completely. If it goes awry, at best the BTEP can be removed. If, however, cells of the BTEP migrate to other parts of the body and generate unwanted secondary effects elsewhere, or if biomolecules affect other cells than the BTEPs', mere reversion of the procedure may be pointless to solve the newly generated problem.

16.3.4 Value and validity

Whenever a trial is considered there ought to be at least strong indications that the BTEP will be efficacious and that its findings will contribute to a better understanding of bone tissue engineering. Otherwise there are no arguments to introduce it (Emanuel *et al.*, 2000). To establish the therapeutic value of the BTEP, existing methodologies can and must be applied. These will enhance the reliability of the trial's outcome. But while these tests may indicate an improvement in the participant's healing and condition, they will not inform us of the regenerative mechanisms behind these improvements. It is equally important for tissue engineering that trials should not solely aim at therapeutic goals, but that they should indeed contribute to a more profound understanding of the working mechanisms of BTEPs and of regeneration *in situ* by answering some fundamentally new questions: is there regenerative action *in vivo*, how does it take place, and is the introduction of the active construct and the interaction with the receiver's body safe? (Roberts *et al.*, 2002; Hollander *et al.*, 2006) To achieve these goals, criteria to determine the extent, quality and mode of operation of the regeneration need to be established. For the participants' wellbeing and to reduce the risks, it is also advisable that this assessment uses non-invasive methods as much as possible (Pancrazio *et al.*, 2007).

One of the main challenges for trials with BTEPs is therefore to establish a fitting methodology that clearly sets the aims of the trial, tests their achievement rigorously and allows us to define whether and how the knowledge gained in one trial can be transferred to other domains of tissue engineering and/or to therapeutic settings. Standardisation of procedures and of the analysis of results, definition and justification of inclusion and exclusion criteria of both BTEPs and participants are all necessary elements (Jakobsen *et al.*, 2005). The lack of a well developed methodology devalues the validity of the research and raises questions concerning the respect for and protection of participants. The inherent variability of the BTEPs and the dynamic generated by the BTEP may also have a negative effect on the ability to generalise results and may limit their external validity. The small number of participants that one can expect to be eligible for most trials and the absence of long-term outcomes from the first BTEP-trials will also preclude a confident extrapolation of trial results to a larger population. The lack of acknowledged parameters will also hamper the determination of cut-off points for the trial. The inherent variability of products and interactions may also interfere with the interpretation of tests and trial results and of adverse events: the cause of an adverse event and its importance for future application of other BTEPs may be hard to determine. Lastly, the surgeon's skills (Lilford *et al.*, 2004) as well as post-operative events and therapy can influence the outcome of the whole process.

Given these manifold variables and uncertainties, the development of good methodologies, procedures and protocols with validated outcome measurements will be essential to expand the domain of tissue engineering further, especially but not exclusively in the domain of clinical trials with BTEPs.

16.3.5 Efficacy, safety and risk

Clinical research can be justified only when the potential risks to the trial participant are minimised, the potential benefits to individual subjects are enhanced and the potential benefits to individual subjects and society are proportionate to or outweigh the risks (Emanuel *et al.*, 2000). A suspicion of equipoise with regard to a specific trial has to exist in order to justify it. It must be unclear at the start which of two treatments is the best for the patient under the given circumstances: applying the BTEP or an established intervention (Freedman, 1987).

Successful regeneration will be greatly beneficial for the patient, returning him or her to greater functionality and postponing the need for further interventions or even making them redundant. If however the attempted regeneration fails, especially when other therapies are available – even when they are theoretically 'second best' to tissue engineering – the intervention may turn into a hazard. One of the challenges in bone tissue engineering clinical trials is therefore the identification, weighing and minimisation of risks. These risks are partly unknown owing to our lack of understanding of the long-term evolution of the BTEP in the body and of the induced regeneration of human tissue *in vivo*. A number of potential hazards and approaches to minimise them can nevertheless be identified (Farrugia, 2006; Halme and Kessler, 2006). First, criteria for cell choice and cell quality need to be established. This does not only concern the choice of the cell type (ES, MSC, fully differentiated cells), but also the choice of cell donor or cell line. Second, there is the potential alteration in the genetic make-up during cell culture and expansion and the presence of unwanted cell types or contaminants in the administered BTEP. Standard treatments to enhance safety, such as sterilisation or irradiation, may not be applicable. Establishing good tissue practices and good manufacturing practices will consequently be crucial for the successful development of BTEPs (EMEA, 2002; EMEA, 2003).

Third, the evolution of the BTEP in the body must be monitored and controlled in order to detect and prevent undesired cell migration, propagation or (de)differentiation and not to evoke rejection or inflammatory responses by the host's body. All these new risk factors come on top of more 'common' risks associated with cell culturing and surgery. There has been so far little attention to the assessment of these 'common' risks in trials with BTEPs, or to the influence of boundary conditions on the action of BTEPs (Kuijer *et al.*, 2007; Lumelsky, 2007).

While many of the risks cited here are also present in other medical technologies, it is the complexity of tissue engineering that leads to an inflation of uncertainties, perhaps even provoking new emergent risks caused by hitherto unencountered interactions of various processes going on in the

BTEP and between BTEP and recipient. This will make the risk assessment for BTEPs in these initial stages extremely difficult to perform. Both the assessibility and the magnitude of the risks challenge us. Never before has an intervention been undertaken that depends on such complex interactions between the product and the recipient and in which such a large amount of variables are present. Keeping in mind that the intervention does not involve critically ill persons for whom no alternative exists, very strong arguments have to be made that risks have been assessed adequately, with regard to their kind, and realistically, with regard to their magnitude.

16.4 Informed consent in clinical trials

16.4.1 Introduction

The obligation to obtain informed consent from prospective participants as their formal authorisation to include them in the trial, after they have been engaged in an informed consent procedure, is an essential protective measure (Emanuel *et al.*, 2000). Asking for informed consent requires participants to be provided with understandable information in an appropriate way about the product, the purpose of the research, its procedures, potential risks, benefits and alternatives and their rights and responsibilities as a participant. For clinical trials in the European Union, these data are extensively listed (The European Parliament and the Council, 2001; European Commission, 2006). The complexity of tissue engineering and the many uncertainties inherent in the early development and application of BTEPs aggravate this duty to inform. Explaining to the layperson, not only the complexity, but also the possible risks in a field as new as tissue engineering is challenging.

Three components should be specifically addressed in the informed consent procedure: the surgery, the use of specific cells and the risks and benefits connected with the BTEP itself. It would be misleading to present to the prospective participant the implant of a BTEP as another surgical intervention, similar to existing interventions, while it is in fact based on a new paradigm with another scope and other intentions than existing interventions, and with specific risks. Adverse events may, for instance, not be occurring at or be restricted to the implant site, yet the BTEP may be the prime cause. The trial participant therefore has a right to know to what extent he or she is protected and insured and how adverse events will be dealt with. Also, given the possible negative outcomes, back-up and containment mechanisms have to be considered before the BTEP's application (European Group on Ethics, 2004). If countermeasures are not available, the participant should know this. This obligation also includes the duty to inform trial participants of newly discovered risks or benefits and inform them of the results of earlier clinical research (Council of Europe, 2005).

16.4.2 Surgery

Bone tissue engineering trials require surgery. Trial participants are mainly concerned about the way the proposed intervention will have an impact on their health and quality of life (Newton-Howes *et al.*, 1998; McGaughey, 2004; El-Wakeel *et al.*, 2006). So while the surgery is ancillary to the main aim of the trial, which is testing the efficacy and safety of the BTEP, it may entail risks and discomforts for the patient. The construction of the BTEP may even increase some of the risks and consequences of implant-associated infections (Kuijer *et al.*, 2007). The presence of the BTEP in the trial does not absolve the investigator from giving all relevant information concerning the surgery and the foreseeable risks of both BTEP and control.

16.4.3 Use of specific cells in the bone tissue engineered product

The implant of allogeneic or xenogeneic material not only has a physiological effect on the recipient in that it is hoped that it will result in a beneficial evolution of his or her condition; it may also have cultural, religious or other relevance for the prospective participant. Consequently a discussion on the origin of the cells in the BTEP should be included in the informed consent process. The issue's relevance is exemplified by the debate in the European Parliament on the regulation of advanced therapy medicinal products where the ethical implications of the incorporation of specific cell types in BTEPs raised more concerns than any other subject (EurActiv.com, 2007).

Whenever products containing allogeneic, xenogeneic or embryonic stem cells become available, the theatre for the discussion on the acceptability of these cell types is likely to move from the public arena to the surgery. If, for example, the use of BTEPs containing ES is legally allowed in a country, this does not automatically imply that all prospective participants will consent to receiving them. They retain the right not to take part in the trial without explaining why. Yet to be able to decide about this, they have to be informed about the composition of the BTEP.

Additionally, the manipulation of human derived, freely donated material in an environment that is driven by instrumental or commercial values is a worrying development to some, as is clear from the growing body of literature on this subject and from the positions taken by, for example, the French and the German national ethics councils (CCNE (France) and Nationaler Ethikrat (Germany), 2003; CCNE, 2007).

If culture media and scaffolds used in BTEPs contain non-human animal derived material, this may also elicit queries from trial participants. Some persons reject all animal derived products, or products derived from animals considered to be unclean or sacred, even when religious leaders often take a more moderate stance (Daar, 1994; Rosner, 1999).

Those who do not share these conscientious objections may not be aware of the weight these issues carry for others and providing this information may seem to make the informed consent process too cumbersome to be practical. Also, many prospective participants will not be familiar enough with the science behind the trial to inquire spontaneously on these issues. Yet if the autonomy of all trial participants, irrespective of their religious, ethical or philosophical allegiances and respect for their opinon are the fundamental principles underpinning informed consent, it is clear that this information should be given to prospective participants, even if this makes the process more elaborate. Not providing this information could be regarded as a breach of the investigator's duty of care toward the trial participant or as a form of paternalism (Enoch *et al.*, 2005). The limited knowledge of lay persons, the ethical connotations of these issues and the delicacy of the subject warrant that the composition of the BTEP is discussed before obtaining informed consent and that conscientious objections are taken seriously.

16.4.4 Communicating risks and benefits

We have already explored the risks and benefits associated with tissue engineering and the need for investigators to be in equipoise. But not only does one have to be in equipoise as a researcher, one has also to present the various issues to trial participants in order to allow them to make up their minds. Given our limited knowledge of both risks and benefits and given that there often is no general consensus about what actually is the gold standard among existing therapies, this calculus will be extremely difficult. In determining whether there is equipoise in the use of BTEPs, both risks and benefits are clearly taken to a higher level.

In *ex vivo* tissue engineering such as bone tissue engineering a new kind of trade-off has to be made in dialogue with the prospective participant: against the enormous benefit stand potentially large risks, probably even unknown emergent risks owing to the process of regeneration that have never been encountered before. What is more, some adverse events may only become apparent after the trial. Considering the complexity and the newness of *ex vivo* tissue engineering, the problematic assessment of risks and benefits and the availability of reliable alternatives, trial designers and investigators will have to demonstrate convincingly to participants that the benefits of the BTEP-treatment will be at least as good as the existing treatment, while the risks involved in applying the BTEP will not exceed those of the conventional treatment. If the risks exceed those of conventional treatment, it is reasonable to expect that the proposed benefits are very likely to be realised and that they would render the increased risks acceptable.

16.4.5 Enhancing participants' autonomy

If we want to enable prospective participants to decide autonomously whether or not to participate, we have to start by acknowledging that the elements mentioned above may diminish this autonomy. Enhancing the autonomy of the trial participant is consequently desirable.

(1) A considerate amount of energy should be put into informing prospective participants. This remains first and foremost the task of the study team (Flory and Emanuel, 2004). The use of audio visual material and new media could prove beneficial as many persons do not understand abstract or highly specialised language. The use of audio visual material in the informed consent procedure was beneficial in a number of cases (Rossi *et al.*, 2005; Hutchison *et al.*, 2007; Strevel *et al.*, 2007). (2) One could consider the development of questionnaires to find out whether candidates actually understand what has been explained to them. (3) Given the complexity of the process, persons asked to participate should be encouraged to seek advice from independent but knowledgeable persons who can assist them in their decision making process (Flory and Emanuel, 2004; Joffe *et al.*, 2001). These 'independent thirds' can advise on different issues that may be worrying, be they of an ethical, philosophical or more technical or scientific nature. These 'independent thirds' can range from other physicians or nurses helping participants to understand the regenerative character of the BTEP, the technique of the intervention or rehabilitation processes, to persons versed in the ethical issues that are associated with the use of specific cell types. The chain of events that leads to surgery may have to be adapted in order to allow and encourage this consultation, but this should not be an impediment to the trial itself.

Providing potential participants with all the information and giving them ample time to discuss the elements of the trial with a third party will engender trust. Keeping in mind that trust is more easily squandered than it is regained (Bok, 1995), the importance of trust in BTEPs trials should not be minimised (Kass *et al.*, 1996) and every effort should be made to ensure that confidence in trials is not betrayed in order to prematurely promote one BTEP to the detriment of a promising development in medicine.

16.5 Follow-up of trial participants

The interaction between the BTEP and the body will result in the gradual acceptance by the body of the 'foreign' BTEP through which it gradually loses its 'foreignness'. This is a long-term process that may continue well beyond the duration of the trial. These events, especially adverse events, will still have to be identified and analysed (van Zuijlen *et al.*, 2001; Wood *et al.*, 2006; European Parliament, 2007).

Trials alone will therefore not suffice to make comprehensive projections about the future safety, efficacy and quality of the therapy, neither will they enable researchers fully to appreciate the long-term change in quality of life. Extrapolations of data gathered during trials will allow some long-term prognoses, but these will always contain a degree of uncertainty. The actual long-term effects can only be judged during the follow-up process. As has been pointed out by the National Institute for Clinical Excellence (NICE) for one of the few well researched clinical applications of tissue engineered products – autologous cartilage implants – the use of these products has to be considered as part of an ongoing clinical trial, because of uncertainties about the long-term effectiveness and the potential adverse effects of the procedure. A similar argument could be applicable to BTEPs.

One could consider the trial as an integrated part of the chain of production, testing and application of BTEPs. This approach allows us to integrate various findings. Information gathered from clinical trials and from the post-clinical trial phase can lead to an adjustment of the culture conditions of the BTEP in order to provide a better adapted BTEP for the specific application. It might therefore be useful to think of BTEPs as 'therapies under control' or of 'technology under investigation' (Wasiak *et al.*, 2006). This also implies that governance of post-trial events needs to be established (Trommelmans *et al.*, 2007b).

16.6 Access to therapy

16.6.1 Introduction

If BTEPs eventually become available for therapy, their actual application will not solely depend on the clinical evidence but also on other factors, including the evaluation of the economic viability of these products (McAteer *et al.*, 2007) and their reception by end users, both surgeons and patients. These products will unquestionably be very expensive, which implies that the decision to apply them will also have repercussions for health care organisations (Bock *et al.*, 2003). Besides the economic aspects, the ethical (and political) issue of the just distribution of health care is at stake. If we want to uphold the principle that those most in need of a specific treatment should be able to get it, whatever its cost and regardless of the patient's financial resources, we will have to apply some reimbursement strategy. But the presence of living, donated cells in BTEPs again adds new ethical issues on top of the already difficult exercise of determining who will have access to these BTEPs.

16.6.2 Biological perspectives

The access of the individual patient to a compatible BTEP will depend first and foremost on the availability of compatible cells for their construction

(Faden *et al.*, 2003). When the BTEP contains autologous cells, there is of course no compatibility problem. The issue is, however, crucial in allogeneic BTEPs. Choosing BTEPs that are less histocompatible, or that are for other reasons less suited, will increase the risks attached to the BTEP and place an extra burden on the recipient of the BTEP in the form of the need for life-long immunosuppressive medication or other negative side effects. Determining how strong the match between the cells in the BTEP and the donor needs to be in the case for allogeneic BTEPs (Caplan, 2007) and how the availability of cells will be secured, will be necessary. This implies that the specific cell choice for the construction of the BTEP and the regulation and conduct of cell sourcing will have an impact on the number of people who will eventually be able to receive a biologically compatible BTEP.

Yet it will always be in the best interest of the recipient that the BTEP is as compatible as possible. This can only be achieved if (1) the variety of donors is large, (2) BTEPs are constructed using appropriate cells and (3) the donated cells are accessible to all who might benefit from them. Otherwise discrimination on the basis of histological characteristics is unavoidable. Consequently, efforts should be made to establish mechanisms that allow for the efficient and safe procurement and distribution of cells from all groups in the population, including populations that have so far not been reached or that have been reluctant to participate in donation schemes. They should be made aware of the consequences of their absence in the donation process.

Experiences of organ donation, umbilical cord blood banking and bone marrow registries indicate that there are large disparities between social, religious and ethnic groups with regard to their willingness to participate in donation schemes. The reasons for this non-participation may vary, but ultimately lead to an underrepresentation of some groups of the population in cell banks and therefore also to a shortage of histocompatible cells, tissue and organs for treatment of these groups.

Differences in the willingness to donate need to be anticipated, if we do not want to reproduce these disparities for BTEPs (Ballen *et al.*, 2002; Faden *et al.*, 2003). Equally, strategies to address the needs of minority groups will have to be initiated from the very design of cell banks on. If those most in need of BTEPs should be able to get a compatible product, the establishment of public stem cell banks seems the most obvious option. The organisation of cell repositories, however, also has economic consequences. Creating a cell repository that is accessible to a large number of people, with a large number of samples, requires a specific approach and, above all, a large investment and will probably be funded differently than a repository aimed at the storage of privately donated samples for autologous use (Faden *et al.*, 2003).

16.7 Conclusion

Developing BTEPs and introducing them in clinical trials and therapy raises a number of ethical challenges, partly owing to the complexity of the process of tissue engineering and of the tissue engineered product itself, partly owing to the introduction of living, heavily manipulated cells in the dynamic construct. Cells are not merely biological matter but they continue to refer to the bodies they were once a part of. In tissue engineering, cells also become the bearer of various kinds of value and the core of several, sometimes entirely new and complex relationships between a large number of stakeholders. Sometimes these ethical challenges may be answered by the application of trusted principles, but on some occasions the aggregation of the challenges will be larger than the sum of its parts and will require our creativity in reassessing our methods of resolving ethical dilemmas in order to maintain the fundamental principles of ethical conduct in science and medicine: the preservation of human dignity and well being and the application of the principle of justice in the context of this fast changing medical development.

In this chapter we have outlined how some of the characteristics of bone tissue engineering influence the safeguarding of fundamental ethical principles, what the ethical objections and problems of the development and application of BTEPs are, and how these issues may be addressed. It is however far too early in the development of bone tissue engineering to come to definitive conclusions about what should and should not be done. As we have already remarked in the introduction, ethicists can analyse these issues and their ramifications, but will not be able to provide simple answers to complex questions. The complexity and the speed with which tissue engineering is developing require that we are constantly aware of the fundamental ethical values that might be harmed in this research and that we look for ways to safeguard them.

16.8 References

Ahsan T and Nerem R (2005), 'Bioengineered tissues: the science, the technology, and the industry', *Orthod Craniofac Res*, **8**(3), 134–40.

Andrews L and Nelkin D (2001), *Body Bazaar. The Market for Human Tissue in the Biotechnology Age*, Crown, New York.

Anon (2006), 'UK centre offers cheap IVF in return for research eggs', *Nature*, **442**, 498.

Ballen K, Hicks J, Dharan B, Ambruso D, Anderson K, Bianco C, Bemiller L, Dickey W, Lottenberg R, O'Neill M, Popovsky M, Skerret D, Sniecinski I and Wingard J (2002), 'Racial and ethnic composition of volunteer cord blood donors: comparison with volunteer unrelated marrow donors', *Transfusion*, **42**, 1279–84.

Bock A-K, Ibaretta D and Rodriguez-Cerezo E (2003), *Human Tissue-engineered Products. Today's markets and future prospects. EUR21000EN*, Joint Research Centre-Institute for Prospective Technological Studies, Brussels.

Bok S (1995), 'Shading the truth in seeking informed consent for research purposes', *Kennedy Inst Ethics J*, **5**(1), 1–17.

Caplan A (2007), 'Adult mesenchymal stem cells for tissue engineering versus regenerative medicine', *J Cell Physiol*, **213**, 341–7.

CCNE (Comité Consultatif National d'Ethique) (France) and Nationaler Ethikrat (Germany) (2003), *Opinion No 77: Ethical Problems Raised by the Collected Biological Material and Associated Information Data: 'Biobanks', 'Biolibraries'*, http://ec.europa.eu/research/biosociety/pdf/opinion_77.pdf.

CCNE (National Consultative Ethics Committee for Health and Life Sciences) (2007), *Opinion (No. 93) Commercialisation of human stem cells and other cell lines,* http://www.ccne-ethique.fr/docs/en/avis093.pdf.

Check E (2006), 'Ethicists and biologists ponder the price of eggs', *Nature,* **442**, 606–7.

Council of Europe (2005). '*Additional Protocol to the Convention on Human Rights and Biomedicine, concerning Biomedical Research'*, http://conventions.coe.int/treaty/en/Treaties/Html/195.htm

Daar A (1994), 'Xenotransplantation and religion: the major monotheist religions', *Xeno*, **2**, 61.

Delvigne A and Rozenberg S (2002), 'Epidemiology and prevention of ovarian hyperstimulation syndrome (OHSS): a review', *Human Reprod Update*, **8**(6), 559–77.

Devolder K and Savulescu J (2006), 'The moral imperative to conduct embryonic stem cell and cloning research', *Camb Q Healthc Ethics*, **15**(1), 7–21.

Dickenson D (2007), *Property in the Body: Feminist Perspectives,* Cambridge University Press, Cambridge.

Dizikes P (2007), 'Reluctance of egg donors stymies Harvard efforts'. *The Boston Globe*, Boston, June 7.

El-Wakeel H, Taylor G and Tate J (2006), 'What do patients really want to know in an informed consent procedure? A questionnaire-based survey of patients in the Bath area, UK', *J Med Ethics*, **32**(10), 612–16.

Emanuel E, Wendler D and Grady C (2000), 'What makes clinical research ethical?' *JAMA*, **283**(20), 2701–11.

EMEA (2002), *ICH Topic E6 (R1). Guideline for Good Clinical Practice. Step 5. Note for guidance on good clinical practice. CPMP/ICH/135/95,* http://www.emea.europa.eu/pdfs/human/ich/013595en.pdf.

EMEA (2003), *Concept Paper in Development of Good Manufacturing Practices Guidance for Gene Therapy and Somatic Cell Therapy Medicinal Products* EMEA/INS/GMP/3379/03. http://www.biosafety.be/GT/Regulatory/EMEA_337903en.pdf

EMEA, Committee for Medicinal Products for Human Use (2007), *Guideline on Requirements for First-in-man Clinical Trials for Potential High-risks Medicinal Products. Draft. 112* EMEA/CHMP/SWP/28367/2007 Corr, http://www.emea.europa.eu/pdfs/human/swp/2836707en.pdf.

Enoch S, Shaaban H and Dunn K (2005), 'Informed consent should be obtained from patients to use products (skin substitutes) and dressings containing biological material', *J Med Ethics*, **31**(1), 2–6.

EurActiv.com (2007), MEPs drop ethical debate in gene-therapy vote. 31-5-2007, http://www.euractiv.com/en/health/meps-drop-ethical-debate-gene-therapy-vote/article-161342.

European Commission. Health and Consumer Protection Directorate-General (2002),

Opinion on the State of the Art concerning Tissue Engineering. Adopted by the scientific committee on medicinal products and medical devices on 1st October 2002 Doc. SANCO/SCMPMD/2001/0006Final, http://ec.europa.eu/health/ph_risk/committees/scmp/documents/out37_en.pdf.

European Commission. Enterprise and Industry Directorate-General. Consumer Goods. Pharmaceuticals (2006), *Detailed Guidance on the Application Format and Documentation to be submitted in an Application for an Ethics Committee Opinion on the Clinical Trial on Medicinal Products for Human Use. Revision 1.* ENTR/CT2, http://ec.europa.eu/enterprise/pharmaceuticals/eudralex/vol-10/12_ec_guideline_20060216.pdf.

European Group on Ethics (2004), *Report of the European group on Ethics on the Ethical Aspects of Human Tissue Engineered Products,* http://ec.europa.eu/european_group_ethics/docs/humantissueprod_en.pdf.

European Parliament (2007), Regulation (EC) No 1394/2007 of the European Parliament and of the Council of 13 November 2007 on advanced therapy medicinal products and amending Directive 2001/83/EC and Regulation (EC) No 726/2004 (Text with EEA relevance), http://eur-lex.europa.eu/LexUriServ/LexUriServ.do?uri=OJ:L:2007:324:0121:0137:EN:PDF.

Faden R, Dawson L, Bateman-House A, Mueller Agnew D, Bok H, Brock D, Chakravarti A, Gao X.-J, Greene M, Hansen J, King P, O'Brien S, Sachs D, Schill K, Siegel A, Solter D, Suter S, Verfaillie C, Walters L and Gearhart J (2003), 'Public stem cell banks: considerations of justice in stem cell research and therapy', *Hastings Cent Rep*, **33**, 13–27.

Farrugia A (2006), 'When do tissues and cells become products? Regulatory oversight of emerging biological therapies', *Cell Tissue Bank*, **7**(4), 325–35.

Flory J and Emanuel E (2004), 'Interventions to improve research participants' understanding in informed consent for research: a systematic review', *JAMA*, **292**, 1593–601.

Freedman B (1987), 'Equipoise and the ethics of clinical research', *N Engl J Med*, **317**(3), 141–5.

Giannoni P, Crovace A, Malpeli M, Maggi E, Arbico R, Cancedda R and Dozin B (2005), 'Species variability in the differentiation potential of *in vitro*-expanded articular chondrocytes restricts predictive studies on cartilage repair using animal models', *Tissue Eng*, **11**(1/2), 237–48.

Gordijn B (2004), *Medizinische Utopien. Eine ethische Betrachtung,* Vandenhoeck and Ruprecht, Göttingen.

Halme D and Kessler D (2006), 'FDA regulation of stem-cell-based therapies', *N Engl J Med*, **355**(16), 1730–35.

Healy L, Hunt C, Young L and Stacey G (2005), 'The UK Stem Cell Bank: its role as a public research resource centre providing access to well-characterised seed stocks of human stem cell lines', *Adv Drug Deliv Rev*, **57**(13), 1981–8.

Hollander A, Dickinson S, Sims T, Brun P, Cortivo R, Kon E, Marcacci M, Zanasi S, Borrione A, De Luca C, Pavesio A, Soranzo C and Abatangelo G (2006), 'Maturation of tissue engineered cartilage implanted in injured and osteoarthritic human knees', *Tissue Eng*, **12**(7), 1787–98.

Hutchison C, Cowan C, McMahon T and Paul J (2007), 'A randomised controlled study of an audiovisual patient information intervention in informed consent and recruitment to cancer clinical trials', *Br J Cancer*, **97**, 705–11.

Jakobsen R, Engebretsen L. and Slauterbeck J (2005), 'An analysis of the quality of cartilage repair studies', *J Bone Joint Surg Am*, **87**, 2232–9.

Joffe S, Cook E, Cleary P, Clark J and Weeks J (2001), 'Quality of informed consent in cancer clinical trials: a cross-sectional survey', *Lancet*, **358**(9295), 1772–7.

Kass N, Sugarman J, Faden R and Schoch-Spana M (1996), 'Trust, the fragile foundation of contemporary biomedical research', *Hastings Cent Rep*, **26**(5), 25–9.

Krampera M, Pizzolo G, Aprili G and Franchini M (2006), 'Mesenchymal stem cells for bone, cartilage, tendon and skeletal muscle repair', *Bone*, **39**(4), 678–83.

Kuijer R, Jansen E, Emans P, Bulstra S, Riesle J, Pieper J, Grainger D and Busscher H (2007), 'Assessing infection risk in implanted tissue-engineered devices', *Biomaterials*, **28**(34), 5148–54.

Landecker H (2007), *Culturing Life. How Cells became Technologies*, Harvard University Press, Cambridge, MA.

Launis V (2002), 'Human gene therapy and the slippery slope argument in medicine', *Med Health Care Philos*, **5**, 169–79.

Lenoir N (2008), 'Europe confronts the embryonic stem cell research challenge', *Science*, **287**, 1425–7.

Lilford R, Braunholtz D, Harris J and Gill T (2004), 'Trials in surgery', *Br J Surg*, **91**, 6–16.

Lumelsky N (2007), 'Commentary: Engineering of Tissue Healing and Regeneration', *Tissue Eng*, **13**(7), 1393–8.

McAteer H, Cosh E, Freeman G, Pandit A, Wood P and Lilford R (2007), 'Cost-effectiveness analysis at the development phase of a potential health technology: examples based on tissue engineering of bladder and urethra, *J Tissue Eng Regen Med*, **1**(5), 343–9.

McGaughey I (2004), 'Informed consent and knee arthroscopies: an evaluation of patient understanding and satisfaction', *Knee*, **11**(3), 237–42.

National Commission for the Protection of Human Subjects of Biomedical and Behavioral Research (1979), *The Belmont Report*, US Government Printing Office, Washington DC.

Newton-Howes P, Bedford N, Dobbs B and Frizelle F (1998), 'Informed consent: what do patients want to know?', *N Z Med J*, **111**(1073), 340–2.

Nuffield Council on Bioethics (2001), *Stem cell therapy: the ethical issues*, http://www.nuffieldbioethics.org/go/ourwork/stemcells/publication_304.html.

Outka G (2002), 'The ethics of human stem cell research', *Kennedy Inst Ethics J*, **12**, 175–213.

Pancrazio J, Wang F and Kelley C (2007), 'Enabling tools for tissue engineering', *Biosens Bioelectron*, **22**, 2803–11.

Pontifical Academy for Life (2000), *Declaration on the Production and the Scientific Use of Human Embryonic Stem Cells*, http://www.vatican.va/roman_curia/pontifical_academies/acdlife/documents/rc_pa_acdlife_doc_20000824_cellule-staminali_en.html.

Rawls J (1971), *A Theory of Justice*, Harvard University Press, Cambridge, MA.

Roberts S, McCall I, Darby A, Menage J, Evans H, Harrison P and Richardson J (2002), 'Autologous chondrocyte implantation for cartilage repair: monitoring its success by magnetic resonance imaging and histology', *Arthritis Res Ther*, **5**, R60-R73.

Rosner F (1999), 'Pig organs for transplantation into humans: a jewish view', *Mt Sinai J Med*, **66**(5/6), 314–19.

Rossi M, Guttmann D, MacLennan M and Lubowitz J (2005), 'Video informed consent improves knee arthroscopy patient comprehension', *Arthroscopy*, **21**(6), 739–43.

Salgado A, Coutinho O and Reis R (2004), 'Bone tissue engineering: state of the art and future trends', *Macromol Biosci*, **4**, 743–65.

Stocum D (1998), 'Regenerative biology and engineering: strategies for tissue restoration', *Wound Repair Regen*, **6**(4), 276–90.

Strevel E, Newman C, Pond G, MacLean M and Siu L (2007), 'The impact of educational DVD on cancer patients considering participation in a phase I clinical trial', *Support Care Cancer*, **15**, 829–40.

Tawqeer R, Salacinski H, Hamilton G and Seifalian A (2004), 'The use of animal models in developing the discipline of cardiovascular tissue engineering: a review', *Biomaterials*, **25**, 1627–37.

The European Parliament and the Council (2001), *Directive 2001/20/EC of the European Parliament of the Council of 4 April 2001 on the approximation of the laws, regulations and administrative provisions of the Member States relating to the implementation of good clinical practices in the conduct of clinical trials on medicinal products for human use. 2001/20/EC,* http://eudract.emea.europa.eu/docs/Dir2001-20_en.pdf.

The European Parliament and the Council (2004), *Directive 2004/23/EC of the European Parliament and of the Council of 31 March 2004 on setting standards of quality and safety for the donation, procurement, testing, processing, preservation, storage and distribution of human tissues and cells,* http://eur-lex.europa.eu/LexUriServ/LexUriServ.do?uri=OJ:L:2004:102:0048:0058:EN:PDF.

Titmuss R (1997), *The Gift Relationship: from Human Blood to Social Policy,* LSE, London.

Trommelmans L, Selling J and Dierickx K (2007a), *Ethical Issues in Tissue Engineering, European ethical-legal papers no 7,* Centre for Biomedical Ethics and Law, Leuven. www.cbmer.be

Trommelmans L, Selling J and Dierickx K (2007b), 'A critical assessment of the directive on tissue engineering of the European union', *Tissue Eng*, **13**(4), 667–72.

UNESCO, International Bioethics Committee (2001), *The Use of Embryonic Stem Cells in Therapeutic Research. Report of the IBC on the ethical aspects of human embryonic stem cell research*, BIO-7/00/GT-1/2 (Rev.3), http://unesdoc.unesco.org/images/0013/001322/132287e.pdf.

van Zuijlen P, Vloemans J, van Trier A, Suijker M, van Unen E, Groenevelt F, Kreis R and Middelkoop E (2001), 'Dermal substitution in acute burns and reconstructive surgery: a subjective and objective long-term follow-up', *Plast Reconstr Surg*, **108**, 1938–46.

Waldby C and Mitchell R (2006), *Tissue Economies. Blood, organs and cell lines in late capitalism*, Duke University Press, Durham and London.

Wasiak J, Clar C and Villanueva E (2006), 'Autologous cartilage implantation for full thickness articular cartilage defects of the knee', *Cochrane Database of Syst Rev*, Issue 3. Art. No.: CD003323.

Wood J, Malek M, Frassica F, Polder J, Mohan A, Bloom E, Braun M and Coté T (2006), 'Autologous cultured chondrocytes: adverse events reported to the United States food and drug administration', *J Bone Joint Surg Am*, **88**, 503–7.

World Medical Association (1997), 'Declaration of Helsinki', *JAMA*, **277**, 925–6.

Index